NUTRITION

Eighth Edition

MARGARET S. CHANEY

**Professor Emeritus of Home
Economics,
Connecticut College**

MARGARET L. ROSS

**Professor of Nutrition
Emeritus,
Simmons College**

**HOUGHTON MIFFLIN COMPANY
BOSTON**

New York

Atlanta

Geneva, Ill.

Dallas

Palo Alto

Printed in the U.S.A.

Library of Congress Catalog Card Number: 76–151636

ISBN: 0–395–12425–5

Preface

Our knowledge of the nutrients and the metabolic processes they undergo in the body to maintain health and promote growth continues to expand through the findings of research. However, there is a gap between the scientific knowledge of nutrition and its application. Malnutrition and undernutrition are still grave problems throughout the world, both in developing countries and in the developed countries, including the United States. Education in the application of nutrition knowledge is urgently needed, particularly in light of the rapidly expanding world population and the threat of food-population imbalance.

Today's student of nutrition has the responsibility of acquiring the most recent and accurate information on nutrition and of applying this knowledge in both personal living and the professional field. The eighth edition of *Nutrition* has been prepared for this purpose. It has been completely revised and largely rewritten. The material on "Nutrition During Some Periods of the Life Cycle" has been reorganized and expanded into two chapters, one on "Nutrition During Infancy," the other on "Nutrition During Childhood, Adolescence and the Later Years." Consideration is given to such topics as over- and undernutrition, the relation of diet to dental health, space feeding, radioactivity in foods, imbalance of nutrients, low-cost foods, and the world food situation. The literature was thoroughly reviewed in preparation of this revised edition. The most recent material available and new figures and tables are used throughout the book.

As in earlier editions, the text deals with the individual's health as related to food and the body's ability to use it. The emphasis is on normal nutrition and the interrelationships of nutrients. Although discussion of nutrition during disease is not included in detail, certain pathological conditions in which diet is of primary importance are mentioned.

The material is treated from a scientific standpoint, and some knowledge of organic chemistry and physiology is assumed. To serve its proper function as a text on nutrition, the book sets an authoritative standard for good health and supports it by experimental evidence. The references at the end of each chapter are the investigations mentioned in the text; those which involved human subjects were given preference.

Books and journals which may be useful in supplementing and expanding information discussed in the text are listed in the Appendix. Appendix tables include one which gives the nutritive values for common household measures of more than 600 foods, as revised in 1970 by the Agricultural Research Service, United States Department of Agriculture. Also, a list of food composition tables for use in the United States and one for use in other parts of the world are included in the Appendix.

Grateful acknowledgment is given to Nancy G. Bergman, home economics editor of Houghton Mifflin Company, who assisted in the preparation of the manuscript and who gave many critical and constructive suggestions upon reading it. In addition, the authors sincerely appreciate the assistance of many other individuals and organizations who granted permission for reproduction of tables and figures, supplied pre-publication data, and gave helpful suggestions.

Margaret S. Chaney
Margaret L. Ross

Contents

Nutrition and Health

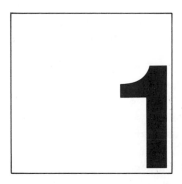

Today the great contributions of the science of nutrition to the health and welfare of all people are facts accepted without question by both professional and lay groups. Nutrition terminology is now included in everyday vocabulary; polyunsaturates, amino acids, and vitamin B_{12} join the ranks with calories, iron, and vitamin D in common usage on television and radio, in newspapers and popular magazines, and in daily conversation. Nutrients originally thought of as required solely to prevent such diseases as beriberi, scurvy, and rickets now are appreciated as being necessary because of their relationship to buoyant health, vitality, and longevity. When they are well fed, today's children are taller and sturdier and reach maturity at an earlier age than children of previous generations. Today adults do not show as early signs of aging, nor are they as susceptible to many of the diseases previously considered health hazards.

THE ROLE OF NUTRITION IN THE WORLD'S FUTURE

Nutrition is a worldwide problem (1). There are still millions of people in the world who are starving and underfed due to lack of food, lack of knowledge, and lack of facilities. In 1968 in the developing countries, not including the Communist bloc, there were approximately 350 million children under six years of age and 338 million from seven to 14 years old. Schaefer (2) estimated that 50 per cent of the younger children and 30 per cent of the older children were seriously malnourished. Such nutritional impairment may lead to permanent retardation in physical and possibly in mental development (3), to widespread disease, and high death rates.

Because nutrition research has demonstrated the relationships of nutritional status to health, vigor, and achievement, far-sighted leaders of many nations are seeking information and assistance in solving their urgent problems. Three international organizations, actively interested in nutritional aspects of health, stand ready to help. The Nutrition Committee of the Food and Agriculture Organization of the United Nations (FAO) is especially concerned with nutritional problems related to production, distribution, and consumption of food. The Nutrition Section of the World Health Organization (WHO), also of the United Nations, has as a primary obligation investigation of conditions related to clinical aspects of nutrition. The United Nations Children's Fund (UNICEF) was established to better health standards of children in needy areas. UNICEF provides medical care for mothers, and milk, vaccine, and medicine for children. The Agency for International Development of the United States (AID) also contributes much toward better nutrition for people in developing countries. Some of the specific problems of international nature met by these organizations will be mentioned later.

The Nutrition Program of the United States Public Health Service (USPHS), formerly the Secretariat of the Interdepartmental Committee on Nutrition for National Defense (ICNND), was designated in 1967 to study conditions within the United States. A survey, known as the National Nutrition Survey (NNS), was undertaken to assess the incidence and location of malnutrition in this country. Procedures were formulated (4), and expert consultant committees were appointed to aid in evaluating the findings. Guidelines for interpreting biochemical data were based on those employed by the ICNND (5). Low-income areas of ten states were selected for the initial phase of the study. Preliminary data reported from most of these states should not be considered as indicating malnutrition and should not be considered as typical of any state or group. Unexpected findings of some shortcomings include nutritional diseases thought to have been wiped out in this country, such as goiter, rickets, night blindness, and kwashiorkor. One of every three children under six years was anemic. Among those ten years and older, 96 per cent had an average of ten missing, decayed or filled teeth.

Food technology is making tremendous advances on problems of agriculture and transportation of fresh produce, its processing, packaging, and storing. This knowledge provides benefits of immeasurable value to the consumer. Chemical food additives, now comprising a long list, may also be desirable; they may supply lacking nutrients in controlled amounts or prevent food spoilage, or, by enhancing color and flavor, increase the quality of the dietary. On the other hand, if used indiscriminately, some food additives may be harmful. As a means of protecting the consumer, the United States Food and Drug Administration (FDA) has formulated standards of identity, quality, and fill of container for some food products and makes periodic inspections of food. In 1958 a Food Additives Amendment became law, and in 1960, a Color Additive Amendment.

The FDA has established standards for vitamin and mineral supplements, for enrichment of bread and certain grains, and for fortification of milk products, margarine, and salt. Regulations also have been established for foods for special dietary uses. These include foods for control of body weight, foods for regulation of sodium or carbohydrate intake, infant foods and formula preparations, and hypoallergenic foods. In 1966, the FDA published tentative new regulations which amended and revised those in force (6). However, none of these regulations will become effective until after completion of public hearings on the many objections filed.

The possibility of harm by the accidental or indirect addition of certain chemicals to foods through the use of pesticides has caused concern. Many scientists believe that with the proper controls against dangers resulting from indiscriminate use of these chemicals, such compounds may serve as a boon to agriculture by providing opportunities for improved food production. This conclusion was verified in a study by Duggan and associates (7) who determined the amounts of the toxic residues in foods ready for consumption. Twelve groups of 82 foods were included: dairy products; meat, fish, and poultry; grains and cereal products; white and sweet potatoes; leafy vegetables; legumes; root vegetables; garden fruits; other fruits; oils, fats, and shortenings; sugar and adjuncts; and beverages. The quantities and kinds used to provide a two-week total diet sample were analyzed and 25 different residues were found. In all cases the amounts of the residues were very small and substantially lower than established tolerances. In another approach (8), the storage of pesticide chemicals in the body was measured quantitatively. The amounts found were below the tolerance levels set by the FDA and were not considered hazards.

Food faddism and nutrition quackery have been called the biggest racket in the health field. The press, radio, and television present much factual material to the public, but a considerable amount of this may be biased. Food fads may play havoc with human nutrition to the extent that they may counteract the benefits of today's scientific knowledge. Some fads promote an excessive use of certain foods to the exclusion of others and may be detrimental in that the result is a deficiency of essential nutrients. Another type of fad puts undue stress on the virtue of certain supplements; such products as multivitamin and mineral concentrates may perform vital roles for persons who cannot eat properly or do not utilize nutrients well, but these compounds are not considered essential for the healthy individual. Other fads are based on the idea that certain combinations of foods are harmful when eaten at the same meal. This is generally accepted as a false idea; in fact, nutritionists favor combinations of foods since they complement one another and in some cases aid in utilization of nutrients. The unwise use of pills in weight reduction may cause serious harm to the body. Some drugs cause a feeling of satiety, some depress the appetite, and others stimulate metabolism. Common sense should make the intelligent individual analyze the ideas involved in a food fad before accepting it.

Radiation exposure as a result of nuclear fallout is a hazard of modern times. Of the several radionuclides known to be present in food, strontium and cesium are important from a health standpoint; iodine[131] is of less concern because of its short half-life. Strontium[90] is a more serious problem because the metabolism of strontium and calcium are closely related (9).

In order to measure the amount of strontium[90] in a food, either accumulated directly as on the leaves of a plant or indirectly through the soil, a "strontium unit" is employed; this is defined as a picocurie* of strontium[90] per gram of calcium. Analyses are made at regular intervals to determine the current content of strontium[90] in food, and the average total in the diet of different age groups is also calculated. The Federal Radiation Council has set up Radiation Protection Guides, not as indicators of danger, but to govern normal peacetime practices—the belief being that the figures listed are definitely much lower than those which would constitute a hazard. For strontium[90] the guides provide for 200 picocuries per day. In Washington, D.C., in August, 1962, the average daily intake per person was estimated at 25.9 picocuries of strontium[90]. Dairy products supplied one-half to two-thirds of this strontium[90]; grain products, about one-eighth. Much of the fallout material is lost when the outer leaves of vegetables are discarded, the product washed, or the grain milled. The ratio of strontium[90] in the cow's milk is about one-tenth of that in her feed. Because of the relatively large proportion of radionuclide found at times in milk, it might seem that this food should be used less. However, this is not advised since milk is an excellent source of calcium and a reduction in intake of milk would increase the strontium[90] to calcium ratio in the total diet. Ways are being studied for reducing the content of radiostrontium in milk in the event of an emergency. A process developed by the United States Department of Agriculture (USDA) can remove more than 90 per cent of radioactive strontium from milk. The ratio of strontium[90] to calcium in both animal and human tissues (including bone and muscle) is approximately one-fourth of that in the diet.

In a study (9) conducted to determine possible nutrient changes when milk was treated to remove 90 per cent of the strontium it was found that there was no loss of vitamin A, riboflavin, pantothenic acid, folic acid, vitamin B_{12}, calcium, magnesium, sodium, phosphorus, or iron. Thiamin, niacin, and vitamin B_6 were reduced by 50, 27, and 15 per cent, respectively. However, milk does not furnish large amounts of these three vitamins; the treated milk was found to have no untoward effects on the growth and general wellbeing of rats and pigs.

* A picocurie is one-millionth of one-millionth of a curie, the curie being the amount of radioactivity produced by 1 gm. of radium.

APPROACHES TO THE STUDY OF NUTRITION
IN RELATION TO HEALTH

Quantitative analyses of food may be carried out in the laboratory.
Since food plays a primary role in nutritional status, information on the
composition of the foods incorporated in the diet is considered essential
background material. Great progress has been made in quantitative
determinations of the nutrients; chemical, fluorometric, and biological
techniques have been and are being perfected. As a result there are
available today many data for the nutrients in foods, in both comparatively large and in microscopic amounts (10).

Research on the effects of processing, storage, and cookery is of great
value in assaying the nutrients in food as actually eaten; this is especially
important for the nutrients that are soluble in water or affected by heat,
oxidation, and chemicals. Knowledge is being acquired about the percentages of foods which are digested and available for use by the body;
impairment in digestion may greatly affect the utilization the body may
make of the nutrients. The table of food composition in the Appendix
(page 435) has been brought up-to-date through current knowledge
secured in the laboratory. This table, prepared by the Agricultural Research Service (ARS) of the USDA, was revised in 1970 (11).

*Calculations are tabulated of available food supplies and their con-
sumption assessed in dietary surveys.* The USDA furnishes yearly estimates of the food available in this country. To obtain these figures, the
total amounts of food produced in the United States are combined with
the amounts carried over from the year before and with imported foods.
From this total are deducted the amounts of food exported, those left
over at the end of the current year, those used by the armed forces,
those used for nonfood purposes, and an estimate of the amounts lost
in distribution channels. The figures secured represent economic consumption, not physiological ingestion. A quarterly publication of the
Economic Research Service (ERS) entitled *The National Food Situation*
gives this information. From the tables of "apparent civilian per capita
consumption of major food commodities," comparisons may be made of
year-to-year trends in food levels; nutrient consumption in the United
States as a whole can be estimated from these data.

Detailed studies of food consumption in households in cities and
rural areas of the United States have been made by the ARS. The fifth
and most recent of these studies covered the period April, 1965,–March,
1966, and gives seasonal data (12). The survey included a total of
approximately 15,000 housekeeping households in the Northeast, North
Central, South, and West, which were grouped by regions as urban,
rural nonfarm, and rural farm. In the spring of 1965 about 7500 households were investigated and in each of the three following seasons,
2500 other households were visited. Trained interviewers collected data

which included kinds, quantities, and costs of foods used at home and of meals and snacks away from home during the seven days preceding the interview. Other data used to classify the families included family income, and age, education, and employment of the homemaker. Since data were secured on foods as they came into the kitchen, the figures represent economic consumption, not physiological. The spring survey also included information on a day's food intake of family members, thus supplying for the first time on a national basis data on food intakes and nutrient content of the diets of men, women, boys, girls, and infants. Some of the results of this survey will be mentioned later as they pertain to specific nutrients.

Studies on animals have applications for human beings. Rats, guinea pigs, and dogs have been used for years in nutrition experiments. Today chemical tests have been perfected and are preferred for certain types of studies such as the determination of vitamin values; microbiological procedures, in which bacteria or molds are used, have also been developed. There are many advantages in the use of these objective determinations. However, animals still are essential in certain types of studies, such as those which investigate the effects of lack or imbalance on the body, and those which concern interrelationships between nutrients. Much can be learned with animals without endangering human beings and with a saving of time, money, and effort. An example is the well-known long-time series of studies by Sherman and his co-workers on many generations of rats, bred and controlled so that their life histories were similar, and selected so that variables were eliminated to a great extent. In one such study, in which the proportion of milk in the ration made the only difference, the larger amount of milk was found to favor successful bearing and rearing of the young, rapid growth, early maturity, and postponement of old age. Due to the orderly and long-time research on rats Sherman (13) could say:

> We now have good scientific evidence that such nutritional improvement of life can begin before birth or at practically any time after, that in early life it can mean improvement of mental as well as physical growth and development, and that this earlier maturity can be followed by a longer period and a higher plane of full adult capacity with superior attainment and performance over a longer career, and a lower percentage of years of dependence. Much of what we have thought to be attributable to heredity or fate we now find to be amenable to nutritional improvement. Both heredity and nutrition are now known to be major factors in determining the length of normal lives (pp. v and vi).

WAYS TO EVALUATE THE NUTRITIONAL STATUS
OF HUMAN BEINGS

Different goals may be set as the basis for nutritional studies. Sinclair (14) has listed five degrees of nutritional status: (1) excess nutriture when an excessive supply of food results in impaired function or defective structure; (2) normal nutriture when the nutrients promote desirable function and structure and there is a sufficient supply of reserves; (3) poor nutriture when function and structure are unimpaired but reserves are inadequate; (4) latent malnutriture which implies impaired function or structure but not to the extent that disease is easily detected; (5) clinical malnutriture when a definite disease is caused by the lack. The boundaries between these states are not clear cut; either extreme may cause death. As indicated in Sinclair's gradations of nutriture, there are four stages in the development of a poor condition—inadequate consumption of food, a decrease in the body's reserves, impairment in function, and anatomical lesions. These stages may be detected by the use of different criteria. If the day-to-day supply of food just balances the need, the nutriture still may be poor. Body reserves known to be sufficient in ordinary adult life may not satisfy during stress, such as blood donation or the period of childbearing; rate of excretion may be affected by the amount of a nutrient found in the tissues. What is considered adequate may not be optimal, nor may it suffice over several generations even when the individual shows no ill effects during his own lifetime. It is important to determine which of these criteria is the basis for judgment before applying the results to another situation (15).

The dietary standards set by the United States, Great Britain, and Canada illustrate this point. The recommended dietary allowances used in the United States are planned to supply a large enough margin above average body requirements to care for the variations which may occur in practically all individuals in the general population. These recommended allowances may not apply to specific individuals and are not considered large enough to supply the nutrients needed by persons who are diseased or are in traumatic stress. The table of Recommended Dietary Allowances (RDA) revised in 1968 by the Food and Nutrition Board (FNB) of the National Academy of Sciences—National Research Council (NAS—NRS) is included in the Appendix (16). By comparison, the figures recommended by the Committee of Nutrition of the British Medical Association are amounts sufficient or more than sufficient for the nutritional needs of practically all healthy persons in the population. The figures set by the Canadian Council on Nutrition are thought to be adequate to maintain health in the majority of Canadians.

Table 1-1 gives the standards for males in these three countries, Norway, and Japan. Those for Norway are described as being somewhat higher than average requirements; the allowances for Japan are believed to be sufficient to establish and maintain a good nutritional state in typical individuals.

The FDA has established levels, known as Minimum Daily Requirements (MDR), for certain vitamins and minerals, and these levels form the basis for labeling regulations (see p. 431, Appendix). These levels, promulgated in 1941, have not been altered except for a revision

Table 1–1

Comparison of the Dietary Standards of Five Countries

Nutrients	United States[1] Male, 70 kg.	United Kingdom[2] Male, 65 kg.	Canada[3] Male, 72 kg.	Norway[5] Male, 70 kg.	Japan[6] Male, 56 kg.
Energy, kcal	2800	3000	2850	3400	3000
Protein, gm.	65	75	48[4]	70	70
Calcium, gm.	0.8	0.5	0.5	0.8	0.6
Iron, mg.	10	10	6	12	10
Vitamin A, IU	5000	2475[7]	3700	2500[8]	2000[8]
Thiamin, mg.	1.4	1.2	0.9	1.7	1.5
Riboflavin, mg.	1.7	1.7	1.4	1.8	1.5
Niacin Equiv., mg.	18	18	9[8]	17	15
Ascorbic Acid, mg.	60	30	30	30	65

[1] Recommended Dietary Allowances, Seventh Revised Edition. Washington, D.C.: FNB, NAS-NRC Publ. 1694 (1968).
[2] Recommended Intakes of Nutrients for the United Kingdom. Report 120, Department of Health and Social Security, London (1969).
[3] Dietary Standards for Canada. *Canadian Bull. Nutr.* 6 No. 1 (1964).
[4] Dietary Standards for Canada. Protein Revision. *Canadian Nutr. Notes, 25:*71 (1969).
[5] Evaluation of Nutrition Requirements, State Nutrition Council, Norway, 1958.
[6] Nutrition in Japan, Ministry of Health and Welfare (1965).
[7] Figure converted from 750 mg. retinol equivalents. One retinol equivalent equals 3.33 IU of retinol.
[8] For the preformed vitamin only.

of the riboflavin requirement and addition of a requirement for niacin. These were chosen to indicate a minimal standard below which demonstrable signs of deficiency would be produced. There has been much misunderstanding of the MDR and some confusion between them and the RDA (17). Therefore the FDA proposed in the 1966 revision of the regulations for foods for special dietary use that they be replaced by recommended allowances adapted from information in RDA.

A physical examination is usually the first step in diagnosis. Sinclair in his discussion on assessment of human nutriture shows the relationships of nutrition to health by the following diagram:

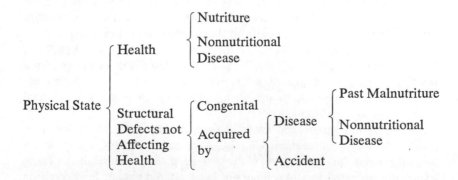

This indicates the complex nature of a bodily condition and the difficulty with which a diagnosis may be made. Fortunately, there are symptoms of malnutrition which serve as a guide to the state of nutrition. Some of the deficiency symptoms will be referred to in later chapters. Often the clinical signs are not specific and may result from factors other than diet. Furthermore, malnutrition may be provoked by nondietary factors such as infection or faulty digestion and elimination, or it may result from a multiple nutrient deficiency. To complicate matters still more, the time involvement in the onset and development of deficiency diseases may vary greatly. For these reasons, the physical examination should never be used as conclusive evidence as a means of evaluating nutritional status.

Weight is related to nutriture but is not a reliable gauge for diagnosis. Weight was once considered to be a reliable indication of nutriture. Today it is realized that the desirable weight of a person depends not only on his height and age but also on his bone structure, muscular development, and body fat content. No two people are alike and tables which give weight for height, age, and sex tend to give averages, secured from a large number of cases. It is more difficult to state the ideal. For men and women 25 years and over, the average weight at 25 is considered the desirable weight (Table 1-2) (18). According to the Metropolitan Life Insurance Company, weight is apt to increase with age even in adult life; for instance, between the ages of 30 and 50, short women tend to gain 13 or 14 pounds, or more than 10 per cent of their weight.

Life insurance studies show that overweight people, especially men, are more prone to serious illness and are poorer surgical risks than are those of desirable weight. This is especially true for those past 40 and for those who are considerably overweight. Among the problems associated with overweight are heart, circulatory, and kidney disorders, and diabetes. Gall bladder and liver disorders and a lowered resistance to infection are also more common among the overweight.

For young people still in their twenties a little extra weight does no harm and may be beneficial. Table 1-2 is for people 25 and over. To estimate weights for young women between the ages of 18 and 25 a "rule of thumb" method is given, 1 pound being subtracted for each year under 25 from the limits for each height. Thus a girl of 18 who has a medium frame and measures 5 feet 4 inches should weigh from 106 to 119 pounds.

For children of medium build a weight 7 to 10 per cent above the average is considered desirable. A table commonly used for children is given in the Appendix. Rate of growth of children is thought to be a more accurate measure of good nutriture than is a single weight figure that meets the amount desired at a set time. Today the Wetzel grid is

Table 1–2

Desirable Weights for Men and Women of Ages 25 and Over*†‡

WEIGHT IN POUNDS ACCORDING TO FRAME (IN INDOOR CLOTHING)

Height§		Small Frame		Medium Frame		Large Frame	
Feet	Inches	Men	Women	Men	Women	Men	Women
4	10	—	92–98	—	96–107	—	104–119
4	11	—	94–101	—	98–110	—	106–122
5	0	—	96–104	—	101–113	—	109–125
5	1	—	99–107	—	104–116	—	112–128
5	2	112–120	102–110	118–129	107–119	126–141	115–131
5	3	115–123	105–113	121–133	110–122	129–144	118–134
5	4	118–126	108–116	124–136	113–126	132–148	121–138
5	5	121–129	111–119	127–139	116–130	135–152	125–142
5	6	124–133	114–123	130–143	120–135	138–156	129–146
5	7	128–137	118–127	134–147	124–139	142–161	133–150
5	8	132–141	122–131	138–152	128–143	147–166	137–154
5	9	136–145	126–135	142–156	132–147	151–170	141–158
5	10	140–150	130–140	146–160	136–151	155–174	145–163
5	11	144–154	134–144	150–165	140–155	159–179	149–168
6	0	148–158	138–148	154–170	144–159	164–184	153–173
6	1	152–162	—	158–175	—	168–189	—
6	2	156–167	—	162–180	—	173–194	—
6	3	160–171	—	167–185	—	178–199	—
6	4	164–175	—	172–190	—	182–204	—

* Courtesy of the Metropolitan Life Insurance Company, New York, 1969.
† For girls between 18 and 25, subtract 1 pound for each year under 25.
‡ To ascertain desirable nude weights women should subtract 2 to 4 pounds, men, 5 to 7 pounds.
§ Heights given with shoes on; 1-inch heels for men, 2-inch heels for women.

used to sort out the children who have failed or are failing to develop normally (19, 20). Wetzel, a pediatrician, has listed nine physique channels, ranging from the very fat to the very thin body. By using height-weight data in the Wetzel grid method, the child's record throughout his growth period may be plotted. The grid technique, according to Wetzel, permits the investigator to visualize the character of an individual child's growth and development and to assay in a reliable manner, by means of a continous record, his progress in relation to his natural capacity and the expected performance.

It is sometimes difficult to ascertain which kind of frame a person has. This is one reason why figures in height-weight tables should not be used to judge the state of health. It is thought that very slender or small-boned persons may be healthy and resistant when their weight is near the lower limit of the weight range, and very large-boned persons may safely stay at the upper limit of the range. However, extremes in weight may not be compatible with good health, and individuals should regulate their diets and activities to stay within reasonable weight ranges. Since disease and defects may be the cause of failure to gain or lose in the case of children or failure to maintain desired weight in the case of adults, a medical examination may be advised.

The terms "linear" and "lateral" are often used to designate the slender and stocky types. Many examples of each may be seen. However, any given person may have inherited some characteristics of both types, thus complicating weight prediction. The tall, slender person with narrow head, small chest capacity, long limbs and trunk, slender bones, and little reserve adipose tissue tends to be proportionally light for his stature, in contrast to the stocky individual with round head, short and thick neck, limbs, and trunk, broad thorax, and ample store of fat. Associated with these anatomical differences are certain physiological characteristics which influence the ability to put on weight. The linear type is apt to have poor circulation, a slow-emptying stomach, short intestinal tract, and poor assimilation; the lateral build with opposite extremes tends to be overnourished.

The fact that build is inherited is shown in the common observation that thinness and stoutness run in certain families, but it is not an excuse for the emaciated person of thin build or the obese stocky individual. Other inherited tendencies are less easily proved. There is little evidence that one person uses his food more completely than another, a statement frequently used as an excuse by the individual who will not make an honest effort to lose or gain. Glandular abnormalities may be inherited and, in the case of underactivity of the thyroid, adrenal, pituitary, or sex glands, the person may tend to corpulence, but such instances are quite rare and account for few of the many problem cases. More often the condition which is laid at the door of inheritance is merely the continuance of faulty habits of living from one generation to another, as a close analysis of the likes and dislikes of grandmother, mother, and child will show. In fact, the seemingly unexplainable cases of overweight and underweight nearly always may be traced to habits of sleep, exercise, and diet.

Food habit and diet records can serve as general indications of nutriture. In such studies, groups of homemakers, school children, or students in college nutrition classes may be asked to supply information about their daily habits of eating, elimination, exercise, sleep, and foods eaten—preferably over a period of seven days. The information usually is recalled and, if the subjects are intelligent and cooperative, the data provided may be very useful. But obviously, many errors can result such as failure to recall all food eaten and confusion in estimating amounts in servings. Such studies may be useful tools in classroom health teaching, but the results can be considered only general guides

A Daily Food Guide

MEAT GROUP

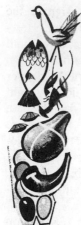

Foods Included

Beef; veal; lamb; pork; variety meats, such as liver, heart, kidney.

Poultry and eggs.
Fish and shellfish.
As alternates—dry beans, dry peas, lentils, nuts, peanuts, peanut butter.

Amounts Recommended

Choose 2 or more servings every day.
Count as a serving: 2 to 3 ounces of lean cooked meat, poultry, or fish—all without bone; 2 eggs; 1 cup cooked dry beans, dry peas, or lentils; 4 tablespoons peanut butter.

VEGETABLE-FRUIT GROUP

Foods Included

All vegetables and fruits. This guide emphasizes those that are valuable as sources of vitamin C and vitamin A.

paragus tips; raw cabbage; collards; garden cress; kale; kohlrabi; mustard greens; potatoes and sweetpotatoes cooked in the jacket; spinach; tomatoes or tomato juice; turnip greens.

Sources of Vitamin C

Good sources.—Grapefruit or grapefruit juice; orange or orange juice; cantaloup; guava; mango; papaya; raw strawberries; broccoli; brussels sprouts; green pepper; sweet red pepper.

Fair sources.—Honeydew melon; lemon; tangerine or tangerine juice; watermelon; as-

Sources of Vitamin A

Dark-green and deep-yellow vegetables and a few fruits, namely: Apricots, broccoli, cantaloup, carrots, chard, collards, cress, kale, mango, persimmon, pumpkin, spinach, sweetpotatoes, turnip greens and other dark-green leaves, winter squash.

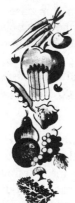

Amounts Recommended

Choose 4 or more servings every day, including:
1 serving of a good source of vitamin C or 2 servings of a fair source.
1 serving, at least every other day, of a good source of vitamin A. If the food chosen for vitamin C is also a good source of vitamin A, the additional serving of a vitamin A food may be omitted.
The remaining 1 to 3 or more servings may be of any vegetable or fruit, including those that are valuable for vitamin C and for vitamin A.
Count as 1 serving: $\frac{1}{2}$ cup of vegetable or fruit; or a portion as ordinarily served, such as 1 medium apple, banana, orange, or potato, half a medium grapefruit or cantaloup, or the juice of 1 lemon.

Figure 1–1

A Daily Food Guide. (*From* Nutrition, *Food at Work for You, Home and*

MILK GROUP

Foods Included

Milk—fluid whole, evaporated, skim, dry, buttermilk.

Cheese—cottage; cream; Cheddar-type, natural or process.
Ice cream.

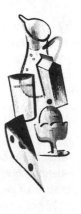

Amounts Recommended

Some milk every day for everyone.
Recommended amounts are given below in terms of 8-ounce cups of whole fluid milk:

Children under 9___	2 to 3	Adults_____	2 or more
Children 9 to 12____	3 or more	Pregnant women___	3 or more
Teen-agers_____	4 or more	Nursing mothers___	4 or more

Part or all of the milk may be fluid skim milk, buttermilk, evaporated milk, or dry milk.

Cheese and ice cream may replace part of the milk. The amount of either it will take to replace a given amount of milk is figured on the basis of calcium content. Common portions of cheese and of ice cream and their milk equivalents in calcium are:

1-inch cube Cheddar-type cheese = ½ cup milk
½ cup cottage cheese   = ⅓ cup milk
2 tablespoons cream cheese   = 1 tablespoon milk
½ cup ice cream   = ¼ cup milk

BREAD-CEREAL GROUP

Foods Included

All breads and cereals that are whole grain, enriched, or restored; *check labels to be sure.* Specifically, this group includes: Breads; cooked cereals; ready-to-eat cereals; cornmeal; crackers; flour; grits; macaroni and spaghetti; noodles; rice; rolled oats; and quick breads and other baked goods if made with whole-grain or enriched flour. Bulgur and parboiled rice and wheat also may be included in this group.

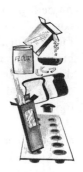

Amounts Recommended

Choose 4 servings or more daily. Or, if no cereals are chosen, have an extra serving of breads or baked goods, which will make at least 5 servings from this group daily.

Count as 1 serving: 1 slice of bread; 1 ounce ready-to-eat cereal; ½ to ¾ cup cooked cereal, cornmeal, grits, macaroni, noodles, rice, or spaghetti.

OTHER FOODS

To round out meals and meet energy needs, almost everyone will use some foods not specified in the four food groups. Such foods include: unenriched, refined breads, cereals, flours; sugars; butter, margarine, other fats. These often are ingredients in a recipe or added to other foods during preparation or at the table.

Try to include some vegetable oil among the fats used.

Garden Bulletin, No. 1, Family Fare, Separate 1, December, 1968.)

to possible nutritional status. Information tabulated this way may be compared with a standard such as the daily food guide (21) (Figure 1–1) and scored on the basis of points or percentage.

The dietary study gives more exact data on food intake. In contrast to dietary recall studies and the food consumption survey described on page 11 is the A.P. (as purchased) or inventory study. Such studies are carried on over a long period of time with a homogeneous group in an institutional setting where the food served is the same in type for everyone. A quantitative record of all food purchased or contributed during the study is kept along with an inventory of food on hand at the beginning and end of the study. Waste losses are either estimated or determined. Standard food composition tables are used to determine the nutrient content of the diet. This type of study permits comparison of groups of people as to age, sex, activity, etc.

More exact data may be obtained for individuals by means of the E.P. (edible portion) dietary study. Results of the A.P. dietary study, as well as dietary surveys and available food supply tabulations, indicate calorie content of the group diet but do not show the calorie consumption of a given person. The A.P. dietary study assumes that each member consumes his share of the food on the table. The E.P. dietary study, on the other hand, investigates the food as served to each person at the table and involves weighing all food. In-between-meal food is recorded; corrections are made for waste. Aliquot samples may be burned in the bomb calorimeter or calculation may be made using food composition tables. A shortcoming of the E.P. dietary study is that only the present diet is accounted for, whereas past faulty food intake may be the cause of poor nutriture. Also, when a food composition table is the basis for the calculations, the data may vary considerably from those of the food actually eaten; this is especially true in combinations of foods (22).

Biochemical tests are related to specific nutrients and to specific body functions. In conjunction with a study of nutrient intake, investigations may be carried out to determine how the body utilizes one or more of the nutrients. The levels of specific nutrients in blood, urine, or other body tissues, or blood values for hemoglobin, alkaline phosphatase, or pyruvic acid may be determined by chemical analyses. Assessment may measure the ability of various parts of the body to perform their functions, such as the relationship of visual acuity to vitamin A, heart function to thiamin, capacity for muscular work to energy intake, or blood clotting to vitamin K. In addition, the condition of the teeth and gums, the thyroid gland, bones, or the gastrointestinal tract where lesions may occur are frequently evaluated in nutritional status studies. If norms and ranges of normality have been determined and if the conditions of the test procedure are strictly followed, such data as may be secured tend to give valuable information which aids early diagnosis of deficiency. Many examples of this approach to nutritional status will be found in later chapters. If only one method of studying nutriture were to be used, biochemical tests would be the choice. Since these tests may indicate a deficiency before physical symptoms are recognized, the findings are especially valuable in assessing suboptimal nutrition. However, they may be misleading since the values may be affected by present dietary customs. Too, body reserves of the different nutrients vary greatly both in size or reserve supply and in time required to indicate depletion.

Approaches to nutritional assessment vary depending on the purposes of the studies and the population groups surveyed. Five studies illustrate this. A first example is the coordinated research program carried on under the direction of the USDA and State Agricultural Experiment Stations from 1947 through 1958. The nutritional status of children, adolescents, and adults in 39 states of this country was investigated. Physical examinations, biochemical analyses of blood and urine, self-selected dietaries which included seven-day records of food intake, dental examinations, and x-rays of bones and teeth were conducted. The methods used were sufficiently comparable to permit common interpretation. Special studies in some of the experiment stations investigated essential amino acids, vitamin C utilization, blood cholesterol, carotene as a source of vitamin A, and blood riboflavin. A bulletin entitled *Nutritional Status U.S.A.* (23) summarizes the results of this cooperative project.

A different approach to the problem of nutrient needs is shown by another example of coordinated research carried on in nutrition research laboratories of home economics departments in four universities: Alabama, Minnesota, Nebraska, and Oklahoma. Details of this study are given in *The Metabolic Response of Young Women to a Standardized Diet* (24). Thirty college women served as subjects. The standardized diet was constructed so as to keep the intake of essential nutrients at fairly constant levels over extended periods and to vary the level of one nutrient only during certain periods. The core diet, a combination of common foods, was planned to be palatable and to provide low levels of most of the nutrients; it was supplemented by synthetic and purified products in controlled amounts. Ranges in metabolic response to the various nutrients were determined. Data gained from this study concerning calcium, phosphorus, and nitrogen balances and the urinary excretion of riboflavin will be given in later chapters.

The third type is demonstrated by a series of studies begun in 1947 and still continuing under the direction of Horwitt and co-workers (25) at the Elgin State Hospital, Elgin, Illinois. The subjects used in each phase of the investigation—thiamin, riboflavin, niacin and tryptophan, and tocopherol—were carefully selected from several hundred male patients on the basis of chronicity of mental illness, good physical condition, emotional stability, cooperativeness, and desirable food habits. Basic diets, planned to be adequate in all respects except that of the specific nutrient being studied, have been varied to avoid monotony and are prepared and administered by trained personnel in the dietary department. In the biochemical research laboratory, chemical, microbiological, and rat growth tests have been conducted to determine the quantitative amounts of nutrients eaten, as well as specific components in blood and urine related to metabolic processes. The number of subjects used, the long periods of time of each study, and the scientifically evaluated and established methods used make this series of projects a valuable addition to today's knowledge of nutrition.

The study by Macy and her associates (26) on the nutritional status of mothers and their infants represents another approach. The large number of subjects included were healthy nonpregnant white women and pregnant white and Negro women who received care from public and private sources in the Detroit area and who had typical uncomplicated gestation. The study evaluated the nutritional status and physiological changes related to the stresses of reproduction by means of clinical observations, medical histories, food intakes, and microchemical determinations of six components of the blood. This very complete and carefully controlled investigation will be discussed in Chapter 14.

The last example of nutrition investigations includes the work begun in 1955 by the ICNND, a committee composed of representatives from seven departments of the United States Government. In 1965 this committee was dissolved and the work continued by the Nutrition Section, Office of International Research, National Institutes of Health. In 1967 the investigations were broadened to include domestic as well as international nutrition studies. It now is known as The Nutrition Program, National Center for Chronic Disease Control, United States Department of Health, Education, and Welfare. In the early years the ICNND conducted epidemiological surveys in 30 developing countries in Latin America, the Middle East, Africa, and the Far East. Identical or similar observations and methods of measurement were used in the dietary and biochemical studies (27, 28). In every case the surveys were conducted by specialists of the host country, assisted by clinicians, biochemists, laboratory technicians, nutritionists, dentists, and food and agriculture specialists from the United States. Variations in food habits and in nutrient intakes were found to result in different nutrition and health problems. Follow-up work conducted in the surveyed countries has indicated some of these problems. Mention will be made later of some of the developing countries surveyed and of the studies now being conducted in the United States.

Methods used in nutrition investigations must be valid. Shortcomings in nutrition studies which may affect the value of the research have been mentioned. Inadequate or inaccurate plans preliminary to the investigation may invalidate the results even before it is begun; its purpose must be carefully stated and reviewed from time to time. The number of subjects needed varies with the breadth or depth of the investigation; they may be chosen at random as fair samples of a large group, or they may be selected with great care to represent a specific type. When feasible, all variables but one should be eliminated. Cooperation, health, and intelligence are desirable traits of the subjects. Standardized methods should be employed. The use of controls and checks is necessary. Reversal-type experiments are performed when possible; in these, the order in which a variant is administered to the subjects is alternated, thus ruling out effects of sequence, time, etc. This complicates and often prolongs the study, but the results should be more reliable. Criteria for appraising the results must be set; objective measurements make the results more reliable. Complete records must be kept and data properly interpreted. Statistical methods of analysis should be applied when possible. The student who has a critical approach to the assessment of nutriture will find that she becomes adept in distinguishing between the logical and the illogical, the true and the false. Knowledge of nutritional needs is incomplete; practices approved today may be found faulty tomorrow. An open mind is a requisite to the man and woman whose interest lies is the science of nutrition.

PROBLEMS

1. Keep a complete record of all food and beverages consumed at and between meals for a seven-day period. Keep track of time and place of each meal and list each food eaten as to kind and amount. Under "kind" specify whether raw or cooked, if fruit or vegetable, and how prepared. For example, a vegetable salad may be made of cooked carrots and beans and raw celery; potato may be fried, mashed, creamed. Amounts should be expressed as definitely and accurately as possible—servings of meats in measurements, servings of vegetables in cups, slices of bread in number and size, etc.
2. Score your diet for each day of the above period and determine your average score for the week. Use the following score card.

Food Selection Score Card for the College Student

Food Group	Amounts Recommended	Credits		Your Daily Score
Milk[1]	4 cups or more	4 cups 3 cups 2 cups 1 cup	25 18 12 6	
Meat[2]	2 servings or more	2 servings, including at least 1 of meat, poultry, or fish 1 serving of any of above 1 serving of another food in meat group	25 15 10	
Vegetable-fruit[3]	4 servings or more	1 serving of citrus fruit 1 serving of dark-green or deep-yellow vegetable 2 servings of any fruit or vegetable	10 10 10	
Bread-cereal[4]	4 servings or more	4 servings 3 servings 2 servings 1 serving	20 15 10 5	
Total Score			100	

[1] Milk group: *maximal score 25.*
  1 cup = 8 oz. of milk.
  Equivalents in calcium value:
    1″ cube of cheddar-type cheese = ⅔ cup of milk.
    ½ cup of cottage cheese = ⅓ cup of milk.
    2 tablespoons of cream cheese = 1 tablespoon of milk.
    ½ cup ice cream = ¼ cup of milk.
[2] Meat group: *maximal score 25.*
  1 serving = 2 to 3 oz. of lean cooked meat, poultry, or fish, all without bone.
  1 serving = 2 eggs.
  1 serving = 1 cup of cooked dry beans, dry peas, or lentils.
  1 serving = 4 tablespoons of peanut butter.
[3] Vegetable-fruit group: *maximal score 30.*
  1 serving = ½ cup of vegetable or fruit or an ordinary size serving.
[4] Bread-cereal group: *maximal score 20.*
  1 serving = 1 slice bread.
  1 serving = 1 ounce ready-to-eat cereal.
  1 serving = ½ to ¾ cup of cooked cereal, rice, macaroni, or cornmeal.
Note: No more than the maximal score for each group may be credited daily.

REFERENCES

1. Virtanem, A. I. Some Central Nutritional Problems of the Present Time. *Fed. Proc., 27:*1374 (1968).
2. Schaefer, A. E. Observations from Exploring Needs in National Nutritional Programs. *Am. J. Pub. Health, 56:*1088 (1966).

3. Frisch, R. E. Present Status of the Supposition that Malnutrition Causes Permanent Mental Retardation. *Am. J. Clin. Nutr., 23:*189 (1970).

4. Schaefer, A. E. The National Nutrition Survey. *J. Am. Diet. Ass., 54:*371 (1969).

5. O'Neal, R. M., *et al.* Guidelines for Classification and Interpretation of Group Blood and Urine Data Collected as Part of the National Nutritional Survey. *Pediat. Res., 4:*103 (1970).

6. Federal Register, December 14, 1966: 31 F.R. 15730.

7. Duggan, R. E., *et al.* Pesticide Residues in Total-Diet Samples. *Sci., 151:*101 (1966).

8. Hodges, R. F. The Toxicity of Pesticides and Their Residues in Food. *Nutr. Revs., 23:*225 (1965).

9. *Review.* Composition of Milk After Removal of Strontium[90]. *Nutr. Revs., 25:*244 (1967).

10. Council of Foods and Nutrition, American Medical Ass. Improvement of Nutritive Quality of Foods. *J. Am. Med. Ass., 205:*868 (1968).

11. Agricultural Research Service, USDA, Consumer and Food Economics Research Division, Nutritive Value of Foods. *Home and Garden Bull.,* No. 72 Rev. (1970).

12. Agricultural Research Service, USDA, Consumer and Food Economics Research Division. Household Food Consumption Survey, 1965–66. Reports 1–10.

13. Sherman, H. C. *The Nutritional Improvement of Life.* New York: Columbia University Press (1950).

14. Sinclair, H. M. The Assessment of Human Nutriture. In Harris, R. S., and Thimann, K. V. (eds.), *Vitamins and Hormones.* New York: Academic Press (1948).

15. Kelsay, J. L. A Compendium of Nutritional Status Studies and Dietary Evaluation Studies Conducted in the United States, 1957–1967, *J. Nutr., 99,* no. 1, Supp. I, Part II, Sept. 1969.

16. Food and Nutrition Board, NAS-NRC. *Recommended Dietary Allowances, Revised 1968.* NAS-NRC Publ. 1694, Washington, D.C. (1968).

17. Miller, D. F., *et al.* Chronologic Changes in the Recommended Dietary Allowances. *J. Amer. Diet. Ass., 54:*109 (1969).

18. Metropolitan Life Insurance Co. *Four Steps to Weight Control.* New York: Metropolitan Life Insurance Co. (1966).

19. Grueninger, R. M. *Don't Take Growth for Granted.* Illustrated Lecture Notes: Physical Growth, School Health, The Wetzel Grid. Cleveland: NEA Service Inc. (1961).

20. Wetzel, N. C. Physical Fitness in Terms of Physique, Development, and Basal Metabolism, with a Guide to Individual Progress from Infancy to Maturity. A New Method of Evaluation. *J. Am. Med. Ass., 116:*1187 (1941).

21. Consumer and Food Economics Research Division and Human Nutrition Research Division, ARS, USDA. Food at Work for You. *Home and Garden Bull.,* No. 1, Family Fare Separate 1 (1968).

22. Groover, M. E., *et al.* Problems in the Quantitation of Dietary Surveys. *J. Am. Med. Ass., 201:*8 (1967).

23. Morgan, A. F. (ed.), *Nutritional Status U.S.A.* Berkeley: Calif. Agr. Expt. Sta. Bull. 769 (1959).

24. Leverton, R. M., *et al. The Metabolic Response of Young Women to a Standardized Diet.* USDA Home Econ. Research Rept. No. 16 (1962).

25. Horwitt, M. K., *et al. Investigations of Human Requirements for B-Complex Vitamins.* NAS-NRC Publ. 116, Washington, D.C. (1948).

26. Macy, I. G., *et al.* Physiological Adaptation and Nutritional Status During and After Pregnancy. *J. Nutr., 52,* Supp. 1:1 (1954).

27. Interdepartmental Committee of Nutrition for National Defense, National Institutes of Health. *Manual for Nutrition Surveys,* 2nd ed. Bethesda, Md. (1963).

28. Wilson, C. S., *et al.* A Review of Methods Used in Nutrition Surveys Conducted by the ICNND. *Am. J. Clin. Nutr., 15:*29 (1969).

Food, the Source of Energy

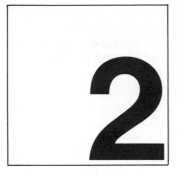

The belief that food consisted of a single universal principle, however various its form, was held for centuries. Magendie, the French physiologist (1783–1855), first clearly defined the differences in the nutritive values of the three foodstuffs, protein, fat, and carbohydrate, thereby opening a field of research concerning the extent to which each class of food could serve as a source of energy. The work of Liebig (1803–1873) in the field of organic chemistry established the elementary composition of protein, but it was accompanied by misconceptions as to its role in nutrition. During the last part of the nineteenth century the term "balanced ration," meaning a desirable proportion between carbohydrate, fat, and protein, was much discussed. The body's need for inorganic salts was also considered an important problem, and various combinations were suggested which, when used in a purified diet, would support growth. In 1906 Hopkins, of Cambridge University, showed that a diet of pure protein, fat, carbohydrate, and minerals could not promote growth in young animals, but that some alcohol-soluble organic substance in milk would furnish the missing material. A little later, Osborne and Mendel, and McCollum and Davis, verified Hopkins' findings and proved there were at least two factors involved. This work broadened the field of knowledge of what Mendel termed the "little things" of nutrition, and since then extensive chemical and physiological experiments have been performed, especially on the vitamins. The development of nutrition has thus passed through various phases, the old shading into the new, yet each era possessing a distinctive emphasis. Today special attention is being given to the interrelation and correlation of the many factors involved in energy, protein, mineral, and vitamin metabolism. Multiple deficiencies are the most widespread nutrition problems. For example, in children, when protein deficiency is severe but carbohydrates are plentiful kwashiorkor occurs;

if both protein and calories are lacking, nutritional marasmus results. Either of these diseases may prevent other nutrient lacks from causing acute disturbances. Protein lack may stunt growth to the extent that a low vitamin A intake does not result in xerophthalmia. If the protein intake is increased but vitamin A is not increased, a deficiency of vitamin A becomes evident. Energy, the phase of nutrition first studied, still holds a basic place and new knowledge is continually being gained through experimental work in this field.

FUNCTIONS OF FOOD IN THE BODY

Food builds body tissues. Growth of the body makes a great demand upon the food supply. Much experimental work has shown that alteration of the quality or quantity of food will result in changes in growth. Protein is an important substance in building tissues, but minerals also enter into their structure, often in combination with the protein; an example is iron in the hemoglobin of the blood. Calcium and phosphorus are involved in development of the skeleton and teeth. Although it is not ordinarily considered as such, water is a building material and is indispensable in all body tissues, forming about two-thirds of the total weight. These structural materials are especially needed during the most active growth period, but there is still a demand during later life due to the constant chemical changes in all the cells and tissues which go on as long as the cells live. The highest level of maintenance requires food adequate in kind and amount.

Food regulates body processes. Regulation of the body's activities might seem a less important function, but as scientific study has revealed how amazingly intricate a process the body's mechanism is, the importance of food as a means of controlling its efficiency is also recognized. Few people think of water as a food, but it cannot be replaced by any other substance in either regulation or structure of the body. Similarly, minerals are of great importance in these functions, and vitamins have a special significance. Temperature control of the body is peculiarly the function of water. Other processes in which both water and minerals are largely involved are osmotic pressure, hydrogen ion concentration of tissues, and the solvent power of fluids which affects all the interchanges of metabolic products in the body. Minerals have much influence over nerve irritability and muscle elasticity; for example, the calcium-sodium balance plays a part in the passage of nerve impulses and heart movements. Innumerable experiments have demonstrated that stimulation to growth is particularly affected by vitamins in the diet. The importance of iodine in thyroid gland functioning is doubtless only one of the cases in which a mineral has a vital connection with glandular function.

Food supplies energy. The various functions of food are so interrelated that no single one can be considered more important than the others; all must be provided for adequately in the healthy body. The materials which contain potential energy and compose by far the largest part of the total solids of food are carbohydrates, fats, and proteins. These provide the constant supply of fuel needed for body activity—some of it conscious, much of it without volition. The energy requirement can be met for a limited time by the body's own substance, but for maintenance of health under ordinary conditions, it must be supplied by food intake. In the past the practice of starving a fever was considered wise, but the resulting emaciation made recovery more difficult; today, a large intake of easily digested fuel foods is ordinarily prescribed by the attending physician. The organic foodstuffs do not release their power directly when ingested but generally pass through many chemical changes and ultimately are oxidized in the body cells to carbon dioxide, water, and nitrogenous compounds. This combustion is the source of the energy which permits the body to carry on its activities. The commonly used standard for measurement of the energy value of substances is the calorie. The same term is used to express the body's energy requirement. The unit used in nutritional work is the large calorie or the kilocalorie (kcal) and is the amount of heat required to raise the temperature of 1 kilogram of water 1 degree Centigrade. The small calorie or the gram calorie is one-thousandth of the value of the large unit and is used when minute amounts of heat are to be considered.

Another unit of energy measurement is the joule (1), a unit used in some other scientific fields. The joule has been recommended for international use by the British National Committee for Nutritional Sciences. The 1969 revision of the United Kingdom recommended intakes of nutrients includes columns for both kcal and megajoules (MJ). To convert calories to joules the factor to be used is 1 calorie = 4.184 joules. Some American nutritionists are considering the advisability of this change. However, the FNB has taken no action.

The diet may vary widely in its composition of energy-giving foods. In ordinary living little thought is given to the proportion of the three energy-giving foodstuffs in the diet. Availability and cost, habit, and taste are factors which greatly influence the ratio. The amount of protein in the American diet and the importance of calories in the utilization of this nutrient will be considered in Chapter 6. Protein foods are an expensive source of calories both economically and metabolically and furnish a relatively small part of the day's calories. Carbohydrate, on the other hand, is an economical source of energy and supplies about half the calories in the diet. The sweet flavor of the sugars and the blandness of the starches are other reasons for the large amount of carbohydrates consumed; they are filling foods and have a wide variety of uses in the day's menus. Fatty foods provide the remainder of the calories; they tend to add flavor along with low bulk and high satiety value.

The distribution in the average American diet of the three foodstuffs, in terms of percentage of total calories, is often given as follows: for the adult—carbohydrate, 50–60, fat, 30–40, protein, 10–15; for the child—carbohydrate, 50, fat, 35, and protein, 15. There is considerable deviation in these proportions, however, especially in fat and carbohydrate. Food consumption studies of families in the United States show that the trend from 1909 to 1970 has been from 56 to 46 per cent from carbohydrate, 32 to 42 per cent from fat, while protein has remained relatively constant at 11 to 12 per cent (2). Some recent studies show a continued trend toward keeping carbohydrate intake at lower levels; protein consumption has increased and, in some instances, fat intake has decreased. The latter may be related to concern about atherosclerosis and coronary artery disease.

The proportions of the three energy foodstuffs are influenced by personal taste, income level, and cultural patterns. For example, the pastas that are a staple in the Italian diet, the tortillas favored by Mexicans, and the rice used by Orientals make the diets of these groups high in carbohydrate. By contrast, in Alaska grains are not a common agricultural crop and the Eskimo eats comparatively little carbohydrate. An ICNND survey of Alaskan Eskimos (3) reported that 29.3 per cent of the total calorie intake was from protein, 35.4 per cent from fat, and 35.3 per cent from carbohydrate. A similar study conducted in East Pakistan (4) showed that the calories from protein were 11 per cent of the total, fat, 7 per cent, and carbohydrate, 82 per cent.

FUEL VALUE OF FOODS

The fuel value of a food depends on its chemical composition. It is common knowledge that foods vary in their power to satisfy hunger. This fact may be understood by studying a table of food composition. Foods high in fat are likewise high in calories and those containing much water are, conversely, poor sources of energy. As a general rule, a large amount of water is associated with a proportionately large amount of cellulose, and foods that combine these two foodstuffs may be eaten in generous amounts without increasing the calorie content of the diet very much. On the other hand, a dried fruit or vegetable, although still high in cellulose, will have much fuel value because of its relatively great amount of carbohydrate. Practical application of these facts is made daily. The stenographer chooses a lunch of salad, sandwiches, and tea, but the day laborer prefers meat, fried potatoes, and pie. The long-distance hiker packs a meal of concentrated foods, such as cheese, crackers, dried fruits, and nuts. Chocolate candy, salted nuts, ice cream, cake, and pie are to be avoided by the person who wishes to keep from gaining weight, and if eaten at the end of a large meal they may cause a stuffed, uncomfortable feeling. This is one reason why serving fruit for dessert is desirable.

The cooking of food sometimes materially reduces the amount of fuel available to the body. Frequently a considerable difference in the number of calories is found in food before and after cooking; meat which contains a large amount of fat is a good example. With application of heat, much of the fat melts and runs down into the cooking pan. If this fat is not used in the preparation of gravy or served on the food in some way, the calorie value of the meat as it comes to the table is distinctly less than when it came from the shop. A piece of bacon may lose as much as nine-tenths of its calories when broiled. There may be some loss of soluble nutrients during the cooking of vegetables, but this loss is minimized when small amounts of water are used and if the cooking water is incorporated into gravies and soups.

MEASURING THE ENERGY VALUE OF FOOD

The bomb calorimeter is used to measure the heat of combustion. Some mechanical device is necessary to determine accurately the heat of combustion of substances. The bomb calorimeter made by Berthelot and modified by Atwater and his co-workers is used in research projects. In an experiment, a weighed portion of the food whose calorie value is to be determined is placed in the bomb; after the bomb is charged with pure oxygen, it is submerged in water. An electrical circuit causes combustion to take place. The heat given off into the water is measured by a thermometer calibrated to one-hundredth degree Centigrade. The rise in temperature of the water and the total heat capacity of the water bath and bomb are determined; it is then possible to determine the energy released by the food burned. The process requires accuracy at every point.

Definite values are obtained when pure foodstuffs are burned. The heat of combustion of a substance is one of its characteristic constants. By burning each of the foodstuffs in a bomb calorimeter, it has been found that carbohydrate has an average fuel value of 4.1; fat, 9.45; and protein, 5.65 calories per gm. Explanation of the differences in energy content exists in the chemical composition of the three materials. In carbohydrate there is enough oxygen in the molecule to combine with all the hydrogen, and only the carbon, present in small proportion, remains to be burned; a correspondingly small amount of heat will be produced. With fats which have little oxygen in the molecule, the carbon and nearly all the hydrogen are oxidized and much heat is evolved. This explains why, weight for weight, butter fat yields more calories than does sugar. In their heat-giving power, proteins lie between fats and carbohydrates, since they contain more oxygen than do the fats. The nitrogen when burned has no fuel value.

THE CALORIC VALUE OF FOOD WITHIN THE BODY

The process of combustion within the body is similar to that in the calorimeter, but there are some significant differences. Oxidation of food in the cells is, on the whole, like the burning of the same material in the laboratory, but it differs in two ways. The first difference is one of incompleteness of digestion in the body, as may be shown by analysis of excreta; the second is an additional loss as a result of incomplete burning within the body. These differences were considered by Atwater and Snell (5), who were the first to develop a system of calculating calorie values. After securing the average fuel values of the three food-stuffs in the calorimeter, they studied the losses which might be˙ expected in the body. They deducted 1.25 calories per gm. of protein since this foodstuff is incompletely oxidized by the human being; an average of 46 determinations on the urine of men consuming mixed diets showed that 1.25 calories represented the heat of combustion of the nitrogenous end products excreted by the body per gm. of protein. No such loss is found when the body oxidizes fat and carbohydrate.

The decrease in fuel value in the body due to incompleteness of digestion was also studied by Atwater and Snell who furnished data concerning the coefficients of digestibility of many common foods. On a typical mixed diet they assumed that the following averages were valid for use: carbohydrate, 98 per cent; fat, 95 per cent; protein, 92 per cent. On multiplying these coefficients of digestibility by the respective calorimeter values, protein having been corrected for incomplete oxidation, they obtained the figures 4, 9, and 4, which are called the physiological fuel values of the three foodstuffs. These factors are considered useful when estimating the fuel value of average American diets, but they are not satisfactory for individual foods or for diets in which the proportions of protein, fat, and carbohydrate differ markedly as they might in diets of other countries.

Specific data should be used to calculate calorie values of individual foods. Rehabilitation problems after World War II emphasized the significant part played by calories, especially in sections of the world where food supplies are limited. Small errors in calculating the energy content of a food could make huge differences in international allocations. As a consequence, the FAO appointed a Committee on Calorie Conversion Factors and Food Consumption Tables to study problems related to energy values. Two bulletins resulted: *Energy-Yielding Components of Food and Computation of Calorie Values,* published in 1947, and *Food Composition Tables for International Use,* in 1949 (6, 7).

Food composition tables have been available for use in America since 1896 when Atwater and Wood first prepared the USDA's famous Bulletin 28. But the most comprehensive set of American tables, Agriculture Handbook No. 8, *Composition of Foods—raw, processed, prepared* by Watt and Merrill (8), first appeared in 1950. A revised edition was issued in 1963. Both the American and FAO bulletins have employed specific data, when available, in calculating caloric value rather than the Atwater and Snell factors.

Coefficients of digestibility of the three foodstuffs vary considerably in different foods. A wheat flour of 70 to 74 per cent extraction has a carbohydrate coefficient of digestibility of 98 per cent, whereas the carbohydrate in a flour of 97 to 100 per cent extraction is only 90 per cent digested (9). The protein coefficient of digestibility of milk is 97 per cent, that of dry beans, peas, and nuts, 78 per cent (see Table 4–1, p. 67). Both the Agriculture Handbook No. 8 and the 1947 FAO bulletin mentioned above give tables of the digestibility factors now known, but more information is needed, particularly for foods used in the developing countries.

Errors in protein calculations exist in the older food composition tables since the protein content of a food was ascertained by multiplying its nitrogen content by 6.25 on the assumption that all proteins contain 16 per cent nitrogen; this is not true. It was also generally considered that all nitrogen in a product was in the form of protein; this is not the case in any food, and in some plant foods the amount of nonprotein nitrogen may be considerable. Little information on this aspect of the problem is available; until it is, food composition tables will use the factor 6.25 except for a few foods listed in the 1947 FAO bulletin. For example, in milk the nitrogen content is multiplied by 6.38, in refined wheat flour, by 5.70, in almonds, by 5.18.

Another problem considered by the FAO Committee is the calorie value of the organic acids which are oxidized in the body. Whereas in general these acids furnish only a small amount of fuel, in fruits and vegetables the contribution may be considerable. The factor 2.45 calories per gm. is used for the organic acids. In lemon juice 6.25 per cent of the total calories comes from the organic acids; in oranges, 6.45 per cent; in cauliflower, 6.54 per cent; in cabbage, 2.29 per cent.

METHODS OF COMPILING DATA ON FOOD VALUES

Data may be secured from tables of food composition. Reference was made in Chapter 1 to the table of food composition in the Appendix. Development of such a table is an involved procedure requiring not only the acquisition of available data but also a critical approach to selection, classification, and interpretation (10). To be acceptable for use, values must be reliable, that is, derived through approved procedures of analysis carried out accurately. Many determinations for each food, made in different locations at different times, are desirable. A single representative value is selected from all the data on hand concerning a food. For example, the calorie value of ground beef varies depending on its fat content, which may range from 2 to nearly 50 per cent; the average amount was found to be 21.2 per cent. Therefore, ground beef with this fat content was selected for use in the food composition table. When several foods are combined, as in a recipe, the nutritive values may vary widely. Whether whole or skim milk is used in a cream soup, cocoa or chocolate used in a beverage, or nuts or raisins added to cookies makes a difference in both calorie value and nutrient values. Merrill, Adams, and Fincher (11) have prepared a bulletin which gives formulas and procedures used in calculating the nutritive values of the home-prepared foods listed in Handbook No. 8.

Food value tables in use today include many nutrients, and work is in progress to secure quantitative information for more. Specific amino acid data are especially important in countries where protein malnutrition is prevalent. Figures on more of the vitamins and minerals will be useful as they become available, but much time and cooperative effort will be required to obtain these data (12). Many tables have already been compiled for foods of various countries (see pages 428–430 for a list of food composition tables). Those by Chatfield and a complete list of references prepared by McMasters (13) may be of special interest to nutrition students and to nutritionists working in other countries.

Short methods for estimating food values are used. At times less exact and accurate information may be sufficient, possibly even preferred. Larger numbers of people may be used if size of servings is estimated rather than weighed; also a more representative sample of subjects and better cooperation may be secured. Time and cost are influencing factors. But it should be remembered that, if sufficient control is not exercised, an investigation may be worthless. Small errors may be very serious.

In the short methods of dietary calculation, average values for groups of foods are used; products with similar nutritive values and functions are combined. Compromise in groupings is necessary because eight or more nutrients are involved and because the same foods, in varying degrees, may be good sources of several nutrients. Leichsenring and Wilson (14), who have formulated a plan for use with foods as eaten by individuals or groups of people, list 42 group classifications. Fewer categories are needed when food as purchased is to be used in computing food values. Eleven groupings are included in the short method used by the USDA in studying food plans for families and institutions, but this grouping is not intended for individual or family dietaries. Hankin and associates (15, 16, 17) have developed and tested on a group of Japanese-American men a short means of dietary calculation for epidemiologic studies based on multiple regression analysis. This method offers promise of decreasing the time and cost of obtaining reliable estimates of nutrient intakes. It involves a procedure for converting quantities of measured foods into equivalent gram weights and a brief questionnaire which ascertains the frequency of ingestion of specified foods by the group being studied.

A mechanical means for processing data pertinent to dietary studies has been developed by the USDA for use with Home and Garden Bulletin No. 72, *Nutritive Value of Foods* (18). This simple computer uses two sets of punched cards, one with the quantities of food consumed, the second with nutritive values per specific unit of food. The two sets are matched by identifying food codes. These cards provide an efficient and economical method for tabulating data.

PROBLEMS

1. Compute the calories in three of the more typical days of the seven-day food intake record which was kept in Problem 1, Chapter 1. Calculate the average daily intake.
2. Calculate the protein, fat, carbohydrate, calories, and cost of several commonly used recipes.
3. Plan a day's diet for a college girl who requires 2000 calories per day. In your plan include the foods listed as essential in the daily diet. Use the score card from Problem 2, Chapter 1.
4. Compile lists of foods high in fat and in calories, and high in water and low in calories to be used by lay persons on reducing diets.

REFERENCES

1. Ames, S. R. The Joule-Unit of Energy. *J. Am. Diet. Ass., 57:*415 (1970).
2. National Food Situation. NFS-134. ERS, USDA (1970).
3. Mann, G. W., *et al.* The Health and Nutritional Status of Alaskan Eskimos, A Survey of the ICNND—1958. *Am. J. Clin. Nutr., 11:*31 (1962).
4. Interdepartmental Committee of Nutrition for National Defense, National Institutes of Health. *Transactions of the Second Far East Symposium on Nutrition, Taiwan 1964.* USA, ICNND National Institutes of Health. Bethesda, Md. (1965).
5. Atwater, W. O., *et al.* Description of a Bomb Calorimeter and Method of Its Use. *J. Am. Chem. Soc., 25:*659 (1903).
6. Food and Agriculture Organization of the United Nations, Committee on Calorie Conversion Factors and Food Composition Tables. *Energy-Yielding Components of Food and Computation of Calorie Values.* FAO, Rome (1947).
7. Chatfield, C. *Food Composition Tables for International Use.* FAO, U.N. Nutritional Studies No. 3, Rome (1949).

8. Watt, B. K., *et al. Composition of Foods—raw, processed, prepared.* USDA, Agr. Handbook No. 8 (Revised 1963).

9. Merrill, A. L., *et al.* Physiologic Energy Values of Wheat. *J. Am. Diet. Ass., 24:*953 (1948).

10. Watt, B. K. Concepts in Developing a Food Composition Table. *J. Am. Diet. Ass., 40:*297 (1962).

11. Merrill, A. L., *et. al. Procedures for Calculating Nutritive Values of Home-Prepared Foods.* ARS, USDA 62-13 (1966).

12. Leung, W. W. Problems in Compiling Food Composition Data. *J. Am. Diet. Ass., 40:*19 (1962).

13. McMasters, V. History of Food Composition Tables of the World. *J. Am. Diet. Ass., 43:*442 (1963).

14. Leichsenring, J. M., *et al.* Food Composition Table for Short Method of Dietary Analysis (2nd rev.). *J. Am. Diet. Ass., 27:*386 (1951).

15. Hankin, J. H., *et al.* A Short Dietary Method for Epidemiologic Studies I. Developing Standard Methods for Interpreting Seven-Day Measured Food Records. *J. Am. Diet. Ass., 50:*487 (1967).

16. Ibid. II. Variability of Measured Nutrient Intakes. *Am. J. Clin. Nutr., 20:*935 (1967).

17. Ibid. III. Development of Questionnaires. *Am. J. Epidemiol., 87:*285 (1968).

18. Thompson, E. M., *et al.* Computers in Dietary Studies. *J. Am. Diet. Ass., 40:*308 (1962).

The Energy Balance

3

The body's appetite center, popularly called the "appestat," is located in the hypothalamus. When this center functions normally calorie intake is regulated so that an adult's body weight may be maintained without special consideration. On the other hand, appetite often fails to function as a perfect gauge, as is shown by the widespread conditions of overweight and underweight.

It might be thought that calorie intake is sure to be optimal when an adult's weight is kept constant, but three questions must be considered before this conclusion is reached. First, is the weight proper and desirable for the individual who, it may be assumed, is in good health? Second, is a change called for in treatment of some diseased condition, such as a fever? Third, from the standpoint of the community or the nation does the individual's calorie intake allow for the most productive labor? The answers to these questions are not simple and are for the most part beyond the scope of this book, but they must be considered in any discussion of energy metabolism.

METHODS FOR ASCERTAINING THE BODY'S ENERGY NEEDS

Respiration studies are given precedence as a means of determining calorie requirement. In days gone by, an individual's energy output often was determined by means of involved balance studies which considered the relationship of intake to output of carbon and nitrogen during a long period of carefully controlled diet. This procedure has been replaced by the more simple and flexible direct and indirect calorimetry. The direct method is similar in principle to the bomb calorimeter determination, but it differs in many details, since it is applied to a living subject. It is the fundamental method and is employed as a check for the indirect devices in more common use. Because it is most frequently used, indirect calorimetry will be considered first. The energy output is not measured directly by heat given off, it is calculated from the oxygen used by the subject during a definite period of time. This is possible because a known amount of oxygen is required to burn a given food and this process has a constant heat equivalent.

Several types of apparatus are used in clinical practice. These measure only oxygen consumption. In basic research, both oxygen and carbon dioxide utilization are ascertained. When the calorie requirement of a person at work is to be determined, indirect calorimetry is used. A machine has been developed for this purpose by Müller and Franz. This consists of a small gas meter that measures the volume of air exhaled and a collection bag the size of a basketball bladder; the entire apparatus weighs less than eight pounds and may be worn during a test. It affords a relatively convenient and inexpensive indirect method of obtaining simultaneously data on total pulmonary ventilation and samples of expired air.

Another development in indirect calorimetry permits continuous and long-term analysis of exhaled gases. Whedon and co-workers (1) have evolved a metabolic chamber for use in such studies. In the room-sized chamber expired air is collected continuously for periods of several hours or several days, and the exact system of analysis permits accumulation of data which indicate minute-to-minute variations in oxygen-carbon dioxide exchange. Air conditioning of the chamber permits control of temperature and humidity over a wide range of environments.

Direct calorimetry is the fundamental method of energy determination. In ascertaining fuel needs of an individual, no other method is as direct as is that involving use of the respiration calorimeter. The general principles of this apparatus are similar to those of the bomb calorimeter in that there is a well-insulated closed chamber, a supply of oxygen for combustion, and a means for measuring the heat evolved by the temperature rise of water.

The first calorimeter which gave accurate determinations on human subjects was made at Wesleyan University, Middletown, Connecticut, by Atwater. Gradually, improvements were devised which permitted more accurate work. The Atwater-Rosa-Benedict calorimeter is accepted today as a reliable type of respiration calorimeter, but because of its great cost only a few machines have been constructed. Fundamental data have been secured in the respiration calorimeter at the Carnegie Nutrition Laboratory. Others are at the Russell Sage Foundation, Cornell University, and Pennsylvania State University. At the latter institution, a respiration calorimeter designed for use in determining the energy requirement of cattle has been adapted for studies on human beings.

Another technique has been applied to direct calorimetry by Benzinger and his associates (2) at the Naval Medical Research Institute at Bethesda, Maryland. This method is considered valuable because of its rapid response to temperature changes and its high degree of precision; it translates the rate of heat transmission from the calorimeter chamber into a varying electrical force which is recorded continuously during a test. Studies on human beings have investigated rapid changes in heat loss as affected by shifts in body position, drafts of air, and drug stimulation.

The amount of creatinine in the urine has been used to measure basal heat production. Work done by Folin and others has established that the amount of creatinine in the urine is an index of muscle mass. If the assumption is true that the total protoplasmic mass, which is largely muscle, is the fundamental source of heat in the body, the creatinine excretion may be used as a measure of the energy metabolism. Talbot (3) has used this means in the study of children's energy needs and considers it valid.

Dietary studies consider actual food intake. The methods of indirect and direct calorimetry described above are somewhat limited in their usefulness because the subject is either lying down or working at a single type of activity during the test. As a means of obtaining a complete picture of daily living, the dietary study is commonly used and is valuable in spite of certain defects to be discussed later. In order to estimate body needs, it is necessary to use a large number of healthy subjects who may be depended on for reliability and cooperation. Careful selection of individuals considered typical of a group is of vital importance for drawing valid conclusions. In the adult, maintenance of body weight over a period of time is indicative of a proper food intake. The child should eat enough for optimal growth. In a dietary study it is assumed that a healthy individual will voluntarily eat day after day the amount of food his body needs. Therefore, voluntary food intake is quantitatively measured over a period of time. The actual caloric value of the food consumed may be estimated by the use of reliable tables of food composition or by burning an aliquot sample in a calorimeter. In conducting a dietary study, between-meal eating presents a problem, not only because of the possibility of incomplete or inaccurate reports of the food consumed, but also because of the difficulty in estimating the calorie value of the product whose composition is not accurately known. Actual study in the calorimeter of an aliquot portion eliminates this source of error. Another difficulty is related to waste; some workers have carefully analyzed this throughout the entire period; others have made chemical determinations at intervals; but the majority have assumed the refuse to be a certain percentage of the total food as purchased.

Studies by Adelson, Delaney, Miller, and Noble (4, 5) made on three groups, two urban and one farm, determined that 7 to 10 per cent of the calorie value of household food supplies were discarded. In the case of fat, the percentage not consumed was greater than that consumed. The study divided the food into seven homogeneous groups for comparison.

Calorie losses varied considerably: meat, poultry, and fish, 17.7 per cent; fats and oils, 8.8 per cent; grain products, 4.7 per cent; sugar and sweets, 1.9 per cent; dairy products, 2.9 per cent; eggs, 3.1 per cent; vegetables, fruits, and nuts, 5.5 per cent.

The type of investigation to be made influences the choice of method. Four methods of determining energy needs of the body have been discussed: indirect calorimetry employing respiration apparatus; direct calorimetry investigations; creatinine measurement; and dietary studies. Although the results of each method express heat production, the means by which the problem is attacked vary definitely in complexity, in time involved for the test, and in ease of operation as well as in the accuracy of results secured. The great original cost of a direct calorimeter, the intricacy of its manipulation, and the number of technicians required limit its use. In the past it was used to secure fundamental data and to check the reliability of the results obtained by other methods. Swift and co-workers (6, 7) used both direct and indirect calorimetry in a study of heat production of men; they found close agreement between the results with the two methods.

In the dietary study the use of chemical analyses or of calorimetric determinations gives more accurate results in calculating the calorie intake than does the use of proximate composition tables. When carefully done on a large group, over a long period of time, with control of waste and adequate knowledge of health conditions, the data secured are of value in setting a standard for comparable groups. Frequently the dietary study is conducted, not to set standards for energy, but to determine whether or not the group in question is receiving calories equivalent to their predicted requirement.

As a means of determining basal metabolism, the respiration apparatus has long held a prominent place, and today it is used to some extent to measure the effect of various activities on calorie requirement. For the research worker, it is a practical method, but it must be remembered that for accuracy of data all tests must be carefully controlled and checked and the apparatus must be calibrated and kept in good condition.

THE PART BASAL METABOLISM PLAYS IN ENERGY METABOLISM

Basal metabolic processes are continuous in the body. The term "activity" is often thought of as meaning voluntary movement, but it is really much broader, since internal body activity is continuous throughout life. Among the involuntary processes concerned with metabolism are respiration, circulation, glandular activity, and the maintenance of muscle tonus. These are termed the "basal metabolic processes." In respiration the lung action goes on automatically and rhythmically. The blood circulates through the arteries, veins, and capillaries, day and night without ceasing; every contraction of the heart forces out approximately five ounces of blood, a daily total of 4000 gallons. Glands of internal secretion, for the most part, involuntarily carry on their functions, and considerable energy is required for their work. The kidneys are filters which operate continually, and the intestinal tract, even when no food is being digested, contracts and relaxes rhythmically. These functional activities involved in circulation, respiration, and glandular action explain approximately one-fourth of the fundamental or basal requirement. The greater part of the basal needs is the result of oxidation processes in the resting tissues. Through these, muscular tonus, an activity of inestimable importance to health, is maintained. All these processes involve work which in turn requires fuel. As a matter of fact, more than one-half of the body's total fuel needs for a moderately active person arise from these involuntary activities.

In the 1968 revision of RDA the term "resting metabolism" is used in place of basal metabolism. The FNB defines resting metabolism as the metabolism of a person in a normal life situation while at rest, with normal body temperature. It includes the specific dynamic action of meals and is an average minimal metabolism for the night and the periods of the day when there is no exercise and no exposure to cold. The Board states that, in actual practice, there is more interest in the energy requirement of resting metabolism than in that of basal metabolism.

The basal metabolic rate is determined under standard conditions. When certain factors are consistently controlled, it has been found that the energy demands are nearly constant in the same individual from day to day and in different healthy individuals of the same sex, age, and body build. Thus it is important to know what conditions must be regulated to secure comparable results. The basal metabolism is measured when a person is lying quietly in a relaxed condition, awake, in a post-absorptive state (12 to 14 hours after the last meal), and at a comfortable temperature.

Tests made indicate that in the majority of cases 30 minutes of rest in bed are necessary to secure relaxation; consequently, one-half to one hour of rest is a procedure preliminary to running a basal metabolism test. However, since the stimulating effect of strenuous work may persist for as much as five or six hours, it is desirable to avoid active exercise before a determination is made. An early morning hour is frequently used because at this time the body is more completely relaxed. Nervous as well as muscular relaxation is necessary; nerve activity will increase contraction of skeletal muscles which in turn increases the rate above basal. A half-hour of rest on the bed will do little toward attaining the desirable physical state if fear or excitement over the experience is not reduced; for this reason the first test made on a subject is apt to give higher than normal figures.

The test is made when the body is in a post-absorptive condition because food increases the rate. This is another reason morning is usually chosen for the determination, but Bauer and Blunt (8) have shown that the noon hour may be used, provided only a light breakfast is eaten. In their studies the morning meal contained not more than 470 calories and 14 gm. of protein and was eaten at least four hours before the metabolism observation was made. Under such conditions the oxygen consumption varied on an average of only 0.6 per cent from that observed before breakfast. Since it is frequently easier to secure subjects for experimental work later in the day than in the morning, they suggest use of the noon hour for the basal period.

A uniform, comfortable room temperature is another necessary condition for basal determinations, since an extreme may cause shivering or perspiring which will increase the metabolic processes.

In clinical practice chemical procedures usually are substituted for the basal metabolism test. Since the basal metabolic rate is affected by thyroid activity, certain tests involving iodine compounds may be used to measure normalcy. The level of protein-bound iodine (PBI) or of butanol-extractable iodine (BEI) in the blood may be determined. Good correlations with basal metabolism tests have been obtained with both these methods in subjects not receiving iodine treatment. However, with patients on iodine therapy the BEI determination is recommended since it measures only the iodine bound to protein, whereas the PBI determination also measures the free iodine in the blood. Another technique involves determining the amount of a measured dose of radioactive iodine in the thyroid gland at the end of 24 hours. Still another method measures the binding affinity of the serum proteins for thyroid hormones. In this procedure the triiodothyronine uptake on a resin sponge is determined. This method is reliable even when the subject has been taking iodine medication.

BASAL METABOLISM PREDICTIONS AND ACTUAL FIGURES

The body's surface area is most commonly used as the basis for predicting an individual's basal rate. Table 3–1 gives the standards based on surface area for ages three to 75, and Figure 3–1 gives a nomograph by which surface area may be ascertained when weight and height are known. This method of determination was developed by DuBois (9); the fact that heat loss from the body is directly proportional to skin surface explains the general acceptance of this method for estimating basal rate.

Other methods of predicting the basal metabolic rate are also used. Weight and standing height were proposed as the basis for basal metabolism predictions by Harris and Benedict (10). The results of this method compare favorably with those of DuBois. A rough approxima-

Table 3–1

Basal Metabolism Standards: Man*†

Age	Males	Females	Age	Males	Females
yrs.	cal. per sq.m. per hr.	cal. per sq.m. per hr.	yrs.	cal. per sq.m. per hr.	cal. per sq.m. per hr.
3	60.1	54.5	26	38.2	35.0
4	57.9	53.9	27	38.0	35.0
5	56.3	53.0			
6	54.0	51.2	28	37.8	35.0
7	52.3	49.7	29	37.7	35.0
			30	37.6	35.0
8	50.8	48.0	31	37.4	35.0
9	49.5	46.2	32	37.2	34.9
10	47.7	44.9			
11	46.5	43.5	33	37.1	34.9
12	45.3	42.0	34	37.0	34.9
			35	36.9	34.8
13	44.5	40.5	36	36.8	34.7
14	43.8	39.2	37	36.7	34.6
15	42.9	38.3			
16	42.0	37.2	38	36.7	34.5
17	41.5	36.4	39	36.6	34.4
			40–44	36.4	34.1
18	40.8	35.8	45–49	36.2	33.8
19	40.5	35.4	50–54	35.8	33.1
20	39.9	35.3			
21	39.5	35.2	55–59	35.1	32.8
22	39.2	35.2	60–64	34.5	32.0
			65–69	33.5	31.6
23	39.0	35.2	70–74	32.7	31.1
24	38.7	35.1	75+	31.8	
25	38.4	35.1			

* From Boothby, in *Handbook of Biological Data,* 1956. W. S. Spector, editor. Reprinted courtesy W. B. Saunders Co., Philadelphia.

† These values are smoothed means of basal calories per sq.m. per hr. from the three largest and most authoritative sets of standards. The British standards (Robertson and Reid) are based on 987 males and 1323 females; the Mayo Foundation standards (Boothby, Berkson, and Dunn) are based on 639 males and 828 females; the Carnegie Nutrition Laboratory standards (Harris and Benedict) are based on 136 males and 103 females.

tion of the basal rate sometimes used is 1 kcal per kg. of body weight per hour.

When total body weight is used to determine basal fuel needs, no distinction is made between composition of muscle, fat, and water. It is in muscle that practically all the cell activity and oxygen consumption takes place, and therefore the amount of this tissue, frequently spoken of as lean body mass, is recognized as a more significant indicator than total body weight. Miller and Blyth (11) studied 48 college students who had a wide range of body fat (2.7 to 44 per cent), a wide range of lean body

Figure 3–1

Chart for determination of surface area. (From Boothby, Berkson, and Dunn, in Studies of the Energy Metabolism of Normal Individuals: A Standard for Basal Metabolism, with a Nomogram for Clinical Application. Am. J. Physiol., 116:468 [1936]. Reprinted by permission.)

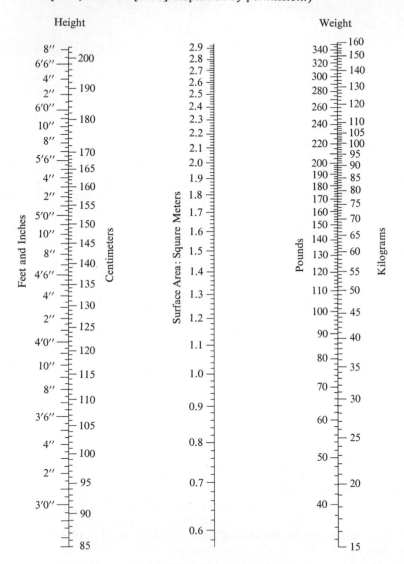

mass (40 to 90 kg.), and normal thyroid activity. These workers found that all individuals, lean or plump, had the same metabolic rate per unit of lean body mass. As yet there is little use of this method of predicting the basal rate, due to comparatively few studies on lean body mass. Keys (12) advocates use of the value of 4.4 ml. O_2 per minute per kg.

of fat-free body weight of both males and females 20 to 60 years of age to indicate the expected basal metabolic rate. Young and co-workers (13) at Cornell University have studied basal oxygen consumption in order to predict lean body mass in young women. They have proposed the formula:

LBM (kg.) = 16.270 + 0.1354 basal oxygen in ml./minute.

To predict lean body mass, however, they believe that the use of skin-fold and body weight data is the preferred method.

Comparison is made of actual and predicted metabolism. Because of its help in diagnosis and its significance as a measure of physical fitness, the basal metabolism test may be included as a routine part of a complete physical examination. In determining how to assess test results, it is first important to be satisfied that the data secured are not high because the subject is inexperienced and consequently apprehensive or overly zealous. Familiarity with the apparatus favors relaxation of mind and muscle, with the result that more reliable figures may be obtained than from a first-run test. Some workers advocate use of the lowest figure secured from two or three tests, if these results agree within 5 per cent. Others take the mean of all tests performed on an experienced subject.

It is common practice to express the relationship of actual and predicted basal metabolism in terms of percentage. When this is done, a deviation of 10 per cent usually is assumed to be normal, although 15 per cent plus or minus the predicted figure sometimes is accepted. Of 127 normal cases studied by Boothby and Sandiford (14), 99.3 per cent were within the range of −15 to +15, and 92.1 per cent were within the −10 to +10 range. If the result of a basal metabolism test is outside the range accepted by the physician, the person will be considered as having abnormal metabolism and will be treated accordingly.

The prediction standards which have been in use are thought to be too high. Actually the standards set are not truly basal since the subjects tested are awake and the body is not as completely relaxed as it would be if the test were not being conducted. According to Keys, who has made thousands of measurements on many different series of men, the Boothby, Berkson, and Dunn (15) standards overestimate true basal metabolism by about 10 per cent. Data have been obtained which show that, on the basis of body surface, the female has an average basal rate lower than that of the male; they associate this with woman's higher proportion of body fat.

Robertson and Reid (16) in 1952 compiled a table of basal metabolism standards for normal people in Britain. Their figures, resulting from 2310 determinations, are about 10 per cent lower than those generally advocated for use in this country because they are based on the lowest results on the third day of testing, in contrast to American data based largely on first tests. The latter may be called "clinical," the former, "physiological" standards, indicating their usefulness in clinics and for research purposes, respectively.

FACTORS WHICH INFLUENCE THE BASAL RATE

Body composition must be considered. The importance of actively functioning tissue in energy metabolism has been mentioned. In muscle, oxidation processes constantly go on and these increase the person's fuel needs to a very great extent. The more athletic type of individual with more muscle will have greater requirements; the fat flabby type with more storage tissue will have less. This explains the greater fuel needs of the average man over the average woman, but sex, per se, probably is not an influential factor. According to Benedict (17), the athlete's basal rate will be 5 per cent higher than the nonathletic person's.

Other factors play a role by affecting the activity of the body cells. Rate of growth is an important factor in stimulating cell activity; the general statement may be made that the greater the growth the higher will be the basal metabolism. An increment may be expected during infancy, adolescence, pregnancy, and lactation; information concerning these special periods will be considered under each related chapter. Here cellular activity in the average adult is the point at issue.

There have been many investigations on women to determine the effect of the menstrual cycle on basal metabolism. Consensus is that there is a tendency toward rise in metabolism before menstruation and a decrease on the first days of the period. It is not known whether these results are caused by increasing and diminishing glandular activity or by nervous strain resulting in muscular tension which may be at its height prior to the menstrual flow. In general, the variation noted is small and may be ignored when considering the time for making a basal determination.

There is a decrease in metabolism with age which, between the twentieth and the sixtieth years, may amount to 20 per cent. Whereas this decrease is on the whole uniform and gradual, in old age the rate diminishes more rapidly, due probably to lessening of muscle tonus and the slowing down of the body processes.

Basal metabolism determinations were made by Blunt and Bauer (18) on 18 college women who ranged from 18 to 26 per cent underweight, but no significant differences from their predicted figures were observed. A two-day E.P. dietary study showed that as the girls made their usual food selection, the average daily intake was 1830 calories per girl per day. Ten subjects were eating less than 1800 calories daily, six of them, between 1800 and 2000 calories. These amounts were considered hardly enough for the girls' daily needs and by no means sufficient for the desired gain in weight. Probably a stimulation of appetite and an increased food consumption are all that is necessary to bring the uncomplicated case of an underweight adult to normal. Underweight children may have a very high basal rate due to the relatively high proportion of muscle tissue, the body fat having been depleted early in malnutrition.

Recovery from disease in which there has been wasting of body tissue involves greater body needs and an increased basal metabolism. This is only a temporary rise and the body soon adjusts itself to its former level. Conditions of disease itself may affect the metabolic rate. Fever, which is associated with many disorders, greatly increases the calorie requirement. DuBois (9) states that for each degree Centigrade rise in body temperature there is an average increase of 10 per cent in basal metabolism; for each degree Fahrenheit rise, a 7 per cent increase. Certain glandular disorders raise or lower the needs of the body at rest; the thyroid gland is most closely associated with energy metabolism. Excess secretion will result in a marked increase in energy output, at times as much as 100 per cent over the expected rate, whereas a decreased secretion may lower the oxygen consumption markedly. Some clinics use the respiration apparatus to detect thyroid malfunction. Obesity uncomplicated by glandular disturbance has no effect on metabolism, but when it is related to thyroid or gonad insufficiency the basal rate may be definitely low. When there is hyperfunction of the adrenal glands, the energy requirement is raised.

The basal rate is affected by climate but not to any extent by race. Climate is a factor in determining the basal metabolic rate. Lower basal figures are associated with warmer environmental temperatures. Keys estimates a depression of the rate by 5 to 10 per cent in warm, and by 10 to 15 per cent in really hot climates. It might be thought that in cold regions the increase would be of the same magnitude. Actually only a slight acceleration is noted, due probably to housing which tends to overcome the potential effects of the cold. However, shivering may increase the resting metabolic rate by 50 to 100 per cent.

As environmental temperature increases the basal rate tends to decrease. It was found that lean men in the tropics have a basal heat production about 7 per cent below that of lean American men of the same weight.

The possibility of a racial factor has been investigated by numerous workers for many years. Today it is generally agreed that any differences which may be found are due very slightly, if at all, to racial differences. The seasonal variations noted in the Japanese and thought by some of their research workers (19) to be due to a racial factor are also associated with differences in environmental temperatures, diet, ability to relax, and amount of physical exertion.

FACTORS WHICH AFFECT THE BODY'S TOTAL ENERGY REQUIREMENT

Activity increases the need above the basal rate. Muscular activity, more than any other body process, is concerned in raising the fuel needs above those of a body at complete rest. Many investigations have been conducted to determine the energy expenditure involved in various activities; both direct and indirect calorimetry techniques have been used in these studies. With these fundamental research studies, standards have been set which are useful in predicting the fuel needs of a person according to his activity. Table 3–2 shows the wide variations to be expected in the day's needs as caused by different forms of exercise. What the figures in Table 3–2 do not indicate is the degree of intensity with which different people do a similar task. In using these data, too, it must be remembered that the actual time spent in an activity such as dancing may be much less than the hours spent at the dance; failure to allow for the less strenuous interim activity may exaggerate the energy requirement.

Richardson and McCracken (20) measured the energy expenditures of six subjects while they were lying down in bed, sitting, and standing quietly. Using the Müller-Franz respirometer, a total of 132 tests was made for each body position, and mean values determined. They found sitting required 10.2 per cent more fuel than lying down, and standing required 5.6 per cent more than sitting.

In studies of energy expenditure while walking, Richardson and McCracken found that at 108 and 120 steps per minute the calories used per hour were 3.9 and 12.9 per cent more, respectively, than those used at a rate of 96 steps per minute. In calories per hour, knee-bending used 29 per cent more fuel than trunk-bending. It has been assumed that less energy is used when sitting to perform household tasks over short periods of time than when standing, but according to Richardson and McCracken this is not true.

Elliot and co-workers (21) at the Ohio Agricultural Experiment Station found that in making a bed, its height from top of mattress to floor was a significant factor; the fuel used decreased when the height of the bed was raised from 20 to 30 inches. In the same laboratory it was demonstrated that ascending stairs required an average of 1.561 calories per minute and descending stairs, 1.336 calories; the pitch of the stairs made no difference in this experiment.

When a basal metabolism apparatus is used, the subject must be awake to cooperate. It has been customary to deduct 10 per cent from the "awake" figures when estimating energy expenditure during the sleeping hours. However, it is known that there is considerable variation in the amount of energy used during sleep, depending on the degree of

Table 3–2

The Energy Cost of Activities (Exclusive of Basal Metabolism and Influence of Foods) *†

Activity	Cal. per kg per hr	Activity	Cal. per kg per hr
Bedmaking	3.0	Piano playing (Mendelssohn's	
Bicycling (century run)	7.6	Song Without Words)	0.8
Bicycling (moderate speed)	2.5	Piano playing (Beethoven's	
Boxing	11.4	Appassionata)	1.4
Carpentry (heavy)	2.3	Piano playing (Liszt's	
Cello playing	1.3	Tarantella)	2.0
Cleaning windows	2.6	Reading aloud	0.4
Crocheting	0.4	Rowing	9.8
Dancing, moderately active	3.8	Rowing in race	16.0
Dancing, rhumba	5.0	Running	7.0
Dancing, waltz	3.0	Sawing wood	5.7
Dishwashing	1.0	Sewing, hand	0.4
Dressing and undressing	0.7	Sewing, foot-driven machine	0.6
Driving car	0.9	Sewing, electric machine	0.4
Eating	0.4	Singing in loud voice	0.8
Exercise		Sitting quietly	0.4
Very light	0.9	Skating	3.5
Light	1.4	Skiing (moderate speed)	10.3
Moderate	3.1	Standing at attention	0.6
Severe	5.4	Standing relaxed	0.5
Very severe	7.6	Sweeping with broom,	
Fencing	7.3	bare floor	1.4
Football	6.8	Sweeping with carpet sweeper	1.6
Gardening, weeding	3.9	Sweeping with vacuum	
Golf	1.5	sweeper	2.7
Horseback riding, walk	1.4	Swimming (2 mi per hr)	7.9
Horseback riding, trot	4.3	Tailoring	0.9
Horseback riding, gallop	6.7	Tennis	5.0
Ironing (5 lb iron)	1.0	Typing, rapidly	1.0
Knitting sweater	0.7	Typing, electric typewriter	0.5
Laboratory work	2.1	Violin playing	0.6
Laundry, light	1.3	Walking (3 mi per hr)	2.0
Lying still, awake	0.1	Walking rapidly	
Office work, standing	0.6	(4 mi per hr)	3.4
Organ playing (⅓ handwork)	1.5	Walking at high speed	
Painting furniture	1.5	(5.3 mi per hr)	8.3
Paring potatoes	0.6	Walking down stairs	‡
Playing cards	0.5	Walking up stairs	§
Playing ping pong	4.4	Washing floors	1.2
		Writing	0.4

*From C. M. Taylor and O. F. Pye, *Foundations of Nutrition*, 6th ed. New York: Macmillan, 1967. Reprinted by permission.

† To obtain total energy expenditure, add 1.1 calorie per kg per hr for each activity.

‡ Allow 0.012 calorie per kilogram for an ordinary staircase with 15 steps, without regard to time.

§ Allow 0.036 calorie per kilogram for an ordinary staircase with 15 steps, without regard to time.

relaxation during the time in bed and on the type of activity and muscular tension before going to bed. Sometimes a hood is used in this test. This permits continuous determination of oxygen consumption (and carbon dioxide production) during sleep; no mouthpiece is used and the subject can alter his body position somewhat while asleep. Buskirk and associates (22) have concluded that the 10 per cent deduction from the basal rate to represent the caloric cost of sleep may be inappropriate and that for an average value during sleep, the basal metabolic rate is more representative.

The factor of nervous activity, both of the brain center and of the branching system of nerves, is of interest from the standpoint of energy requirements, but it is more difficult to study than is muscular activity. Nervous tissue is of small magnitude, composing not more than 2 per cent of the body weight. A very delicate technique, however, has been developed to measure the energy requirement of nerve tissue. It has been found by means of a pair of extremely sensitive galvanometers that, as a result of a 10-second stimulation, a single nerve impulse caused an initial rise in temperature of 0.0000001°C., and that in the recovery phase nine times as much heat was given off. It is evident from these figures that the increase in total metabolism due to oxidation in the nerves is infinitesimal. This positive proof of a nerve metabolism similar to that of muscle metabolism stimulated other scientists in this field, and today it is known that the different types of nerve tissue have different rates of oxygen consumption, that of gray matter being much more than that of white matter.

Benedict and Benedict (23) have approached the problem in a different way. In a study of six subjects they compared the total energy output during intense mental effort with that of complete muscular and mental repose. They found that sustained activity of the mind noticeably accelerated the heart rate, made the respiratory movements irregular, and caused almost overpowering fatigue of mind and body. Of course, the test involved more or less nervous strain, yet the results showed that the increase in oxygen consumption was very small and represented only a 3 to 4 per cent rise in heat production. Since this would be the equivalent of only about 10 calories of additional energy for a period of 3 hours of concentrated study, the experiment demonstrates that the energy requirement of mental work is a matter of theoretical rather than of practical interest.

In considering practical problems, it is important to remember that although the increase in energy requirement due to nervous and mental effort is small, there may be considerable increase in muscular activity as the result of nervous stimulation. This secondary muscular activity may account for the different heat output when the same type of task is performed by two people, one high-strung and emotional, the other calm and relaxed; it may be this factor which causes one girl to be underweight while her sister carries excess pounds. Nervous or emotional unbalance which causes the hands to make continual fluttering motions or to toy with pencil or beads, the tendency to be easily startled by noises which are commonly unnoticed, the shivering manifested by some individuals when others show no such reaction—innumerable situations in daily living—exact their toll in the realm of energy. Proper muscular and nervous control is as much a part of the nutrition program as is the calorie intake.

Food influences the total calorie requirement. Lavoisier and Rubner in their classical experiments on calorimetry demonstrated that ingestion of foods caused an increase in heat production. This energy consumed as food is utilized in the production of heat and is known as specific dynamic action (SDA). Originally this was associated largely with the protein in the diet. It is known that when protein, fat, and carbohydrate are fed singly to a fasting subject different effects are noted, with protein causing by far the greatest increase in heat production. However, on a mixed diet the total effect is much less than that obtained by adding the individual effects. From a practical point of view the total diet must be considered. Only about 6 per cent of the energy value of the dietary intake is consumed by SDA. The amount varies with the level of calorie intake and is markedly decreased after fasting and after starvation. Two concepts for explaining the SDA (24) are being investigated. The first is that it is a result of a deficiency or an imbalance in the diet. The second is that, in the metabolism of foods eaten in excess of body needs, energy is wasted when glucose is converted for storage into glycerol and fatty acids, and amino acids are synthesized into peptides. In these conversions the high energy products of digestion are changed into storage compounds of low energy value and a waste of energy results.

The control of body temperature is a continually operating factor. The body temperature of a warm-blooded animal is kept at its normal level, for man about 98.6°F., by external and internal means. The external means and most of the internal are physical, and since the physical involves less wear and tear of body tissues, it is preferable to chemical regulation. External control of body temperature is affected by climate with all its variations in temperature, humidity, and air currents which, through their interrelations, provide all degrees of comfort and discomfort known to man. External control of body temperature is further affected by clothing, housing, and heating and cooling devices. As civilization has advanced, man has made ever greater use of these means. House construction differs greatly by regions. For example, in the North additional wall insulation and storm windows are required for heat conservation. House heating has been a constantly developing science until today America is known for the excessive heat in its buildings. Systems for efficiently cooling and ventilating buildings are now also common.

The type of clothing used must be recognized as a means of regulating heat loss or retention. In hot weather fabric of light weight and open mesh facilitates radiation of heat from the body. White or a light color helps to prevent absorption of the sun's rays. To keep the body warm, fabric with fibers that enmesh the air provides insulation against loss of heat from the body. This effect may be enhanced by a fleecy layer such as is often found on coats and blankets. Since houses are so well heated today, the heavy wool garments worn by our ancestors have been discarded, and additional layers of clothes are worn outdoors. The chief concern is sufficient protection from the cold which increases the body's demand for fuel.

Ease of control of body temperature is influenced somewhat by conditions of the body itself. In cold weather the person of optimal weight has an advantage over the thinner type, since a well-developed layer of subcutaneous fat acts as an efficient insulator against heat losses. Likewise the fatter person is at a disadvantage when it is hot and must control his exercise habits to prevent accumulation of heat which is not easily dissipated from his body.

Physical activities of the body are so closely related to the chemical regulation that the two must be considered together. Whatever the activity may be, it will necessitate an energy equivalent, and the required calories must be supplied either from additional food or from body tissue. This is a serious matter for the person who is underweight and who does not eat enough food, for he cannot afford to lose body tissue. The oxidation which results from all bodily movement is the chemical control which regulates temperature. These movements may be voluntary or involuntary. The former include walking rapidly, running, stamping feet, or rubbing hands. When such exercise is not taken or proves insufficient, the body attempts involuntarily to meet the extra demands upon it. Shivering occurs. When the environmental temperature is high, perspiration forms and its evaporation provides an effective cooling mechanism.

STANDARDS USED FOR THE DAILY ENERGY REQUIREMENT

Recommendations for calorie requirement have been based on occupation. Many experiments have been performed by using the methods described earlier in this chapter. From these studies, authorities such as Voit, Atwater, Tigerstedt, and Langworthy tabulated results according to occupation or general type of activity. These standards are no longer considered valid, for several reasons. First, any occupation includes a number of activities which vary from job to job in actual percentage of time spent as well as in intensity of work. Second, energy expenditure is influenced not only by the work done but also by the body weight—a factor which was ignored in setting up standards according to occupation. Third, modern technology has brought about changes in energy involved in a piece of work so that today fewer heat units are expended per hour of work than were in the past. Fourth, the work week now consists of fewer hours than it did when the standards were set. Ignoring these factors is apt to result in a gross overestimation of energy needs.

Estimations of energy requirements are based on the results of actual studies. Scales of calorie needs have been based on the factorial method, on food consumption investigations, and on dietary studies. In the first method, an estimate of energy expenditure is calculated from the individual's basal metabolic rate; the calories used during the hours of work and play, which involves keeping activity records; and the energy used in connection with SDA. The assumption is made that the energy output when accompanied by maintenance of body weight is indicative of the body's requirement.

The other methods mentioned above and first referred to in Chapter 1, when done on a large scale, give an indication of the intake of groups of people. If the nutritional status of these people has been diagnosed as good, it might be assumed that the supply equals the need. This assumption may not be accurate since more or less food may be consumed without immediate or clear-cut effects on the people concerned.

These methods of estimating energy needs hold many chances of error which will be evident to the student. Because of the large numbers of people studied and the controls used, the results may be found useful in relation to group needs but should not be relied on for prescribing for an individual.

Standards for energy requirements have been issued. In 1940 the FNB was established to advise the federal government on nutrition as it related to national defense. The need for dietary standards was recognized and a survey made of the evidence at hand. Based on the judgment of more than 50 nutrition authorities, formulations were developed of daily allowances adequate for maintenance of good nutrition in the United States population. The seventh revision was made in 1968 (25) (see table in Appendix p. 432). In 1950 the Nutrition Committee of FAO set up a Committee on Calorie Requirements (26) to define principles and make general recommendations which may be adapted to needs of persons in all parts of the world. A second report of this committee was issued in 1957.

The International and United States standards have certain similarities, but there are differences in the recommendations and in the rules for application in this country. Both standards give calorie requirements at the physiological level for healthy persons. Both describe a "reference" man and a "reference" woman and use them as the basis from which may be derived comparative requirements of people who differ in body size, age, and climatic environment. This man and woman are described as healthy, free from disease, and physically fit.

In the FAO plan both are 25 years old; the man weighs 65 kg., the woman, 55 kg. They live in the temperate zone at a mean external temperature of 10° C. (50°F.). In the United States, the "reference" man and woman are 22 years of age, weigh 70 kg. and 58 kg., respectively; the environmental temperature is estimated to be 20°C. (68°F.). The FNB has used these latter figures in preparing the RDA and adjusted calculations when necessary.

The "reference" man and woman eat an adequate diet and neither gain nor lose weight. The man's occupation consists of work which is neither sedentary nor hard physical labor. The woman's activities include either household work or a light industrial position.

In the FAO standards, the man's calorie requirement is given as 3200 per day, the woman's, as 2300. Since the activity pattern stated by the FAO is considered to be excessive for the average American, the 1968 revision of the RDA lists 2800 and 2000 calories, respectively, for the American "reference" man and woman. Adjustments are made for variations in activity, body size, age, and climate. It is assumed that most Americans are occupied in light physical activity. Examples of a day's typical activities suggested by the FNB are shown in Table 3–3. If the occupation entails heavy work, the energy expenditure may be greatly increased.

Increase in body size calls for greater kcal allowances than are indicated for the "reference" man and woman. For the adult who is neither

Table 3–3

*Examples of Energy Expenditures by Reference Man and Woman**

		Man		Woman	
Activity	*Time (hr)*	*Rate (kcal/min)*	*Total*	*Rate (kcal/min)*	*Total*
Sleeping† and reclining	8	1.1	530	1.0	480
Sitting‡	7	1.5	630	1.1	460
Standing§	5	2.5	750	1.5	450
Walking‖	2	3.0	360	2.5	300
Other#	2	4.5	540	3.0	360
			2,810		2,050

* Recommended Dietary Allowances, Seventh Revised Edition. Washington, D.C.: FNB, NAS-NRC Publ. 1694 (1968).
† Essentially resting metabolic rate.
‡ Includes normal activity carried on while sitting, e.g., reading, driving automobile, eating, playing cards, and desk or bench work.
§ Includes normal indoor activities while standing and walking intermittently in limited area, e.g., personal toilet and moving from one room to another.
‖ Includes purposeful walking, largely outdoors, e.g., home to commuting station to work site, and other comparable activities.
Includes intermittent activities in occasional sports, exercises, limited stair-climbing, or occupational activities involving light physical work. This category may include weekend swimming, golf, tennis, or picnics using 5 to 20 kcal/min for a limited time.

over- nor underweight, adaptation of kcal allowances may be based on weight. However, overweight persons tend to be less active than non-obese persons, and this may compensate for the increased energy cost of carrying the extra weight. On the other hand, the estimation of calorie requirement on a weight basis may be too low for underweight individuals.

Weight gain after 22 years tends to be fatty tissue. Therefore the FNB recommends that the so-called desirable* weight at age 22 should be maintained throughout the rest of life. Adjustments for calorie needs according to age of adults are advised. It is known that the resting metabolic rate declines approximately 2 per cent per decade of adult life and that there is a probable decrease in physical activity after early adulthood. Therefore the FNB proposes the following reductions in calorie allowances:

> 5 per cent between ages 22 and 35
> 3 per cent per decade between ages 35 and 55
> 5 per cent per decade between ages 55 and 75
> 7 per cent for age 75 and beyond

Little calorie adjustment is thought necessary for a decrease in temperature when the body is protected with adequate clothing, central heating, and heated transportation. Similarly, environmental conditions such as insulation, air conditioning, and limitation of activity are likely to prevent increases in calorie needs during warmer weather. When active exercise is carried on at a temperature between 20° and 30°C. (68° and 86°F.), it is recommended that calorie allowances be increased by at least 0.5 per cent per degree temperature rise. In this range the body temperature and the metabolic rate tend to increase, and extra energy is expended in an effort to maintain normal body temperature.

MEETING THE BODY'S NEED FOR FUEL

Wide variations in calorie consumption occur throughout the world. The problems involved in feeding an ever-expanding world population are great, especially in less developed regions. For many people, obtaining sufficient calories to sustain life is a major concern. USDA, Foreign Economic Administration Report No. 191, 1964, estimated that 92 per cent of the Latin-American people were living on diets which failed to supply the recommended calorie intake. At approximately the same time (1965), according to the survey made of the nutritive value of the diets of people in the United States, all age-sex groups except the 15- to 17-year-old girls had calorie intakes of 89 per cent or more of the recommended allowance; for the latter age group, the energy intake averaged 87 per cent.

---

* Desirable weight is defined by the FNB as the average weight of individuals of a given sex and height at age 22.

The main sources of the calorie supply vary widely in different regions of the world. In North America a high percentage of the total calorie intakes comes from animal products, fats, and oils, while in Asia, Africa, Eastern Europe, and the U.S.S.R., calories are obtained mainly from grain products, roots, and tubers.

The effects of low calorie intake on output of work have been studied. Estimations of deterioration of output at different levels of calorie deficit have been reported. If the percentage of output during hard work is 100 on an intake of 3600 calories, it will be 82 at 3300 calories, 66 at 3000 calories, and 44 at 2500 calories. These estimates may be too high, but they show what might happen to industry when diets are restricted in calories.

A detailed study of semistarvation and its rehabilitation was begun by Keys and co-workers (12) at the University of Minnesota in 1944. Thirty-six healthy young men who were conscientious objectors volunteered for the study and lived in a controlled environment throughout the year's investigation. During a control period of three months in which the diet was considered adequate, the men were put through a battery of tests; among these were x-rays, electrocardiographs, basal metabolism determinations, tests on the treadmill, endurance tests, and hemoglobin in the blood. During the next six months the men were on a famine diet, low in calories, protein, vitamin A, and riboflavin. The battery of tests was repeated and at the end of the period when the men showed many signs of deficiency, such as edema, anemia, weakness, and depression, a three-month rehabilitation test was started. In the control period the average calorie intake per man per day was 3492. The famine diet of 1800 calories produced weight losses of about 25 per cent. In the three months of rehabilitation the men were divided into four groups and received extra calories in amounts of 0, 400, 800, and 1200 calories daily. Tests showed that certain physiological changes lowered the calorie requirements of the men. Voluntary curtailment of activity as well as a reduction in energy utilization in proportion to loss of body weight accounted for two-thirds of the calorie saving. The basal rate fell 31 per cent, partly due to less active body tissue, partly to less intense metabolic work per unit of tissue; the work of the heart decreased by 50 per cent. This study suggested what may be expected during periods of famine and war.

According to the USDA, civilian food supplies in the United States in 1969 furnished 3270 kcal per person per day and are expected to supply 3290 kcal in 1970 (27). Clearly, lack of calories is no problem among American people as a whole. The dietary surveys reported in *Nutritional Status U.S.A.,* which are based on seven-day food records of 5664 healthy boys and girls and 3670 men and women, show average calorie intakes that are on the whole only slightly lower than the amounts recommended in the 1968 RDA.

Among other studies conducted to determine calorie consumption is an investigation (28) which combined the inventory and counter-service of two dining halls catering largely to men students of Brandeis University and the Harvard University Graduate School of Business Administration. Store issues, invoices, and quantitative data on recipe and yield weights and measures were recorded, as well as amounts of foods served and plate waste. Standard composition tables were used to calculate calories and selected nutrients, expressed in terms of theoretical average intake per person per day. No information was obtained concerning between-meal snacks. At the Brandeis University dining hall, the calories consumed were calculated as 3352 per man per day; at the Harvard University dining hall, 2934 calories.

Detection of caloric deviations is important. In advanced cases of deviation due to low or excess in calorie intake, the clinical symptoms detected during a physical examination may indicate the trouble. In less severe situations, an approximation of caloric well-being is often approached by comparing actual body weight with a standard and success or failure in improving the condition may be judged by the ability to gain or lose weight.

In treating a person who deviates widely from his expected weight, it is especially important to consider the amounts of tissue found in different body compartments as well as the total weight. Studies have been conducted to determine the percentages of body fat, lean body mass, extracellular fluids, and bone minerals. Among the methods used to study these body compartments are densitrometry, which is related to specific gravity; body water measurements, estimated on the dilution principle; subcutaneous fat, measured by skinfold or by soft tissue x-rays; basal metabolism; skeletal weight, determined from x-rays of bone diameters; and K^{40} content of the body, using a whole body scintillation counter. This last method involves a technique for estimating lean body mass that is useful also in other fields of nutrition. The counter, designed to measure very small amounts of radiation which emanate from the body, is relatively simple to use, takes only a short time, and is non-traumatic to the subject.

The amount of body fat in men and women differs widely. According to Keys, in healthy young men 12 per cent of the body is fat and anything less than 9 per cent represents malnutrition. Young and co-workers (29), using several methods of study, have determined that approximately 29 per cent of the weight of young women is fat. These workers have developed a practical equation for predicting specific gravity, which is considered a reliable indirect method of estimating body fatness. The equation is based on a single skinfold measure (at the mid-abdominal line halfway between the umbilicus and pubis) and the percentage of standard or average weight.

$$\text{Specific gravity} = 1.0884 - .0004321\, x_1 - .0003401\, x_2$$
$$x_1 = \text{skinfold} \qquad x_2 = \text{standard weight}$$

An equation for determining lean body mass, based on basal metabolism, was given earlier in this chapter (see page 39). Such studies as these, involving the various compartments of the body, introduce a challenging approach to the study of weight control.

An investigation based on data collected by 26 life insurance companies, which is reported in *Build and Blood Pressure Studies, 1959* (30), showed that weight tends to increase with age—in women at a later age than in men. According to this investigation, 1 in 5 adult males and 1 in 4 adult females are 10 per cent or more above average weight; 1 in 20 men and 1 in 9 women weigh 20 per cent or more above the average. The data also show that actual weights for persons over age 30 are from 15 to 25 pounds more than the desirable weights. The average weight maintained during the twenties is thought to represent the desirable weight for persons over 30.

Mortality rates increase with overweight conditions, primarily because of cardiovascular-renal diseases, but also because of diabetes mellitus and diseases of the digestive tract, the biliary tract, and the liver. The studies just mentioned warn that the mortality is one-third higher in men who are 10 per cent or more overweight than in men with desirable weights. Mortality rates are less high for overweight women than for men, but both health and mortality are adversely affected by overweight (31).

REGULATION OF BODY WEIGHT

Food intake has a definite relationship to body weight. Since weight within a certain range is considered a sign of well-being, the intelligent person who finds himself outside his range will attempt to gain or lose as the case warrants. His first consideration should be the quantity and quality of his food intake. If weight is above the optimal predicted for his build, the amount of food eaten should be reduced so the body fat may be burned for some of the energy expenditure; this limited intake may cause a sensation of hunger for a few days until the body is adjusted to its new level. On the other hand, the undernourished adult needs to store muscle and fat much as does the child, and so the food supply must be large enough to permit increment of tissue as well as maintenance. The underweight person should try to eat some additional food at each meal after he feels satisfied; by this means he may increase his capacity for food and, at the same time, gain in weight. According to Macy and Hunscher (32), success or failure in growth of children may result from a difference of as few as 10 calories per kg. of body weight. Research (33) indicates that a diet which supplies a calorie deficit of 1000 per day is roughly equal to a loss of two pounds per week. A greater loss than this is considered unwise.

Although appetite is the regulatory mechanism between intake and requirement, in many cases it does not function perfectly. The obese person must learn to curb his appetite and be guided by reason, while the undernourished should stimulate his desire for food in every way possible.

Quality as well as quantity must be considered in relation to the energy requirement. For the moderately overweight subject the only alteration in the diet may be the elimination of pie, cake, ice cream and other rich desserts, candy, salad dressings, and cream. Milk, either whole or skim, valuable for its calcium, should be included; because of their contribution of minerals and vitamins, potatoes may be given preference over bread. For the more obese a strict diet should be adhered to and there should be an even greater cut in calories than indicated above. Such a diet eliminates calorie-rich foods and includes large amounts of those vegetables and fruits which contain much water and cellulose and which supply vitamins and minerals to regulate body processes. The proportion of carbohydrate to fat must be considered because some carbohydrate is essential for the complete oxidation of fat. Associated with marked loss in weight, there may develop acidosis and digestive upsets, susceptibility to heart trouble, tuberculosis, anemia, and a lowered resistance to infection. Therefore, constant supervision of a doctor is advised.

More calories consumed than expended results in weight gain. It is well known that not all obese persons may succeed in reducing. Success is more likely if the condition is recognized in its early stages, and if the subject is emotionally well-adjusted and has a strong enough desire to lose weight so that he will adhere to a reducing schedule. Emotional and mental support from an interested person are great aids. The excuses an obese individual may give for failure to lose weight are apt to have little scientific basis. Hypothyroid disturbance in which the basal rate is low is likely to be associated with retention of excess water rather than with excess body fat. An error in metabolism resulting in increased lipogenesis may make the process of reducing more difficult. Some authorities now recommend a total fast of 24 to 48 hours at the beginning of the reducing program to break the abnormal metabolic pattern. This must be done under careful supervision.

For the underweight person who desires to gain, the recommended dietary regime is opposite that of the obese. Vegetables and fruits in moderation are needed for their bulk, minerals, and vitamins, but emphasis is on concentrated high calorie foods such as cream, butter, whole milk, nuts, eggs, and cheese. The difficulty in digesting some of these foods, particularly rich sauces and desserts, means a tax on body efficiency, and thus they may have to be served sparingly. A thin person's appetite is often poor, and when he forces his intake, appetite fails him. In such a case it is better to work on measures for increasing the desire for food; thiamin-rich foods such as wheat germ may stimulate the appetite and indirectly aid in the consumption of a liberal diet.

Several types of reducing diets have been advocated. The logical way to reduce involves cutting down on calories while maintaining an otherwise adequate diet with a wide variety of protective foods. While this is the safest procedure, it requires more will power than a specific reducing diet. There are many such diets, and most can be discarded because they are so limited in variety of foods that they are not apt to be adequate in nutritive value. Several others have a more scientific basis.

Any one of the three organic foodstuffs may be emphasized in a reducing diet plan; the main point is to have a calorie deficit and at the same time to supply a nutritionally balanced diet which the subject finds practical and satisfactory to follow over the required period of time, and even throughout life. Jolliffe (34) advocated a diet containing 1 gm. of high value protein per kg. of body weight per day, less than 30 per cent of the calories as fat, and a minimum of 50 gm. of carbohydrate. The high protein regime is popular and has several points in its favor; foods high in protein also tend to contain considerable iron, phosphorus, and the B-complex vitamins, which along with the protein make for a well-built and regulated body; this diet has satiety value. However, it is expensive; also it seems probable that the calorie intake will be so low that much of the protein will be burned for fuel rather than be used to maintain muscle tissue. The specific dynamic action of protein has in the past been considered sufficient to justify its liberal inclusion in a reducing diet, but this effect is no longer considered significant.

A low-fat or low-carbohydrate diet, high in protein and low in calories, has been used to treat obesity; this type of diet was found to result in an increase in insensible weight loss. Studies made by Cederquist and associates (35) at Michigan State University and by Young (36) at Cornell University have included diets in which 50 per cent or more of the calories were furnished by fat; in both investigations subjects were overweight college women. With a diet containing a moderate amount of fat, it was found that loss of weight could be accomplished without an accompanying hunger, excessive fatigue, or tendency to regress after the experiment was completed. Flabbiness of tissues and looseness of skin did not accompany the weight loss.

In the past decade formula diets have become popular. These use preparations planned to supply approximately 900 calories, composed of about 30 per cent protein, 20 per cent fat, and 50 per cent carbohydrate, supplemented with minerals and vitamins. To the lay person, the formula diet may seem an easy way to limit intake and cut calories. However, most nutritionists advise eating a wide variety of foods but limiting intake of those high in calories. The formula diet may tend to forestall the urge to eat just a little more. If used for limited periods, or perhaps as one of the three meals, it may have value, but is not advocated for a long-time regime. This type of diet does not help a person learn the components of an adequate diet and form normal eating patterns (37).

Activity plays a role in weight control. Strenuous exercise should be avoided by the underweight person and an attempt made to refrain from becoming hyperexcitable. Worry and tenseness result in greater muscle strain and thereby cause a demand for additional calories. It is important that the underweight conserve energy and have adequate rest and sufficient sleep. Often, too, a lighter study load for the student or an hour of assistance for the busy homemaker will relieve tension sufficiently to cause improvement in weight (38).

The role of physical exercise in a weight reduction program is also important (39). Buskirk and co-workers (40) studied six obese patients over a two-to-nine-month period during which time caloric intake and physical activity were quantitatively controlled. Energy expenditures of three subjects were measured in the metabolic chamber, and in all six subjects nitrogen and calorie balance and body composition determinations were made at regular intervals. The calorie contents of the diet, feces, and urine were measured in the bomb calorimeter. Subtraction of energy expenditure and calories lost in feces and urine from the calorie intake gave energy balance figures. It was found that a daily walking schedule of one to three hours clearly contributed to a negative calorie balance and loss of body weight during the period when calorie restriction was moderate, about 80 per cent of the maintenance level. When the calorie intake was 1000 or less per day, the contribution made by the exercise was less evident.

Mayer (41) has listed the comparative energy expenditures, in excess of that of sitting, during some activities recommended for the overweight person. Expressed in terms of calories per hour they are: walking, 100 to 500 calories depending on the speed; swimming, up to 685; climbing, up to 885; skating, up to 685; cycling, up to 585. Mayer approves of regular exercise as a sound preventive measure. He found that the onset of obesity in elementary and secondary school boys and girls tends to occur during the winter months when outdoor activity often is reduced. In an investigation of young people's eating and exercising habits he found that the obese actually eat significantly less but also exercise less actively.

Other factors may affect food intake and body weight. Of course, whether the object is to gain or to lose, regularity of meals and thorough mastication of food are habits to be instilled for the preservation of good health.

Meal spacing should be considered in any weight reduction regime. Three meals a day, each containing adequate protein, with no snacks between, are usually advocated. Some authorities advise dividing the daily food intake into small portions, to be eaten as six to eight meals a day. Multiple feedings are thought to minimize lipogenesis, and also, by maintaining the blood sugar level, to reduce hunger pains. Of course when this reducing method is followed, the quality of the diet is important. Chocolate nut sundaes or malted milks furnishing about 400 calories, or chocolate bars of 200 calories can help to add pounds.

Between-meal lunches are frequently recommended by physicians and nutrition workers for underweight persons. This procedure is open to several questions. First, does the supplementary lunch affect the appetite for the regular meal so that less total food will be eaten? Is a high quality diet maintained? Sometimes even though the snacks supply the required extra calories, interest is lessened in the next meals so that such foods as milk and vegetables are left untouched. The additional meals lose their value if either the amount or kind of total daily intake is impaired. Finally, there is a question concerning the wisdom of overworking the digestive tract; it may be better to consume the food in three rather than in four meals. In many cases, however, a fourth meal will result in a gain in weight with no apparent harm to the body.

Another factor to be considered is a person's attitude toward food. Lack of appetite frequently may be remedied by a change in diet, an adjustment more easily made than one in the psychological reaction toward food. However, dislikes can be overcome by will power and perseverance. A small serving at first, variety in the manner of preparation, or a combination of a liked with a disliked food are helpful methods of securing a pleasurable response to the food. Of secondary but significant importance are such factors as cleanliness, fresh air, and freedom from infection.

The atmosphere at meal time is another consideration. Attractive table service and pleasant conversation contribute to total satisfaction leading to good appetite and proper food consumption.

Special problems may arise. Before starting any regime planned to bring about weight change a person should have a thorough physical examination and a detailed tabulation of food consumption. Disease may be the cause or effect of poor nutritional status and, if present, may complicate the treatment. Considerable time may be necessary to rehabilitate after semistarvation. According to Keys, a person who has lost up to 30 per cent of his body weight may with proper care be returned to normal in six months. Food may be concentrated so that many calories occupy a comparatively small bulk and at the same time not be excessively rich or sweet. Occasionally intravenous feeding is prescribed for the very underweight, emaciated person; in this case a fat emulsion is considered the best carrier of calories. In oral feeding also, fat prescriptions may be advocated; an emulsion of 40 per cent peanut oil and 10 per cent glucose, with a calorie value of 4 per ml., has been found palatable and well tolerated by 141 patients.

The contributions to the daily diet made by one combination of foods are shown in Table 3–4. All the dietary allowances have been met. At first

Table 3–4
Nutrients Furnished by Foods Selected from the Daily Food Guide

Food	Weight gm.	Measure	Food Energy kcal.	Protein gm.	Calcium gm.	Phosphorus gm.	Iron mg.	Magnesium mg.	Vitamin A Value IU	Vitamin D IU	Ascorbic Acid mg.	Thiamin mg.	Riboflavin mg.	Niacin mg. equiv.	Vitamin B6 mg.	Vitamin B12 μg.
Milk, whole	488	2 cups	320	18	0.58	0.45	0.2	63	700	200	4	0.14	0.82	4.4	0.20	1.95
Cocoa, whole milk[1]	250	1 cup	245	10	.30	.27	1.0	61	400	100	3	.10	.45	2.2	.10	.98
Eggs, scrambled[1]	128	2 eggs	220	14	.10	.24	2.2	16	1380	138	0	.10	.36	4.0	.13	2.20
Beef, roast	85	3 oz.	165	25	.01	.21	3.2	24	10	0	—	.06	.19	7.3	.44	1.85
Lima beans, immature	170	1 cup	190	13	.08	.21	4.3	82	480	0	29	.31	.17	4.6	.15	—
Lettuce, loose leaf	50	2 lge. leaves	10	1	.03	.01	.7	6	950	0	9	.03	.04	.8	.03	—
Potato, baked	99	1 medium	90	3	.01	.06	.7	12	Trace	0	20	.10	.04	2.3	.09	—
Applesauce	255	1 cup	230	1	.01	.01	1.3	13	100	0	3	.05	.03	.1[3]	.08	—
Banana[2]	175	1 medium	100	1	.01	.02	.8	39	230	0	12	.06	.07	.8[3]	.61	—
Raisins (on cereal)	41	¼ cup	120	1	.03	.04	1.5	14	8	0	1	.05	.03	.2[3]	.10	—
Orange juice	187	¾ cup	90	2	.02	.03	.2	19	413	0	90	.17	.02	.8	.05	—
Toast, white, enriched	22	1 slice	70	2	.02	.02	.6	6	Trace	Trace	Trace	.06	.05	1.0	.01	Trace
Bread, white, enriched	50	2 slices	140	4	.04	.05	1.2	11	Trace	Trace	Trace	.12	.10	2.0	.02	Trace
Oatmeal	240	1 cup	130	5	.02	.14	1.4	50	0	0	0	19	.05	1.1	.05	—
Margarine	20	4 pats	140	Trace	.00	.00	.0	0	680	0	0	—	—	—	.05	—
Total			2260	100	1.26	1.76	19.3	416	5351	438	171	1.54	2.42	31.6	2.06	6.98
Recommended Allowance for Girl 16–18 years[4]			2300	55	1.3	1.3	18	350	5000	400	50	1.2	1.5	15	2	5
Recommended Allowance for Girl 18–22 Years[4]			2000	55	.8	.8	18	350	5000	400	55	1.0	1.5	13	2	5

[1] Recipe from Procedures for Calculating Nutritive Values of Home-Prepared Foods. Washington, D.C.: ARS, USDA, Pub. 62–13, March 1966.
[2] Weight and measure apply to A.P. figures.
[3] Figure for niacin used.
[4] Recommended Dietary Allowances, Seventh Revised Edition. Washington, D.C.: FNB, NAS–NRC Publ. 1694 (1968).

Sources of data:
Phosphorus and Magnesium: Handbook No. 8.
Niacin equivalent: Table 12–5, text.
Vitamin B6 and Vitamin B12: Pantothenic Acid Vitamin B6 and Vitamin B12 in Foods, ARS, USDA, Home Economics Research Report No. 36, August 1, 1969.
Other nutrients: Table A–3, text.

glance it might seem wise to decrease some amounts or eliminate some foods. However, this would be likely to result in a deficit in those nutrients already close to the border. For example, raisins, bread, and cereal add significantly to iron; eggs, lettuce, and margarine, to vitamin A value. Without the orange juice, ascorbic acid would be very low; the banana contributes markedly to vitamin B_6.

Fasting has been recommended as a means of weight reduction in grossly obese patients who have not responded to other treatment methods (42). Such therapy is effective because the accumulation of ketone bodies in the blood stream depresses the appetite. This method of reducing is not approved since the body loses more protoplasmic tissue and fluid than it does fat (43) and since after fasting there tends to be rapid weight gain. A semistarvation diet of 500 to 600 calories daily is sometimes used (44). It consists largely of protein, most of which is used for energy. If this very low calorie regime is used, the subject should be under a physician's care.

Drugs are sometimes used indiscriminately in weight control regimes. Included may be thyroid extract, digitalis, amphetamines, barbiturates, and prednisone. The FDA currently is accumulating evidence as to the use and dangers of these drugs, and it seems probable that they may be eliminated from use as reducing medications. Their effects vary from stimulating metabolism to depressing appetite; they may have serious side-effects and be habit-forming. Only in cases of extreme weight deviation and under the close supervision of a physician should they be used, and then only for a short time.

The effect of weight reduction on mineral and nitrogen metabolism is an important consideration. Young found that retentions of calcium, phosphorus, and nitrogen were poorer during weight reduction, irrespective of whether the diet was higher or lower in fat content. Leverton and Gram (45), also working with obese young women, found less efficient metabolism of calcium and phosphorus during weight loss.

Scheck and associates (46) determined the nitrogen, calcium, phosphorus, and sodium balances of five obese men, during periods of full calorie intake, starvation, and refeeding. The starvation period lasted 18 to 40 days; during this time extremely negative nitrogen and phosphorus balances and less extremely negative calcium balances occurred. In the refeeding period when the diet contained 600 calories, 35 gm. protein, 500 gm. sodium, and varying small amounts of calcium and phosphorus, the nitrogen and mineral balances improved, indicating rebuilding of body stores.

Consolazio and co-workers (47) initiated studies to determine minimal calorie and nutrient needs during periods of limited food supply. It was found that a diet of 400 calories from carbohydrate was better than a starvation diet in reducing protein catabolism, maintaining water balance, decreasing electrolyte excretion, and preventing ketosis. However, losses of water and protein still were significant and electrocephalogram tracings were abnormal. Without minerals in the diet urinary excretion of minerals was reduced drastically. With mineral supplementation mineral balance was maintained except for potassium. The extreme dietary restrictions used in this study might be necessary for the military when resupply was impossible but were considered inadequate for active men even for short periods.

Water need not be limited in the reducing diet. According to Barborka (48), it should be taken according to the person's usual habits; salt also should not be restricted unless there is excessive fluid retention.

PROBLEMS

1. Make an analysis of all facts necessary in the diagnosis of malnutrition in an underweight child or adult. Select an actual case where one or more of the factors discussed in this chapter limits the attainment of good health and describe in detail your procedure in the treatment of the individual.
2. Calculate the predicted basal metabolism for your actual and your average weight.
3. Keep a detailed record of your activities for the 24 hours of each of two days, as to type of activity, time of day, and time spent in hours and minutes. Classify your activities for each day according to those listed in Table 3–2. Make suitable substitution for any not in the table. Using the appropriate per kilogram factors, determine your energy requirement per kilogram and per total body weight. Explain any difference between the 2 days. Determine your average requirement per day.
4. Compare the average energy requirement determined by means of your activity record with the average calorie intake calculated in Problem 1, Chapter 2. Recommend changes which would make your diet adequate for energy.
5. Plan two reducing diets, each of approximately 1200 calories. One should be low in carbohydrate, the other, low in fat. How nearly does each meet the nutrient standards of the RDA?

REFERENCES

1. Whedon, G. D. New Research in Human Energy Metabolism. *J. Am. Diet. Ass., 35:*682 (1959).
2. Benzinger, T. H., *et al.* Human Calorimetry by Means of the Gradient Principle. *J. Appl. Physiol., 12:*Supp. 1 (1958).
3. Talbot, N. B. Basal Energy Metabolism and Creatinine in the Urine. *Am. J. Dis. Childr., 52:*16 (1936).
4. Adelson, S. J., *et al.* Household Records of Foods Used and Discarded. *J. Am. Diet. Ass., 39:*578 (1961).
5. Adelson, S. J., *et al.* Discard of Edible Food in Households. *J. Home Econ., 35:*633 (1963).

6. Swift, R. W., *et al.* The Utilization of Dietary Protein and Energy as Affected by Fat and Carbohydrate. *J. Nutr., 68:*281 (1959).

7. Swift, R. W., *et al.* The Effect of High versus Low Protein Equicaloric Diets on the Heat Production of Human Subjects. *J. Nutr., 65:*89 (1958).

8. Bauer, V., *et al.* Effect of a Small Breakfast on the Energy Metabolism of Children. *J. Biol. Chem., 59:*77 (1924).

9. DuBois, E. F. *Basal Metabolism in Health and Disease,* 3rd ed. Philadelphia: Lea & Febiger (1936).

10. Harris, A., *et al. A Biometric Study of Basal Metabolism in Man.* Washington, D.C.: Carnegie Institution of Washington (1919).

11. Miller, A. T., *et al.* Lean Body Mass as a Metabolic Reference Standard. *J. App. Physiol., 5:*311 (1953).

12. Keys, A., *et al. The Biology of Human Starvation.* Minneapolis: University of Minnesota Press (1950).

13. Young, C. M., *et al.* Basal Oxygen Consumption as a Predictor of Lean Body Mass in Young Women. *J. Am. Diet. Ass., 43:*125 (1963).

14. Boothby, W. M., *et al.* Basal Metabolism. *Physiol. Revs., 4:*69 (1924).

15. Boothby, W. M. *et al.* Studies of the Energy Metabolism of Normal Individuals: A Standard for Basal Metabolism with a Nomogram for Clinical Application. *Am. J. Physiol., 116:*468 (1936).

16. Robertson, J. D., *et al.* Standards for the Basal Metabolism of Normal People in Britain. *Lancet, 272:*940 (1952).

17. Benedict, F. G. Basal Metabolism Data on Normal Men and Women (Series II), with Some Considerations of the Use of Prediction Standards. *Am. J. Physiol., 85:*607 (1928).

18. Blunt, K., *et al.* The Basal Metabolism and Food Consumption of Underweight College Women. *J. Home Econ., 14:*171 (1922).

19. Yoshimura, M., *et al.* Climatic Adaptation of Basal Metabolism. *Fed. Proc., 25:*1169 (1966).

20. Richardson, M., *et al. Energy Expenditure of Women Performing Selected Activities.* USDA, Home Econ. Research Rept. No. 11 (1960).

21. Elliot, D. E., *et al. Energy Expenditures of Women Performing Household Tasks.* Wooster: Ohio Agr. Expt. Sta. Bull. *939* (1963).

22. Buskirk, E. R., *et al.* Human Energy Expenditure Studies in the National Institute of Arthritis and Metabolic Diseases Metabolic Chamber. II. Sleep. *Am. J. Clin. Nutr., 8:*602 (1960).

23. Benedict, F. G., *et al. Mental Effort in Relation to Gaseous Exchange, Heart Rate, and Mechanics of Respiration.* Washington, D.C.: Carnegie Institution of Washington, Publ. 446 (1933).

24. Griffith, W. H., *et al.* Present Knowledge of Specific Dynamic Action. *In Present Knowledge in Nutrition,* 3rd ed. New York: Nutrition Foundation (1967).

25. Food and Nutrition Board, NAS-NRC. *Recommended Dietary Allowances,* 7th ed. Washington, D.C.: NAS-NRC Publ. 1694 (1968).

26. Food and Agriculture Organization of the United Nations, Second Committee on Calorie Requirements. *Calorie Requirements.* FAO Nutritional Studies No. 15, Rome (1957).

27. National Food Situation. NFS-134. ERS, USDA (1970).

28. Myers, M. L., *et al.* Foods Consumed by University Students. *J. Am. Diet. Ass., 43:*336 (1963).

29. Young, C. M., *et al.* Predicting Specific Gravity and Body Fatness in Young Women. *J. Am. Diet. Ass., 40:*102 (1962).

30. Society of Actuaries. *Build and Blood Pressure Studies, 1959.* Metropolitan Life Insurance Co. Statistical Bull., Jan. 1960.

31. Marks, H. H. Influence of Obesity on Morbidity and Mortality. *Bull. N.Y. Acad. Med., 36:*15 (1960).

32. Macy, I. G., *et al.* Calories—A Limiting Factor in the Growth of Children. *J. Nutr., 45:*189 (1951).

33. Wohl, M. G. Obesity. *In* M. B. Wohl and R. S. Goodhart (eds.), *Modern Nutrition in Health and Disease,* 4th ed. Philadelphia; Lea and Febiger (1968).

34. Jolliffe, N. (ed.), *Clinical Nutrition,* 2nd ed. New York: Harper & Row (1962).

35. Cederquist, D. C., *et al.* Weight Reduction on Low-Fat and Low-Carbohydrate Diets. *J. Am. Diet. Ass., 28:*113; 213 (1952).

36. Young, C. M. Weight Reduction Using a Moderate-Fat Diet. *J. Am. Diet. Ass., 28:*410; 529 (1952).

37. American Medical Association, Council on Foods and Nutrition. Formula Diets and Weight Control. *J. Am. Med. Ass., 176:*439 (1961).

38. Grande, F. Energetics and Weight Reduction. *Am. J. Clin. Nutr., 21:* 305 (1968).

39. Bradfield, R. B., *et al.* Effect of Activity on Caloric Response of Obese Women. *Am. J. Clin. Nutr., 21:*1208 (1968).

40. Buskirk, E. R., *et al.* Energy Balance of Obese Patients During Weight Reduction. *Ann. N.Y. Acad. Sci., 110:*1918 (1963).

41. Mayer, J. The Physiological Basis of Obesity and Leanness. *Nutr. Abstr. Revs., 25:*597;871 (1955).

42. Bolinger, R. E., *et al.* Metabolic Balance of Obese Subjects During Fasting. *Arch. Intern. Med., 117:*3 (1966).

43. Lawlor, T., *et al.* Metabolic Hazards of Fasting. *Am. J. Clin. Nutr., 22:*1142 (1969).

44. Drenick, E. J. Weight Reduction with Low-Calorie Diets—Practical Management. *J. Am. Med. Ass., 202:*118 (1967).

45. Leverton, R. M., *et al.* Further Studies of Obese Young Women During Weight Reduction: Calcium, Phosphorus and Nitrogen Metabolism. *J. Am. Diet. Ass., 27:*480 (1951).

46. Scheck, J., *et al.* Mineral and Protein Losses During Starvation. *J. Am. Diet. Ass., 49:*211 (1966).

47. Consolazio, C. F., *et al.* Metabolic Aspects of Calorie Restrictions: Nitrogen and Mineral Balances and Vitamin Excretion. *Am. J. Clin. Nutr., 21:*803 (1968).

48. Barborka, C. J. Present Status of the Obesity Problem. *J. Am. Med. Ass., 147:*1015 (1951).

GENERAL REFERENCES

49. Johnson, O. C. Present Knowledge of Calories. *In Present Knowledge in Nutrition,* 3rd ed. New York: Nutrition Foundation (1967).

50. Keys, A., *et al.* Body Weight, Body Composition and Calorie Status. *In* M. B. Wohl and R. S. Goodhart (eds.), *Modern Nutrition in Health and Disease,* 4th ed. Philadelphia: Lea and Febiger (1968).

51. Mayer, J. Physiology of Hunger and Satiety: Regulation of Food Intake. *In* M. G. Wohl and R. S. Goodhart (eds.), *Modern Nutrition in Health and Disease,* 4th ed. Philadelphia: Lea and Febiger (1968).

Carbohydrates

In many parts of the world and especially among people of low income levels, carbohydrates occupy an unusually large and important place in the dietary; they may even prevent death from starvation. This is because they are the major dietary source of energy. But for many Americans carbohydrates are considered mainly as a means of making meals more appetizing. Some persons avoid this foodstuff because it adds excessive calories; others do so as a means of preventing or treating such disorders as dental caries and diabetes. Limitation in use by diabetic patients is a problem for the therapeutic dietitian. Relationships between dietary carbohydrates, lipid metabolism, and coronary heart disease are being studied.

THE CHEMISTRY AND OCCURRENCE OF CARBOHYDRATES

Carbohydrates vary in their chemical and physical nature. The carbohydrates differ widely in their make-up. The simple sugars or monosaccharides of interest from a nutritional point of view are the hexoses, glucose, fructose, and galactose; they are soluble in water and are readily diffusible (Figure 4–1). The disaccharides—sucrose, maltose, and

Figure 4–1
Structural formulas of monosaccharides

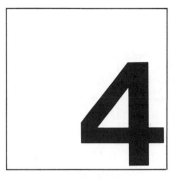

lactose—listed in order of their solubility in water are also diffusible. Each of these is composed of two simple sugars and in each case one of the two is glucose; the other is fructose, glucose, or galactose, respectively (Figure 4–2). Hydrolysis by acid or enzyme easily takes place (Figure 4–3).

Figure 4–2

Structural formulas of disaccharides

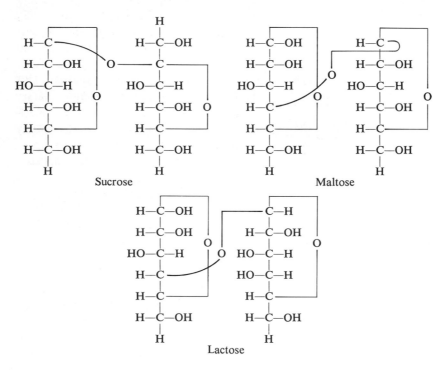

Sucrose   Maltose

Lactose

Figure 4–3

Synthesis and hydrolysis of a disaccharide

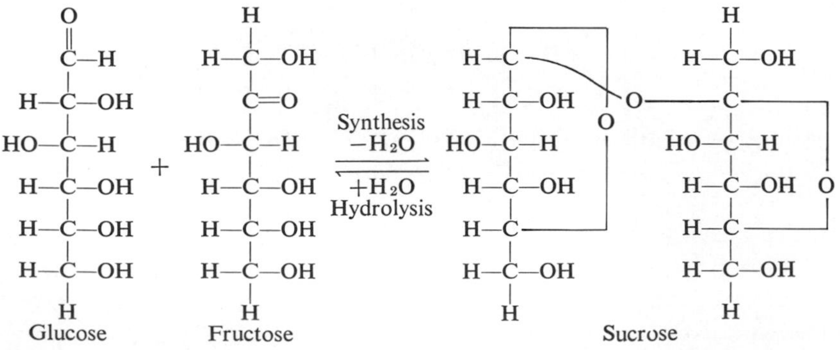

Glucose   Fructose   Sucrose

The polysaccharides include starch, the dextrins, glycogen, and the celluloses. They are complex compounds of high molecular weight composed of varying numbers of glucose molecules linked together in long chains. The characteristics of a polysaccharide are determined by the number of glucose units it contains and their arrangement within the polysaccharide molecule. Polysaccharides tend to be insoluble in water and are broken down in various degrees. Heat, acid, and enzymes act on starch to form dextrin, and eventually, by hydrolysis, glucose is formed. Dietary glycogen is negligible in amount; this compound, sometimes referred to as animal starch, is formed within the body and is stored in the liver and muscles. Cellulose, the polysaccharide found commonly in plant foods, is very insoluble. Although cellulose, like starch, is composed of many glucose molecules, the structure is different—it is made up of β-linkages. The human body contains no enzyme which enables hydrolysis of cellulose to take place.

There are many food sources of the carbohydrates. The table of food composition in the Appendix shows comparative carbohydrate values of many foods. With the exception of lactose and glycogen, the carbohydrates come from plant sources. Among the most common examples are fruits, which supply glucose, fructose, and sucrose, table sugar, which supplies sucrose, and the grain products, which supply starch. Most unrefined plant products contain cellulose. Commercial processes involved in refining remove this polysaccharide to varying degrees.

Sugar is commonly used as a food additive. This is largely to enhance the flavor of the product, but if enough is incorporated, sugar acts as a preservative.

Endogenous carbohydrate may be secured from both fats and proteins. While the principal supply of carbohydrate for body use comes from dietary or exogenous sources, it is well known that some glucose is synthesized within the body. In the breakdown of fat, protein, and carbohydrate, 2- and 3-carbon fragments may be formed, and these may be built into simple sugar. Approximately 10 per cent of dietary fat and approximately 50 per cent of dietary protein may be transformed into carbohydrate in this way. It is believed that only the glycerol fraction of fats and certain amino acids can be used for glucose synthesis. This information is of special significance to the diabetic patient and must be considered in calculating his diet.

THE BODY'S NEED FOR CARBOHYDRATE

Dietary carbohydrate is the major source of energy. Although all three of the organic foodstuffs are used to supply fuel for the body's work, it is well known that carbohydrate plays the most important role; the sun is known to be the source of this energy. In Chapter 2, the use of carbohydrate as a valuable source of fuel was mentioned. If dietary carbohydrate is deficient in amount, more protein is converted into fuel. When this occurs, the body may not have sufficient protein available for use as a muscle builder. Therefore, carbohydrate is considered to have a protein-sparing action. Likewise in the extreme restriction of carbohydrates, fats may be metabolized rapidly and be accumulated in the blood stream in incompletely oxidized or ketone form, a condition which leads to acidosis. Carbohydrates in amounts as low as 100 gm. per day act to conserve water and electrolytes; this has been observed when obese persons on a very low calorie diet fail to show a weight loss (1) for a time.

Various parts of the body benefit specifically from carbohydrates. Carbohydrate is stored in the liver as glycogen. Studies with animals have shown that these glycogen stores serve as detoxicating agents and increase the animals' ability to resist the deleterious effects of the various poisons. Carbohydrate is especially important in cardiac muscle where a constant supply of fuel is vital. In some cardiac patients, high carbohydrate therapy has been employed to prevent hypoglycemia; this treatment may be used when the glycogen stores are poor. Glucose is the sole source of fuel for the brain and nervous system and is necessary if they are to function normally. Galactosides (composed of galactose, a fatty acid, and a nitrogen base) are also present in the brain and nervous tissue and are essential.

The following examples show special functions of specific carbohydrates: cellulose aids in elimination; lactose and, to a lesser degree, other carbohydrates aid in synthesizing some of the B-complex vitamins; lactose serves in utilization of calcium and other minerals.

DIGESTION, ABSORPTION, AND METABOLISM OF CARBOHYDRATES

Carbohydrates are broken down and absorbed within the digestive tract. Mastication makes the foods eaten available for the physical and chemical changes necessary for use by the body. Various enzymes work in different areas of the digestive tract to promote breakdown of carbohydrates. The enzymatic digestion of starch begins in the mouth. It is continued in the stomach, where hydrochloric acid aids in hydrolysis, and then is continued in the small intestine, where digestion is practically completed.

The monosaccharides are in forms which favor absorption without any preliminary body reactions, whereas the more complex products must be broken down. It has been assumed that the hydrolysis of the disaccharides is carried out completely in the lumen of the intestines, but studies on human beings by Dahlquist and Borgstrom (2) indicate that breakdown may also occur in the cells of the mucous membrane of the small intestine. These investigators have shown that the site for the absorption varies, with lactose being absorbed in the duodenum and proximal jejunum, maltose, in the jejunum and proximal ileum, and sucrose, in the distal jejunum and ileum. They found also that lactose is very efficiently absorbed and utilized.

As for cellulose, no enzymatic changes occur in the human body. However, mastication cuts the fibers into small sections and the stomach acid may soften them. Absorption of water by cellulose during the passage through the intestinal tract increases bulk and stimulates peristalsis. None of these physical changes results in the hydrolysis of cellulose.

The completeness of the digestion of carbohydrates, expressed as coefficient of digestibility, varies with the food source (Table 4–1).

Table 4–1
*Digestibility of Protein, Fat, and Carbohydrate: Man**

	Coefficient of Apparent Digestibility†		
Foodstuff	*Carbohydrate* per cent	*Protein* per cent	*Fat* per cent
Animal food products			
Meat, fish		97	95
Milk, milk products	98	97	95
Eggs	98	97	95
Cereal products			
Cornmeal			
Whole ground	96	60	90
Degermed	99	76	90
Macaroni, spaghetti	98	86	90
Oatmeal, rolled oats	98	76	90
Rice			
Brown	98	75	90
White or polished	99	84	90
Wheat			
97–100 per cent extraction	90	79	90
85–93 per cent extraction	94	83	90
70–74 per cent extraction	98	89	90
Fats, animal or vegetable			95
Fruit	90	85	90
Legumes and nuts	97	78	90
Other vegetables	85	65	90
Potatoes	96	74	90
Sugar	98		

* Compiled from *Composition of Foods—raw, processed, prepared.* Agricultural Handbook No. 8, ARS, USDA, Revised 1963.
† Values are expressed in per cent which represents the grams of protein, fat, or carbohydrate apparently digested per 100 gm. of the same nutrient ingested as part of the food listed. Quantity digested is taken as that quantity of the nutrient ingested but not subsequently found as such in the feces. Values are for foods as commonly prepared for ingestion. (Nutrient intake minus nutrient in feces)/(nutrient intake) × 100 = coefficient of apparent digestibility.

Two methods of absorption are thought to occur. One already referred to is diffusion, resulting from osmotic processes which permit absorption of simple sugars into the blood stream. The other type of absorption involves chemical combination of the sugars with phosphorus and occurs during passage through the intestinal wall; when the compound enters the blood stream the phosphate releases the sugar.

The metabolism of carbohydrates proceeds in the liver and other body tissues. Glucose is carried in the blood stream to the liver. In the presence of the enzyme hexokinase and a high energy phosphate complex, adenosine triphosphate (ATP), glucose is phosphorylated to glucose-6-phosphate, then to glucose-1-phosphate, and finally to glycogen. This polysaccharide is found in muscle tissue as well as in the liver. Some of the glucose-6-phosphate may be degraded to lactate, pyruvate, and possibly other 3-carbon fragments.

For carbohydrate metabolism to proceed normally, several B vitamins as well as the minerals, magnesium and phosphorus, are required. Nicotinic acid, riboflavin, thiamin, vitamin B_6, and pantothenic acid function as coenzymes, and magnesium and phosphorus, as cofactors in the chemical reactions involved in the metabolism of carbohydrates. Actually only a small proportion of glucose is stored as glycogen, maybe 100 to 150 gm. Aside from its detoxicating effect, glycogen serves as an emergency fuel and as a stabilizing factor in maintaining the blood sugar level. Most of the glucose is oxidized to carbon dioxide and water; some is converted into fatty acids, and some combines with free amino groups to form amino acids. To maintain a desirable concentration of glucose in the blood, the hormone insulin is essential; it not only converts glucose into glycogen but also later causes oxidation of glucose by the tissues. Epinephrine, thyroxin, and glucagon also affect carbohydrate metabolism.

The normal level of blood sugar during fasting is 70 to 90 mg. per 100 ml. of blood. This level rises sharply for one-half to one hour after administration of a test dose of sugar, and if the subject has a normal sugar tolerance, it will fall to the original level by the end of two hours.

Thornton and Horwath (3) used 12 college students in determining the effect of breakfast on blood sugar levels. The low level which followed an overnight fast rose markedly when breakfast was fed. If another meal was not given five hours later, the blood glucose level continued to fall. This drop below the fasting level may be reflected in physiologic inefficiency. This study suggests the importance of meals with short intervals between. Quantitative determinations of blood sugar are routine laboratory procedures and form the basis for diagnosis of diabetes. Another routine test determines the presence or absence of sugar in the urine. Urinary sugar may be detected in conditions other than diabetes, and, if noted, more exact diagnostic procedures should be performed.

RELATIONSHIP BETWEEN INTAKE OF CARBOHYDRATES AND
NUTRITIONAL STATUS

Carbohydrate-rich foods tend to occupy a large proportion of the day's diet. Throughout the world there tends to be a large consumption of grain products, and more of the total calories are derived from carbohydrate than from fat or protein. One main factor affecting consumption is the availability of food. Inhabitants of tropical countries raise many crops, grown during much of the year. On the other hand, those living in very cold climates may have to rely largely on fish or meat. Other factors of great significance throughout most of the world are poverty and lack of tillable land. Grains may occupy a disproportionate place in the diet when the economic level is low.

In recent years, people living in the United States have tended to eat less of the natural grain products and have placed more emphasis on sweets, ready-to-eat cereals, mixes, and bakery products. Figure 4–4

Figure 4–4
Percentage changes in supplies of carbohydrates from 1889 through 1969. (Drawing prepared by Dr. M. A. Antar.)

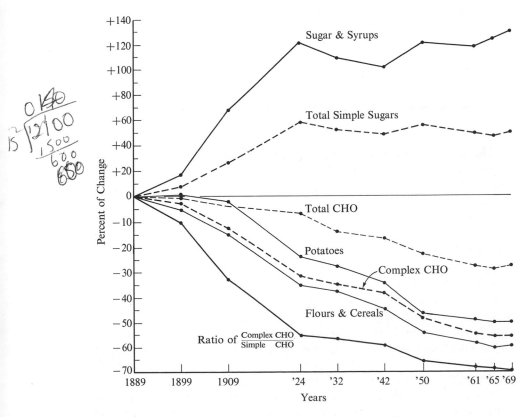

shows changes in carbohydrate supplies over a period of 80 years. The data used in preparing the figure were secured from government sources and represent retail food market supplies available in the United States; they are expressed as percentages of the values of 1889 (4). From then to 1969, total available carbohydrate decreased about 28 per cent. However, for cereal products and potatoes the decreases were 60 per cent and 50 per cent, respectively, while the supplies of sugars and syrups increased by 130 per cent. A slight drop in use of sugars occurred during the Depression and World War II.

In 1970, according to the USDA (5), 46 per cent of total calories were derived from carbohydrate. Table 4–2 gives the per cent of carbohydrate furnished by starch and the sugars, from 1909 to 1970.

Table 4–2

Carbohydrate Available per Capita per Day in the United States and Per Cent Furnished by Starch and Sugars*

Year	Carbohydrate gm.	Starch %	Sugars %
1909–1913	492	68.3	31.7
1925–1929	476	58.7	41.3
1935–1939	436	56.8	43.2
1947–1949	403	52.4	47.6
1957–1959	374	49.6	50.4
1965	374	48.8	51.2
1970[1]	381	47.7	52.3

* National Food Situation. NFS–134. ERS, USDA (1970).
[1] 1970 preliminary.

The use of noncaloric sweetening agents increased from 1.7 lb. per capita in 1957 to 7.2 lb. in 1967. Sixty to 70 per cent of the total food use of these products has been in soft drinks and dry beverage bases. Cyclamates have been more popular than saccharin. Recent research on rats showed that large amounts of cyclamates may result in cancer. As a precaution, the FDA banned the unrestricted use of cyclamates, effective February, 1970 (6, 7).

Foods containing carbohydrates tend to affect elimination. As the cellulose content of a food increases and the bulk of the mass in the intestines becomes greater there is a tendency to stimulate peristaltic activity. This speeds elimination. Extremes in amounts of the undigested materials may cause either diarrhea or constipation. Individuals vary in the amount of roughage needed for regularity and in the tonus of the muscles which control the passage of materials through the gastrointestinal tract.

Most of the gas-forming foods are carbohydrate in nature; these include lactose, honey, molasses, beans, cabbage, cauliflower, onions, and spinach. Formation of gas in the digestive tract affects both the bulk and consistency of the feces. Many fruits and some vegetables contain a considerable amount of organic acid; this stimulates intestinal motility. Buttermilk, which contains lactic acid, also stimulates the activity.

There is no recommended allowance for carbohydrate, but excessive intake is considered unwise. Despite the importance of carbohydrate in meeting the body's needs, no standard for intake has been set. This is true largely because of the body's ability to intraconvert the three organic foodstuffs. A person may adjust to a diet very low in carbohydrate. However, the FNB states that, for individuals accustomed to normal diets, 100 gm. of carbohydrate per day appear to be the minimal amount needed to avoid ketosis and use of protein for fuel.

The importance of a well-balanced diet is emphasized throughout this text. Habitual and wide deviation, especially relating to carbohydrate, may have serious effects on well-being. A lack of carbohydrate may result in malnutrition. Hypoglycemia may cause serious metabolic disturbances in the body. On the other hand, an excess of carbohydrate, especially in the form of sugar, may result in such disorders as obesity, dental caries, or diabetes. Several investigators have shown that blood lipids are higher on diets containing sucrose than on those containing starch and that the serum triglycerides are affected more by carbohydrates than is cholesterol (8, 9, 10). Work by Antar and associates (11) indicates a synergistic effect between dietary sucrose and animal fat. They used 15 hyperlipoproteinemic patients, fed diets high in saturated fat and cholesterol. When sucrose was substituted for starch as 40 per cent of the total calories serum cholesterol, phospholipid, and triglyceride levels increased significantly. These increases were not noted when the patients' diets were high in polyunsaturated fats and low in cholesterol.

It is generally considered that the amount of sugar in the diet of most Americans is not sufficient to have an adverse effect on their serum lipids so that no change in the type of carbohydrate in the diet is warranted from the standpoint of coronary heart disease (12).

A probable indirect effect of a rich diet in sweets should be mentioned. A disproportionate intake, especially between meals, is apt to limit the consumption of other foods which would supply more protein, minerals, and vitamins; one of the so-called deficiency diseases might then result.

PROBLEMS

1. Calculate the grams of carbohydrate in the food intake records used in Problem 1, Chapter 2. Carry decimals to one place.
2. Determine the amount of carbohydrate you obtained from sugars. How much of this was eaten between meals?

REFERENCES

1. Bloom, W. L. Carbohydrates and Water Balance. *Am. J. Clin. Nutr.,* *20:*157 (1967).

2. Dahlquist, A., *et al.* Digestion and Absorption of Disaccharides in Man. *Biochem. J., 81:*411 (1961).

3. Thornton, R. H., *et al.* Blood Glucose Levels as Influenced by Either One or Two Meals. *J. Am. Diet. Ass., 52:*214 (1968).

4. Antar, M. A., *et al.* Changes in Retail Market Food Supplies in the United States in the Last Seventy Years in Relation to the Incidence of Coronary Heart Disease, with Special Reference to Dietary Carbohydrates and Essential Fatty Acids. *Am. J. Clin. Nutr., 14:*169 (1964); personal communication, 1971.

5. National Food Situation. NFS-134. ERS, USDA (1970).

6. Rubini, M. E. More on Cyclamates. *Am. J. Clin. Nutr., 22:*229 (1969).

7. *Cyclamate Sweeteners.* NFS 130, p. 27, ERS, USDA, November, 1969.

8. Lopez, A., *et al.* Some Interesting Relationships Between Dietary Carbohydrates and Serum Cholesterol. *Am. J. Clin. Nutr., 18:*149 (1966).

9. Hodges, R. W., *et al.* Dietary Carbohydrates and Low Cholesterol Diets: Effects on Serum Lipids of Man. *Am. J. Clin. Nutr., 20:*198 (1967).

10. Stare, F. J. Dietary Fats and Carbohydrates, Blood Lipids and Coronary Heart Disease. *Am. J. Clin. Nutr., 20:*149 (1967).

11. Antar, M. A., *et al.* Interrelationship Between the Kinds of Dietary Carbohydrate and Fat in Hyperlipoproteinemic Patients. *J. Atherosclerosis Res., 11:*191 (1970).

12. Grande, F. Dietary Carbohydrates and Serum Cholesterol. *Am. J. Clin. Nutr., 20:*176 (1967).

GENERAL REFERENCES

13. Hardinge, M. G., *et al.* Carbohydrates in Foods. *J. Am. Diet. Ass., 46:*197 (1965).

14. Hodges, R. E. Present Knowledge of Carbohydrate. *In Present Knowledge in Nutrition,* 3rd ed. New York: Nutrition Foundation (1967).

15. Levine, R. Role of Carbohydrates in the Diet. *In* M. S. Wohl and R. S. Goodhart (eds.), *Modern Nutrition in Health and Disease,* 4th ed. Philadelphia: Lea & Febiger (1968).

The
Lipids

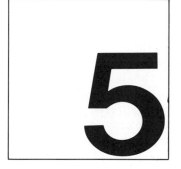

Fat, used to designate a type of food, is an everyday word for the lay person. The nutrition student is apt to refer to the lipids, a more inclusive term for the fats and fatlike substances that compose this class of nutrients. Neutral or true fats, which are organic esters or triglycerides of fatty acids and glycerol, constitute by far the largest part of the lipid group, but other lipids are also important in nutrition. The compound lipid lecithin, found in all cell protoplasm as well as in foods, contains glycerol, two fatty acids, phosphoric acid, and choline. Among the derived lipids are the free fatty acids, alcohols, the sterols—cholesterol and ergosterol, hydrocarbons such as the carotenoids, and the fat-soluble vitamins. Most of the discussion in this chapter will center around the neutral fats, certain of the fatty acids termed "essential," and cholesterol. The fat-soluble vitamins and carotenoids are considered in Chapter 11.

For many years the disadvantages of fat in the diet have taken precedence over the advantages. Dietary fat has been associated with calories, body fat with obesity. Skin rashes have been considered the result of excessive fat in the diet, and many infants have been placed on skim or partially skim milk formulas in an effort to prevent this trouble. The kind and amount of dietary fat and the amount of dietary cholesterol influence the concentrations of cholesterol and triglycerides in the blood. High levels of these components of the blood tend to lead to an increased incidence of coronary heart disease. Because of these relationships, consumption of foods high in fat may be restricted, sometimes to an undesirable extent.

On the other hand, butter or margarine is added generously to cooked vegetables for added flavor, cream is served with desserts, and oils are used in salad dressings. Frying may be a preferred method of cooking for some foods since both flavor and color may be improved by this use of fat. Because of its low bulk, extra fat may be incorporated in the diet of the undernourished person.

Certain of the fatty acids have been designated as essential for skin health, growth, and reproduction in animals and also, it is assumed, in man. Some advantages of unsaturated over saturated fatty acids in the diet have been demonstrated. Today the relationship of the amounts and types of fat in the diet to the maintenance of good health is being studied extensively.

THE CHEMISTRY AND SOURCES OF THE LIPIDS

The lipids vary considerably both in composition and structure. They occur naturally in both animal and plant foods and vary widely in physical and chemical characteristics. When separated from the surrounding tissues with which they usually are associated, most natural fats and oils are found to consist of approximately 98 to 99 per cent triglycerides; the remaining very small part is composed of monoglycerides, diglycerides, free fatty acids, phospholipids, and an unsaponifiable fraction.

Neutral fat, an ester of fatty acids and glycerol, is a mixed glyceride containing a variety of fatty acids; butter has been found to contain at least 69 fatty acids, all existing as triglycerides (1). The length of the carbon chain of fatty acids varies. Butyric acid contains only four carbon atoms, whereas stearic acid and oleic acid each contain 18, and arachidonic acid, 20. Figures 5–1 and 5–2 give the formulas for palmitic acid and linoleic acid. Figure 5–3 shows the synthesis and hydrolysis of a mixed glyceride. The physical characteristics of a neutral fat are affected by the size of the fat molecule and by the amount of saturated and unsaturated fatty acids it contains. In general, the more saturated the fat and the higher the molecular weight, the more solid it will be. A completely saturated fat is a rarity; mutton tallow is an example of a highly saturated fat. Lard and chicken fat are less firm. The oils differ from fats

Figure 5–1

A saturated fatty acid—palmitic acid

$$CH_3—(CH_2)_{14}COOH$$

Figure 5–2

An unsaturated fatty acid—linoleic acid

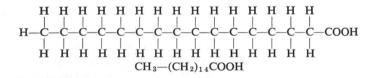

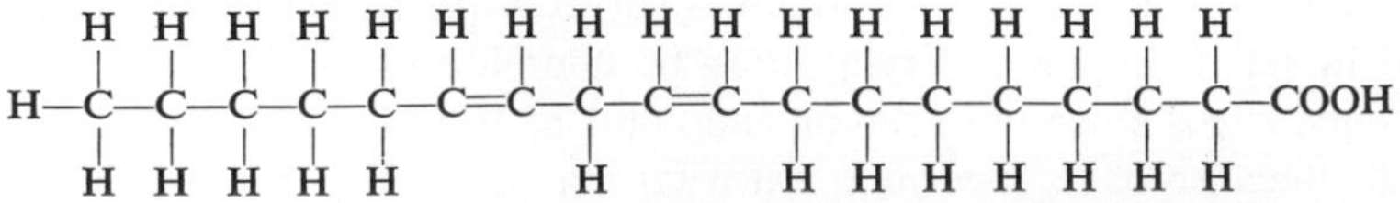

$$CH_3—(CH_2)_4—CH{=}CH—CH_2—CH{=}CH—(CH_2)_7—COOH$$

Figure 5–3

Synthesis and hydrolysis of a triglyceride.

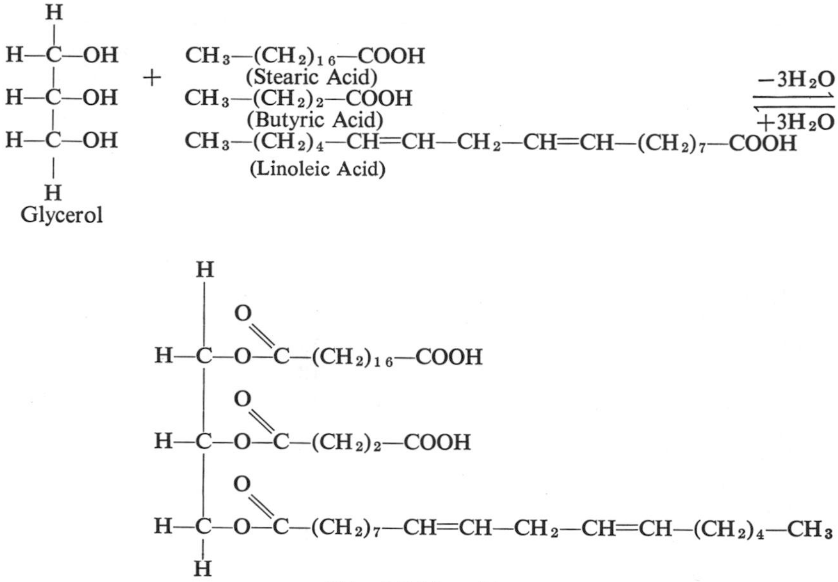

$$
\begin{array}{c}
\text{H} \\
| \\
\text{H—C—OH} \\
| \\
\text{H—C—OH} \\
| \\
\text{H—C—OH} \\
| \\
\text{H} \\
\text{Glycerol}
\end{array}
\quad + \quad
\begin{array}{l}
CH_3\text{—}(CH_2)_{16}\text{—COOH} \\
\text{(Stearic Acid)} \\
CH_3\text{—}(CH_2)_2\text{—COOH} \\
\text{(Butyric Acid)} \\
CH_3\text{—}(CH_2)_4\text{—CH=CH—CH}_2\text{—CH=CH—}(CH_2)_7\text{—COOH} \\
\text{(Linoleic Acid)}
\end{array}
\quad
\begin{array}{c}
\xrightarrow{-3H_2O} \\
\xleftarrow{+3H_2O}
\end{array}
$$

$$
\begin{array}{l}
\qquad\quad \text{H} \\
\qquad\quad | \\
\qquad\quad\quad\;\; \text{O} \\
\qquad\quad\quad\;\; \diagdown \\
\text{H—C—O—C—}(CH_2)_{16}\text{—COOH} \\
\qquad\quad | \\
\qquad\quad\quad\;\; \text{O} \\
\qquad\quad\quad\;\; \diagdown \\
\text{H—C—O—C—}(CH_2)_2\text{—COOH} \\
\qquad\quad | \\
\qquad\quad\quad\;\; \text{O} \\
\qquad\quad\quad\;\; \diagdown \\
\text{H—C—O—C—}(CH_2)_7\text{—CH=CH—CH}_2\text{—CH=CH—}(CH_2)_4\text{—CH}_3 \\
\qquad\quad | \\
\qquad\quad \text{H}
\end{array}
$$

Mixed Triglyceride

in being liquid at room temperature and, as a class, they contain more unsaturated fatty acids. There are marked differences in the amounts of saturated and unsaturated fatty acids in commonly used fats and oils (Table 5–1).

Only about 5 per cent of the fatty acids in naturally occurring fats are shorter than myristic acid, C_{14}. Coconut oil is an exception. Approximately 50 per cent of its fatty acid content is lauric acid, C_{10}.

Of the saturated fatty acids, the most common are stearic, palmitic, and myristic; of the unsaturated, oleic. The latter is a monounsaturated fatty acid with one double bond in the molecule. Three polyunsaturated fatty acids (PUFA) which occur naturally are linoleic, linolenic, and arachidonic; these are di-, tri-, and tetraenoic acids having two, three, and four double bonds, respectively. Fish oils with four, five, and six double-bond acids belong to this group. Many isomers of the unsaturated acids occur naturally in fats and oils but none of these can be counted on to replace the essential fatty acids in nutritive value (2).

Other terms used in discussing the structure of fatty acids are the *cis* and the *trans* forms. In most fatty acids the configuration of the molecule is the *cis* form in which the molecule is folded back on itself about each double bond; less common is the unfolded or *trans* form. There is some evidence that the *trans* form is of less value to the body. This configuration is found to a greater extent after hydrogenation, a widely prac-

Table 5–1

Selected Fatty Acids in Some Fats and Oils*
EXPRESSED AS 100 GM. EDIBLE PORTION

Food	Total Fat	Total Saturated Fatty Acids	Unsaturated Fatty Acids	
			Oleic	Linoleic
	gm.	gm.	gm.	gm.
Butter	81	46	27	2
Cooking fats:				
Vegetable fat	100	23	65	7
Animal and				
vegetable fat	100	43	41	11
Lard	100	38	46	10
Margarine A[1]	81	18	47	14
Margarine B[2]	81	19	31	29
Salad and cooking oils:				
Corn oil	100	10	28	53
Cottonseed oil	100	25	21	50
Olive oil	100	11	76	7
Peanut oil	100	18	47	29
Safflower oil	100	8	15	72
Sesame oil	100	14	38	42
Soybean oil	100	15	20	52

* Compiled from *Composition of Foods—raw, processed, prepared.* Agriculture Handbook No. 8, ARS, USDA, Revised 1963.
[1] Margarine A, first ingredient named on label: hydrogenated or hardened fat.
[2] Margarine B, first ingredient named on label: liquid oil.

ticed commercial procedure which involves incorporation of hydrogen into the fat molecule, with zinc as a catalyst. The fat or oil is made more solid; the degree of firmness attained is determined largely by the number of double bonds which have been converted into single bonds. This is accompanied by the lowering of the iodine number* of the fat and the raising of its melting point. In this partial hydrogenation the chemical changes which occur lessen the essential fatty acid activity of the fat.

The lipids occur in many foods but vary widely in quantity and quality. In some foods the fat is visible, as in butter, cream, and salad oils, and it may be easily separated, like the suet from a piece of steak. But the fat is invisible in foods such as egg yolk, cheese, and wheat germ. It is said that from one-third to one-half of the fat eaten is in visible form.

* The iodine number expresses the ability of a fat to combine with iodine and is in proportion to the number of double bond fatty acids in the chain; the higher the iodine number, the greater is the degree of unsaturation; for example, corn oil, 115 to 124; lard, 50 to 65; mutton tallow, 32 to 45.

When invisible it is more difficult to judge by appearance the amount of fat present, although in some foods a greasy or oily texture can be observed.

Although the fats from different sources show different proportions of fatty acids and different physical characteristics, these can be altered to some extent. For example, by controlling the hog's feed it is possible to produce a firmer body fat and lard; likewise, the linoleic acid content of lard can be altered from a low per cent to one-third of the total fatty acids by changing the diet. Human and cow's milk contain approximately the same amount of fat but the two milks differ in quality. More linoleic acid and fewer fatty acids of low molecular weight are found in human milk and from 6 to 9 per cent of the calories come from linoleic acid. A cow's milk formula for an infant contains about 1 per cent of its calories as linoleic acid.

The food composition table in the Appendix gives for many foods the content of total lipids and the fatty acids, both saturated and unsaturated, including oleic and linoleic. Table 5–1 gives information on the amount of linoleic acid in some animal fats and plant oils. Miljanich and Ostwald (3) determined the amounts of four fatty acids in ten "newer" brands of margarine, sold and bought primarily because of their content of linoleic acid and high ratio of polyunsaturated to saturated fatty acids. They found large differences in amount of linoleic acid and ratio. They suggest the value to consumers of labels which state these facts.

Foods vary widely in phospholipid content. Approximately one-third of the lipid in egg yolk is phospholipid; liver is also a good source. Storage fats and oils contain very little phospholipid. Animal sterols, mainly cholesterol, occur in all animal fats; egg yolk and butter are rich sources. Glandular organs and brain tissue also contribute much cholesterol. Sources of the four fat-soluble vitamins will be mentioned in Chapter 11. Specific data on composition are given in Table A–4, Appendix, and in supplementary Food Composition Tables, pp. 428–430.

In food processing, changes may take place. Home cooking methods are thought to have little, if any, effect on the nutritive value of fats, although too high a temperature in frying foods may cause changes which retard digestion. Proper storage of fats and oils and of foods rich in these materials is important and should be planned to prevent rancidity; a cold temperature and the absence of oxygen are desirable for this.

Today commercial food processors may add antioxidants to their products and thereby lengthen the time food may be kept from becoming rancid; such practices are used with the hydrogenated fats, potato chips, peanut butter, food mixes, etc. Other processors may add lecithin because of its emulsifying property.

Mono- and diglycerides are used to improve the physical properties of the products in which they are incorporated; for example, in margarine they act as emulsifiers, in ready-to-bake products, they tenderize, in ice cream and confections, they prevent "weeping (4)." Additives such as these, in amounts controlled by federal regulations, are considered safe from the standpoint of health. However, their use in a food product must be stated on the label.

Filled milk, available in many markets, is made by combining fats or oils other than milk fat with other milk solids. Hydrogenated coconut oil, which is high in saturated fatty acids and low in essential fatty acids, is commonly used for this purpose (5).

As has been noted, hydrogenation has a significant bearing on the PUFA content of the fat, with a decrease occurring as the fat becomes more solid. To combat this loss some margarine manufacturers combine a lightly hydrogenated fat with a liquid oil. The product is called a "special" margarine and contains a relatively larger proportion of PUFA.

PREPARATION OF LIPIDS FOR USE IN THE BODY

Digestion and absorption take place first. Although some digestion of fat may occur in the stomach, most of it takes place in the intestines. Bile emulsifies the fat and puts it into a form which permits more complete hydrolysis by intestinal and pancreatic enzymes. Fats are broken down to fatty acids, glycerol, and monoglycerides. Bile salts and choline help in emulsifying these hydrolyzed compounds, producing micelles which are absorbed through the brush border of the intestinal mucosa. During the absorption process the fatty acids, glycerol, and monoglycerides are resynthesized into triglycerides.

The short-chain and the unsaturated fatty acids are absorbed faster than those with the opposite characteristics. Short-chain fatty acids and glycerol are absorbed directly into the portal circulation. Long-chain fatty acids, phospholipids, cholesterol, and esters are absorbed into the lymph circulation. From 90 to 95 per cent of dietary fat is ordinarily made available for use by the body. Fully saturated fats are rather poorly absorbed. Data on the coefficients of digestibility of some common foods are shown in Table 4–1, p. 67. If the rate of passage through the intestinal wall is unusually slow, especially when the intake is large, absorption may not take place fast enough to prevent excessive loss in the feces. On the other hand, with a comparatively slow rate the period of satiety after a meal is prolonged, thus preventing hunger pains. Hydrogenation is not thought to retard absorption. The amount of cholesterol absorbed varies depending to some extent on the diet; if fed alone, cholesterol is poorly absorbed but in the presence of oleic acid it may be 50 per cent absorbed.

The lipids are transported by lymph and blood. Since the lipids are not soluble in water, the triglycerides and cholesterol esters are combined with protein to form lipoproteins. The least soluble of these, the chylomicrons, pass into the lacteals, then into the thoracic duct and the circulating bloodstream. In the lymph and plasma the chylomicrons cause a milky appearance. This condition clears rapidly and the fat of the chylomicrons is taken up largely by the liver where it is made into β-lipoproteins of low density and then secreted into the plasma. High density α-lipoproteins are also formed in the liver. The amount of the α-lipoproteins in the blood remains fairly constant, but that of the β-lipoproteins varies considerably; also there is more cholesterol in the β-lipoproteins. Cholesterol esters are converted to bile acids in the liver, re-excreted into the small intestine, and then re-absorbed. This enterohepatic cycle of bile acids and cholesterol regulates synthesis of cholesterol in the liver. The varying degrees of absorption and of biosynthesis may partly explain the fact that restricting the amount of cholesterol in the diet may not be relied on to lessen serum cholesterol.

Oxidation, synthesis, and storage occur in the body. Acetate is the end product in the breakdown of fats. This compound combined with coenzyme A (acetyl coenzyme A or "active acetate") (CoA) is also the building block for fats. These metabolic processes are enzymatic and concern the phospholipids and cholesterol as well as the triglycerides and fatty acids. Anabolism and catabolism of fats occur in most body tissues, in the muscles as well as in the organs. By stepwise addition or subtraction of two-carbon fractions, the length of the fatty acid chain can be altered; also, saturation and some desaturation may take place.

Whereas most mammals, including man, can synthesize most fatty acids, they cannot form linoleic acid, a fatty acid necessary for good nutrition. Therefore, as previously mentioned, this fatty acid is termed essential in the diet. Provided linoleic acid is present, and also vitamin B_6, man can synthesize arachidonic acid. The third fatty acid sometimes included in this group, linolenic acid, is a precursor of long-chain fatty acids containing five or six double bonds, not of arachidonic acid. Linolenic acid promotes growth but does not appear to cure the dermal symptoms of fat deficiency. For these reasons, the current trend is not to include arachidonic and linolenic acids as essential fatty acids.

It has been demonstrated that the location of the double bond relative to the carboxyl end of the fatty acid chain is significant in determining if an unsaturated fatty acid can be effective in treating an essential fatty acid deficiency. Polyenoic 17-carbon fatty acids with a double bond at the sixth or ninth carbon from the carboxyl end of the fatty acid chain were found to be nearly as effective as linoleic acid in curing skin symptoms of essential fatty acid deficiency.

Storage of fat, largely as triglycerides, takes place within the body more readily than does that of most other nutrients. Adipose tissue is not only a storage substance, it also removes and deposits fat from the blood and builds fat from glucose. If an individual is in calorie balance, no residue is deposited, but if the calorie intake is excessive, the fat accumulates subcutaneously and around body organs. Control of this condition was discussed in Chapter 3.

Liver cells may accumulate large amounts of fat, especially if lipotropic factors are lacking. If the accumulation is large enough, fatty cysts are formed and may eventually cause cirrhosis. Choline is one of the lipotropic factors which aids in the normal removal of fat from the liver; inositol and methionine have similar functions. These substances, more than fat itself, are probably very important in the treatment of human liver disease. A low protein diet favors retention of fat in the liver.

Interest has developed in the presence of ceroid pigment (6) in tissues which have been injured during nutritional imbalances. This pigment results from the oxidation and peroxidation of polyunsaturated fats, with the formation of insoluble long-chain polymers. A high intake of polyunsaturated fat and/or a low intake of vitamin E favors ceroid formation at the site of any local accumulation of lipid. Ceroid is found in human atheromatous aortas and coronary arteries. Under some circumstances it may interfere with the normal process for dissolving blood clots.

THE BODY'S NEED FOR THE LIPIDS

Neutral fat plays several roles, the most important being to supply energy for body needs. Fat is a component of all body tissues and is necessary for life processes. Fat is oxidized in the body cells to supply the energy the body uses all the time. The body activities which require energy were discussed in Chapter 3. The greater concentration of energy in fat than in carbohydrate and protein was explained in Chapter 2. The enzymatic mechanism whereby fats are broken down to give energy is being studied. According to Lehninger (7), oxidation of the fatty acid molecule involves four reaction cycles, and for each adenosine triphosphate (ATP) is a key agent.

The body can synthesize fat and can convert both carbohydrate and protein into fat; these processes go on, even when the body is not receiving enough calories, in order to furnish living tissues the required fat. The mammary gland makes fat, the specific kind being adapted in quantity and quality to the young of the species.

As stated previously, the body can store fat efficiently and in quantity, the reserve to be called on when needed to supply fuel. Stored fat is often considered to be inert material but research using radioactive C^{14} shows that there is a considerable turnover of fat when the subject is in calorie equilibrium. The layer of subcutaneous fatty tissue serves as insulation and tends to maintain a constant body temperature during periods when the environmental temperature changes. The cushions of fat stored around the vital organs and in other strategic positions protect the body from external harm. If these stores are depleted too rapidly, as during a drastic weight reduction regime, these organs may be injured.

The fat in the diet serves as a carrier of the fat-soluble vitamins and may aid in the body's utilization of them and (or) their precursors. It is thought that these vitamins and the PUFA are used more efficiently if other fat is also present. Fat helps in the utilization of carbohydrate and protein; it serves as a protein sparer.

Dietary fats contribute palatability and satiety to the menu. Many flavors and aromas in foods are fat-soluble and are found dissolved in small amounts of oils or fats present in foods; these contribute much to the palatability of the meal. The table fats, cooking fats, and salad oils also are flavor-producers and the homemaker incorporates them in her menus to encourage the appetite.

The food fats also have satiety value and may prevent excessive calorie consumption. The use of a moderately high fat diet as a means of weight reduction was referred to in Chapter 3; since fat takes a comparatively long time to digest, hunger pangs are delayed.

PUFA play important roles. In animal experiments it has been demonstrated that certain fatty acids are necessary for normal growth and reproduction, for skin health, and for the utilization of fat. Lack of linoleic acid and arachidonic acid caused scaliness of skin; this structural change was accompanied by an increased water permeability of the cells. Linolenic acid was found to promote growth but did not have a curative effect on the skin condition that the other two fatty acids did. Oleic acid and the saturated fatty acids do not demonstrate these roles. Neither do the polyunsaturated fish oils mentioned earlier in this chapter.

Evidence of the need of these fatty acids by the human being has been demonstrated by studies of eczema in formula-fed infants. In the past it was customary to treat skin disorders in infancy and childhood by removing fat from the diet. However, it was noted that such children were benefited when the diet contained lard or certain vegetable oils, and on analyzing the serum for fatty acids, Hansen (8) found that the infants with eczema had plasma fatty acids with a comparatively low iodine number. Further studies showed that when the linoleic acid content of the diet was very low the di- and tetraenoic acids in the serum were also very low. As previously mentioned, human milk contains more linoleic acid than cow's milk. This eczema condition therefore might be expected to be more prevalent in formula-fed than in breast-fed babies.

Potent serum cholesterol-lowering power is shown by linoleic acid and arachidonic acid and also by linolenic acid and the unsaturated fish oils. In this function the ratio of the saturated fatty acids to the PUFA in the diet is an important consideration.

The PUFA are necessary for maintenance of normal capillary permeability and fragility in the rat; when lacking, both morphologic and metabolic changes occur in many organs of many animal species.

A relationship is known to exist between the level of PUFA in the body and the vitamin E requirement. Vitamin E functions as an antioxidant, while PUFA with their double bonds increase the susceptibility of body fat to autoxidation. When intake of PUFA is increased, there is greater need for the vitamin; this problem will be discussed in more detail in the vitamin E section of Chapter 11.

Cholesterol and the phospholipids have special functions. These lipids, in conjunction with proteins, are used to build cell membranes and intracellular structures. As a component of myelin, they play an important role in the nervous system. Lipoproteins are found in both plasma and cellular tissue. Biologically active sterols are essential for the secretions of some of the endocrine glands. The function of cholesterol as a precursor of vitamin D will be discussed in the vitamin D section of Chapter 11.

RELATIONSHIPS OF THE LIPIDS TO CORONARY HEART DISEASE

Coronary heart disease is a common disorder today. Cardiovascular disease is the main cause of death in the United States today (9). Arteriosclerotic heart disease, the most common type, has increased in rate while other heart diseases, such as hypertension, rheumatic heart disease, and cerebrovascular disease, have decreased. Other countries having high death rates from heart ailments are Australia, Canada, New Zealand, Scotland, and South Africa (whites only). Among the low death rate countries are those in northwestern Europe, Italy, and Japan. In the United States the death rate increases with age in all racial and sex groups. Males are much more susceptible to the disease than are females. Because of the prevalence of heart disease many studies are being conducted on both prevention and treatment (10, 11).

The amount and kind of lipids in the diet affect serum cholesterol content. The average serum level of cholesterol is 220 to 230 mg. per cent in middle-aged men in the United States. Among peoples with low incidence of heart disease, the level may be 180 mg. per cent or lower. At birth the serum level is quite low and it rises gradually to the age of puberty. From then to 20 or 22 years there is a more rapid rise, then a less rapid rise reaching a peak in men at age 50 to 55, in women, at age 60 to 65. Obese young women were found by Davis (12) to have higher serum cholesterol levels than the nonobese. During an eight-week weight reduction period which limited calorie intake but made no effort to control cholesterol intake the serum cholesterol levels of the obese decreased an average of 81 mg. per cent.

The diet most often recommended to lower serum cholesterol is one low in saturated fatty acids, with an increase in the proportion of poly-unsaturated acids, and low in cholesterol (13). The amounts of starch and sugar in the diet also should be considered because of the synergistic effect of sucrose and animal fats (14).

It is suggested that polyunsaturated fatty acids promote the esterification of cholesterol and put it into an easily utilized form. The ratio in the diet of PUFA (linoleic, linolenic, arachidonic, and the fish oil acids) to the saturated acids is known as the P/S ratio. A ratio of 0.5 or over is thought to be satisfactory. Beef fat, butter fat, and coconut oil are examples of fats with a P/S ratio of less than 0.3; chicken fat, lard, and the common types of margarine have a range of 0.5 to 1.0; "special" margarines and shortenings with a minimum degree of hydrogenation range from 1.2 to 2.0. It is not difficult to attain a ratio of 0.5 or over on an ordinary diet that contains the recommended amounts of milk, meat, and eggs with salad oils and margarine helping to balance the proportions.

When PUFA intake is low or lacking, the transport of cholesterol is retarded and thus it accumulates in the blood serum and walls of the blood vessels.

In a study made in Norway (15) on 412 males who had survived myocardial infarction, 206 were placed on a diet containing approximately 39 per cent of the total calories as fat. Of these fat calories, 8.4 per cent came from saturated fatty acids, 20.6 per cent from polyunsaturated, and 10 per cent from monounsaturated fatty acids. The cholesterol intake was low, averaging 264 mg. daily. The other 206 men were left on their usual unrestricted diets. At the end of three months the average serum cholesterol level of the treatment group was lowered from 296 to 244 mg. per cent, of the control group, from 296 to 285 mg. per cent. In the five-year follow-up period the treatment group had less new myocardial infarctions, in both number and severity. The development rate of these manifestations was closely related to the level of serum cholesterol.

To test the hypothesis that diet can prevent coronary heart disease a Diet-Heart Feasibility Study was conducted by the National Heart Institute of the American Public Health Service (16). It covered a two-year period and involved approximately 2400 middle-aged men living in five urban centers. The subjects lived at home and were free of coronary heart disease, diabetes, and other metabolic disorders. Diets were planned for each participant by a nutritionist and consisted of fat-modified foods specially manufactured and available at specified food centers. The diets varied in total fat and in polyunsaturated fatty acid content; three dietary modifications were given under a double-blind pattern. This study demonstrated that diets which reduced total fat, saturated fatty acids, and cholesterol can be made acceptable to large numbers of people. The overall reduction in blood cholesterol was 11 per cent.

Following this study another investigation (17) was conducted on some of the men living in the Boston area who had participated in the National Diet-Heart Study. The purpose of this study was to determine whether the men could continue to follow fat- and cholesterol-controlled diets which incorporated foods available commercially when nutrition instruction was given. In this instruction and encouragement program a nutritionist spent an average of 30 minutes for each of six clinic visits per year. It was found that, with proper nutrition education, patterns of food consumption could be altered when the foods were purchased in the local market, and that the diets so changed were helpful in reducing serum cholesterol levels. The final report of the National Diet-Heart Study Group was made in 1968 (19). Plans for implementing the program have been made (20).

Serum triglycerides are affected by the carbohydrates in the diet. Chapter 4 included a brief discussion of this relationship. If the substitution of carbohydrate for fat is large, serum triglycerides may be increased and this in turn may influence the content of serum cholesterol (21). More significant than an increase in total carbohydrate is the proportion of sucrose to starch. According to Hodges (10) the level of serum triglyceride taken in a fasting subject should be 110 mg. per cent. Hypertriglyceridemia is more apt to occur among obese persons and those with a diabetic tendency (10).

The effect of exercise has been studied. Physical activity may be beneficial in reducing the serum cholesterol level. In a ten-week study (22) on 86 young men, grouped as to whether they were active or inactive and whether they were lean, muscular, or obese, treadmill running was used to measure the amount of exercise. The greatest reductions in serum cholesterol were noted in the obese-active subjects. There were no significant changes in weight or diet which might have accounted for the cholesterol change. According to Mayer (23) a person who does not exercise is less able to tolerate a high-fat diet, particularly if it is composed of saturated fats.

THE CONSUMPTION OF FAT—ACTUAL AND DESIRABLE

Wide variations occur in the amount of fat consumed. In some countries of Asia, Africa, and Latin America the intake of fat is only about one-third as much as that in the United States, and this fat is largely of vegetable origin. There tends to be a much lower concentration of cholesterol in the serum of people in these areas and the mortality rate from heart diseases also is less.

Records of fat consumption in the United States show an upward trend over the years, expressed in terms of both weight and percentage of total calories. The Consumer and Food Economics Research Division, ARS, USDA, estimates that the total fat available per capita per day has increased from 125 gm. in 1909–1913 to 155 gm. in 1970. In 1909–1913, 83 per cent of the total fat came from animal sources, 17 per cent, from plant sources. In 1968, 65 per cent came from animal sources, 35 per cent, from plant sources. In 1968, 35 per cent of the total available fat came from meat, fish, and poultry, 13 per cent, from dairy products excluding butter, and 13 per cent, from butter and lard. Plant sources of fats and oils supplied 28 per cent of the total fat (24).

Data have been tabulated on the use of saturated fatty acids, oleic acid, and linoleic acid. Friend (25) states that whereas the levels of total saturated fatty acids and oleic acid have changed little since 1947–1949, that of linoleic acid has risen steadily and was in 1970 more than double that for 1909–1913. The rise has been rapid during the last 16 years (Table 5–2). The increase in linoleic acid is due largely to greater use of salad and cooking oils than was the practice in the early years of this century. Antar, Ohlson, and Hodges (26) investigated changes in the United States between 1909 and 1969 in the supplies of total fat, cholesterol, and saturated and polyunsaturated fatty acids. Figure 5–4 shows these changes expressed in percentage deviations

Figure 5–4

Percentage changes in supplies of total fat, cholesterol, and fatty acids from 1909 through 1969. (Drawing prepared by Dr. M. A. Antar.)

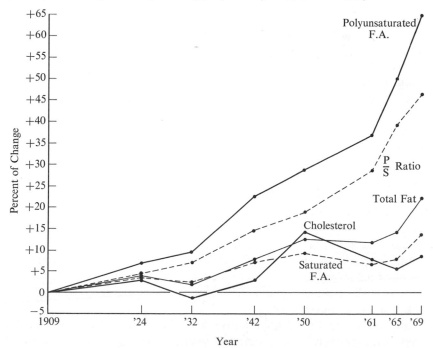

Table 5–2

Fatty Acids Available Per Capita Per Day and Percent of Total Nutrient Fat Accounted for by Fatty Acids, Selected Periods*

Year	Fatty acids			Total nutrient fat	Share of total fat from fatty acids		
	Total saturated	Unsaturated[1]			Total saturated	Oleic acid	Linoleic acid
		Oleic acid	Linoleic acid				
	gm.	gm.	gm.	gm.	%	%	%
1909–13	50.3	51.5	10.7	125.2	40.2	41.1	8.5
1925–29	53.3	55.2	12.5	134.6	39.6	41.0	9.3
1935–39	52.9	54.5	12.7	133.0	39.8	41.0	9.5
1947–49	54.4	58.0	14.8	141.1	38.6	41.1	10.5
1957–59	54.7	58.2	16.6	143.2	38.2	40.6	11.6
1965	53.9	58.8	19.1	144.8	37.2	40.6	13.2
1970[2]	55.5	62.8	22.8	155.2	35.8	40.5	14.7

* National Food Situation, NFS-134. ERS, USDA. (1970).
[1] Major unsaturated fatty acids. Oleic is mono-unsaturated and linoleic is poly-unsaturated.
[2] Preliminary.

since 1909. In their calculations, these investigators included both the main fat sources and the fats from vegetables and cereal products. It is interesting to note the great increase in use of the unsaturated acids in contrast to the lesser and more variable changes in total fat, saturated fatty acids, and cholesterol. Because of this increase of unsaturated acids in the diet, the P/S ratio has increased markedly. In a study by Osborn and Ohlson (27) of the typical diet of the professional staff at the State University of Iowa Hospitals, 41.2 per cent of the 2800 calories consumed came from fat; an average of 3.4 per cent of the calories came from linoleic acid.

Recommendations have been made concerning fat intake. As has already been stated, most nutrition authorities do not recommend a drastic decrease in the fat intake of healthy individuals. This position is taken, first, because of the important roles the lipids play in human metabolism, second, because proof of a causal relationship between a high-fat diet, high serum cholesterol, and increased prevalence of coronary heart disease is lacking, and third, because in obesity the significant factor is not fat but calories. The FNB does believe that many Americans will profit from a moderate reduction in total fat intake and some replacement of saturated fats by unsaturated fats. Foods such as milk, meat, poultry, fish, and eggs should be included in the dietary because of the other nutrients they contain.

Facts relating to the quantitative need for the essential fatty acids have been verified by experimental work and are generally accepted.

Growth, and freedom from skin lesions, may be secured if from 1 to 3 per cent of the total calories comes from dietary linoleic acid. This amount does not appear to present a problem except in the case of infants and small children whose diet consists of milk only. Hansen and co-workers (8) recommend that linoleic acid supply 3 per cent of the calories in an infant's formula. The question of the ratio of polyunsaturated to saturated fatty acids was discussed earlier in the chapter.

Fat is only one of the many factors which affect nutrition. It must be remembered that fat is an essential nutrient and plays many positive roles in the human body. These facts sometimes are forgotten in the controversies over possible harmful effects. It is not within the province of this book, which relates primarily to normal nutrition, to consider disease in detail. The relationship of dietary fat to body weight was discussed in Chapter 3, since this problem is primarily one of food and nutrition. Some other disorders have less clear-cut relationships.

Atherosclerosis has been mentioned in this chapter as it may be related to the lipids in the diet. Many other factors may be involved, including heredity, protein, carbohydrate, calorie balance, choline, vitamin B_6, magnesium, calcium, and exercise.

There seem to be many unsolved problems related to cholesterol, atherogenesis, and coronary artery disease. Changes in the diet, while overcoming one disorder, may unbalance the food intake in other respects and thus do not improve the nutritional status of the person. The consensus among nutrition research workers at this time is that it is premature to advise drastic alterations in the fat intake of healthy individuals.

PROBLEMS

1. Calculate the grams of fat in the food intake records used in Problem 1, Chapter 2. Carry decimals to one place.
2. Compare the amounts of fat you received from animal and from plant sources.
3. Using one or more of the references (p. 000, Appendix), which gives data concerning fatty acid composition of foods, determine as completely as possible the content of saturated fatty acids, oleic, and linoleic acids in one day of your dietary record.

REFERENCES

1. Hashim, S. A. Medium-Chain Triglycerides—Clinical and Metabolic Aspects. *J. Am. Diet. Ass., 51:*221 (1967).
2. Aaes-Jørgensen, E. Unsaturated Fatty Acid Isomers in Nutrition. *Nutr. Revs., 24:*1 (1966).
3. Miljanich, P., *et al.* Fatty Acids in Newer Brands of Margarine. *J. Am. Diet. Ass., 56:*29 (1970).

4. Food and Nutrition Board, NAS-NRC, Food Protection Committee. *The Safety of Mono- and Diglycerides for Use as Intentional Additives in Foods.* Washington, D.C.: NAS-NRC Publ. 251 (1960).

5. Rubini, M. E. Filled Milk and Artificial Milk Substitutes. *Am. J. Clin. Nutr., 22:*163 (1969).

6. Hartroft, W. B., *et al.* Present Knowledge of Ceroid Pigment. *In Present Knowledge in Nutrition,* 3rd ed. New York: Nutrition Foundation (1967).

7. Lehninger, A. L. Oxidative Phosphorylation. *Sci., 128:*450 (1958).

8. Hansen, A. E. *et al.* Role of Linoleic Acid in Infant Nutrition. *Pediat., 31:*171 (1963).

9. Hundley, J. M. Heart Disease: Recent Trends in Morbidity and Mortality. *J. Am. Diet. Ass., 52:*195 (1967).

10. Hodges, R. E. Dietary and Other Factors which Influence Serum Lipids. *J. Am. Diet. Ass., 52:*198 (1968).

11. Connor, W. E. Dietary Sterols: Their Relationship to Atherosclerosis. *J. Am. Diet. Ass., 52:*202 (1968).

12. Davis, E. Y. Serum Cholesterol and Lactate Dehydrogenase Patterns of Young Women. *J. Am. Diet. Ass., 53:*32 (1968).

13. Turpeinen, O., *et al.* Dietary Prevention of Heart Disease. *Am. J. Clin. Nutr., 21:*255 (1968).

14. Antar, M. A., *et al.* Interrelationships Between the Kinds of Dietary Carbohydrates and Fat in Hyperproteinemic Patients. *J. Ather. Res., 11:*191 (1970).

15. Leren, P. The Effect of Plasma Cholesterol Lowering Diet in Male Survivors of Myocardial Infarction, A Controlled Clinical Trial. *Acta. Med. Scand., 180:*Suppl. 466 (1966).

16. Brown, H. B. The National Diet-Heart Study. Implications for Dietitians and Nutritionists. *J. Am. Diet. Ass., 52:*279 (1968).

17. Remmell, P. S., *et al.* A Dietary Program to Lower Serum Cholesterol. *J. Am. Diet. Ass., 54:*13 (1969).

18. The National Diet-Heart Study Research Group. The National Diet-Heart Study Final Report. *Circul.* 37:Supp. No. 1 (1968).

19. Alfin-Slater, R. B. Diet and Heart Disease. *J. Am. Diet. Ass., 54:*486 (1969).

20. Zukel, M. C. Revising Booklets on Fat-Controlled Meals. *J. Am. Diet. Ass., 54:*20 (1969).

21. Albrink, M. J. The Significance of Serum Triglycerides. *J. Am. Diet. Ass., 42:*29 (1963).

22. Campbell, D. C. Influence of Diet and Physical Activity on Blood Serum Cholesterol of Young Men. *Am. J. Clin. Nutr., 18:*79 (1966).

23. Mayer, J. Obesity, Cardiovascular Diseases and the Dietitian. *J. Am. Diet. Ass., 52:*13 (1968).

24. Call, D. L., *et al.* Trends in Fat Disappearance in the United States 1909–13 to 1965. *J. Nutr., 93:* Supp. 1 (1967).

25. National Food Situation. NFS–134, ERS, USDA (1970).

26. Antar, M. A., *et al.* Changes in Retail Market Food Supplies in the United States in the Last Seventy Years in Relation to the Incidence of Coronary Heart Disease, with Special Reference to Dietary Carbohydrates and Essential Fatty Acids. *Am. J. Clin. Nutr., 14:*169 (1964). Personal Communication, 1971.

27. Osborn, M. O. *et al.* Fatty Acids in Hospital Menus. *J. Am. Diet. Ass., 43:*533 (1963).

GENERAL REFERENCES

28. Alfin-Slater, R. B., and Aftergood, L. Absorption and Metabolism of Lipids. *In* M. G. Wohl and R. S. Goodheart (eds.), *Modern Nutrition in Health and Disease,* 4th ed. Philadelphia: Lea and Febiger (1968).

29. Food and Nutrition Board. Dietary Fat and Human Health. Washington, D.C.: NAS-NRC Publ. 1147 (1966).

30. Mead, J. F. Present Knowledge of Fat. *In Present Knowledge in Nutrition,* 3rd ed. New York: Nutrition Foundation (1967).

Protein

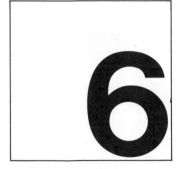

Although the problem of total food intake is of great importance in its relationship to good health, that of quality is of even more concern. It is a well-accepted fact that to build and repair the various body tissues the specific components which make up these parts must be provided. Muscle, nerve, bone, blood, each has a definite structure with varying amounts of protein, minerals, water, fat, carbohydrate, and other constituents, and unless these foodstuffs are supplied in sufficient quantity the body will feel the lack. Protein, after water, composes the greatest proportion of the body tissues and is an indispensable constituent of every living cell. The body's protein needs are met primarily by amino acids, but also by other forms of dietary nitrogen. Today the overall nitrogen picture is being considered as it relates to both quantity and quality of protein and to efficiency in utilization of the various sources.

In the United States protein is supplied largely from animal sources. Meat, poultry, and fish have always been popular in the diet of adult and child alike; they are important foods since they not only make a meal more appetizing but also promote a high plane of nutritional well-being. The high nutritive value of eggs and milk is evidenced by the fact that they serve as the sole source of nourishment during the periods of greatest growth, as in the embryo of the chick and in the first months of life of most mammals.

The prevalence of protein malnutrition and its serious consequences are well recognized today in many technically underdeveloped countries of the world. Among the more general signs of hypoproteinosis in human beings are poor growth, lack of resistance to infection, and a high mortality rate. The more specific syndromes in which protein deficiency is involved are kwashiorkor, pellagra, edema, and certain liver diseases. In many parts of the world the production of foods high in animal protein is greatly limited, transportation and storage facilities are inadequate, purchasing power is low, and prejudice against some foods is an almost insurmountable barrier. Research is being carried on under the auspices of the FAO, WHO, and UNICEF to investigate possibilities for use of protein foods that are indigenous to specific countries; these include fish flour, soy products, ground nut or peanut flour, sesame flour, cottonseed flour, and coconut protein.

In this country investigations are being made concerning improvement of grains through genetic and environmental modifications, combinations of plant sources of protein as a way to improve the total amino acid content, and supplementing the inadequate but available dietary with lacking amino acids or nonspecific nitrogen. Reference will be made later in this chapter to some of these studies.

FUNCTIONS OF PROTEINS AND AMINO ACIDS

Protein is essential in building tissue. In 1828 the word "protein" was coined from a Greek verb meaning "to take first place" to describe the nitrogenous substance which had been found in body tissue. Today the structure and maintenance of function in protoplasm are known to depend on many factors. The prominence of this foodstuff is still recognized; it is the most abundant of the body's organic compounds and is the substance composing to a large extent its soft tissues. At those times in life when growth occurs, the protein requirement for building is necessarily large; thus in the case of the fetus, infant, and child, increment of cellular tissue is to be expected. In the nursing mother secretion of milk makes great demands.

However, all living cells undergo constant changes throughout their entire life span and constantly need renewal. Unlike fat, protein is not stored as reserve material in special compartments of the body when the intake exceeds the need. When the food intake is lacking in nitrogen, however, certain tissue proteins may be depleted to contribute amino acids to a metabolic pool; these proteins may be considered labile reserves. In the body the relatively dispensable proteins in skeletal muscle, parenchymatous organs, and serum albumin contribute more to the pool; liver proteins also are easily depleted. Those of the brain and nerves are comparatively resistant to depletion and those of the heart and kidneys are intermediary. These amino acids permit rapid and continuous interchange of nitrogenous compounds between the cells and the surrounding fluids. This pool insures a balance between the nitrogenous products of synthesis and breakdown; only on depletion of the reserves would a deficiency become serious.

The constancy of the nitrogen content of the fat-free body has been demonstrated in animals under conditions of deprivation and of varying protein intake. It is assumed that this condition applies to the human being also; the average figure is 2 per cent nitrogen in the body of the infant and 3 per cent in the adult body. The body tissue ordinarily associated with protein is muscle. However, nitrogen is incorporated in other body tissues. Bone is usually considered in its relation to calcium and phosphorus, but it also contains a fairly high percentage of protein; it is known that dietary sources of protein are essential in the normal bone development. In young pigs fed a diet deficient in protein, the longitudinal growth of the long bones was greatly retarded; when radiographs of these bones were made, they showed structural changes in cartilage and trabeculae. It is thought that similar bone abnormalities seen in chronically ill children may be related to protein deficiency.

Although it was first assumed that all forms of protein were similar in composition, about 1901 Emil Fischer proved that protein was composed of amino acids, differing in type, arrangement, and quantitative relationships. In a protein the amino acids are linked by a peptide bond with the amino group of one amino acid joined to the carboxyl group of another amino acid. In the synthesis of protein one molecule of water is released as each two amino acids are joined, whereas in the breakdown of protein, as in digestion, one molecule of water is added as each two amino acids are split (Figures 6–1 and 6–2). Among the 22 known

Figure 6–1
Empirical formula for an amino acid (R = a carbon and amino acid radical of varying length.)

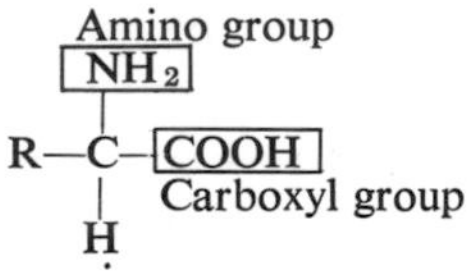

Figure 6–2
Peptide bond formation and breakdown in the synthesis and hydrolysis of a protein

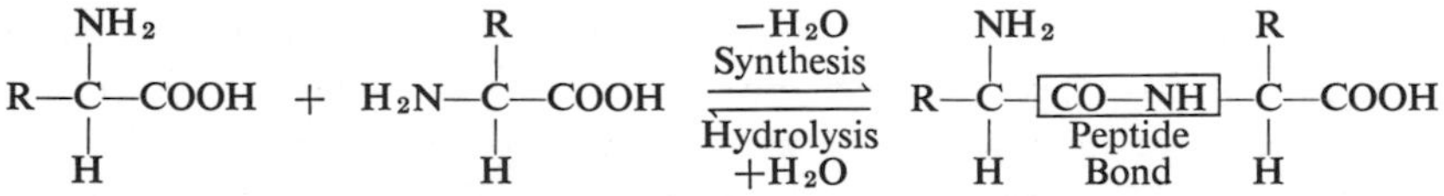

to be physiologically important, eight are termed essential for the human being. These are: leucine, isoleucine, lysine, methionine, phenylalanine, threonine, tryptophan, and valine. They must be provided in the diet since they cannot be synthesized in the body at a rate sufficient to meet the needs for growth and maintenance. Rose and co-workers (1, 2), who fed healthy men purified diets containing adequate amounts of all nutrients except a single amino acid, proved that a pronounced negative balance of nitrogen resulted from omission of any one of the essential amino acids. The subjects also showed marked signs of anorexia, fatigue, and nervous irritability, symptoms which were relieved when the lacking amino acid was replaced. Omission of either histidine or arginine had no effect on nitrogen equilibrium in the adult. Histidine has been shown to be essential for growth of infants and arginine also may be regarded as essential for infants since the body cannot manufacture it with proper speed.

The nonessential amino acids are also important for maintenance and growth, but they may be formed within the body from intermediary products of carbohydrate and fat metabolism and from nitrogen derived either from amino acids such as glycine and glutamic acid or from inorganic ammonium salts. Scrimshaw (3) suggests that when the essential amino acids are supplied in the proportion in which they are found in whole egg they need furnish only about one-fourth of the total nitrogen required by the young adult. The remaining three-fourths could come from nonspecific nitrogen. However, this ratio of nitrogen from the essential amino acids of animal protein to nonspecific nitrogen is not effective in improving the protein quality of vegetable mixtures.

The ratio of nonessential to essential amino acids is considered important in evaluating the quality of a protein. The dividing line between the two groups of amino acids is not sharp. For example, since the nonessential amino acid tyrosine cannot be formed in the body but is newly formed from the essential amino acid, phenylalanine, about 50 per cent of the phenylalanine requirement can be provided by tyrosine. Further, cystine may take the place of about 30 per cent of the methionine requirement. In nature the amino acids occur in a great variety of combinations as protein.

An adequate or complete protein is one which contains sufficient amounts of the essential amino acids to promote life during growth of the young, maintenance, and reproduction; an inadequate protein is one which lacks sufficient quantity of one or more of the essential amino acids so that a poor bodily condition results.

The relative amounts of nitrogen supplied by the essential and nonessential amino acids are sometimes used to indicate the quality of the protein.

When high quality proteins are consumed, less quantity is needed than when they are of poor quality. Since different sources of protein contain varying amounts of the different amino acids, the proteins work more efficiently together than when separate. This is referred to as supplementary value.

Protein is a source of energy. Protein is so commonly thought of as a tissue-builder that it is given only secondary consideration as a source of energy. Since most adults eat more protein than is needed for repair processes and for the manufacture of vital body compounds, and since the adult does not ordinarily store protein, this nutrient may function as a source of energy. It has been demonstrated experimentally during fasting and when the diet contains insufficient carbohydrate and fat for fuel that the quantity of protein available for tissue growth or repair is reduced. When either carbohydrate or fat or both are increased, the use of protein as fuel is lessened or ended and nitrogen excretion is diminished. Even when the diet supplies sufficient carbohydrate and fat for energy, the addition of more of either may cause actual storage of nitrogen. The protein-sparing action of carbohydrate is increased if carbohydrate is fed simultaneously with protein. As a result the time of digestion and the rate of amino acid absorption are prolonged, and the supply of easily available precursors for synthesis of nonessential amino acids is enhanced.

Protein has regulatory functions. This foodstuff is important as a regulator of osmotic pressure and water balance within the body. It also helps maintain one of the body's most important constants, a hydrogen ion concentration very close to that of water. At first thought, it might seem impossible for the body tissues to maintain a fixed reaction, which is slightly basic, when the diet varies so widely in reaction and, on metabolism, forms such large amounts of carbonic and other acids. However, the constancy of reaction is maintained by several delicately controlled mechanisms which are discussed in Chapter 13. The proteins are important in this connection, since they are amphoteric substances which can combine with acid or base and serve as buffers when an excess of a compound of the opposite reaction is present. In the blood, hemoglobin and oxy-hemoglobin and their alkaline salts permit transportation of oxygen to the cells and carbonic acid from them, thus preventing an accumulation of this acid in the tissues. Van Slyke has estimated that the adjustments between oxy-hemoglobin, the stronger acid, and hemoglobin, the weaker, are responsible for the removal of from 92 to 97 per cent of all the carbon dioxide taken from the tissues. The serum proteins, present in smaller concentration, also serve as regulators in the blood stream.

Vital body compounds are nitrogenous in nature. Nitrogenous materials play an important role as precursors of body hormones as well as builders of muscle tissue. For example, hormones elaborated by the pituitary gland are protein in nature. The structure of the enzyme catalase found in all body organs, in greatest concentration in the liver and red blood cells, has been determined by Schroeder (4). It consists of 2020 amino acid building blocks.

Phenylalanine is required in the synthesis of both thyroxin and adrenaline; the insulin molecule contains 12 per cent cystine. Likewise the digestive enzymes and those concerned in oxidation-reduction activity are proteins. Too, some of the substances associated with immunologic and antigenic reactions are nitrogenous in nature; for example, globulin of the blood serum and chromatin in the cell nucleus are proteins.

Methionine, the precursor of cystine, is found as part of the protein in muscle and in glandular and epithelial tissue; this amino acid also supplies methyl groups found in creatinine and choline. Tryptophan and the vitamin niacin are associated with prevention of pellagra and, within limits, are used interchangeably by the body. Hemoglobin, one of the essential proteins of the blood, is made up of a globulin and hematin; the latter, containing four pyrrole rings, is thought to be derived largely from the dispensable amino acid, glycine. Glutathione (a tripeptide of cystine, glycine, and glutamic acid) is present in small amounts in all active tissues and is important in oxidation-reduction reactions in plants and animals.

On decarboxylation, histidine yields histamine which has a significant biological role. Threonine, when choline is present in the diet, is known to have a lipotropic effect, preventing deposition of excess fat in the liver. The original claim that lack of arginine decreased the number of spermatozoa in the seminal fluid was not confirmed in Rose's experiments (1, 2).

PREPARATION OF DIETARY PROTEIN FOR USE BY THE BODY

Digestion of protein is carried on in the stomach and intestines. Because there are no protein-splitting enzymes in saliva, hydrolysis of protein begins in the stomach; here hydrochloric acid aids in the breakdown. Enzymes in the pancreatic and intestinal juices complete the process and amino acids are the end products. The various gastrointestinal enzymes attack the peptide linkages at different rates, depending on the chemical nature of the amino acids which participate in formation of the peptide bond; some of the linkages are particularly resistant to enzyme action. As was stated on page 26, approximately 92 per cent of dietary protein is digested. Table 4–1 (page 27) gives the coefficients of digestibility of the protein of some common foods. Products of plant origin bound with cellulose are less completely digested, while those of animal origin with little or no connective tissue are more completely hydrolyzed. The average time for digestion lies between that of carbohydrate and that of fat.

Absorption of amino acids occurs largely in the small intestine. Studies using S^{35}-labelled proteins indicate that, of the total amount of foodstuff eaten, 11 per cent is absorbed by the stomach wall, 60 per cent, by the small intestine, and 28 per cent, by the colon. This absorption is more than a simple diffusion process and involves an active function of the walls of the tract. The highly specialized cells of the mucosa are capable of selecting and rejecting particles of molecular size; absorption of the different amino acids may vary in rate depending on quantity and quality of the amino acids and on other dietary factors. It has been demonstrated that vitamin B_6 is needed in this active transfer. After passing through the walls of the digestive tract, the amino acids are picked up by the circulating blood stream and transported to the liver and to various body tissues.

Metabolism of the amino acids may involve several processes. In the body tissues amino acids may be synthesized, deaminized, or decarboxylated. If synthesis is to proceed efficiently, both essential and non-essential amino acids must be available simultaneously and in sufficient amount. The sources of the amino acids may be exogenous or endogenous. Synthesis of amino acids and protein goes on constantly to care for the growth, repair, and maintenance of body tissues. The turnover rates, determined by means of tagged amino acids, vary considerably among the various body proteins, ranging from a few days for serum proteins, to months for muscle proteins, to several years for certain types of collagens. Synthesis is regulated by deoxyribonucleic acid (DNA), a compound which controls the structure of a specific protein. The code secured from DNA is carried to the site of protein synthesis by a polymer of DNA called messenger ribonucleic acid (RNA).

Products from the intermediary metabolism of fats and carbohydrates may combine with free amino acid groups by means of a process called transamination to form nonessential amino acids.

In catabolism the amino group is usually split off; this process, known as deamination, occurs largely in the liver. Most of the nitrogen freed from these amino groups and not utilized in the transamination process forms urea which is excreted in the urine; some is eliminated in the form of uric acid and creatinine. Catabolism may involve decarboxylation in which carbon dioxide is split off and active amines are formed; histamine is such a product. Amines also are frequently produced in the intestines by bacteria and may react as toxins. Normally the intestinal wall and the liver act to detoxicate them.

ESTIMATION OF THE REQUIREMENT FOR PROTEIN

Protein values may be studied by analysis of foods for nitrogen and amino acid content. Because foods contain varying amounts of nitrogen and varying amounts and kinds of amino acids, all of which will affect the body's need, it is important to have a quantitative measure of nitrogen and amino acids found in foods. Chemical analysis will give nitrogen content. To convert nitrogen into protein the nitrogen content is multiplied by the factor 6.25. As was explained in Chapter 2, this factor is not applicable to all proteins, but the factor 6.25 is approved for general comparisons.

Microbiological assays and chromatographic methods are used in studying the amino acids in foods. The microbiological method requires use of specific organisms. When standardized techniques are employed and interfering substances are eliminated, this method agrees well with the data from chemical analyses. Column and gas liquid chromatography, a more recently developed means for determining the amino acid content of a food, provides data on amino acid content. These methods will predict the potential value of a protein but they do not necessarily indicate the biological value. Among the methods used in studying protein requirement are nitrogen and amino acid balance studies, creatinine output in the urine, albumin in the serum, essential and nonessential amino acid patterns in blood plasma, and tissue and plasma enzyme levels. However, more work must be done before the value of any of these methods for assessing human protein requirements is fully understood.

Nitrogen balance studies on human beings are used in studying requirements. These studies ascertain the least amount of protein required to keep an adult in nitrogen equilibrium. Determinations are made of the nitrogen contained in the food eaten and that excreted from the body. Such studies (5) are time-consuming and expensive and require special precautions if the results are to provide a reliable basis for conclusions.

There must be a long pre-experimental period to allow for adjustment to any changes in protein intake. If the subject has been accustomed to eating more protein than in the experimental diet, the nitrogen excreted will be greater at first than if he had been ingesting less. During the study period a weighed amount of a uniform diet should be consumed by the subject. The food must be planned to furnish adequate carbohydrate and fat for energy in order to spare protein for its primary function. It is also important to supply the needed vitamins and minerals. Calorie and water intake should be constant throughout, and protein should be kept the same in quantity and quality during each test period. Factors such as age and sex are considered in selecting the subjects; the state of health is important, especially as it relates to absence of infection. Cooperation is essential since the participants must be relied upon for accuracy in recording consumption of food and collection of excreta. Both urine and feces are collected quantitatively throughout the period, and in very exact studies perspiration is taken into account. Losses through the skin and in connection with the growth of hair, skin, and nails have been estimated as 0.8 mg. of nitrogen per basal calorie per day; the losses through the skin are greater when environmental temperature and humidity are high.

From the data obtained by analysis of food and excreta, the subject's nitrogen balance is calculated. If the figure approximates zero, it might be thought that the amount of protein eaten corresponds to the minimum. This is not the case, however. Since an adult does not store protein, the excretion of nitrogen, until a slight negative balance persists, will be equal to the nitrogen of the food at any level of intake above the minimum. The experiment must be repeated with progressively lower amounts of protein, keeping the calories covered by adequate carbohydrate and fat until a slight negative balance persists. A point slightly above this figure represents the minimum requirement for the particular protein used in the study. The arduousness of conducting studies on the minimum amount required for balance probably accounts for the very small number of studies made on human beings in which the protein came from a single source.

Amino acid balance studies also have been made. Rose and co-workers (1, 2) made investigations to determine quantitative needs; while keeping seven of the amino acids constant in amount, the eighth was gradually lowered until the minimal level for equilibrium was reached. During a period of 12 years they conducted 45 human experiments on eight amino acids, using from 17 to 42 young men with each amino acid. Rose recommends that the minimal values be doubled to give safe amounts. Such data as these make it feasible to evaluate specific proteins or diets in terms of their ability to fulfill human requirements.

Since the beginning of these experiments on men, several laboratories have investigated the amino acid requirements of women, using some variations in procedure. Leverton and co-workers (6) reported on threonine, valine, tryptophan, phenylalanine with and without tyrosine, and leucine; Swendseid, Williams, and Dunn (7) on the sulfur-containing amino acids and isoleucine; and Reynolds and co-workers (8), on lysine, methionine, and cystine. The needs of women have been found to be somewhat less than those of men. A reassessment of the lysine and tryptophan requirements of young women has been reported by Fisher and co-workers (9). On intakes of approximately 5 gm. nitrogen per day the requirements for both these amino acids were in the range of 50 mg. per day, figures considerably lower than those set in earlier studies. These workers explain the differences in requirements by the lower levels of other essential amino acids provided in their experimental diets compared to those used in the early studies. It should be remembered that these figures represent minimal requirements for balance and do not include nitrogen needed to fulfill other functions of protein; for young women of child-bearing age the minimal figure is far from safe.

A factorial method is recommended for ascertaining protein requirement. This method involves determining the obligatory losses of nitrogen from the body; these losses are indications of necessary replacements. Both the FAO/WHO Expert Group and the FNB base their recommendations for protein requirement on these losses through urine, feces, skin, sweat, hair, and nails. Of the routes of loss, that via the urine is the greatest. It is known that throughout a wide range of nitrogen intakes a subject is kept in equilibrium by adjustment in the output of urine and that below a certain level the loss of nitrogen becomes greater. To determine this point the subject is put on a protein-free diet, adequate in calories. Under these conditions the minimum level is found at which the urinary output will fall before the body will be actually depleted of nitrogen. At this point the loss of nitrogen through urine is called the basal or the endogenous excretion.

From studies on many animals it has been determined that the output of nitrogen in the urine is related to the basal metabolic rate; this has been estimated to be about 2 mg. nitrogen per basal kcal. Since it is simpler to determine the basal metabolic rate than the basal nitrogen excretion, the former data are used in estimating urinary loss.

In the feces the obligatory loss of nitrogen on a protein-free diet is 0.4 mg. nitrogen per basal kcal, or about 20 per cent of the urinary endogenous loss. This fecal nitrogen comes largely from digestive juices and secretions and from desquamated epithelial cells of the tract.

Nitrogen losses from skin, hair, and nails are estimated to be 0.56 gm. per square meter of surface area in the male and 0.37 gm. in the female. Minimal loss of nitrogen through sweat is about 0.36 gm. per day; under extreme conditions, this loss can be ten times as great. The lower surface area loss by the female is considered to be offset by a small nitrogen loss during menstruation. Using the data available the FNB has set 0.8 mg. nitrogen per basal kcal to cover the losses from skin, sweat, hair, and nails. When the three routes of obligatory loss are totalled the result is 3.2 mg. nitrogen per basal kcal, or 20 mg. ideal protein (N $\times$ 6.25). Assuming that the basal metabolic rate of the reference man is 1750, the minimal daily requirement for protein is 35 gm. This figure is not used to express the recommended dietary allowance.

THE RECOMMENDED DIETARY ALLOWANCE

The recommended allowance is more than the estimated minimal requirement. The minimal requirement, based on the amount of dietary protein necessary to replace losses of nitrogen, assumes that the individual is average and the protein is ideal in quality and its utilization is complete. These conditions are not to be expected. Variability in physiological reaction among individuals is normal and this variability must be considered when the allowance is applied to an individual instead of to a population group. Hussein and co-workers (10) studied urinary and fecal losses in 100 young men to determine the degree of variation to be expected. The men were fed a diet adequate in calories but lacking in protein for 14 to 16 days. Minimum nitrogen excretion occurred in six to eight days, and during the rest of the time individual variations were measured. The variation in urinary nitrogen loss expressed per kg. body weight was about 14 per cent of the mean, or when calculated per kcal, 18 per cent. The variation in fecal loss was greater but the loss in feces was so much less than in urine that the total nitrogen loss in urine plus feces varied only slightly. The FNB adds 30 per cent to the obligatory loss figure, assuming this will cover variability needs of practically all persons.

In the United States and some other countries where animal proteins are plentiful and where there is a tendency to consume a great variety of foods, the quality of protein is likely to be good and its utilization efficient. However, even here, differences in intake are to be expected due to financial status, availability of the food supply, and personal preference; both bodily and dietary factors may affect utilization. The FNB includes a quality-correction factor of 70 per cent to care for these differences. This brings the recommended dietary allowance of the 70 kg. reference man to 65 gm. of protein per day and that of the 58 kg. reference woman to 55 gm. per day, or approximately 0.9 gm. per kg. of body weight. This figure is slightly lower than that used for many years, based on the nitrogen balance studies conducted by Sherman and other investigators.

Protein allowances have been set for infants, children, and pregnant and lactating women. For the infant during the first year of life the recommended allowance is based on the composition of human milk or a formula which simulates human milk. This amounts to 1.8 gm. protein per kcal. For children over one year the maintenance protein level has been increased to allow for growth gains. It is assumed that body weight gain is 18 per cent protein. During pregnancy an additional 10 gm. protein per day have been added for growth of fetus and placenta, and other material tissues. It is estimated that approximately 950 gm. of protein are deposited during the last six weeks of pregnancy. If the mother nurses her baby her additional need is determined by her daily milk secretion, estimated to be 850 to 1200 ml. Human milk contains an average of 1.2 gm. protein per 100 ml. milk. The recommended allowance for the lactating woman is 75 gm. per day, assuming that the quality of protein in her diet is not always ideal.

EVALUATION OF PROTEIN AND AMINO ACIDS

Animals are used to determine biological values. Early investigations by such scientists as Osborne and Mendel, McCollum, and Sherman are of historical interest, for their experiments on the rat form the basis of much of modern practice. These investigators used a standard technique to study the effects of various proteins on weight gain of young rats. Osborne and Mendel (11) found that both quality and quantity of protein in the diet are important. In studies on rats they demonstrated that growth was retarded on an adequate diet containing 9 per cent casein, a protein that is considered complete, while normal weight gain resulted when the casein level was increased to 18 per cent. Addition of small amounts of cystine to the lower protein diet corrected its deficiency, indicating that cystine was not present in casein in large enough ratio to supply the animal's amino acid needs when the intake of this protein was on a comparatively low level. An even more severe stunting of growth was found when rats were fed 4 per cent casein in place of 18 per cent.

In recent years much work has been done on the effects of lack and of supplementation of specific amino acids in the diet. Harper and associates (12) showed that amino acid imbalance, which results in growth depression, can be produced when a diet low in protein is supplemented with a mixture of amino acids that lacks the specific indispensable amino acid which is the limiting factor in the dietary protein. Their studies with the proteins fibrin (deficient in histidine) and casein (low in threonine) showed that depression in the growth rate of rats is caused by adding amino acid mixtures lacking histidine to a fibrin diet, or lacking threonine to a casein diet. The extent of the growth depression appeared to be related directly to the degree of the imbalance. They found in other studies that growth and food intake are lowered in rats fed a diet low in protein but containing an excess of an essential amino acid. This growth depression was overcome by supplementing the diet with the most limiting amino acid.

Evaluation studies are being made on human beings. Today balance studies are made to compare the values of specific sources of nitrogen and amino acids as to quantity, quality, and sources, and as to the proportions in which the amino acids occur in foods and in the diet. When specific purified amino acids are incorporated in a test diet additional nonspecific nitrogen may be needed. Kies and co-workers (13, 14) have shown that nitrogen retention was improved when glycine and diammonium citrate were added to a diet in which corn or rice supplied a suboptimal amount of protein. Scrimshaw and associates (15) compared the replacement value of a mixture of nonessential amino acids with that of glycine and diammonium citrate in the diet of 21 young men. Skim milk furnished 90 per cent of the protein and the rest came from oatmeal. Twenty and 25 per cent of the protein were replaced isonitrogenously by either the nonessential amino acid mixture or the glycine and diammonium citrate and the effect on urinary nitrogen and sulfur excretion and on fasting plasma amino acid concentration was noted. At the 25 per cent replacement level the nonessential amino acids appeared to be a more effective source of nonspecific nitrogen. When the total nitrogen intake was sufficient Kies and co-workers (16, 17) found lysine to be the first limiting factor in both corn and rice. It has been found, also, that two foods containing incomplete proteins when fed simultaneously favored better retention of nitrogen than did either food fed alone (18). This is demonstrated when corn and beans, staple foods in Central America, are used together.

The superiority of animal over plant proteins is generally recognized. Since much of the world has access to only small amounts of animal protein, investigations have been made to evaluate wheat protein as a substitute. In a study by Bolourchi and co-workers (19) nitrogen equilibrium was maintained in 12 young men fed a diet containing 11.8 gm. nitrogen, of which 90 to 95 per cent came from white flour, the remainder from fruits and vegetables. It is generally conceded today that adults can meet their protein requirements if they meet their calorie requirements by consuming enough grain products such as rice, corn, or wheat. The child, with greater proportional needs, cannot do this.

Plasma amino acids are studied as a means of evaluating proteins. Swendseid and co-workers (20, 21) investigated the post-absorptive plasma of men who were in nitrogen equilibrium on a diet containing 45 gm. of well-balanced protein. They found that the concentrations of the amino acids were relatively constant and that the ratio of essential to nonessential amino acids in the plasma also was constant. When the nitrogen in the diet was doubled the amino acid proportions and ratios were not altered. However, on a low protein intake the plasma concentration of the essential amino acid, valine, was significantly reduced, whereas the concentrations of the essential amino acid, methionine, and of the nonessential amino acids, glutamine-aspargine, glycine, and alanine, were significantly increased. The ratio of essential to nonessential amino acids was markedly reduced. Swendseid regards this low ratio as an indication of poor nutritional status. In Bolourchi's study (22) to evaluate wheat flour, blood urea concentrations were determined; levels were found to be half those of the control period when animal proteins were fed. Application of this finding may be of value in the dietary treatment of some renal disorders.

Methods of scoring have been devised. In 1957 a standard called The Provisional Pattern was set by the FAO. This pattern is based on the minimal requirements of essential amino acids of human beings. Other patterns useful in comparing food values have been set up based on the amounts of essential amino acids found in whole egg, human milk, and cow's milk. Table 6–1 shows these four patterns. Studies made on young women by Swendseid, Harris, and Tuttle (23, 24), and by Kirk, Metheny, and Reynolds (25) have compared the FAO pattern with those of egg protein, and of milk and peanut proteins, respectively. Both groups of investigators found that in the FAO pattern there was too high a proportion of tryptophan in relation to the other amino acids. It is also thought that methionine is too high and lysine may be slightly high. When adjustments for these three amino acids are made in the FAO pattern it resembles those of egg and human milk. The FAO/WHO Expert Group favors use of either the egg or human milk pattern as a reference. If the

Table 6–1

Essential Amino Acids in 1957 FAO Provisional Pattern and in Milk and Egg Protein mg. of Amino Acid Per Gm. of Total Nitrogen*

Amino acid	1957 FAO provisional pattern	Cow's milk	Human milk	Hen's egg
Isoleucine	270	407	411	415
Leucine	306	630	572	553
Lysine	270	496	402	403
Total "aromatic" amino acids	360	634	652	627
Phenylalanine	180	311	297	365
Tyrosine	180	323	355	262
Total sulfur-containing amino acids	270	211	274	346
Cystine	126	57	134	149
Methionine	144	154	140	197
Threonine	180	292	290	317
Tryptophan	90	90	106	100
Valine	270	440	420	454
Total essential amino acids	2016	3200	3127	3215

* Protein Requirements, Report of a Joint FAO/WHO Expert Group, WHO Technical Report Series No. 301. Geneva (1965).

1957 Provisional Pattern is used the Expert Group does not recognize tryptophan as unity but expresses the essential amino acid proportions in terms of mg. per gm. of nitrogen. This is known as the E/T ratio, which is the proportion of the total nitrogen derived from essential amino acids.

The A/E ratio is sometimes used. This gives the mg. of one essential amino acid per gm. of the total essential amino acids. The E/N ratio gives the proportion of essential amino acids to nonessential amino acids; this latter ratio is used in studies on blood plasma. The chemical or protein score was one of the first means used to compare foods as to quality. It measures the extent to which a food supplies its most limiting amino acid. Table 6–2 gives data on the amino acid content of 30 food products and designates the amino acid most likely to be the limiting factor in relation to the calculations of the FAO Provisional Pattern.

Several formulas have been devised for use in evaluating protein in the diet. These are based on specific laboratory procedures. Among these are BV (Biological Value), PER (Protein Efficiency Ratio), NPU (Net Protein Utilization), NBI (Nitrogen Balance Index), and

Table 6-2

Essential (and related) Amino Acids in the Provisional Pattern of Amino Acids in Selected Foods (mg. of Amino Acid per gm. of Nitrogen), Protein Scores, and Biological Values*§

Item	Iso-leucine	Leucine	Lysine	Phenyl-alanine	Tyro-sine	Sulfur-Containing Acids		Threo-nine	Trypto-phan	Valine	Protein Score	Biological Value	
						Total	Methio-nine					Grow-ing Rat	Human Adult
Provisional Amino Acid Pattern	270	106	270	180	180	270	144	180	90	270	100		
Milk (cow's)	407	630	496	311	323	211†	154	292	90	440	78	90	62, 79, 100, 43, 51
Egg	428	565	396	368	274	342	196	310	106	460	100	87	94, 97
Casein	402	628	497	334	367	215†	190	272	85	448	80	69	68, 64, 70
Egg albumin	403	556	372	392	271	397	245	275	90	486	100	97	91, 91
Beef muscle	332	515	540	256	212	237	154	275	75†	345	83	76	67, 80, 84, 75
Beef heart	317	558	513	283	232	217†	149	288	81	360	80	74	
Beef liver	327	577	468	315	234	226†	147	302	94	393	84	77	
Beef kidney	304	542	453	294	232	208†	128	278	92	365	77	77	
Pork tenderloin	320	462	515	240	225	233†	156	292	80	302	86	79	
Fish	317	474	549	231	159	262	178	283	62†	327	70	75	94
Oats	302	436	212†	309	213	211	84	192	74	348	79	66	88, 89
Rye	253	398	244	285	209	277†	89	190	76	301	80		60, 60
Rice	322	535	236	307	269	222	142	241	65†	415	72		67, 67, 88
Corn meal	293	827	179	284	385	197	117	249	38†	327	42	54	24‡
Millet	374	583	190†	247		430	254	254	80	445	70	56	
Kaoliang	351	834	178†	420	128	205	93	223	70	381	66	56	
White flour	262	442	126†	322	174	192	78	174	69	262	47	52	42, 40, 45, 67, 70

Wheat germ	269	412	344	208	200	*165†*	99	333	56	322	61	75	89
Wheat gluten	261	426	*107†*	308	192	223	100	151	60	264	40	40	42, 42
Groundnut flour	258	376	217	315	226	*150†*	56	169	70	306	56	54	56, 83
Soy flour	333	484	395	309	201	*197†*	86	247	86	328	73	75	65, 71, 81
Sesame seed	300	500	*159†*	460	244	317	181	182	93	216	59	71	
Sunflower seed	296	402	*195†*	275	149	197	95	209	78	313	72	65	
Cottonseed meal	236	368	269	325	164	*188†*	88	221	74	308	70	64	91
Potato	260	304	326	285	*99†*	159	87	237	72	339	56	71	60, 80, 71, 79
Navy bean	358	541	460	347	245	*126†*	64	274	58	379	47	38	46, 46
Peas	336	504	438	290	245	*157†*	77	230	74	317	58	48	56, 90
Sweet potato	283	345	293	355	281	*219†*	119	324	115	484	81	72	64
Spinach	275	461	367	295	*127†*	239	115	285	101	352	70		
Cassava	118	184	310	133	98	*60†*	22	136	131	144	22		

* *Protein Requirements*. FAO of the United Nations, Committee on Protein Requirements. FAO Nutritional Studies No. 16 (Rome) 1957.

'§ Figures for amino acid content are taken from M. L. Orr and B. K. Watt, *Amino Acid Content of Foods*, Home Economics Research Report No. 4, USDA, (1957).

† This item is lowest in relation to the provisional pattern of amino acids and is the basis for the protein score of the food.

‡ Low figure probably due to a leucine-isoleucine imbalance.

NDpCal% (Net Dietary Protein Calories per cent). BV is defined as the proportion of absorbed nitrogen that is retained in the body. PER measures body weight gain in relation to weight of protein eaten but does not consider utilization. NPU expresses nitrogen retention in relation to intake; this is the most commonly used index. As this index number decreases the protein requirement increases. NBI expresses the rate of increase in nitrogen retention with respect to intake and in most circumstances is equivalent to the protein's biological value. NDpCal% represents the proportion of dietary calories supplied by protein, corrected for efficiency of protein utilization, expressed as a percentage of the total calorie intake. More detailed discussion of the various indices may be found in Evaluation of Protein Quality, Publication No. 1100 (26) of the National Academy of Sciences—National Research Council.

FACTORS TO BE CONSIDERED IN SETTING THE RECOMMENDED
DIETARY ALLOWANCES

Dietary factors other than protein influence the body's use of protein. Reference was made on page 97 to the need for sufficient calories so that protein may not be used as a source of energy. It has been stated also that carbohydrate and fat are important because their products of intermediary metabolism combine with nitrogenous materials to form amino acids within the body. The minerals and vitamins are also important in that they affect normal growth and development. Among the more critical of these are potassium, phosphorus, and niacin.

The time factor influences nitrogen utilization. Geiger (27) found that an animal may not grow well even when he receives adequate amounts of all the amino acids; unless the amino acids or supplementary proteins are fed simultaneously, growth retardation results. This indicates a limited ability of the body to store amino acids as such, in which case their supplementary action would not be evident. Leverton and Gram (28) advise consideration of distribution of quantity and kind of protein among the three meals as a means of securing the best retention of nitrogen; 14 college women on a controlled diet had better nitrogen retention when eight ounces of milk were given at breakfast than when no animal protein was included at this meal. The significance of the time factor will be most apparent in relief feeding and in emergency diets in which the protein is less adequate.

Studies have been made on the effects of heat and radiation as used in the processing of foods; it has been shown that heat treatment of protein may either improve or retard the utilization of protein. For example, heat helps in processing soybean flour, partly because it makes methionine more available and partly because raw soybeans contain trypsin-inhibitors which may both retard growth and hinder digestion. Another example of the beneficial effect is in egg white which contains ovomucoid, a trypsin-inhibitor which heat destroys.

On the other hand, heat treatment may retard digestion, depending on the length of time and degree of temperature used. It is now thought that the lower biological value of a heated protein is due less to actual destruction of the amino acid and more to a chemical change which results in a retarded rate of enzymatic digestion so that the needed amino acid is not present in the blood stream in time to be synthesized into new tissue. It has been shown that lysine is less available when the food containing it is cooked in a pressure cooker. In bread baking the loss of lysine has been associated with the browning of the crust; toasting and drying of baked bread also result in a further loss of the amino acid. It has been advocated that bread be fortified with lysine to make up for these losses. It is also known that reducing sugars may combine with some of the amino acids at high temperature to form products resistant to hydrolysis by enzymes; toasting flaked and puffed cereals may lower the value of their proteins but moist heat is not detrimental. Milk proteins may be damaged by overheating, especially when milk sugar is present, but the processes applied in pasteurization, evaporation, canning, and cooking fresh milk do no harm. Sterilization by radiation at the rate of 3 million rep* gamma has been shown not to affect the biological value of beef proteins but did reduce by 8 per cent the biological value of milk proteins; it has been suggested that radiation may damage the sulfur-containing amino acids.

Certain conditions of the body may affect the need for protein. Growth, pregnancy, and lactation have been mentioned briefly; they will be discussed in greater detail in Chapters 14, 15, and 16. In recovery from malnutrition and from wasting diseases, and in treatment of hypochromic anemia, additional protein is needed, and the common practice is to increase the protein supply and at the same time to administer easily digested foods. After injuries, burns, and surgery, nitrogen losses are to be expected and this catabolic tendency may continue for a period of weeks. If these conditions are accompanied by protein deficiency, delayed healing of tissues, shock, infection, and malnutrition may be evident. Adequate amounts of dietary protein as well as calories may materially reduce nitrogen loss.

Increased susceptibility to infection may be explained by a depletion of protein reserves and an inability to make the antibody globulin because of lack of the essential amino acids. This is another indication of the importance of high-quality protein during illness.

Today it is realized that nitrogen should be included in the solutions

* Rep, or roentgen equivalent physical, is a measure of radiation absorbed per gram.

given intravenously to surgical patients. When mixtures containing only water, carbohydrate, and electrolytes are administered, a negative nitrogen balance and loss of body weight results. It has been shown (29) that when intravenous solutions supply adequate calories and are supplemented with protein, nitrogen and body weight losses are minimized.

The stresses of everyday living caused by extreme cold, worry, minor pain, and tension may result in increased urinary nitrogen excretion. This loss may vary greatly from person to person and in different population groups. The FAO/WHO Expert Group recommends that 10 per cent be added to the obligatory loss figure to care for stress.

Muscular activity is not a factor of practical concern. The common conception that muscular activity is carried on at the expense of muscle tissue and therefore necessitates an increase in protein intake has not been proved by scientific investigation. Casual observation of the effects of such activities as football or prize-fighting or of even less strenuous exercise shows that muscle is thereby enlarged, not worn away. But it is not evident whether this protein storage is the result of work or of the subsequent greater appetite and increased food intake. In a series of carefully controlled respiration calorimeter tests, Atwater secured quantitative data on this problem, information which may be applied in a practical manner. He found that muscular work which increased the calorie requirement of his subjects by 97 per cent resulted in only 4 per cent more nitrogen excretion. These experiments indicate that any tendency to deplete protein, as denoted by nitrogen loss, is balanced by development of body tissue. They also show that calorie intake is a matter of greater concern to the laborer than is increased protein. Meat three times a day may appeal to the palate, but it is no more necessary for the man working in the field than for his wife performing her household tasks. The "training tables" for athletes frequently have supplied a high protein intake to football players, but today this practice is not considered essential.

MEETING THE DAILY ALLOWANCE FOR PROTEIN

Much information is available concerning food sources of protein and amino acids. The food composition table in the Appendix gives data on the protein composition of the edible part of approximately 600 foods in common use in the United States. Nearly 2500 items are included in the 1963 revision of *Agriculture Handbook No.* 8; data are given in 100 gm. portions and one-pound purchases.

Another government bulletin by Orr and Watt (30) gives data for the 18 amino acids found most frequently in over 200 food items, expressed in terms of grams of each amino acid per gram of total nitrogen, and in terms of grams of each amino acid per 100 gm. of food. From this bulletin the FAO Committee on Protein Requirements has compiled information concerning the more significant amino acids in 30 food products (Table 6–2). The list includes some foods not commonly used in this country but of special interest to persons in the underdeveloped countries. This table also gives the provisional amino acid pattern and information on protein scores and biological values. The protein score is a scheme for using a reference pattern in evaluating food sources; it gives egg protein a score of 100, and other foods in Table 6–2 were assigned scores which show the percentage of the limiting amino acid that is most lacking. Oats may be used as an illustration. The lysine value of oats is 212 (figure with a dagger symbol since it is the limiting factor); the provisional pattern of amino acids gives 270 for lysine so the protein score is 79. The biological value figures listed in this table are expressed in terms of both the growing rat and the human adult and have been determined in actual studies.

Foods of plant source tend to furnish less adequate protein. Most cereals and millets are deficient in threonine as well as lysine; corn is also deficient in tryptophan. Legume proteins which are good sources of lysine and threonine are lacking in the sulfur-containing amino acids and tryptophan. Peanut proteins lack methionine as well as lysine and threonine. Green peas and green leafy vegetables lack methionine.

Dietary surveys and studies indicate how much protein is eaten. The protein intake of individuals in the United States has increased since the beginning of the century and is now considerably above the minimal recommended allowances. Data from the Household Food Consumption Survey (31) conducted in the spring of 1965 shows that the average consumption of protein per person per day in the United States was 106 gm. and that 95 per cent of the households met or exceeded the RDA. Meat, fish, and poultry supplied approximately 42 per cent of the protein; milk, and milk products, 20 per cent; egg, 6 per cent; grains, 20 per cent, with the remaining 12 per cent supplied by fruits, vegetables, and miscellaneous food items.

The dietary studies reported in *Nutritional Status U.S.A.* (32) indicate that the protein intakes of men, boys, and girls at all ages were for the most part greater than the 1968 revised recommended allowances. The intakes of women also exceeded the recommended allowances throughout most of life; however, after age 65 there was a significant drop. For 446 families in Kansas and Ohio, the protein eaten averaged 104 and 108 gm. per person respectively; this intake amounted to slightly over 10 per cent of the total calories. Among 730 low-income rural families in five southern states, the protein intake was less than in the Kansas and Ohio groups, and Negro families in the South ate less protein than did the white families.

Studies (33) of the protein recommended for the armed services indicate the importance federal authorities give to this nutrient. A majority of the troops in the Army, at home and abroad, are fed an A ration, composed of fresh foods, or convenience foods readily available in any market. The meals, prepared by standard recipes, follow a master menu. A study was made by Canham and associates (34) of the food consumption of men in 12 mess halls at four Army camps during the period 1963–68. The average intake of protein per man per day was 126 gm. In May, 1970, these workers conducted a survey of the nutrient intake of women in an Army Corps Center. During a 12-day period the average daily intake of protein was 94 gm. per female per day.

More exact investigations give data which relate protein and amino acid intakes to the requirement. Reynolds and co-workers (35) investigated the self-chosen diets of 12 women and determined nitrogen balance and essential amino acid content of their intakes during 28 periods. Table 6–3 shows the relationship between intake and minimal requirements for

Table 6–3

*Amino Acid Intakes of Women on Self-Chosen Diets**

Essential amino acid	Intake		Minimal requirements of women for essential amino acids
	Women in nitrogen balance	Women in negative nitrogen balance	
	gm. per day	gm. per day	gm. per day
Isoleucine	1.62 – 5.73	1.15 – 4.88	0.450
Leucine	4.83 – 7.35	3.37 – 6.25	0.620
Lysine	3.25 – 7.17	1.70 – 5.85	0.400
Methionine	0.83 – 2.54	0.67 – 2.03	0.290
Cystine†			(0.250)
Phenylalanine	2.88	1.53 – 4.03	0.220
Tyrosine†			(0.900)
Threonine	1.44 – 3.44	0.97 – 3.02	0.310
Tryptophan	0.44 – 1.28	0.25 – 0.91	0.160
Valine	3.20 – 4.58	2.51 – 5.98	0.650
Total nitrogen	8.20–15.20	4.50–14.40	10.000

* Reynolds, M. S., *et al.* Nitrogen Balances and Amino Acid Content of Self-Selected Diets. *J. Am. Diet. Ass., 29:*359 (1953).
† Not an essential amino acid.

the eight essential amino acids. In all instances the intakes were in excess of the women's minimal needs; leucine, lysine, and valine were present in the largest amounts, methionine and tryptophan in the lowest. In 15 of the 28 balance periods the women were in negative balance despite an apparently adequate protein intake. This condition was associated with low calorie diets. Reynolds states that the amino acids were well distributed throughout the three daily meals and that there was no deficiency of any of the essential amino acids. It is possible that this unexpected situation might be the result of some other nutrient lack or an imbalance.

In the study (36) on the metabolic response of young women to a standardized diet, referred to in Chapter 1, the 30 college women were fed for seven five-day periods a diet containing approximately 11 gm. of nitrogen daily. The amino acids in this diet were well proportioned in relation to one another and more than met minimal requirements of amino acids for women. Daily retentions of all the women averaged 1.60 gm. nitrogen and ranged from 0.36 to 2.61 gm. None of the subjects were in negative balance, but from one-third to one-half of them retained less than 1 gm. nitrogen daily; it was concluded that this protein intake provided approximately the amount required for balance.

Balance studies were conducted at the Universities of Wisconsin, Illinois, and Indiana in cooperation with the Bureau of Home Economics and Human Nutrition of the USDA on 136 women who were over 30 years old; they ate self-selected diets during seven- to ten-day periods. Nitrogen retention was not secured unless an average of 66 to 70 gm. of protein was eaten daily by the women up to the age of 69, and 59 gm. by those over 70 years; at least 1800 calories daily were required for nitrogen retention.

Research has also been conducted in which specific amino acid intakes were investigated. At the University of Wisconsin, studies on varying amounts of methionine and cystine indicated that on intakes of 0.29 gm. of methionine and 0.5 gm. of cystine daily all of 13 women subjects were in balance; it is thought important to consider both these sulfur-containing amino acids in determining the requirement of either. Further Wisconsin studies were conducted on minimal lysine requirements; nitrogen balance was maintained by 14 women when 0.4 to 0.5 gm. of lysine was eaten daily. This is a small amount compared with that found in the usual American diet. Studies made on valine at the University of Nebraska Experiment Station indicated that nitrogen balance could be secured equally well when 0.23 to 0.53 gm. of the amino acid was supplied either in corn or in purified form.

Several methods are being used to improve the quality of the protein in the diet. Because of the practical importance attached to the quality of dietary protein, especially in the developing countries, considerable research is being conducted to develop acceptable, nutritious, and inexpensive products from the food sources available. New products may be especially important because of indications that there may be a lessening surplus of dry skim milk. One line of approach is concerned with combinations of foods (37). Scrimshaw and associates have developed Incaparina, composed of whole ground sorghum grain, cottonseed flour,

Torula yeast, calcium carbonate, and vitamin A. Another combination is L'aubina, developed in Beirut under the direction of Sebrell; it is made from chick peas and parboiled wheat plus small amounts of dried skim milk, and bone ash. It is intended for use in North Africa, the Middle East, India, and Pakistan. Preschool children in Beirut have thrived when L'aubina was used to supplement their deficient diet. Peanut protein isolate, developed in India, is made into a vegetable milk or is added to buffalo milk to make an acceptable product. CSM, a corn-soy-milk mixture fortified with essential minerals and vitamins, at a cost of about eight and one-half cents per pound, is being distributed in some areas by USAID in collaboration with the USDA. It is estimated that 100 gm. of CSM will furnish, besides a high protein food, from one-third to one-half of the calories needed by a two-year-old child, and one-half to three-quarters of the vitamin and mineral requirements.

The improvement of grains provides a second approach to this problem. At Purdue University (38, 39) a genetic strain of corn called Opaque-2 was developed. In this corn the inadequate protein zein was reduced to half its usual concentration and the glutelin content was doubled. There is about a 50 per cent increase in lysine and tryptophan and the balance between leucine and isoleucine is improved due to a decrease in leucine. Opaque-2 corn was first tested on young rats, later on preschool children, men, and women. In the human adult, nitrogen equilibrium was attained on 300 gm. of Opaque-2 corn, when fed as the principle source of protein; this amount of corn is commonly consumed in some areas.

Improvement in amino acid content of corn can be achieved by artificial defoliation of the corn plant at certain stages of development. Scientists at the University of Nebraska found that corn defoliated by hail or frost had a significantly higher crude protein content; further study showed that all amino acids except tryptophan increased when development was arrested at either the blister or milk stage (40).

A third approach to the problem of quality improvement involves changing an unpalatable flavor or texture to produce a more attractive product. Soy beans are used as human food only in limited quantity. At General Mills soy protein isolates which contain approximately 95 per cent protein have been spun into fine filaments and then, by addition of a flavor or color, have been made to resemble chicken, ham, or beef. Tests have shown that these preprocessed foods are acceptable and nourishing (41). Fish protein concentrate has been made from species of fish not acceptable for human consumption; extraction of most of the oil results in a bland odorless product which contains about 80 per cent protein of high biological value (42). Algae are seldom used as food even though their amino acid content warrants their use. In experiments in which color and flavor were altered, algae were found to be acceptable; they are particularly effective in supplementing rice protein (43). This algae-rice combination resulted in nitrogen retention similar to that when fish, soybean, or egg was fed as the source of protein.

A common method of improving protein quality involves addition of one or more purified amino acid to a protein indigenous to the area. Wheat, the grain used largely as the main source of protein in many countries, is limited in lysine. Therefore some authorities advocate a mandatory worldwide program of lysine supplementation (44). Before this method is approved many investigators recommend that a large-scale well-controlled study be conducted on preschool children in areas throughout the world to determine if the supplementation will affect growth and development, morbidity and mortality (45). The Committee on Amino Acids of the FNB has reviewed available data on lysine fortification of wheat flour and has evidence that for young children the minimum lysine requirement cannot be met by unfortified wheat (46). However, since there is conflicting evidence as to the need for lysine fortification of wheat for adults the Committee has endorsed investigations of the feasibility of supplementing wheat for entire populations.

A simple protein rule may be followed. Neither the 0.9 gm. per kg. standard nor that expressed in terms of calories is easily followed by the lay person, and formulating the standard in terms of specific foods is helpful. Thus it helps to plan for adequate protein intake in terms of specific foods. If the average daily menu includes milk, meat, fish or poultry, cheese or eggs, some cereal products and some legumes, the protein need probably is well met. Other foods, such as fruits and vegetables, supply small amounts of protein and add to the desirable daily intake.

A limited food budget necessitates careful consideration of the proportion to be spent for protein. When the amount of money to be spent is restricted, it is difficult to secure a palatable and adequate diet, and the homemaker whose knowledge of food values is slight needs assistance in purchasing. Various social agencies, confronted with the problem of advising families on minimal financial expenditure, have planned low-cost dietaries and market orders. USDA specialists are also ready to help and have issued bulletins which suggest a week's food supply for families living at different income levels. Table 6–4 gives a week's food needs for a low-cost plan for a family consisting of parents ages 22 to 35, a girl of nine, and a boy of 11. Calculations have been made of the various nutrients in this food list. Table 6–5 gives figures for the energy and protein values of the various groups or classes of food and the percentage of the total furnished by each class. In this low-cost dietary, animal products and legumes supply more than two-thirds of the protein, grain products, more than one-fifth.

Table 6–4

A Week's Low-Cost Food Needs for a Family of Four*

Milk, cheese
  6 qt. whole milk
  3 qt. skim milk
  2 14½ oz. cans evap. milk
  ¾ lb. dry skim milk
  ¾ lb. cheddar cheese

Meat, fish
  3 lb. chuck beef, boneless
  3 lb. hamburger
  3 lb. pork shoulder
  1 lb. beef liver
  ¼ lb. salt pork
  1¼ lb. cod steak

Eggs
  25

Dry beans, nuts
  ⅔ lb. dry white beans
  6 oz. peanut butter
  ⅓ lb. shelled peanuts

Dark-green & deep-yellow vegetables
  1 lb. carrots
  1 lb. broccoli
  1½ lb. sweet potatoes

Citrus fruit, tomatoes
  5 medium size oranges
  1 #2 can tomatoes
  1 46-oz. can orange juice, un-
    sweetened
  ½ 46-oz. can grapefruit-orange
    juice, sweetened

Other vegetables & fruits
  10 lb. potatoes
  2½ lb. cabbage
  2 lb. celery
  3 lb. onions
  1 lb. beets
  1¾ lb. iceberg lettuce
  1 lb. green snap beans
  2 lb. rutabagas
  3 lb. apples
  2 lb. bananas
  ½ lb. raisins
  1 lb. canned applesauce

Grain products
  6 lb. enriched bread
  2 lb. whole wheat bread
  1 lb. family flour, enriched
  1 lb. whole-meal wheat cereal

  ½ lb. macaroni, enriched
  ½ lb. rice, white, enriched
  ½ lb. corn flakes, enriched
  ½ lb. rolled oats
  ½ lb. graham crackers

Fats and oils
  1¼ lb. margarine
  8 oz. cooking oil
  ½ lb. salad dressing

Sugar, sweets
  1½ lb. granulated sugar
  ½ lb. brown sugar
  ½ lb. table syrup
  ½ lb. molasses

* Adapted from *Family Food Plan Revised 1964*, approved for reprinting December, 1968. ARS, USDA.

DEVIATIONS FROM THE ACCEPTED STANDARDS

There is no adequate proof that a high-protein diet is harmful to a healthy human being. The idea that a steady diet high in protein may be detrimental, resulting in definite metabolic disorders in middle life, has had enthusiastic proponents. Among the first was Chittenden, who believed that his low-protein intake freed him from rheumatism, bilious attacks, and headaches, and improved his appetite and feeling of physical fitness. Experimental work on animals, as well as some clinical investigations, has been interpreted to mean that such disorders as arteriosclerosis,

Table 6–5

*Distribution of Calories and Protein in the Low-Cost Dietary for a Family of Four**

Food Groups	Food energy		Protein	
	kcal.	per cent[1]	gm.	per cent[1]
Milk, cheese	8583	13.1	576.1	23.4
Meat, fish, eggs, legumes	19038	29.1	1120.9	45.5
Dark-green and deep-yellow vegetables	891	1.4	25.9	1.1
Citrus fruit, tomato	1436	2.2	26.4	1.1
Potatoes, other fruits and vegetables	6617	10.1	157.3	6.4
Grain products	17030	26.1	552.8	22.4
Fats, oils	7075	10.9	5.6	0.1
Sugar, sweets	4649	7.1	0.0	0.0
Total for week	65319	100	2465.0	100
Total for day	9331		352.1	
Recommended allowances for day[2]	9300		200.0	

* For description of family see page 113.
[1] Expressed to one decimal.
[2] Recommended Dietary Allowances. Seventh Revised Edition. Washington, D.C.: FNB, NAS-NRC Publ. 1694 (1968).

nephritis, and constipation may be caused by high-protein feeding. However, Keys and Anderson (47) in experiments on physically healthy, schizophrenic men maintained at calorie equilibrium and on a constant fat intake, but with protein intake shifting from low to high and back to low, found no significant change in the serum cholesterol values.

During the past few decades there has been a revolution in the dietetic treatment of kidney diseases. Only in cases where there is retention of the metabolic end products of protein is the protein reduced, and then not below the amount the body will inevitably metabolize. In the more common cases of faulty kidney function in which blood protein is lost through kidney excretion, protein well above ordinary intakes may be prescribed. This helps maintain blood protein and the water balance at the normal level.

The effect of a high-protein diet was studied in two Arctic explorers, Stefansson and Anderson, who lived on a meat diet for one year. Their measured daily intake of protein was 100 to 140 gm., and at one period was as high as 180 gm. Examinations of blood and urine at the end of the study revealed no abnormalities.

The question of protein in relation to cost is also raised. This consideration is often faced by the nutritionist in planning low-cost, adequate diets. In such cases the protein sources must be considered carefully, and the quality as well as the quantity of protein be brought as nearly as possible to the optimal level. Even when the budget is more liberal, false ideas of economy and detrimental effects through its use may curtail the amount of protein in the diet more than is desirable.

The advisability of a low protein intake is questioned. Many studies have shown that diets which contain a small amount of protein also tend to have proteins of low biological value. This and the possibility of inefficiency in utilization of the nutrient are arguments against limiting the amount of protein in the diet. Protein is very important for the desired growth of the young. Both animal experiments and studies of children have shown a stunting in growth reflected in both height and weight when the consumption of protein is low.

There is evidence (48) that protein malnutrition in the first two years of life may result in retardation of psychomotor development. In recent years results of both animal and human studies indicate that severe nutritional deficiency, especially of protein, may have a profound and permanent detrimental effect on mental development, learning ability, and behavior.

It is also thought that efficiency in utilization of protein may decrease with aging. At the same time, in the older person calorie intake is apt to be lower. This makes it somewhat difficult to have enough of the foods high in protein in the day's meals. The results of a low protein diet throughout life may be a greater susceptibility to infection, fatigue and irritability, slower recovery from disease, and retarded healing of wounds and burns. More specific results of low protein intake include liver disorders, anemia, impaired antibody formation, and edema; this latter condition often is associated with war and famine. After the World Wars, undernourished children lost some of their "hunger swelling" when their diets were supplemented with milk and cheese. In macrocytic anemia a liberal protein intake is often advised.

Protein-calorie malnutrition (PCM) is the most common disorder of early childhood occurring in developing tropical countries (49). The two types of PCM are kwashiorkor and nutritional marasmus (Figure 6–3). Varying degrees of severity result in increased susceptibility to infection, physical stunting, permanent brain damage, and a high mortality rate. Kwashiorkor occurs when the diet is very low in protein and includes calories from carbohydrate. In nutritional marasmus the diet is low in both protein and calories. Thus the former disease is the result of an unbalanced diet, the latter, of starvation.

Although a low protein intake is not approved by the majority of nutrition workers in the United States, it is recognized that the body is able to adjust itself to less protein than most individuals consume, and some investigators believe that such a regime is desirable. Hegsted (50), in a study of protein needs during growth, found that relatively small

Figure 6–3

Clinical features of two main severe forms of PCM—kwashiorkor and marasmus—contrasted diagramatically. (From Jelliffe, Child Nutrition in Developing Countries. Washington, D.C.: U.S. Dept. of Health, Education and Welfare, Public Health Service Publ. No. 1822 [1968].)

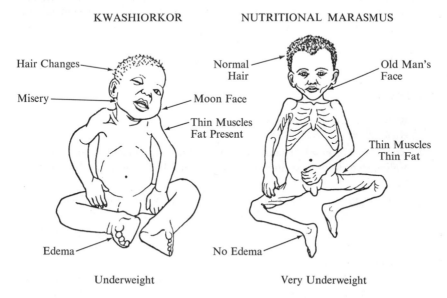

KWASHIORKOR   NUTRITIONAL MARASMUS

Hair Changes
Misery

Normal Hair
Old Man's Face

Moon Face

Thin Muscles Fat Present

Thin Muscles Thin Fat

Edema

No Edema

Underweight   Very Underweight

amounts of protein are deposited in the tissues, and he suggests that the protein required for both growth and maintenance may actually be considerably lower than the allowances recommended by the FNB. Nevertheless, as long as it is possible from the standpoints of availability of supplies and financial resources to secure a liberal amount of protein-high food, and until there is proof of harm to the body from such consumption, a limited protein dietary probably will not receive popular support.

PROBLEMS

1. Calculate the grams of protein in the food intake records used in Problem 1, Chapter 2. Carry decimals to one place. Determine the average grams of protein in your daily diet and the per cent of the total calories from protein. How do these figures compare with the standards given? If your figures deviate more than 20 per cent from the standard, suggest changes.
2. Prepare a table of representative foods, each of which yields 10 gm. of protein. Give name of food, weight in grams, measure, equivalent in average servings, and cost. Compare the portions as to quantity, quality, and cost of protein.

3. Prepare a table of 100 gm. portions of representative foods arranged in order of protein value.

4. Plan an exhibit of one-egg equivalents in protein.

5. Plan a day's diet for a lacto-vegetarian man weighing 65 kg. whose energy requirements is 2800 calories. His food must contain neither meat nor eggs. Be sure that the diet contains 0.9 gm. of protein per kg. of body weight and that it includes the foods, except meat and eggs, listed as essential in the daily diet. Use the score card from Problem 2, Chapter 1.

REFERENCES

1. Rose, W. C. The Amino Acid Requirements of Adult Man. *Nutr. Abstr. Revs., 27:*631 (1957).

2. Rose, W. C., *et al.* The Amino Acid Requirements of Man. XV. The Valine Requirements; Summary and Final Observations. *J. Biol. Chem., 217:*987 (1955).

3. Scrimshaw, N. S. Nature of Protein Requirements. Ways They Can Be Met in Tomorrow's World. *J. Am. Diet. Ass., 54:*94 (1969).

4. Schroeder, W. A., *et al.* The Amino Acid Sequence of Bovine Liver Catalase: A Preliminary Report. *Arch. Biochem. Biophy., 131:*653 (1969).

5. Sherman, H. C. Protein Requirement of Maintenance in Man and the Nutritive Efficiency of Bread Protein. *J. Biol. Chem., 41:*97 (1920).

6. Leverton, R. M., *et al.* The Quantitative Amino Acid Requirements of Young Women. *J. Nutr., 58:*59, 83, 219, 341, 355 (1956).

7. Swenseid, M. E., *et al.* Amino Acid Requirements of Young Women Based on Nitrogen Balance Data. *J. Nutr., 58:*495, 507 (1956).

8. Reynolds, M. S. Amino Acid Requirements of Adults. *J. Am. Diet. Ass., 33:*1015 (1957).

9. Fisher, H., *et al.* Reassessment of Amino Acid Requirements of Young Women on Low Nitrogen Diets. I. Lysine and Tryptophan. *Am. J. Clin. Nutr., 22:*1190 (1969).

10. Hussein, M. A., *et al.* Variations in Endogenous Nitrogen Excretion in Young Men. *Fed. Proc., 27:*485 (1968).

11. Osborne, T. B., *et al.* The Comparative Nutritive Value of Certain Proteins in Growth and the Problem of Protein Minimum. *J. Biol. Chem., 20:*351 (1915).

12. Harper, A. E., *et al.* Some New Thoughts on Amino Acid Imbalance. *Fed. Proc., 23:*1087 (1964).

13. Kies, C. V., *et al.* Effect on Nitrogen Retention of Men of Varying the Total Dietary Nitrogen with Essential Amino Acid Intake Kept Constant. *J. Nutr., 85:*260 (1965).

14. Kies, C. V., *et al.* Effect on Nitrogen Retention of Men of Altering the Intake of Essential Amino Acids with Total Nitrogen Held Constant. *J. Nutr., 85:*139 (1965).

15. Scrimshaw, N. S., *et al.* Partial Dietary Replacement of Milk Protein by Nonspecific Nitrogen in Young Men. *J. Nutr., 98:*9 (1969).

16. Kies, C. V., *et al.* Effect of Nonspecific Nitrogen Supplementation on Minimum Corn Protein Requirement and First-limiting Amino Acid for Adult Men. *J. Nutr., 92:*399 (1967).

17. Kies, C. V., *et al.* Time, Stress, Quality, and Quantity as Factors in the Nonspecific Nitrogen Supplementation of Corn Protein for Adult Men. *J. Nutr., 93:*377 (1967).

18. Chen, S. C., *et al.* Nitrogenous Factors Affecting the Adequacy of Rice to Meet the Protein Requirements of Human Adults. *J. Nutr., 92:*429 (1967).

19. Bolourchi, S., *et al.* Wheat Flour as a Source of Protein for Adult Human Subjects. *Am. J. Clin. Nutr., 21:*827 (1968).

20. Swendseid, M. E., *et al.* Plasma Amino Acid Levels in Young Subjects Receiving Diets Containing 14 or 3.6 g. Nitrogen per Day. *Am. J. Clin. Nutr., 21:*1381 (1968).

21. Swendseid, M. E., *et al.* Plasma Amino Acid Levels of Men Fed Diets Differing in Protein Content, Some Observations with Valine-Deficient Diets. *J. Nutr., 88:*239 (1966).

22. Bolourchi, S., *et al.* Wheat Flour, Blood Urea Concentration and Urea Metabolism in Adult Human Subjects. *Am. J. Clin. Nutr., 21:*836 (1968).

23. Swendseid, M. E., *et al.* Egg Protein as a Source of the Essential Amino Acids. *J. Nutr., 68:*203 (1959).

24. Swendseid, M. E., *et al.* Nitrogen Balance Studies with Subjects Fed the Essential Amino Acids in Plasma Pattern Proportions. *J. Nutr., 79:* 276 (1963).

25. Kirk, M. C., *et al.* Nitrogen Balances of Young Women Fed Amino Acids in the FAO Reference Pattern, the Milk Pattern, and the Peanut Pattern. *J. Nutr., 77:*448 (1962).

26. Food and Nutrition Board, Committee on Protein Malnutrition. *Evaluation of Protein Quality.* Washington, D.C.: NAS-NRC Publ. 1100 (1963).

27. Geiger, E. The Role of the Time Factor in Protein Synthesis. *Sci., 111:* 594 (1950).

28. Leverton, R. M., *et al.* Nitrogen Excretion of Women Related to the Distribution of Animal Protein in Daily Meals. *J. Nutr., 39:*57 (1949).

29. Levey, S. Reduction of Nitrogen Deficits in Surgical Patients Maintained by Intravenous Alimentation. *Nutr. Revs., 24:*193 (1966).

30. Orr, M. L., *et al. Amino Acid Content of Foods.* USDA, Home Econ. Research Rept. No. 4 (1957).

31. Agricultural Research Service, USDA Consumer and Food Economics Research Division. *Food Intake and Nutritive Value of Diets of Men, Women, and Children in the United States, Spring 1965.* ARS 62–18 (1969).

32. Morgan, A. F. (ed.), *Nutritional Status U.S.A.* Berkeley: Calif. Agr. Sta. Bull. 769 (1959).

33. Mehrlich, F. P. Current Status of Garrison and Combat Feeding in U.S. Army. Bethesda, Md.: Natl. Institutes of Health, Third Far East Symposium on Nutrition, p. 251, Feb. 1967.

34. Personal communication from Col. John B. Canham, MC, U.S. Army Medical Research and Nutrition Laboratory, Fitzsimons General Hospital, Denver, Colo.

35. Reynolds, M. S., *et al.* Nitrogen Balances and Amino Acid Content of Self-Selected Diets. *J. Am. Diet. Ass., 29:*359 (1953).

36. Leverton, R. M., *et al. The Metabolic Response of Young Women to a Standardized Diet.* USDA, Home Econ. Research Rept. No. 16 (1956).

37. Scrimshaw, N. S. Meeting Tomorrow's Protein Needs. *J. Am. Diet. Ass., 54:*94 (1969).

38. Clark, H. E. Nitrogen Balances of Adults Consuming Opaque-2 Maize Protein. *Am. J. Clin. Nutr., 20:*825 (1967).

39. Clark, H. E. Meeting Protein Requirements of Man. *J. Am. Diet. Ass., 52:*475 (1968).

40. Fox, H. M. Protein Possibilities for a Hungry World. *International Agriculture Series 7.* St. Paul: University of Minnesota, Institute of Agriculture (1967).

41. Koury, S. D., *et al.* Soybean Proteins for Human Diets? *J. Am. Diet. Ass., 52:*480 (1968).

42. Roels, O. A. Marine Proteins. *Nutr. Revs., 27:*35 (1969).

43. Lee, S. K., *et al.* Supplementary Value of Algae Protein in Human Diets. *J. Nutr., 92:*81 (1967).

44. Howe, E. E. *et al.* Amino Acid Supplementation of Protein Concentrates as Related to the World Protein Supply. *Am. J. Clin. Nutr., 16:* 321 (1965).

45. Hegsted, D. M. Amino Acid Fortification and the Protein Problem. *Am. J. Clin. Nutr., 21:*688 (1968).

46. Goldsmith, G. A. Interests and Activities of the Food and Nutrition Board. *J. Am. Diet. Ass., 53:*222 (1968)

47. Keys, A., *et al.* Dietary Protein and the Serum Cholesterol Level in Man. *Am. J. Clin. Nutr., 5:*29 (1957).

48. King, C. G. Frontiers in Nutrition: Research, Education and Action. *J. Am. Diet. Ass., 53:*222 (1968).

49. Jelliffe, D. B. *Child Nutrition in Developing Countries: A Handbook for Fieldworkers.* Washington, D.C.: U.S. Dept. of Health, Education, and Welfare, Publ. No. 1822 (1968).

50. Hegsted, D. M. Protein Requirement in Man. *Fed Proc., 18:*1130 (1959).

GENERAL REFERENCES

51. Albanese, A. A., and Orto, L. A. The Proteins and Amino Acids. *In* M. G. Wohl and R. S. Goodhart (eds.), *Modern Nutrition in Health and Disease,* 4th ed. Philadelphia: Lea & Febiger (1968).

52. Brown, W. D. Present Knowledge of Protein Nutrition. In *Present Knowledge in Nutrition,* 3rd ed. New York: Nutrition Foundation (1967).

53. Joint FAO/WHO Expert Group. *Protein Requirements.* Geneva: WHO, Technical Report Series No. 301. FAO Nutrition Meetings Report Series No. 37 (1965).

54. Food and Agriculture Organization of the United Nations, Committee on Protein Requirements. *Protein Requirements.* FAO Nutritional Studies No. 16, Rome (1957).

55. Food and Nutrition Board, Committee on Amino Acids. Evaluation of Protein Nutrition. Washington, D.C.: NAS-NRC, Publ. 711 (1959).

56. Food and Nutrition Board, Committee on Protein Malnutrition. *Evaluation of Protein Quality.* Washington, D.C.: NAS-NRC Publ. 1100 (1963).

Calcium
and
Phosphorus

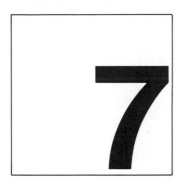

Just as a building needs a strong foundation of cement or stone and a framework firm enough to guard it from destruction by wind and rain, so must the body have a sturdy skeletal structure in order to carry its weight well and to protect its internal organs. A well-built, substantial framework is not only necessary as a safeguard for health, it also makes for a well-shaped and correctly poised body. To attain the proper bone development necessary for physical perfection, the two minerals calcium and phosphorus are essential; other minerals, some of the vitamins, and protein also play important roles in building and maintaining the bone structure. If these nutrients are lacking during the growth period, the result will be a stunted and deformed body, a frail structure. If the deficit occurs after growth is completed, the external effects will be less noticeable.

Important as calcium and phosphorus are to bone development, these minerals have an equally significant and delicate part in regulation of the body's internal activities. The rapid movement of radiocalcium from blood to interstitial space and bone indicates the fine control of this mineral within the body.

Some adults can remain in calcium equilibrium on a wide range of intakes; this ability of the body to adjust is an example of adaptation and serves as a safeguard for survival. Balance on a low intake indicates that the need for calcium is so great that endogenous calcium is reused. The level of calcium in the serum must be kept within certain limits if body functions are to be carried on normally. Absorption of calcium in the human being is not complete. Factors affecting absorption are considered very important in maintaining calcium balance. These and other problems will be discussed in this chapter.

CALCIUM AND PHOSPHORUS IN THE BODY IN RELATION
TO THEIR FUNCTIONS

These minerals are the chief elements in building the skeletal structures of the body. The young woman who weighs 125 pounds will have in her body about 2 pounds of calcium and 1¼ pounds of phosphorus; the body of the man weighing 150 pounds will contain about 2¼ and 1½ pounds, respectively, of the two minerals. These amounts represent 1.5 and 1 per cent, respectively, of the total weight. Approximately 99 per cent of the calcium is in the bones, largely as multiple apatite, forms of calcium phosphate, soluble with difficulty. By means of autoradiographs and using Ca⁴⁵, Henry, Kon, and Tomlin (1, 2) have investigated bone development with special reference to calcium metabolism. They describe two groups of processes. The first is growth by accretion of mineral at certain areas of the surface and resorption at other areas; the second, growth of interstitial tissue involving calcium uptake. This latter means of growth is a nonreversible accumulation; an example is the dentine which shows very small uptake when compared with cortical bone. Proof is given in the work of Bauer, Aub, and Albright (3) that bone contains calcium not only as structural material, but also, to a smaller extent, as active, metabolizing material in the trabeculae—lace-like structures situated throughout the bones and in close contact with the blood stream. The trabeculae are responsible, to a great degree, for the relative constancy of the blood calcium and explain the fact that a lack of calcium in the diet does not show promptly in decalcified bones. In extreme conditions of calcium lack or in hormone imbalance the bone shaft may be depleted; however, a temporary shortage will be cared for by the more available storehouse in the trabeculae.

The natural eruption of the teeth occurs during the growth period. Ordinarily the first teeth appear at about the fifth month and the temporary set is completed by age three. The first permanent teeth are the six-year molars, called "posts," since their function is to preserve the shape of the jaw. Gradually the 20 baby teeth are replaced by the permanent ones which started to form even before birth. The mineral content of this part of the skeletal structure is of great importance because a well-built tooth is better able to grind and cut, and because decay, accelerated by poor calcification, endangers the health of the whole body. However, as Kon and his associates indicated in their work with radioactive calcium, the teeth are not drained of the mineral as easily as are bones and, in the adult, are affected only slightly, if at all, by a shortage of the mineral in the diet. Microscopic studies may give evidence of lack of calcium while the tooth is being formed.

Calcium and phosphorus in body fluids and soft tissues perform other functions. The normal concentration of calcium in the blood of the adult human being ranges from 9 to 11 mg. per 100 ml., that of inorganic phosphorus, 3 to 4 mg. per 100 ml. The average values for children are 10 to 11 mg. of calcium and 5 to 6 mg. of inorganic phosphorus per 100 ml. of blood. About half the blood calcium is bound with protein in a nondiffusible state; the rest is in the ion form. The protein-bound calcium acts as a reserve, available when needed to help maintain the normal calcium ion concentration of the blood. On the other hand, the calcium ion aids largely in coagulation of the blood. It is thought to liberate thromboplastin from the blood platelets; this in turn reacts with prothrombin to form thrombin which is essential in blood clotting. Since the blood coagulates slowly when the calcium ion concentration is low, many hospitals use the routine pre-operation procedure of intravenous injection of a calcium salt. Other factors besides calcium are involved in blood coagulation. The calcium ion in body fluids also functions to regulate the beating of the heart; for maintenance of a rhythmic beat, calcium must be in proper concentration with sodium, potassium and magnesium. Studies by Herbert and coworkers (4) have demonstrated that calcium may have a role in absorption of vitamin B_{12} from the intestinal tract.

The parathyroid glands help regulate the level of calcium in the serum; this level may drop to 6 or 7 mg. per cent when the glands are removed, or it may increase if they are hyperactive. Several parathyroid hormones function in this regulation. Parathormone controls the level in the serum directly by acting on the bone and indirectly by affecting excretion of phosphate by the kidneys. Other parathyroid hormones, calcitonin and thyrocalcitonin, also play a part in calcium metabolism (5). It has been suggested that calcitonin synthesized in the laboratory may be useful in treating bone disorders such as osteoporosis and in reducing the time involved in healing bone fractures. The kidneys also assist in maintaining the serum level, sometimes permitting the reabsorption of as much as 99 per cent of the calcium passing through the tubules, again excreting excesses of calcium which may have been released by bone resorption.

The calcium content of the soft tissues is somewhat lower than that of the blood. Here calcium is a constituent of intercellular cement where it functions to make a nondispersible medium. This mineral also helps maintain normal cell permeability, thus aiding in osmotic pressure control. The calcium ion regulates contractility of muscle and delays fatigue, probably by increasing the muscle's oxygen content. The mineral also takes part in nervous system activity, transmitting nerve impulses over neuro-muscular junctions. In the rat severe calcium deficiency results in muscular weakness and collapse. Paralysis of the hind legs, associated with abnormal posture and gait, may be observed. The life span is reduced and the mortality rate is greatly increased. These extremes are seldom, if ever, seen in the human being.

From 20 to 30 per cent of the body's phosphorus is found in the fluids and soft tissues. It is a constituent of every cell, where it serves many vital functions; it is essential for anabolic and catabolic reactions in the body where phosphorus, as ATP, plays a role in high energy bond formation. Part of the phosphorus occurs in organic form, in such compounds as phospholipids, phosphoproteins, nucleoproteins, phosphoric acid esters of carbohydrates, and in several complex vitamin-enzyme systems. The phosphorus-containing nucleoproteins are essential in cell division, in reproduction, and in the transfer of hereditary characteristics. One of these nucleoproteins, DNA, is thought to control the activities of all the inheritable processes of the cell.

Part of the phosphorus is in the form of inorganic phosphate; here it acts as a buffer and helps regulate the hydrogen ion concentration of the body. Inorganic phosphorus also functions in regulation of osmotic pressure and in secretion and excretion. Other minerals, including sodium and potassium, participate with calcium and phosphorus in the proper functioning of the body's fluids and soft tissues.

When phosphorus deficiency is severe, the needs of the cellular soft tissues are cared for at the expense of the skeleton; the bones become thin and low in mineral content and osteoporosis develops. However, as in the case of calcium, the teeth are relatively unaffected.

THE ABSORPTION OF CALCIUM AND PHOSPHORUS

Calcium and phosphorus are not completely utilized. The two minerals occur in foods in both organic and inorganic forms. In the intestine, organic compounds are hydrolyzed, freeing the inorganic salts which are ready to be absorbed. The physiological mechanism which controls absorption of calcium is thought to be an active transport process. The phosphates are more readily absorbable and this is probably a diffusion process.

The FNB assumes that under normal conditions there is a 40 per cent absorption of calcium. For this degree of absorption vitamin D must be present. When this vitamin is lacking, there is little or no absorption of this mineral; the urine will contain only negligible amounts and most of the calcium will be found in the feces. Research studies indicate that a vitamin D-induced calcium-binding protein found in the intestinal mucosa plays a role in calcium transport (6). The way in which vitamin D functions in this activity is being investigated. On a normal mixed diet a healthy adult may eliminate daily 125 mg. or more of calcium in the feces and 175 mg. in the urine. The FNB estimates that the "reference" adult is likely to lose only about 20 mg. of calcium through sweat daily, although under environmental conditions which produce active perspiration, considerable calcium may be lost in sweat (7). Minor losses also occur through hair and nails.

Phosphorus is not dependent on vitamin D for its absorption. Less work has been done on the absorption of phosphorus than of calcium, and it is assumed that conditions favoring utilization of calcium will also favor phosphorus. Studies have shown that losses of phosphorus through the skin are relatively minor.

The body's need for calcium affects its utilization. It is logical to assume that calcium will be used in greater quantity and more efficiently when the skeletal tissues demand it. This is the basis for the greater allowances during periods of growth. Bronner and Harris (8) studied the absorption of Ca^{45} by adolescent boys and adult men and found that the boys had higher retention values due to bone formation. As intake of the mineral increased, however, the per cent absorbed decreased; when the body's needs had been met, there was less bone salt formation and more resorption. Macy (9) found that when children who were in an unsaturated state of calcium were fed a liberal supply of calcium and phosphorus, they had high rates of retention compared to children whose mineral intake had been safeguarded by long-time consumption of a quart of milk daily. The degree of saturation of skeletal tissues cannot be detected by observing external body characteristics or by qualitative tests.

During gestation when the need for minerals is increased, there tends to be more efficient utilization. In certain diseases and during aging, calcium metabolism is affected. These will be discussed later.

Several other factors influence absorption of these minerals. Both food calcium and phosphorus and the minerals as they occur in the digestive juices are sources of these substances in the blood stream; it has been estimated that from 0.3 to 0.8 gm. of calcium is secreted daily into the gastrointestinal tract. Conditions which are favorable for absorption of dietary calcium and phosphorus also affect that of the mineral in the secretions and explain why fecal excretion may be higher than intake on a low-calcium diet.

Since more work has been done on calcium than on phosphorus, the former mineral will be emphasized in this discussion. As indicated, vitamin D and the parathyroid hormones play important roles in calcium absorption. Other factors which are not considered as significant will be discussed briefly. In experiments with rats dietary lactose has been shown to enhance calcium utilization; the comparatively slow rate of absorption throughout the small intestine is thought to be the reason for the superiority of lactose over the monosaccharides. Spencer and co-workers (10) found calcium lactate superior to calcium gluconate in seven out of eight human subjects. With the lactate, balances were more positive due to a slight but consistent decrease in fecal calcium. Using the tracer technique they found that calcium lactate caused an increase in calcium[47] plasma levels and a decrease in calcium[47] excretions.

Research conducted on the rat indicates that lysine promotes calcium absorption, but as was the case of lactose, calcium balances in man were not improved when 10 to 20 mg. of the amino acid were fed (11). Arginine may also play a role in the absorption of this mineral.

Ascorbic acid favors calcium utilization. In 1925 Chaney and Blunt (12) found that orange juice in the diet of children improved their ability to retain calcium and suggested that one reason for this might be its vitamin C content. In 1957 Leichsenring and co-workers (13) demonstrated the value of both orange juice and crystalline ascorbic acid in the absorption of calcium by healthy college women; neither affected phosphorus utilization.

The calcium salts in the digestive tract must be soluble for absorption; since these are not readily soluble in neutral or alkaline medium, most of the absorption occurs in the upper part of the small intestines. Studies have shown that in rachitic animals the contents of the alimentary tract tend to be alkaline throughout; in such cases the bone fails to receive its quota of calcium. In ordinary infant feeding and in rickets, an acid such as lactic or citric may be prescribed as an aid in mineral utilization.

The favorable effects of ascorbic acid, protein, and fat in moderation are credited partly to their acid reaction in the digestive tract. However, it has been found that, when the diet is high in fat, utilization is hindered. This may be due to the formation of insoluble salts of saturated fatty acids (14). Yacowitz (15) showed that an increased calcium intake by human beings free from coronary heart disease resulted in a reduction in serum cholesterol and triglycerides. Even greater decreases were noted in hypercholesterolemic and hypertriglyceridemic persons. Thus calcium may exert a protective action against the development of arteriosclerosis.

The utilization of calcium, present as an oxalate, has been questioned. In work done on rats the calcium of spinach (which contains considerable oxalic acid) was found to be utilized poorly, if at all, and it was assumed that this would apply equally to human beings. Bonner and others (16) conducted 121 five-day balance studies on ten children, five to eight years of age. Calcium utilization on an adequate mixed diet of common foods was compared with that when 100 gm. of puréed spinach were added to the diet. The vegetable did not replace any other source of calcium but added 5 to 7 per cent to the total amount consumed; for the younger children this was 0.8 gm. of calcium, for the eight-year-olds, 1.3 gm. of calcium. Retention of calcium was not significantly altered with the spinach supplement; there was no significant additional loss of calcium in the feces which would have been expected if the insoluble calcium oxalate was excreted. Johnston and co-workers (17) studied calcium retention in six college women, before and after adding spinach to the diet. During three four-week periods the rigidly controlled diet varied only as to the inclusion of spinach; the calcium balances were not altered significantly by the addition daily of 120 gm. of spinach which contained 0.6 gm. of oxalic acid and 160 mg. of calcium. Nutritionists commonly recommend spinach as a valuable food because of the other nutrients it contains but ignore its calcium as a means of helping to meet the day's allowance.

Cocoa, which contains oxalic acid, also has been viewed with skepticism, especially in its use with milk. The implication has been that the utilization of calcium in milk might be lessened if it were combined with cocoa. In experiments on eight young women Bricker and co-workers (18) showed that there was no significant difference in calcium utilization between milk and cocoa-milk beverage. The women were found to have a tolerance for one ounce of dry cocoa a day, an amount which would make approximately six servings of the beverage. Digestive upsets and lack of appetite resulted when more than one ounce of dry cocoa was consumed in a day.

Phytic acid may hinder utilization of calcium. Oatmeal, which is used to a great extent in many dietaries, is high in phytate; farina, on the other hand, contains none. In an experiment on boys performed by Bronner and others (19) the uptake of radioactive calcium on an oatmeal breakfast was only 74 per cent as much as that on a farina meal. Although the interference of phytate in calcium absorption is evident, this problem is not considered significant in this country where the food phytate of the usual diet is small in amount.

The effects of sodium fluoride on calcium absorption have been studied. Some workers, using large amounts of the fluoride, have reported improvement in calcium retention in men; other studies have not demonstrated this effect. Since there is a possibility of undesirable side-effects of large amounts of fluoride Spencer and co-workers (20) gave smaller doses (20.6 mg. per day) for periods of 22 to 42 days. They found no improvement in intestinal absorption of calcium and in calcium balances. However, they suggested that treatment with relatively small doses of fluoride for periods longer than 42 days might be beneficial for patients who have an increased rate of bone resorption.

There is the possibility that an excess of fiber in the digestive tract may, by promoting fecal excretion, decrease the amount of calcium and phosphorus absorbed. This was shown to occur in dogs when large amounts of agar or cellulose flour were fed. Roughage may be expected to have a detrimental effect on calcium absorption only when it increases markedly the rate of peristalsis, thus decreasing the time in the intestinal tract.

The ratio of calcium to phosphorus in the diet is not thought to be of practical significance in relation to the utilization of the minerals. However, when the ratio of the two minerals is greatly unbalanced, the mineral which is smaller in amount is not as well absorbed (21, 22). This problem will be discussed further in the section on vitamin D.

REQUIREMENTS AND RECOMMENDED ALLOWANCES FOR
CALCIUM AND PHOSPHORUS

The balance study is the commonly used method of investigating calcium and phosphorus requirements. The general plan for the balance study has been described (page 97). When calcium is to be investigated by this means, the procedures must be adjusted to conform with research findings. One of these relates to the need for a very long study period in order to make necessary adjustments in relation to the subject's past diets. Most individuals are able to adapt over a period of time to the level of their intake. If calcium intake is high, much of that eaten will be excreted in the feces and the subject appears to be receiving just what he needs; if the amount of calcium is then lowered, there may be a negative balance for a long period, but eventually most subjects will again reach equilibrium. Similar but reverse adaptation may occur over a long period when the intake is shifted from a low to a higher level. In the past the need for the very long period of study was not recognized and the conclusions drawn were not always justifiable.

Other problems recognized in a calcium balance study relate to individual differences in utilization and to the physiological state of the subjects. Obviously, it is important to have many subjects who are healthy and of similar backgrounds in age, sex, nationality, and dietary customs. Nutritional status and emotional stability should be ascertained. The greater significance which may be given to longitudinal studies and to those of long duration is easily understood.

Calcium and phosphorus balances were included in the study (23) of the metabolic response of young women to a standardized diet. On a mean daily intake of approximately 757 mg. of calcium, the balances of the 30 subjects ranged from −138 to +130 mg. and averaged 0; at this level of intake, 14 of the subjects were in negative balance. On a daily phosphorus intake of approximately 950 mg., the range of balances was from −162 to +215 mg.; ten of the women were in negative balance. For the majority of the subjects, the amounts of calcium and phosphorus in the standardized diet were less than in their self-chosen diets, and it seems probable that the negative balances were only temporary, resulting from the short adjustment period allotted in this experiment.

Sherman, whose calcium standards for adults have been used for many years, assumed that man utilized all the calcium he ate. Sherman's minimal requirement figure of 450 mg. per day was increased to 680 mg. by adding a 50 per cent factor for safety. Mitchell and Curzon (24) plotted the calcium balances reported in the literature on 107 subjects, including those studied by Sherman. They found that 9.75 mg. per kg. per day was the calcium requirement for equilibrium. In experiments on over 50 adults conducted by Steggerda and Mitchell (25, 26) at the University of Illinois, the requirement for calcium equilibrium was also found to be approximately 10 mg. per kg. For the man weighing 70 kg. this would be approximately 0.7 gm. of calcium daily.

A study on metabolic patterns of seven- to ten-year-old girls in seven southern states over a five-year period included intake and output data for ten minerals (27). The results are of value in estimating calcium and phosphorus requirements. In all subjects, diets containing a mean of 907 mg. or more of calcium and 1075 mg. or more of phosphorus resulted in positive balances.

In estimating the calcium requirements during growth, another method of study has been used (28). With data taken from the actual weights of children who were growing at acceptable rates over a period from birth to 20 years, Mitchell and Curzon devised a theoretical growth curve. They computed the daily weight gains and the calcium content of these daily weight gains; the calcium calculations were based on the assumption that the skeletal calcium content at birth is 0.8 per cent of the total weight, in the adult, 1.5 per cent. In the curve it is assumed that the gain of skeletal calcium is regular from birth throughout the growth period. The growth requirement as set up is based on the assumption that if requirements for daily bone growth are met, the composition of adult bones will also be attained.

When calcium growth needs and per cent utilization of the mineral are figured, an approximation of the requirement may be deduced by using the following formula:

$$\frac{\text{Calcium needed for growth (in mg.)}}{\text{Per cent utilization of calcium}} \times 100 = \text{requirement for dietary calcium (in mg.)}$$

However, the calcium requirement estimated by this means applies only to children who are growing at an average rate in both height and weight and who from birth have been well nourished with respect to calcium.

The question of how much calcium should be recommended is disputed (29). There is considerable difference of opinion among authorities on the amount of calcium which should be included in the diet. In many parts of the world the customary intake is low but a deficiency disease related to lack of calcium is not known to exist. In some studies it has been found that persons living on minimal calcium intakes had well calcified bones and lost little calcium through the kidneys. In a study made by Hegsted and co-workers (30) on inmates of a penitentiary in Lima, Peru, the average calcium requirement for maintenance was estimated to be between 100 and 200 mg. daily. Walker (31) states that no demonstrable stigmata are found in the people of Africa who are accustomed to a low calcium diet. Nicolaysen, Eeg-Larsen, and Malm (32) quote considerable evidence to show that throughout the world human beings adapt to low calcium levels. It is thought that certain environmental conditions may favor these lower levels. The conclusions of some authorities are indicated by the standards for adults which the FAO and 13 countries have established (Table 7–1).

Table 7–1

Comparative Adult Calcium Standards in Selected Countries and FAO*
EXPRESSED IN GRAMS

Country	Sex		Date of Issue
	Male	Female	
United States	0.8	0.8	1968
FAO	0.4–0.5	0.4–0.5	1962
Australia	0.4–0.8	0.4–0.8	1965
Canada	0.5	0.5	1964
Central America and Panama	0.45	0.45	1966
Colombia	0.5	0.5	1967
Japan	0.6	0.6	1965
Netherlands	1.0	1.0	1961
Norway	0.8	0.8	1958
Philippines	0.5	0.5	1967
South Africa	0.7	0.6	1956
United Kingdom	0.5	0.5	1969
East Germany	0.8	0.8	——
West Germany	0.8	0.8	1962

* Compiled from *Recommended Dietary Allowances,* Seventh Revised Edition. Washington, D.C.: FNB, NAS-NRC Publ. 1694. (1968).

A liberal intake of calcium is recommended in this country. The FNB in its 1968 revision of the RDA continues to approve a daily intake for adults, both male and female, of 0.8 gm. calcium. It bases its decision on the following figures:

Urinary calcium excretion, approximately	175 mg. per day
Endogenous fecal excretion, approximately	125 mg. or more per day
Sweat, approximately	20 mg. per day
Total	320 mg. per day
Assumed absorption	40 per cent
Amount required to maintain equilibrium	800 mg. per day

This liberal intake—one which can readily be achieved in the United States—is possible on the daily ingestion of less than 3 cups of milk; by this means not only calcium but also other nutrients are obtained. To a great extent milk is also responsible for the abundant health and longevity of the residents of the United States and for the low morbidity and low mortality rates.

Van Duyne, Lanford, Toepfer, and Sherman (33) conducted long-term experiments on rats and furnished evidence that a liberal supply of calcium is advantageous. These workers suggest that, within normal bounds, the choice between high and low calcium intake indicates that a liberal consumption of calcium should be expected to contribute both to immediate efficiency and to good health throughout the life span. The unpredictable degree of utilization of the mineral and the possibility of a chronic substandard nutritional status are other arguments for a liberal intake.

There has been some indication that kidney stones are associated with high calcium intakes, but the reports have dealt primarily with persons with ulcers for whom the high milk intake has been accompanied by alkaline therapy. There is considerable evidence that kidney stones are a result of low magnesium intake or of an increased magnesium requirement resulting from an overabundance of dietary calcium and (or) phosphorus. Abnormal deposition of calcium in other soft tissues also has been associated with inadequate magnesium. There are some diseases in which the body does not utilize calcium normally, but removing calcium from the diet has not been shown to be beneficial in these instances.

The phosphorus requirement of the body also has been investigated. Mitchell and Curzon (24), who analyzed phosphorus balances in 23 human beings, concluded that the adult can utilize, on the average, 42 per cent of the phosphorus consumed. Radioactive phosphorus studies also indicate that a large part of the phosphorus ingested is absorbed; on a normal diet, about two-thirds of the dietary phosphorus appears in the urine.

Since bone contains about twice as much calcium as phosphorus it might be thought that the dietary ratio of calcium to phosphorus also should be 2 : 1. However, as has been stated, there is a larger percentage of phosphorus than of calcium in the blood and soft tissues. The ordinary diet in this country contains as much or more phosphorus than calcium. For these reasons the FNB recommends an allowance for phosphorus equal to that for calcium for all ages except the young infant. The ratio of calcium to phosphorus recommended in early infancy is 1.5:1.

At certain times a margin of safety is especially important. Requirements for women are as high as those for men despite the fact that women weigh less. This recognizes the importance of a generous intake in preparation for the child-bearing period. The detrimental effect of poor nutrition on the developing embryo makes an optimal diet before pregnancy especially important for the young woman.

The amounts recommended for the periods of pregnancy and lactation to provide for the growth of the fetus and placenta and for milk production are greater than those for the average adult. The calcium and phosphorus needs during these periods and during childhood will be discussed in later chapters.

The question may be raised as to the needs of the young man and woman of college age. If there has been a consistently liberal intake of calcium throughout the growth period, a decrease in milk consumption to the one pint level may take place at an earlier age than if storage has not been optimal; if the opposite is true, it may be wise to continue the larger amount into early adult life.

The effects of recumbency on calcium metabolism as in protracted illness or on a long space flight are being investigated. Mack and La-Chance (34) got a significant negative coefficient of correlation between bone mass losses and the mean levels of calcium intake after 14 days of horizontal bed rest. However, the bone mass losses decreased as the calcium intake was increased. The urinary and fecal calcium output during bed rest significantly surpassed that during ambulation.

Illness, when accompanied by fever, results in lowered gastric acidity and decreased absorption of calcium, and probably also of phosphorus; chronic respiratory infections and recurrent colds may cause a lowered utilization of calcium over long periods of time. In rickets and osteomalacia, to be discussed in Chapter 11, special consideration must be given to a liberal intake of the bone-forming materials. In parathyroid hypofunction, tetany is caused by a decrease in urinary excretion of phosphorus and an accompanying increase in serum phosphorus and a drop in serum calcium. The therapy frequently recommended includes administration of calcium lactate or gluconate in large amounts several times daily. In hyperthyroidism there may be severe renal damage and bone demineralization; this condition is difficult to detect if the diet is high in phosphorus because this type of diet tends to preserve normal levels of calcium and phosphorus in the serum.

Osteoporosis is associated with a disturbed calcium metabolism, evident in an altered rate of bone formation and bone resorption (35, 36). The disease is quite prevalent among older persons in the United States and in females more frequently than in males. It is thought that a diet inadequate in calcium over a period of years may contribute to the presence and severity of osteoporosis. Treatment of many osteoporotic people with calcium supplements has resulted in calcium retention and improved bone density. Since osteoporosis may be due to calcium lack, the FNB suggests that the recommended daily allowance of 0.8 gm. calcium may allow little margin of safety for some women.

DIETARY SOURCES OF CALCIUM AND PHOSPHORUS

Milk is the best source of dietary calcium; it also contains considerable phosphorus. Anyone who has tried to plan an adequate diet either for an individual or for a family group realizes the difficulty of fulfilling the calcium standard, as set by the FNB, if milk is not included. Milk contains 0.120 per cent of calcium and 0.093 per cent of phosphorus. In a practical way it means more to know that one-third of a cup of milk will give an adult about one-eighth of his calcium requirement for the day. Two and one-half cups will so nearly supply the necessary amount that little or no concern need be felt for the remainder. Milk is also a good source of phosphorus, though not quite as good as of calcium. One-third of a cup of milk contains an amount of phosphorus equivalent to one-tenth of the daily requirement. For the child, with its greater demand for these minerals, three or more cups of milk in an otherwise adequate diet is ample provision.

Several forms of milk are commonly used and since this food is the best source of calcium, the question of the comparative contents must be considered. Steggerda and Mitchell (25) in calcium metabolism studies on human adults found that there is no appreciable difference in the utilization of liquid whole milk, liquid skim milk, milk heated to 160°F. for 30 minutes, homogenized milk, dried milk solids, soft curd milk prepared by base-exchange, and milk to which citric acid or orange juice has been added. To determine whether the growth of children is influenced by the kind of milk they drink, the United States Public Health Service has studied the growth in weight and height of over 3700 children, aged ten months to six years. The subjects were grouped as follows: those who had received no milk except heated milk, including pasteurized, boiled, evaporated, and dried, and those who had received raw milk for more than the latter half of their lives. The average weight and height of the heated milk group were slightly more than were those of the raw milk group, the differences being considered insignificant; a higher incidence of infection-borne diseases was reported among the latter children. This study gives practical proof to the idea that even if there may be some loss of the minerals in the heating process, the effect is insignificant for the child on a mixed diet. Both evaporated and dried milk are often used in infant feeding and have been found to be well utilized. Dried milk in irradiated form has been shown to be effective as a preventive of rickets.

Filled milk differs from whole milk only in that the milk fat is removed and replaced by other fats or oils; therefore filled milk is considered the equivalent of whole milk in mineral content (37). The non-dairy products called imitation milks are not the calcium equivalent of milk.

The calcium content of other foods must be considered. Although milk is the superior source of calcium, certain other foods contain important amounts of this mineral. A piece of cheddar cheese of one cubic inch contains approximately as much calcium as one-half cup of milk; 1 ounce (2 tablespoons) of cottage cheese has only about one-fifth as much calcium as does one-half cup of milk; and an equivalent weight and measure of cream cheese has only two-thirds the calcium of cottage cheese. Eggs are only a fair source of calcium, ten eggs being approximately equal to 1 cup of milk, yet in a country like China where eggs are plentiful and milk is scarce their calcium value is important. It is also important to note that the calcium from eggs is very well utilized by the body.

Some vegetables when eaten in abundance increase the total calcium in the diet but their bulk precludes their use as a main source. Leafy green vegetables as a class are better sources than are the others. However, the amount of an element present is not necessarily a measure of its availability to the body.

Fruit must be considered a source of calcium, the best varieties being orange, grapefruit, and fig. The value of oranges was proved in a balance study made by Chaney and Blunt (12) on two girls. It was found that the retention of calcium, as well as that of phosphorus, magnesium, and nitrogen, was proportionately greater when orange juice was included in the diet than could be explained by the added calcium from the fruit. The presence of ascorbic acid, the basic residue of the orange, and the possible increased acidity of the intestinal tract were suggested to explain the beneficial results secured.

Meats and grains are among the poorest sources of calcium. However, bread may supply considerable calcium depending on the amount of milk in the recipe, and the presence of mold inhibitors, dough conditioners, yeast mixtures, and optional calcium enrichment agents. Butter made from the fat of milk contains negligible amounts of calcium; refined sugar, none. Molasses, on the other hand, supplies a considerable amount of the mineral.

Figure 7–1 compares the amounts of calcium available from five groups of food in the United States. In Europe the common use of liberal

Figure 7–1
Calcium consumption and sources (per capita per day). (From National Food Situation, #126. Washington, D.C.: Economic Research Service, USDA [November, 1968].)

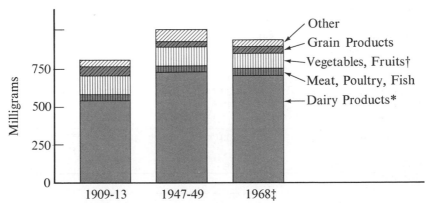

* Excludes butter

† Includes melons, potatoes, sweet potatoes, dry beans, peas, and nuts.

‡ Preliminary

quantities of cheese largely solves the problem of calcium consumption, and it is conceivable that an adult may safely omit milk almost wholly from the diet, provided that a good deal of cheese is included. In the United States a large cheese intake is uncommon.

Many foods other than milk contain liberal amounts of phosphorus. Phosphorus is more generally distributed in both animal and vegetable foods than is calcium. When a variety of foods is eaten there is little reason for concern over the possible lack of phosphorus. Meats are a very good source of phosphorus; fish is even better. The whole grains are superior in phosphorus content to the highly milled products. Eggs are slightly better as a source of phosphorus than of calcium. Dried beans are rich in this mineral and some nuts contain fairly large amounts. Vegetables and fruits on the whole are rather low in phosphorus although they do make some contribution.

A comparison of the different classes of foods in the low-cost dietary demonstrates their relative values as sources of calcium and phosphorus (Table 7–2). This dietary meets the mineral standards because of its content of milk and cheese which, although they furnish only about one-seventh of the calories, provide two-thirds of the calcium and more than one-third of the phosphorus. The grain and the meat groups are much

Table 7–2

Distribution of Calcium and Phosphorus in the Low-Cost Dietary for a Family of Four*

Food groups	Food energy		Calcium		Phosphorus	
	kcal	%[1]	mg.	%[1]	mg.	%[1]
Milk, cheese	8583	13.1	19551	65.3	15020	35.1
Meat, fish, eggs, legumes	19038	29.1	1696	5.7	13473	31.5
Dark-green and deep-yellow vegetables	891	1.4	672	2.2	663	1.6
Citrus fruit, tomatoes	1436	2.2	540	1.8	584	1.4
Potatoes, other fruits and vegetables	6617	10.1	2573	8.6	4135	9.7
Grain products	17030	26.1	3826	12.8	8516	19.9
Fats, oils	7075	10.9	146	0.4	150	0.4
Sugar, sweets	4649	7.1	955	3.2	236	0.6
Total for week	65319	100	29959	100	42777	100
Total for day	9331		4280		6125	
Recommended allowance for day[2]	9300		3700		3700	

* For description of family see Chapter 6, page 113.
[1] Expressed to one decimal.
[2] *Recommended Dietary Allowances,* Seventh Revised Edition. Washington, D.C.: FNB, NAS-NRC Publ. 1694 (1968).

better sources of phosphorus than of calcium. Molasses is responsible for the calcium contributed by the sugar group; this calcium has its origin in lime which is added to the cane juice in the refining process to neutralize acid.

Food preparation may affect the amount of mineral obtained. When foods such as meat and fruits are cooked, their juices are retained as a palatable and nourishing liquid. However, milk and vegetables may suffer from decrease when they are cooked or otherwise prepared for the table. As stated previously, there may be some loss of calcium and phosphorus in the heating of milk. The longer the time used in the heating process, the greater the loss, and this factor seems to be more important than does the degree of heat attained. Since the precipitate which settles to the bottom of the pan is made up largely of calcium phosphates, it is wise to stir the product as it heats to incorporate these salts into the liquid. If the amount of milk in a diet is ample, no concern need be felt over small losses in the preparation of fruits and vegetables, but on low-cost diets the following points are worth consideration. Soaking fruits and vegetables, a step frequently used to prevent darkening and to revive the wilted tissues, involves mineral loss. In the case of dried products the liquid in which the food is soaked should be used in the cooking process, both for improved flavor and for nutritive value. When possible, it is well to cook a vegetable in its "jacket" since a greater proportion of the mineral is found associated with the skin. The size of the pieces in which the food is cut preparatory to cooking should be considered, especially when a large quantity of water is to be used; the thinner the slice and the smaller the piece, the greater will be the loss. Cooking in water causes losses of both calcium and phosphorus, the amount being greater when much water is used; the minerals are found in the cooking water which is drained off.

The common practice of putting a number of vegetables into the soup pot and flavoring the mixture with meat or garlic is valuable in that it conserves the minerals in the food; such a dish should have a larger place in the low-cost American dietary. Today the greater use of salads and many raw vegetables which formerly were cooked has increased the possibility of securing minerals from such sources.

CALCIUM AND PHOSPHORUS CONTENT OF THE AMERICAN DIET

The food supply provides liberal amounts of foods rich in calcium and phosphorus. Dairy products which, excluding butter, provide approximately three-fourths of the calcium in the food supply are produced plentifully in this country. The calcium contribution of various forms of dairy products has changed over the years. Today the American people consume more low-fat fluid milk and less whole fluid milk, more cheese, frozen dairy products, and nonfat dry milk, and less evaporated and condensed milk than they did in the 1940's.

There is a plentiful amount of phosphorus in the food supply. In 1970 dairy products furnished 36 per cent of the total amount of phosphorus available for civilian food consumption; meat, poultry, and fish, 26 per cent; flour and cereal products, 13 per cent; fruits and vegetables, 11 per cent; eggs, 6 per cent; legumes, 6 per cent; miscellaneous, 2 per cent (38).

Studies indicate that the ingestion of calcium is apt to be less than the amount recommended. In the nationwide survey conducted in 1965 it was found that 30 per cent of the diets supplied less than the recommended allowance for calcium. As the annual income increased from less than $3000 to $10,000 and over, the percentage of the diets below the allowance decreased from 36 to 24. Urban households on low incomes tended to use less calcium than did those in rural areas.

The quantity of milk, cream, and cheese (estimated as milk equivalent) consumed per person per week was 8 per cent less in 1965 than in 1955. There was a lower average consumption of milk, cream, and cheese in the South than in other sections of the country but the percentage of diets below the calcium allowance was about the same since the kinds and quantities of grain products supplied more calcium than in other regions. This counterbalanced the lower intake of dairy products.

In coordinated research studies (39) made in 39 states, the calcium intakes of children four to 20 years old and men and women 20 to more than 80 years old were estimated. In both groups the average daily intakes of boys and men were higher than those of girls and women. This was especially evident in teenage girls where there was a wide gap between the recommended allowance and the average intake and in women whose calcium intakes continued to diminish into old age. In women of 70 years and beyond, the daily average was only 0.5 gm. calcium, whereas in men it was 0.82 gm. White (40) has analyzed 24-hour weighed diet composites collected by high school girls and college women. The daily mean dietary calcium intake of the 15 high school girls was 782 mg., that for the 21 college women, 780 mg. Phosphorus mean intakes for the two groups were 933 mg. and 1021 mg., respectively. White found good agreement between the analytical data, secured by emission spectoscopy and data calculated from food composition tables.

Murphy and associates (41) studied the nutrient content of Type A school lunches as served to sixth-graders in 300 schools from 19 states. Aliquots of meals were analyzed for calcium and phosphorus and it was found that the lunches on the average contained 455 mg. calcium and 518 mg. phosphorus. Since a very large number of school children count on this midday meal it is good to know these lunches more than meet the goals of one-third of the RDA. Other minerals will be referred to in Chapter 10.

The low consumption of calcium by some people in the United States, especially by children, is due partly to economic conditions. An inadequate family income accompanied by the cost of fluid whole milk accounts for a considerable number of low-calcium dietaries; this is true despite the fact that, penny for penny, milk furnishes more nutrients than do most other foods. Dried nonfat milk is a valuable addition to the family food supply, especially when the income is low, because it is inexpensive and can be stored without refrigeration. The belief that milk is a food for young children only, and the adult habit of drinking coffee or tea with the meal, are further reasons for the insufficient intake. Some individuals, especially young women on reducing diets, believe that calcium pills may be used as a complete substitute for milk; they do not consider the value of milk in other minerals and vitamins. Education on the importance of milk in the diet and practical aid in menu and recipe planning should result in increased consumption of milk and milk products.

PROBLEMS

1. Calculate the milligrams of calcium and phosphorus in the food intake records used in Problem 1, Chapter 2. Carry decimals to one place. Determine the average milligrams of calcium and phosphorus in your daily diet. How do these figures compare with the standards given? If they are low, make suggestions which will correct the deficiencies.

2. Plan portions of representative foods, each of which yields one-tenth of the day's recommended allowances of calcium and of phosphorus. Record data, giving name of food, weight in grams, measure, and equivalent in average servings. Compare the portions as sources of calcium; as sources of phosphorus.

3. Prepare a table of 100-mg. portions of representative foods arranged in order of calcium value; in order of phosphorus value. List equivalents in average servings.

4. Plan the day's diet for a woman weighing 55 kg. who has an idiosyncrasy for cheese and for milk as a beverage and in cooking. In your plan include the foods, except milk and cheese, listed as essential in the daily diet. Use the score card from Problem 2, Chapter 1. Be sure that the diet is adequate in calcium and phosphorus. The woman's calorie requirement is 2200 and she should have 0.9 gm. of protein per kg. of body weight.

REFERENCES

1. Henry, K. M., *et al.* The Relationship Between Calcium Retention and Body Stores of Calcium in the Rat: Effect of Age and Vitamin D. *Brit. J. Nutr., 7:*147 (1953).

2. Tomlin, D. H., *et al.* The Interstitial Metabolism of Calcium in the Bones and Teeth of Rats. *Brit. J. Nutr., 9:*144 (1955).

3. Bauer, W., *et al.* Bone Trabeculae as a Readily Available Reserve Supply of Calcium. *J. Exptl. Med., 49:*145 (1929).

4. Herbert, V., *et al.* Notes on Vitamin B$_{12}$ Absorption: Auto-immunity and Childhood Pernicious Anemia; Relation of Intrinsic Factor to Blood Group Substance. *Med., 43:*679 (1964).

5. Copp, D. H., *et al.* Evidence for Calcitonin—A New Hormone from the Parathyroid that Lowers Blood Calcium. *Endocrin., 70:*638 (1962).

6. Ebel, J. G., *et al.* Vitamin D-Induced Calcium-Binding Protein. *Am. J. Clin. Nutr., 22:*431 (1969).

7. Consolazio, E. F. Relationship Between Calcium in Sweat, Calcium Balance and Calcium Requirements. *J. Nutr., 78:*78 (1962).

8. Bronner, F., *et al.* Absorption and Metabolism of Calcium in Human Beings, Studied with Ca[45]. *Ann. N.Y. Acad. Sci., 64:*314 (1965).

9. Macy, I. G. *Nutrition and Chemical Growth in Childhood,* Vol. 1. *Evaluation.* Baltimore: Charles C Thomas (1942).

10. Spencer, H., *et al.* Comparative Absorption of Calcium from Calcium Gluconate and Calcium Lactate in Man. *J. Nutr., 89:*283 (1966).

11. Spencer, H., *et al.* Effect of Lysine on Calcium Metabolism in Man. *J. Nutr., 81:*301 (1963).

12. Chaney, M. S., *et al.* The Effect of Orange Juice on the Calcium, Phosphorus, Magnesium, and Nitrogen Retention, and Urinary Organic Acids of Growing Children. *J. Biol. Chem., 66:*829 (1925).

13. Leichsenring, J. M., *et al.* Effect of Ascorbic Acid and of Orange Juice on Calcium and Phosphorus Metabolism of Women. *J. Nutr., 63:*425 (1957).

14. Speckman, E. W., *et al.* Relationships between Fat and Mineral Metabolism—A Review. *J. Am. Diet. Ass., 51:*517 (1967).

15. Yacowitz, H., *et al.* Effects of Oral Calcium upon Serum Lipids in Man. *Brit. Med. J., 1:*1352 (1965).

16. Bonner, P., *et al.* The Influence of a Daily Serving of Spinach or Its Equivalent in Oxalic Acid Upon the Mineral Utilization of Children. *J. Pediat., 12:*188 (1938).

17. Johnston, F. A., *et al.* Calcium Retained by Young Women Before and After Adding Spinach to the Diet. *J. Am. Diet. Ass., 28:*933 (1952).

18. Bricker, M. L., *et al.* The Effect of Cocoa Upon Calcium Utilization and Requirements, Nitrogen Retention and Fecal Composition. *J. Nutr., 39:*455 (1949).

19. Bronner, F., *et al.* Studies in Calcium Metabolism. Effect of Food Phytates on Calcium Uptake in Children on Low-Calcium Breakfasts. *J. Nutr., 54:*522 (1954).

20. Spencer, H., *et al.* Effect of Sodium Fluoride on Calcium Absorption and Balances in Man. *Am. J. Clin. Nutr., 22:*381 (1969).

21. Sherman, H. C. Calcium Requirement of Maintenance in Man. *J. Biol. Chem., 44:*21 (1920).

22. Sherman, H. C. Phosphorus Requirement of Maintenance in Man. *J. Biol. Chem., 41:*173 (1920).

23. Leverton, R. M., *et al. The Metabolic Response of Young Women to a Standardized Diet.* USDA, Home Econ. Research Rept. No. 16 (1962).

24. Mitchell, H. H., *et al. Actualities Scientifiques et Industrielles.* Herman and Company, No. 771 (1939).

25. Steggerda, F. R., *et al.* Further Experiments on the Calcium Requirement of Adult Man and the Utilization of the Calcium in Milk. *J. Nutr., 21:*577 (1941).

26. Steggerda, F. R., *et al.* Variability in the Calcium Metabolism and the Calcium Requirements of Adult Human Subjects. *J. Nutr., 31:*407 (1946).

27. Moyer, E. Z., *et al. Basic Data on Metabolic Patterns in 7- to 10-Year Old Girls in Selected Southern States.* USDA, Home Econ. Research Rept. No. 33 (1967).

28. Holmes, J. O. The Requirement of Calcium During Growth. *Nutr. Abstr. Revs., 14:*597 (1945).

29. Symposium on Effects of High Calcium Intakes. *Fed. Proc., 18:*1075 (1959).

30. Hegsted, D. M., *et al.* A Study of the Minimum Calcium Requirements of Adult Men. *J. Nutr., 46:*181 (1952).

31. Walker, A. R. P. Note to the Editor. *Nutr. Revs., 16:*31 (1958).

32. Nicolaysen, R., *et al.* Physiology of Calcium Metabolism. *Physiol. Revs., 33:*424 (1953).

33. Van Duyne, F. O. *et al.* Life-time Experiments Upon the Problem of Optimal Calcium Intake. *J. Nutr., 21:*221 (1946).

34. Mack, P. B., *et al.* Effects of Recumbency and Space Flight on Bone Density. *Am. J. Clin. Nutr., 20:*1194 (1967).

35. Cohn, S. H., *et al.* High Calcium Diet and the Parameters of Calcium Metabolism in Osteoporosis. *Am. J. Clin. Nutr., 21:*1246 (1968).

36. Lutwak, L. Nutritional Aspects of Osteoporosis. *J. Am. Geriat. Soc., 17:*115 (1969).

37. Bronner, F. Mineral Nutrition and the Problem of Filled or Synthetic Milks. *Am. J. Clin. Nutr., 22:*113 (1969).

38. National Food Situation. NFS-134, ERS, USDA (1970).

39. Morgan, A. F. (ed.), *Nutritional Status U.S.A.* Berkeley: Calif. Agr. Sta. Bull. 769 (1959).

40. White, H. S. Inorganic Elements in Weighted Diets of Girls and Young Women. *J. Am. Diet. Ass., 55:*38 (1969).

41. Murphy, E. W., *et al.* Major Elements in Type A School Lunches. *J. Am. Diet. Ass., 57:*239 (1970).

GENERAL REFERENCES

42. Food and Agricultural Organization of the United Nations. *Calcium Requirements.* FAO Nutrition Mtgs. Rept. Series No. 30 (WHO Technical Rept. Series No. 230). Rome (1962).

43. Hegsted, D. M. Present Knowledge of Calcium, Phosphorus, and Magnesium. In *Present Knowledge in Nutrition,* 3rd ed. New York: Nutrition Foundation (1967).

44. Leitch, I., and Aiken, F. C. The Estimation of Calcium Requirement: A Re-examination. *Nutr. Abstr. Revs., 29:*393 (1959).

Iron

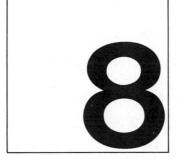

Iron differs from most other nutrients in that comparatively little of the iron intake is absorbed and after use by the body almost all of it is returned to the plasma for reuse. Iron-deficiency is unlikely in the normal male and in the post-menopausal female, except for the older woman who may have reached menopause in a state of iron depletion because of excessive menstrual losses or repeated pregnancies (1). Iron losses from the body of the healthy male are slight; but the young woman loses iron in menstrual blood, and in some seemingly healthy young women this loss can be very high. Iron intake may not be adequate during the child's growth and during the reproductive period. In fact, the state of iron balance may have so narrow a safety margin during periods of infancy, childhood, adolescence, reproduction, and in cases of hemorrhage that, if accompanied by poor diet or poor absorption, hypochromic anemia may occur. Also, continued donations of blood can drain the body sufficiently to cause anemia; frequency of contributions should be controlled by a physician.

Because so many individuals may be in one of these precarious states of iron metabolism, this mineral and its relationship to other nutritional factors involved in the formation of blood are important. Anemia is not easily diagnosed by a cursory inspection of the skin, for both pigmentation and thickness of this tissue may mask the condition. Only measurement of tissue-iron stores and quantitative blood tests will reveal the true state of iron nutriture of an individual.

THE BODY'S NEED FOR IRON

Most of the body's iron is found in the blood. The blood is a complex fluid which supplies food and oxygen to the cells and removes waste products. Its composition is automatically controlled and, under conditions of health, remains quite constant. This circulating medium contains iron as an essential part of its structure, in amounts exceeding that in other body tissues. The total amount of iron in the bodies of healthy men and women may range from less than 2 to more than 6 gm. The actual amount varies with body size, hemoglobin level, and the extent of iron stores (2).

Certain facts learned in physiology should be recalled here. Iron exists chiefly in the erythrocytes of which there are about five million in a cubic millimeter of human blood. These minute discs, only one thirty-two hundredth of an inch in diameter, are produced largely in bone marrow and contain hemoglobin—a compound formed by the union of hematin, an organic compound containing iron, and a basic protein, globin. This complex protein is the respiratory pigment of the blood, and because it can unite with oxygen at certain pressures and release it at lower pressures, it controls the supply of oxygen to the tissues.

Most of the iron in the body is in the hemoglobin of the red blood cells; much smaller amounts, in the plasma. The main function of the iron in hemoglobin relates to carrying oxygen, as a result of which oxidation and reduction processes are carried on within the cells. In the plasma, the fluid part of the blood as distinguished from the corpuscles, a protein compound called transferrin carries iron to the body tissues. This transport system may turn over, each day, from 35 to 40 mg. of iron, that absorbed from ingested food and that from the normal breakdown of red blood cells and from storage depots.

The iron present in the body has been classified as functional or essential iron and as storage iron. Approximately 70–75 per cent is functional. The remaining 25–30 per cent is in storage forms as ferritin and hemosiderin in the liver, bone marrow, and spleen. Of the functional iron, 65–70 per cent is in the hemoglobin of the blood and 4 per cent, in the myoglobin of muscle tissue (3). The remaining 1 per cent is found in the plasma, bound to the iron-transport protein, transferrin, and in enzymes such as cytochrome oxidase and catalase that serve as catalysts in tissue oxidation. These compounds and myoglobin remain in fairly constant amounts. The iron in the storage tissues is diminished first in the case of iron deficiency. When iron stores become depleted plasma iron and hemoglobin levels fall. Therefore, in nutritional status studies early states of iron depletion can be recognized only by determination of serum iron levels and transferrin saturation (plasma iron divided by the iron-binding capacity), and by direct examination of stainable iron in bone marrow (1, 4, 5).

Knowledge of the state of iron stores is essential. In recent years studies (1, 3) of iron metabolism have shown that deficiencies of iron stores frequently exist in infants, young children, and menstruating or pregnant females. These individuals are especially vulnerable to iron-deficiency anemia. Iron store depletion may result also from blood loss due to infections, inflammatory states, or too frequent blood donations. In such instances hemoglobin values may not be altered appreciably (1, 3). However, examination of smears of bone marrow shows hemosiderin content decreased or even absent. In addition, plasma iron values may be found to be less than 50 μg per 100 ml.; normal values are between 70 and 180 μg. per ml. (2). As iron stores decrease, the transferrin iron-binding capacity rises and the transferrin saturation falls from normal values of 20–40 per cent to 5–15 per cent (2).

The normal condition of the blood may be altered. The blood has been studied under both normal and abnormal states to determine its make-up in health and how it is affected by illness. Certain blood tests are a routine part of a complete physical examination. The size and number of red blood cells and the content of hemoglobin permit differentiation of the various types of anemia. According to Wintrobe (6) the average hemoglobin concentration in grams per 100 ml. for men and women in the United States is 16.0 $\pm$ 2 and 14.0 $\pm$ 2, respectively; average red cell count, in million per ccm., 5.4 $\pm$ 0.8 and 4.8 $\pm$ 0.6, respectively.

Hemoglobin levels and erythrocyte counts often are expressed in percentage by comparing the actual with the average or standard. Furthermore, the relationship of these two constituents may be expressed as a color index which is calculated by dividing the percentage of hemoglobin by that of normal red cells. In a healthy individual the index is close to 1.0; in calculations on women subjects Osgood and Haskins (7) found that over 90 per cent of the cases had indices between 0.9 and 1.1. Even in health some range exists among individuals, but when the examination reveals an abnormal color index, the clinician is likely to diagnose the condition as some form of anemia. In addition, the determination of hematocrit (the ratio of packed red cells to volume of whole blood) is often included in routine blood tests and in research studies. Accepted normal values are 46.5 $\pm$ 7.7 per cent for males and 42.4 $\pm$ 8 per cent for females. Radioactive iron also is used as a tracer in many hematological studies.

Occasionally, the serum iron is found to be higher than normal. Disorders in which this condition is noted include pernicious anemia, transfusion hemosiderosis, hemochromatosis, and certain liver disorders. In prolonged excessive iron therapy also an abnormally high iron content in the serum is found. As mentioned previously, nutritional anemia may be due either to an insufficient supply of iron to replace the daily loss or to an otherwise inadequate diet; this anemia is often found among food faddists and people of very low income level. It also is associated with dietary practices found in certain countries such as China, India, and northern Brazil. The South African Bantu are known to ingest 100 to 200 mg. iron daily, most of which comes from the old iron kettles used in food preparation; excessive iron retention results (8).

Loss of blood through hemorrhage as the result of an injury or an operation may reduce the volume to a considerable extent; this also involves a reduction in the hemoglobin and red blood corpuscles. Absorption of fluids from the surrounding tissue soon replaces the volume of the serum; the red blood corpuscles reach their former number before the pigment becomes normal and this results in an unbalanced proportion of the two, and a low color index. Experimental work on both nutritional and hemorrhagic anemias has shown that increased amounts of certain nutrients in the diet have favorable effects. These include protein, copper, ascorbic acid, niacin, vitamins B_6 and B_{12}, folic acid, riboflavin, vitamin E, and pantothenic acid.

THE BODY'S UTILIZATION OF IRON

Studies indicate how much iron is absorbed. Among the methods used to investigate the absorption of the various nutrients, the balance study has been prominent. However, in iron experiments, this method has been used less often than in protein and calcium studies, chiefly because it has been difficult to devise analysis methods sufficiently delicate for its accurate measurement.

Today, radioactive iron has been incorporated in the diet and used to determine the amount of the mineral absorbed. The per cent of radio-iron absorbed may be determined by measuring the unabsorbed radio-activity in the feces, the amount used for hemoglobin synthesis, or the retention of radioactivity by means of a whole body counter (9). The latter method is proving to be a good means of studying iron because only small amounts of the isotope are required and absorption is measured directly without the complications involved in collection of excreta.

Iron ingested largely in the ferric form must be reduced to the ferrous state in the stomach and intestine before it can pass through the intestinal mucosa into the blood stream; the rate of absorption, largest in the duodenum, decreases progressively as the food mass moves through the tract. Among the conditions within the digestive system which may affect the amount of iron absorbed are acid secretion in the stomach and peristalsis rate in the intestines. The hydrochloric acid of the stomach tends to ionize food iron and put it into a soluble state, thus preparing it for absorption. In the past it was thought that the acidity of the stomach secretions played an important role, but studies with radioactive iron indicate that the pH may be of minor significance.

If the rate of peristalsis is average, there should be time for the body to absorb the iron it requires, but in the case of diarrhea, needed iron may be excreted before it can be absorbed. On the other hand, undue retention, as in atonic constipation, may change the iron into an insoluble form and thus prevent its absorption.

As has been stated, only a small part of dietary iron is absorbed—from 5 to 10 per cent by the normal adult, more than 10 per cent by infants and children. In general, the more iron in the diet the more is absorbed, but the percentage absorption is less.

Iron-deficient subjects absorb iron more efficiently than do normal people. Anemia may be related to nondietary as well as to nutritional deficiencies; a detailed discussion of the anemias does not belong in this text. Here the condition will be mentioned only as it relates to absorption; in a later section it will be discussed in terms of dietary treatment. When radioactive iron is injected into the body of a person with hemorrhagic anemia, the iron is utilized more rapidly and completely than it is in normal people; this is true also in patients with nutritional microcytic anemia. It has been demonstrated that, when anemic human beings are fed doses of tagged iron at levels of 0.2 to 1.0 mg., an uptake of from 50 to 90 per cent is customary, in contrast to the 10 per cent absorption in normal persons; this iron is used in erythropoiesis. The body mechanism which controls iron absorption is not clear; ferritin in the mucosal cells probably plays an important role.

Several dietary factors control iron absorption and utilization. In addition to the amount of iron in the diet, other factors influence absorption. The form of the iron may be important. It is generally acknowledged that iron salts which are readily soluble and in a ferrous state are utilized more efficiently by the human being than are the other forms. This is no doubt true when iron is prescribed as a therapeutic measure. However, the differences may not be as important when dietary sources are considered; this was shown in a study of the utilization of various salts used for bread enrichment. Using radioiron[59] incorporated in a bread formula as ferrous sulfate, reduced iron, ferric orthophosphate, or sodium ferric pyrophosphate, Steinkamp and co-workers (10) found that all four compounds were used equally well by the human body.

Different results were reported by Brise and Hallberg (11) in a study in which they used a double isotopic technique to compare the absorption of iron from ferrous sulfate with a number of other iron compounds. Thirty mg. of iron as ferrous sulfate and an equal amount of the iron preparation under investigation were administered. Two different isotopes of iron were used so that the absorption from the preparation under study could be compared to that of ferrous sulfate. They found that absorption from ferrous salts was greater than that from ferric and that many of the ferrous compounds were absorbed about as well as ferrous sulfate.

It is recommended that ferrous iron for therapeutic use be prescribed in three to five divided doses daily, since only a relatively small per cent of any given amount can be absorbed. Also, it should be given when the upper gastrointestinal tract is free of phytates and phosphates which would combine with the iron to make an unabsorbable residue. If given with an infant's meal of milk and cereal, the iron would be less available. Enteric-coated ferrous iron tablets or iron capsules containing delayed release granules are not advised because the absorption of iron is less efficient in the lower part of the small intestine. The oxalic acid of spinach is not a deterrent to the utilization of iron in this food; in an experiment (12) on four young women who ate a diet including 120 gm. of cooked spinach daily (containing approximately 5 mg. of iron) for eight weeks, 13 per cent was absorbed, an amount which compares favorably with that of other foods. Other minerals in the diet help or hinder iron utilization. Phosphates have already been mentioned; the balance of calcium, phosphorus, and iron is without doubt important. While excess phosphate hinders iron absorption, calcium if present in sufficient amount may combine with the phosphates and free the iron for use. An excess of fiber may hinder absorption of iron as it does that of calcium.

Copper is important in the formation and development of the red blood cells; the mineral is thought to work together with iron (13) in reactions which relate to the oxidative enzymes. The importance of copper in the absorption was demonstrated by Hart, Steenbock, Waddell, and Elvehjem (14), who found that young animals made anemic on a milk diet would not respond to iron administration unless a minute amount of copper was included. The copper present in ordinary foods is sufficient for adults and usually for infants; in anemic babies, copper and iron together have proved effective for blood regulation.

Protein is important in blood regeneration. It has been shown (15) that with diets low in protein iron absorption is reduced. Such diets tend to be low in iron also. Increasing the protein in the diet enhances iron absorption, probably because increased amounts of certain amino acids are available (16). A liberal intake of protein by blood donors is recommended. This will be referred to later in this chapter.

Ascorbic acid, an excellent reducing agent, is valuable because it helps change iron into the ferrous form. Vitamin E, also a reducing agent, aids utilization (17). In work on milk-fed anemic rats it was found that there was a consistently higher rate of hemoglobin regeneration when both vitamins C and E were used to supplement ferrous iron than when only the mineral was given or when either one or the other of the two vitamins was used with the iron. Most of the B-complex vitamins are useful in the treatment of the anemias. Folic acid and vitamin B_{12} are of special value in the macrocytic types; riboflavin, niacin, vitamin B_6, and pantothenic acid, in the microcytic. Studies on animals and human subjects have shown that with vitamin B_6 deficiency iron absorption is increased (18), but the iron is not utilized for hemoglobin synthesis. Thus there is a marked increase in iron stores in serum iron levels.

The body conserves iron well. Once absorbed, the mineral is carried by the plasma where it is oxidized to the ferrous state and bound to transferrin. Iron passes quickly into the bone marrow where the red blood cells are formed. The portion not needed for hemoglobin formation is returned to the plasma which carries it to the liver and spleen and to other tissues for storage. This amounts to about 1000 mg. for adult men and to between 200 and 400 mg. in most women. The low iron stores in women are not considered to be a difference in regulation of iron absorption between the two sexes, but rather a reflection of the limitations of iron supply in relation to women's needs (1).

Normal losses of iron from the body of the adult male amount to between 0.5 and 1 mg. per day. It is excreted in feces, urine, and sweat, and some loss results also from shedding of cells from the gastrointestinal and gastrourinary tracts and from integumental cells such as skin, hair, and nails. Under conditions of high environmental temperature and active exercise which induce sweating, considerable iron is lost through the skin. It has been demonstrated by means of radioactive iron that the total amount of iron lost daily may average 0.61 mg. for men, 0.64 mg. for nonpregnant women; of this, 0.2 mg. came from the gastrointestinal tract, 0.4 to 0.44 mg. through dermal losses, under nonsweating situations (19, 20). Menstrual blood loss in individual women is fairly constant from month to month but varies widely between women. In an extensive study conducted by Hallberg *et al.* (21) the average mean menstrual loss was found to be equivalent to an iron loss of about 0.5 mg. per day, with 95 per cent of the women having an iron loss of less than 1.4 mg. per day. It has been suggested that menstruating women on the average lose less than 1 mg. of iron daily.

AMOUNT OF IRON RECOMMENDED FOR THE DAILY DIET

The recommended dietary allowance is higher for women than for men. The 1968 revision of the RDA lists 10 mg. of iron daily for men (22). This figure takes into account a probable loss of 1 mg. iron daily and an absorption efficiency rate of 10 per cent. For females from age ten up to menopause the recommendation is 18 mg. daily, then the amount decreases to 10 mg. The higher allowance is recommended for premenopausal women because they may need as much as 2 mg. of iron daily to maintain iron balance and adequate iron stores (1). The FNB states that if the woman of childbearing age has ingested enough iron to care for her daily needs and for accumulation of iron stores, the recommended 18 mg. should be sufficient to carry her through pregnancy and lactation. However, in light of the calorie recommendations for the pregnant woman and the fact that there are approximately 6 mg. of iron per 1000 kcal in the ordinary mixed diet in the United States, the recommended intakes are beyond the amounts available from diet alone. Therefore, supplemental iron therapy may be necessary for a large segment of the female population. Although it has been demonstrated that dietary iron absorption increases during the latter half of pregnancy in normal pregnant women and even more in those who are iron deficient, they still may need routine administration of medicinal iron (23, 24). The additional calorie allowance during lactation should result in iron intake adequate to meet the needs of this period, particularly since milk contains little iron.

More iron is recommended during growth periods. Young mammals which live on milk for a time after birth are born with a reserve store of iron in the body. This is not true of the guinea pig, which, the first day of life, begins to feed on green leaves. It has been found, through studies on kittens, puppies, and rabbits, that the percentage of iron is greatest at birth and for a time continues to be adequate for the formation of hemoglobin, even though body size increases. In the human species a high erythrocyte count and hemoglobin level at birth also have been demonstrated. Hemoglobin levels of 17 to 20 gm. per 100 ml. of blood at birth fall rapidly to about 12 gm. at four to six months of age, remain rather constant at this level throughout early childhood, and rise to adult levels in late adolescence.

Smith and Rosello (25) found that infants use little dietary iron until four months after birth; they demonstrated this by administering radioactive iron by transfusions to pregnant women and then, for a considerable period of time after delivery, by analyzing the infants' blood to determine the ratio of radioactive iron to hemoglobin iron.

Twins and infants born prematurely show the same high levels of hemoglobin in the blood as do average babies, but the decrease occurs sooner and more rapidly. In such cases the addition of iron should begin earlier. Iron requirements of full-term infants over three months of age can be met by a daily intake of 1 mg. iron per kg. of body weight. Twins and premature infants may need as much as 2 mg. iron per kg. of body weight daily to meet the demands of hemoglobin synthesis, increasing blood volume, and new cell formation (26). The recommended allowances for iron during the first year of life are based on an average need of 1.5 mg. per kg. per day, up to a maximum of 15 mg. daily.

The condition of anemia may affect the need for iron. Hypochromic anemia results from a deficiency of iron in the diet. Developing gradually, this disorder is associated with weakness, a feeling of fatigue, poor appetite, and pallor. Symptoms may also include constipation, lusterless, brittle, and flattened nails, dyspnea on exertion, and achlorhydria. A blood test shows a low hemoglobin level but the red cell count may be within the normal range; serum iron value and transferrin saturation are decreased and iron-binding capacity is increased. Treatment includes administration of iron salts and a diet planned to favor absorption of iron and blood regeneration.

Anemia tends to develop during an infection. This is thought to be due to diversion of the mineral from the blood-forming centers to the liver and spleen, not to failure to absorb iron. Treatment is based on the cause of the infection but diet also is very important.

Hemorrhagic anemia may not be detected for some time, especially when associated with internal bleeding which may occur in peptic ulcer. Excessive loss of blood also may occur during the menstrual period, or from a wound or accident. Too frequent blood donations may result in this type of anemia. For each pint of blood donated approximately 250 mg. of iron are lost from the body. To replace this loss over a period of a year the daily intake should be increased by 0.7 mg. (1, 2). The wisdom of limiting blood donations to no more than six pints in a year is obvious, especially for women. Leverton and co-workers (27) studied 129 college women who were voluntary donors and served as subjects in a controlled feeding program. Their self-chosen diet was supplemented so that they received 50, 75, or 90 gm. of protein daily. At other times supplements of iron, copper, and riboflavin were added in controlled amounts. Most rapid regeneration occurred when the daily diet contained 90 gm. of protein; with this large protein intake one or more of the other supplements gave no added benefit. With the lower levels of protein an increased intake of iron, copper, or riboflavin increased the rate of regeneration, but pre-donation levels were not reached by the end of six weeks. Oral iron therapy, using simple, soluble ferrous salts, is often advocated in treatment of hemorrhagic anemia. For those who cannot tolerate or absorb oral preparations, parenteral administration may be used. Iron dextran, iron sorbitol, and dextriferron are the three best available preparations for parenteral use (2).

Pernicious anemia is not fundamentally a dietary disease. Instead of a shortage of food iron, there is a lack of substance which produces the body or stroma of the red blood cells; the cells are deficient in number and abnormal in shape and size. Because the hemoglobin is relatively high there is a high color index. There is also a deficient gastric secretion. Castle proposed the theory of two factors involved in the prevention and cure of pernicious anemia, an extrinsic one found in foods and an intrinsic one found normally in gastric secretion but lacking in that of the pernicious anemia patient; the intrinsic factor may be stored in the liver. This theory explains the efficacy of liver, liver extract, and stomach extract in curing the dread disease. Vitamin B_{12} is now known as the extrinsic factor. Folic acid has a favorable effect on the faulty blood condition in pernicious anemia but is not effective in treating the abnormalities in the nervous system. Both folic acid and vitamin B_{12} are prescribed in treatment of pernicious anemia.

FOOD SOURCES OF IRON

Certain foods are advised to meet the standard. The requirement for iron should be met in a definite plan, not left to chance and circumstance. Since lean meat furnishes considerable iron, it should be eaten daily; one serving is a reasonable amount and occasionally it should be in the form of liver. Eggs are a valuable source of iron, but milk, the most complete single food, is low in iron and the daily pint recommended for the adult supplies only a very small fraction of the need.

Dried beans, and the molasses added when they are baked, furnish an inexpensive and good source of iron. Dried fruits are another good source. Of the leafy vegetables, parsley is highest in iron content, but it is a negligible source since it is used chiefly as a garnish. In general, the green vegetables, such as spinach and leaf lettuce, are richer sources than are those with little chlorophyll, such as cabbage, celery, and head lettuce;

iceberg, a crisphead variety of lettuce, contains only about one-third as much iron as do the butterhead varieties and escarole.

Roots and tubers generally furnish little iron. However, potatoes, because of their daily consumption, supply a measurable part of the requirement. This is especially true when the whole potato is eaten as it may be when baked or boiled in the skin. Baking chocolate and cocoa are good sources of iron. One tablespoon of cocoa, sometimes used in making one serving of the beverage, contains almost 1 mg. of iron.

Outer layers of grains contain most of the iron, and thus use of the whole product may be recommended. Flour varies considerably in its iron contribution; whole wheat flour has 3.3 mg. iron per 100 gm.; enriched all-purpose flour, 2.9 mg.; unenriched all-purpose flour, 0.8 mg.; cake flour, 0.5 mg. Dark, medium, and light rye flours contain 4.5, 2.6, and 1.1 mg. iron per 100 gm. flour, respectively.

Iron is probably the most difficult of all nutrients to obtain in sufficient amounts in the daily diet. Unless planned carefully, menus which fulfill the requisites according to the four food groups may be lacking in iron. In the low-cost diet referred to in Chapter 6, the meat, egg, and legume group furnish almost two-fifths of the total iron; fruits and vegetables supply almost one-fifth; and the grain products almost one-third. The inclusion of molasses and table syrup as sweets make this food group a real addition to the iron intake (Table 8–1).

Table 8–1

Distribution of Iron in the Low-Cost Dietary for a Family of Four[*]

Food Groups	Protein		Iron	
	gm.	per cent[1]	mg.	per cent[1]
Milk, cheese	576.1	23.4	10.2	2.2
Meat, fish, eggs, legumes	1120.7	45.5	182.3	39.6
Dark-green and deep-yellow vegetables	25.9	1.1	10.3	2.2
Citrus fruit, tomatoes	26.4	1.1	12.8	2.8
Potatoes, other fruits, and vegetables	157.3	6.4	64.5	14.1
Grain products	552.8	22.4	148.2	32.2
Fats, oil	5.6	0.1	0.5	0.1
Sugar, sweets	0.0	0.0	31.4	6.8
Total for week	2465.0	100	460.2	100
Total for day	352.1		65.7	
Recommended allowance for day[2]	200.0		48.0	

[*] For description of family see Chapter 6, page 113.
[1] Expressed to one decimal.
[2] *Recommended Dietary Allowances,* Seventh Revised Edition. Washington, D.C.: FNB, NAS-NRC Publ. 1694 (1968).

Loss of iron in food preparation is a factor to be considered. The recommended allowances for iron seem none too large when one considers the many factors which may decrease the availability of iron from foods. The amount of iron available in cooked vegetables is controlled to quite an extent by the cooking method. A loss may be expected when vegetables are cooked in water; the size of the pieces, amount of water used, and time of cooking are factors to be considered here. Krehl and Winters (28) in their study of the effect of various cooking methods on retention of nutrients in vegetables found the following average retentions of iron in 12 vegetables after cooking:

Pressure cooked (½ cup water)	85.6 per cent
Water to cover	76.7 per cent
Water (½ cup)	86.4 per cent
Waterless	90.4 per cent

Ordinarily, in meat cookery all juices are retained for use in gravy or soups. Elvehjem and Peterson (29) state that beef juice contains 11.8 per cent of the iron present in the original beef. These workers also found that the percentage of iron in orange pulp is greater than in juice; a similar relationship exists with the tomato. This shows the value of serving the pulp as well as the juice of these foods.

ADEQUACY OF IRON IN THE DIET

The amount of iron available in the national food supply does not meet the recommended allowance for all sex-age groups. According to data computed by the Consumer and Economics Research Division, ERS, USDA, the amount of iron available for civilian consumption per capita in 1970 was estimated to be 17.2 mg. per day; this may be compared with 14.5 mg. available in 1935–39 (30). The change is due largely to increased meat consumption, especially beef. The enrichment of bread, flour, and many cereals adds considerable to the daily iron intake. In the 1965 nationwide dietary survey, 41.4 per cent of the iron consumed came from meat, poultry, fish, eggs, dried beans, and nuts, and 31.3 per cent from grains; vegetables furnished about two and one-half times as much as fruits. As stated previously, the average diet in the United States contributes about 6 mg. of iron per 1000 kcal. Considering the recommendations for calories, the normal diets of children under three years, of boys aged 12–14 years, and of premenopausal women cannot be expected to meet the 1968 recommended allowances for iron (31) (Figure 8–1). It was found in the survey that the daily iron intake was more than 30 per cent below the recommended allowances for several groups: girls and women from nine through 54 years, children under three, boys 12–14, persons with annual incomes under $3000, and those living in the South.

Additional enrichment or fortification of foods so that the ordinary mixed diet would provide 10 mg. of iron per 1000 kcal. has been

Figure 8–1

*Iron from one day's diet as per cent of the 1968 recommended daily
allowances. (From Food Intake and Nutritive Value of Diets of Men,
Women, and Children in the United States, Spring 1965, ARS 62–18.
Washington, D.C.: ARS, USDA [1969].)*

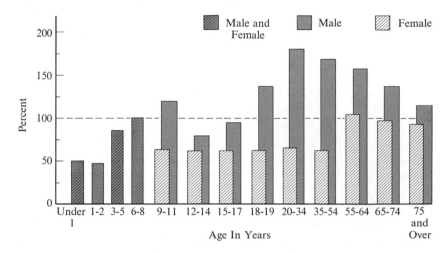

suggested. Such measures should obviate the need for medicinal or supplemental iron preparations. The possibility that increased iron enrichment of foods would result in iron overload for males has been considered. However, the American Medical Association Committee on Iron
Deficiency (1) has stated that 50 mg. of iron per day probably could be
tolerated by males. Further, it is unlikely that many males would consume over 5000 kcal. per day over any lengthy period of time.

Data from studies of large numbers of children and adults in 39 states
indicate that the situation concerning iron intake is quite similar to that
of calcium. Men and boys over 14 years tended to meet or exceed the
recommended allowances, but women were apt to fall short of needs.
Children and adolescents from seven to 14 years and girls up to 18 years
failed to meet the recommended allowances (32). A statistical study
was made of the blood values of about 1500 subjects living in the Northeast. In Maine, Massachusetts, New York, Rhode Island, and West Virginia, the hemoglobin values correlated significantly with both dietary
protein and dietary iron. Among the New York children, boys and
girls up to the age of 12 showed no significant differences in hemoglobin
content of the blood; thereafter the boys' level continued to rise, but
that of the girls declined. In the Western region a very large number of
children and adults were tested for hemoglobin values; different age
groups were studied in different states and then, using all the data
secured, a curve for the whole life cycle was constructed. Throughout
adulthood the hemoglobin level of the men was higher than that of the

women. A high incidence of iron deficiency and of iron-deficiency anemia has been found in infants, adolescents and pregnant women in the United States; women are more likely to show these conditions than men. In a study (33) of the hemoglobin levels of those who applied as blood donors, 12.6 per cent of the women were unable to meet the minimal requirement for hemoglobin set by the American Red Cross, whereas less than 1 per cent of the men were rejected. Another study (26) made on a group of premature infants indicated the prevalence of anemia; if not treated with iron medication this condition continued for the first 18 months of life.

It is now generally recognized that many people, particularly women, are iron deficient although many may not be anemic. Their iron stores are low or depleted. Conscientious efforts must be made to include iron-rich foods in the daily menu and to increase the amounts of iron added to foods by enrichment.

The effectiveness of cereal enrichment has been demonstrated in studies conducted by Burch *et al.* (34) in Bataan. In 1948, prior to rice enrichment, the mean hemoglobin level of the 127 people examined was 10.9 ± 0.24 gm. per 100 ml. of blood; in 1950, after two years of use of the enriched rice, the mean was 12.9 ± 0.18 gm. This increase was attributed to the enriched rice since the diet had not changed significantly in other respects in the two-year period.

PROBLEMS

1. Calculate the milligrams of iron in the food intake records used in Problem 1, Chapter 2. Carry decimals to one place. Determine the average milligrams of iron in your daily diet. How does the figure compare with the standard given? If it is low make suggestions to correct the deficiency.
2. Plan portions of representative foods, each of which yields one-tenth of the day's requirement of iron. Record data, giving name of food, weight in grams, measure, and equivalent in average servings. Compare the portions as sources of iron.
3. Plan a table of 100-gm. portions of representative foods arranged in order of iron value. List equivalents in average servings. Make a graph of these data which could be used for illustrative material.
4. Write menus for three days which a physician could include in dietary instructions to a group of anemic girls in an industrial plant. Using the data secured on average servings, suggest amounts to be eaten daily to supply 20 mg. of iron.

REFERENCES

1. A Report of the Committee on Iron Deficiency, Council on Foods and Nutrition, American Medical Association. *Iron Deficiency in the United States. J. Am. Med. Ass., 203:*407 (1968).

2. Moore, C. V. Iron. *In* M. B. Wohl and R. S. Goodhart (eds.), *Modern Nutrition in Health and Disease,* 4th ed. Philadelphia: Lea and Febiger (1968).

3. Finch, C. A. Iron Metabolism. *Nutr. Today,* 4 #2:2 (1969).

4. Deutler, V. P., *et al. Clinical Disorders of Iron Metabolism.* New York: Grune and Stratton (1963).

5. Bainton, D. F., *et al.* The Diagnosis of Iron Deficiency Anemia. *Am. J. Med., 37:*62 (1964).

6. Wintrobe, M. M. *Clinical Hematology,* 6th ed. Philadelphia: Lea and Febiger (1967).

7. Osgood, E. E., *et al.* Relation Between Cell Count, Cell Volume, and Hemoglobin Content of Venous Blood of Normal Young Women. *Arch. Intern. Med., 39:*643 (1927).

8. deBruin, E. J. P., *et al.* Iron Absorption in the Bantu. *J. Am. Diet. Ass., 57:*129 (1970).

9. Moore, C. V. Iron Nutrition and Requirements. *Ser. Hematol., 6:*1 (1965).

10. Steinkamp, R., *et al.* Studies in Iron Transport and Metabolism. VIII. Absorption of Radioiron from Iron-Enriched Bread. *Arch. Intern. Med., 95:*181 (1955).

11. Brise, H., *et al.* Absorbability of Different Iron Compounds. *Acta Med. Scand., 171:*23 (Supp. 376) (1962).

12. McMillan, T. J., *et al.* The Absorption of Iron from Spinach by Six Young Women and the Effect of Beef Upon Absorption. *J. Nutr., 44:*383 (1951).

13. Matrone, G. Interrelationships of Iron and Copper in the Nutrition and Metabolism of Animals. *Fed. Proc., 19,* No. 2, Part I:659 (1960).

14. Hart, E. B., *et al.* Copper as a Supplement to Iron for Hemoglobin Building in the Rat. *J. Biol. Chem., 77:*797 (1926).

15. Chopra, J. G., *et al.* Anemia in Pregnancy. *Am. J. Pub. Health, 57:*857 (1967).

16. Kroc, D., *et al.* The Influence of Amino Acids on Iron Absorption. *Blood, 21:*546 (1963).

17. Greenberg, S. M., *et al.* Iron Absorption and Metabolism. I. Inter-relationship of Ascorbic Acid and Vitamin E. *J. Nutr., 63:*19 (1957).

18. Frimper, G. W., *et al.* Vitamin B_6-Dependency Syndromes. *Am. J. Clin. Nutr., 22:*794 (1969).

19. Consolazio, C. F., *et al.* Excretion of Sodium, Potassium, Magnesium and Iron in Human Sweat and the Relation of Each to Balance and Requirements. *J. Nutr., 79:*407 (1963).

20. Mitchell, H. H., *et al.* Nutritional Significance of the Dermal Losses of Nutrients in Man, Particularly of Nitrogen and Minerals. *Am. J. Clin. Nutr., 10:*163 (1962).

21. Hallberg, L., *et al.* Menstrual Blood Loss, a Population Study: Variation at Different Ages and Attempts to Define Normality. *Acta Obstet. Gynecol. Scand., 45:*320 (1966).

22. *Recommended Dietary Allowances,* Seventh Revised Edition. Washington, D.C.: FNB, NAS-NRC Publ. 1694 (1968).

23. Hahn, P. F., *et al.* Iron Metabolism in Human Pregnancy as Studied with the Radioactive Isotope Fe^{59}. *Am. J. Obstet. Gynecol., 61:*477 (1951).

24. Apte, S. V., *et al.* Absorption of Iron in Pregnancy. *Am. J. Clin. Nutr., 23:*73 (1970).

25. Smith, N. J., *et al.* Iron Deficiency in Infancy and Childhood. *Am. J. Clin. Nutr., 1:*275 (1950).

26. Gorten, M. K., *et al.* Iron Metabolism in Premature Infants. II. Prevention of Iron Deficiency. *J. Pediat., 64:*509 (1964).

27. Leverton, R. M., *et al.* Blood Regeneration in Women Blood Donors. II. Effect of Protein, Vitamin, and Mineral Supplements. *J. Am. Diet. Ass., 24:*480 (1948).

28. Krehl, W. A., *et al.* Effect of Cooking Methods on Retention of Vitamins and Minerals in Vegetables. *J. Am. Diet. Ass., 26:*966 (1952).

29. Elvehjem, C. A., *et al.* The Iron Content of Animal Tissues. *J. Biol. Chem., 74:*433 (1927).

30. Economic Research Service, *National Food Situation.* USDA, NFS–134 (1970).

31. Agricultural Research Service. *Food Intake and Nutritive Value of Diets of Men, Women, and Children in the United States, Spring, 1965.* USDA, ARS 62–18 (1969).

32. Morgan, A. F. (ed.), *Nutritional Status U.S.A.* Berkeley: Calif. Agr. Sta. Bull. 769 (1959).

33. Hervey, G. W., *et al.* Low Hemoglobin Levels in Women as Revealed by Blood Donor Records. *J. Am. Med. Ass., 149:*1127 (1952).

34. Burch, H. B., *et al.* Nutrition Resurvey in Bataan, Philippines, 1950. *J. Nutr., 46:*239 (1952).

GENERAL REFERENCES

35. Beal, V. A. Iron Nutriture from Infancy to Adolescence. *Am. J. Pub. Health, 60:*666 (1970).

36. Hegsted, D. M. The Recommended Dietary Allowances for Iron. *Am. J. Pub. Health, 60:*653 (1970).

37. Moore, C. V. Iron. *In* M. G. Wohl and R. S. Goodhart (eds.), *Modern Nutrition in Health and Disease,* 4th ed. Philadelphia: Lea and Febiger (1968).

38. Peden, J. C., Jr. Present Knowledge of Iron and Copper. *In Present Knowledge in Nutrition,* 3rd ed. New York: Nutrition Foundation (1967).

39. World Health Organization of the United Nations, Report of a WHO Scientific Group. *Nutritional Anaemias.* WHO Technical Report Series No. 405. Geneva: WHO (1968).

Iodine

Iodine, since its discovery in the thyroid gland in 1895, has been studied with great interest because of its connection with goiter, one of the oldest known disorders. Examination of the paintings of the old masters reveals, especially in portraits of infants, a quite common and marked enlargement at the throat, indicative of the prevalence of this disease years ago. The WHO has estimated that 200 million people over the world are suffering from iodine deficiency resulting in goiter. This disease occurs with varying intensity in almost every country (Figure 9–1). A study (1) made in the Andean region of South America recently indicated that as many as 54 per cent of the population in eight rural villages had goiter and all afflicted had severe iodine deficiency.

The United States was one of the first countries to carry on an extensive program to eradicate goiter through the use of iodized salt, and it has been assumed that the disorder was well under control. However, a preliminary report of the NNS (2) indicates that as many as 5 per cent of the sample examined had enlarged thyroid glands. In one state surveyed it was found that iodized salt was not stocked routinely in many local neighborhood stores, although when it was available there was no price differential. Prevention of goiter by adding iodine to table salt is not an economic problem; it has been estimated that it would cost less than one-fourth of one cent per person per year to supply iodine needs through use of iodized salt. In many sections of the United States iodized salt costs no more than regular salt. Canada has handled the situation by adopting, in 1949, compulsory iodization of table salt. Guatemala and Colombia also have made salt-iodization mandatory. The FNB stands on record as favoring federal legislation on this point in the United States.

The body's need for iodine, the environmental factors which complicate the problem of how much mineral is available, and the conditions which result from an imbalance in the body will be discussed in this chapter.

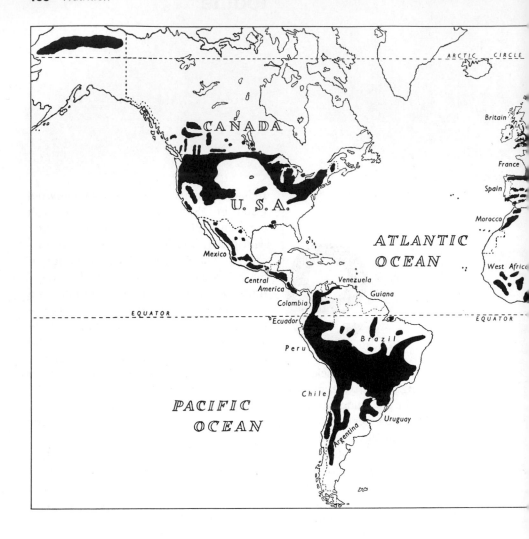

THE METABOLISM OF IODINE AS RELATED TO THE HEALTH OF PEOPLE

Iodine exists in the body in minute amounts and in various forms. The biological importance of iodine far exceeds its amount in the body. It is estimated that the body contains 25 mg. of iodine, about 0.00004 per cent of the total weight. Of this about 10 mg. are in the thyroid gland, the rest in the blood and other tissues. Iodine is taken into the body in the form of inorganic iodides and is absorbed and carried by the blood stream to the thyroid gland where it is greatly concentrated, by a factor of at least 10,000.

Enzymatic processes within the thyroid gland bring about the release of iodide, thyroxin, and triiodothyronine into the blood stream. The

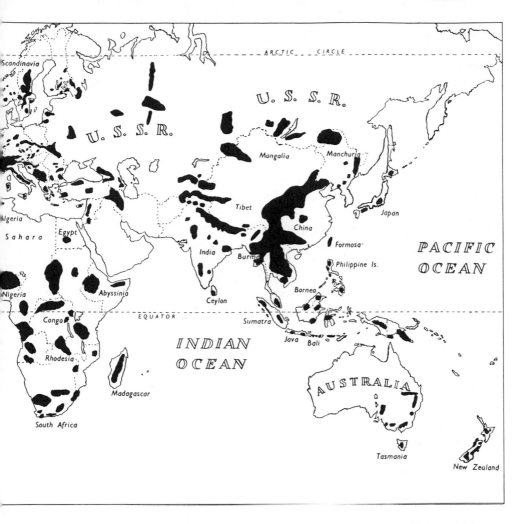

Figure 9–1 *Areas where endemic goiter has been found. World Goiter Map, Chilean Iodine Educational Bureau, London, 1967.*

latter compound is three to four times as active as thyroxin in controlling energy metabolism. Studies made with radioactive iodine show that iodine uptake is very rapid and that the ingested mineral may be returned to the blood within a few hours. The thyroid:serum iodide ratio in a healthy human being is approximately 25:1. In hyperthyroidism the ratio may be greatly increased.

The activity of the thyroid gland has been found to depend essentially on its supply of iodine; if the concentration of the element, normally about 40 mg. per 100 gm. of gland, falls below 10 mg., goiter is likely to develop. This is manifested by hypertrophy of the gland and hyperplasia of the epithelial cells. Thyroid enlargement is caused by the release of a hormone of the pituitary gland in response to a decrease in the circulating thyroid hormones. Atrophy may occur later or a colloid goiter may develop. Nodules may form and become toxic.

Iodine is excreted from the body almost entirely in the urine. The feces contain small amounts of iodine, most of which are derived from thyroxin in the bile.

Iodine is necessary for general health. Thyroxin was isolated by Kendall in 1916. It was not until 1927 that Harrington succeeded in preparing the hormone artificially by synthesis from coal tar products, thus establishing its chemical structure. In the form of thyroxin, iodine regulates energy metabolism, governing the oxidation rate in the cells in relation to the body's changing physiologic needs. Intravenous injection of 1 mg. of thyroxin raises the metabolic rate to some degree and 2 mg. may cause a 20 per cent increase. The potency of this compound and the dangers of its use in excess are very evident.

Iodine is required for normal growth. Acceleration of growth has been secured in both normal and hypothyroid children by the use of thyroid extract as well as by administration of iodine in food. Several foods have been employed as carriers of the mineral in studies of this function of iodine.

The mineral also takes part in reproduction. Problems in breeding animals in areas where there is a lack of iodine are well known, and its use in prophylaxis is accepted as being beneficial. Failure of lactation has been associated with a low intake of iodine, whereas an increased flow of breast milk has accompanied the mineral's inclusion in the diet of nursing mothers.

There are several methods of studying an individual's state of iodine metabolism. The basal metabolism test has long been used in determining whether the thyroid gland is functioning properly; this technique and the applications of the findings to goiter problems were discussed in Chapter 3. But since the basal metabolic rate is regulated by a variety of body processes, other methods of study are more often used in investigating iodine metabolism. One of these is determination of protein-bound iodine (PBI) in the serum. The amount found present is compared with that of a healthy person—three to eight μg. per cent. If the person has received iodine in any form the PBI test is not valid. In this case the BEI test (see chapter 3, p. 36) is preferred as a means of assessing the basal metabolic rate.

The study of urinary excretion of stable iodine furnishes an accepted method of assessing iodine nutriture; it has been used by the ICNND in population surveys. This group determined the iodine content of "casual" urine specimens, expressed in terms of the creatinine content of the sample (3). Urinary iodine is less in goitrous areas than in non-goitrous; fasting also decreases the amount. On the other hand, there is an increased excretion of the mineral in hyperthyroidism, menstruation and pregnancy, and during iodine therapy.

Another procedure used in investigating iodine nutriture measures the uptake of a known amount of radioactive iodine into the thyroid gland during a 24-hour period; the normal or euthyroid uptake is approximately 30 per cent; in hypothyroidism it is less than 10 per cent, in hyperthyroidism, more than 50 per cent.

VARIABILITY IN THE SUPPLY OF IODINE

The natural supply of iodine depends largely on geographical location. Normally, animals secure the necessary iodine from food and water while plants absorb it from the soil. Additional iodine may be furnished to the soil by fertilizers, and this will increase manyfold the amount found in plants. Water may furnish measurable amounts; this was shown in 1923 by McClendon and Williams (4) in analysis of water from various places in the United States.

For the most part, surface waters contain little iodine, although in dry areas the mineral present in salt deposits may appear to some extent at the surface; artesian wells often strike water relatively rich in iodine. As a sole source of the mineral, water, even in the iodine-rich localities, is of comparatively little consequence; for instance, in New Orleans it would require 13 quarts of water to furnish 0.1 mg. of iodine, the amount recommended daily for a child of six to eight years. However, an inverse ratio has been found to exist between the percentage of iodine in water and the incidence of simple goiter. The disease tends to be endemic in mountainous regions, although this does not hold for those of volcanic origin. The Himalayas, Alps, and Pyrenees form goiter areas, as do the Andes Plateau, the Cascade Mountains, and parts of the Appalachian and Rocky Mountain ranges. The river beds of New Zealand, the Thames valley of England, and the St. Lawrence Basin and Great Lakes of the United States are endemic goiter regions. In general, glacial regions are known to contain little iodine.

The iodine content of food is extremely variable. The earliest analyses of foods for iodine were made in 1899, but much of the first work gave questionable data due to the small size of the samples and imperfection of method. A colorimetric technique for determining iodine in food composites first employed by the ICNND is now approved for general use.

There is a wide variation in the iodine content of foods of the same species, and for the same food grown under different soil conditions and in different parts of the world. Jarvis and others (5) of Seattle, in analysis of different species of salmon caught on the West Coast, found a range of from 206 to 405 mg. per kg. on the moist basis; their average figure was 296. The fish at an early stage of maturity contained more iodine than did the spawning salmon; roe were a good source of this mineral.

The canning process did not decrease the amount of iodine. Lobster, clams, and oysters have been shown to be higher than salmon in iodine, but they do not occupy a large place in the dietary; on the other hand, fresh-water fish contain less than do salt-water varieties. Seaweed, the best iodine carrier, is little used as a food in this country, but in Japan, where it is used, goiter is almost unknown (6).

Research has shown that iodine is present in milk but varies from a trace in goitrous areas to 420 μg. per liter in nongoitrous regions. The greater proportion of the iodine is found in the cream layer, the butter fat from 1 liter of milk produced by cows in Minnesota containing 140 μg. of iodine and the skim milk, 12 μg. Orr and Leitch (7) reported that the iodine content of milk was increased five to eight times by adding 0.18 gm. of iodine to the cow's daily ration. Eggs from hens on an iodine-enriched diet are also good sources of iodine.

When various vegetables grown in a given region are analyzed, they are found to differ in iodine content. In general, the leaves of plants contain more iodine than the roots, and vegetables and legumes are richer than fruits. In grains the element is concentrated in the outer layers and is removed in the milling process. Cranberries grown near the sea are comparatively good sources of iodine, containing from 27 to 35 μg. per kg. Since much of the nation's supply of cranberries comes from Massachusetts, this fruit may be considered an important iodine food.

A detailed study by Hercus and Roberts (8) shows the comparative values, expressed in μg. per kg. or per liter, of certain foods in New Zealand. These were tested in their natural state and included: seaweed, 48,000; oyster, 880; sardine, 360; egg, 94; spinach, 48; oatmeal, 30; potato with skin, 22; milk, 20; cabbage, 17; mutton, 10; potato without skin, 10; apple, 6; orange, 2; white bread, 2. These workers also made a few tests on iodine losses in cooking. Spinach and carrots, both raw and cooked for one hour, were analyzed for iodine; spinach decreased from 48 to 18 μg. per kg; carrots, 18 to 14.4. From this they concluded that losses in cooking leafy vegetables were greater than those in roots. They also investigated seasonal variation in iodine content of vegetables and found that they had their maximal amount in autumn and winter. Probably iodine is accumulated during the growth period and is retained in mature tissues.

Vought and London (9) reported a study in which seven categories of foods served at The Clinical Center of the National Institute of Health were investigated. Homogeneous composites of each category were analyzed for iodine content. The median value expressed in terms of μg. per wet kg. are: seafoods, 540; vegetables, 280; meat products, 175; eggs, 145; dairy products, 139; bread and cereals, 105; fruits, 18. In the vegetable category, broccoli, spinach, and turnip greens ranked high.

Data on iodine content of foods usually refers to the raw material. In 1970 Koutras and co-workers (10) published a table (Table 9–1) giving the iodine content of drinking water, milk, and some fully prepared and ready-to-eat food items available in Athens, Greece, and areas where endemic goiter is prevalent. In Greece iodine is not added as a supplement to commercial animal foods or to table salt. This lack and the low iodine content of the soil were suggested as reasons for the comparatively low iodine values determined by these workers. They

Table 9–1

*Iodine Content of Water, Milk, and Food Items**

Food item	Athens				Endemic areas			
	n	Mean	SE	Range	n	Mean	SE	Range
Drinking water, μg/100 ml	12	0.47	0.033	0.35–0.77	163	0.24	0.02	ND–1.0
Cow's milk, μg/100 ml	12	4.15	0.36	7.50–2.60	68	2.5	0.22	ND–9.0
Sheep's milk, μg/100 ml					59	9.4	0.93	1.5–35.3
Goat's milk, μg/100 ml					56	2.2	0.33	ND–15.7
Eggs, μg/egg	15	13.4	3.7	1.8–48.8	19	1.9	0.36	0.5–6.0
Chicken dishes, μg/portion; weight, 240 g (150–500)	16	125.5	42.6	2.7–597.0	16	23.8	10.5	ND–151.0
Meat dishes, μg/portion; weight, 250 g (150–500)	10	6.5	1.9	ND–18.0	16	3.0	0.86	ND–12.3
Fish dishes, μg/portion; weight, 222 g (148–388)	9	63.9	29.6	2.4–158.0				
Legume dishes, μg/portion; weight, 300 g (250–600)	14	3.0	0.7	ND–7.6	16	2.0	1.0	ND–14.3
Greek soft cheese, μg/100 g	15	15.12	1.85	6.7–33.0	15	8.48	1.22	3.6–17.5
Bread, μg/100 g	12	1.56	1.20	ND–14.5	21	0.54	0.25	ND–3.7

SE = standard error. ND = not detectable.
* Koutras, D. A., et al. Dietary Sources of Iodine in Areas With and Without Iodine-Deficiency Goiter. *Am. J. Clin. Nutr.*, 23:-870 (1970).

found substantial amounts of iodine consistently only in foods of animal origin. These investigators advocate universal iodization of household salt because the iodine content of natural foods is barely adequate, even in areas without endemic goiter.

In goitrous sections the iodine content of native foods is too low to be relied on unless the soil is enriched. The problem of studying iodine metabolism is further complicated since some foods are known to be goitrogenic. In 1949, a goitrogenic substance, thiooxazolidone (commonly called goitrin) was isolated from cabbage; this vegetable, rutabagas, and turnips are members of the Brassica family. Goitrin inhibits uptake of iodine by the thyroid gland. Further study on antithyroid compounds in foods has led to the discovery that goitrin is not present in active forms in foods (11). It is formed by enzymatic action from a precursor, progoitrin. At first it was thought that the enzyme that converts progoitrin to goitrin was present in food and could be destroyed by heat, but it is now known that enzymes in the intestinal tract can convert progoitrin to goitrin. Therefore both cooked and raw foods containing these compounds are potentially goitrogenic. Another goitrogen, arachidoside, has been found to be present in the peanut; more is in the red skin than in the nut itself. There is some evidence that a goitrogen occurs in soybeans. In Eastern Nigeria, where the people eat much unfermented cassava which contains cyanogenic glycosides, goitrogenic substances, it has been estimated that up to 60 per cent of the females have goiter (12). No relationship between the incidence of this condition and soil or water was found.

THE AMOUNT OF IODINE CONSUMED AND THAT RECOMMENDED
FOR CONSUMPTION

Dietary studies and surveys give data on iodine intake. Information about the types of salt purchased by households in the United States was obtained for one week in the 1965 dietary survey (13). The percentage of households purchasing all types of salt was lower in 1965 than in 1955 but this is not considered to indicate smaller intake now than formerly. The explanation given is that the purchase of ready-to-eat and convenience foods was greater in 1965 than in 1955. The proportion of households purchasing iodized salt was greater in 1965 than in 1955. In 1965 more than five times as many households purchased the fortified salt than the plain salt. However, many households reporting did not specify the kind of salt used. Probably the choice was left to chance and the figures indicate lack of knowledge about the need for iodized salt.

Variability in iodine content of food complicates the dietary study. In conducting such a study, it is common practice to use tables of food composition which give average or proximate figures. Since the iodine content of foods of different sections of the country vary so widely, this procedure cannot be used unless analyses of the foods utilized in the community are available. Because there are comparatively few data, not many dietary studies have been made.

Vought and London (9), during their investigation of seven categories of foods for iodine content, analyzed the iodine in the diets served for 18 days to 11 patients on metabolic diets at the National Institutes of Health and in 36 meals served to 19 patients on regular house diets. The amount of salt added at the table was determined quantitatively. The range of iodine intake from these diets was found to be wide. For the metabolic patients the amount of iodine varied from 15 to 219 μg. per day, depending on the amount of eggs and milk consumed. In regular house diets the range was 65 to 529 μg. per day, with vegetables and dairy products furnishing the most iodine. The patients chose little seafood or eggs, foods high in iodine. The median amount of salt added at the table was 1.59 gm. per day. If iodized, this would have added 1.22 μg. iodine to the daily intake.

Urinary iodine excretion and thyroid iodine uptake are used more than balance studies to investigate the body's need. Because of the difficulty involved in conducting an iodine balance study only a few have been made. One was conducted by Vought and London (14) on 19 healthy subjects, living in their own homes, over a period of six weeks. In this carefully controlled investigation quantitative intakes and urinary and fecal excretion were determined by chemical assays. The median dietary intake was 128 μg. per day for women and 360 μg. per day for children. The median intake of noniodized salt was 2.75 gm. per day. The drinking water contained 4 to 6.5 μg. iodine per liter and was a negligible source of the mineral. On this intake of iodine the subjects as a group had a slight negative balance (-41 μg. per day), a difference from zero which was not considered significant.

In a study on iodide excretion North and Frazer (15) collected data on 119 patients undergoing thyroid tests. These subjects lived in New Zealand where iodized salt has been available for over 40 years but where little data are available on iodine consumption. Using the iodide excretion level as a fairly accurate measure of intake these investigators estimated that the mean iodine intake of women was about 230 μg. per day, of men, 280 μg. per day, amounts considered well above those needed.

In Thailand, where endemic goiter is highly prevalent, the ICNND made studies on radioactive iodine uptake and on urinary excretion (16). In only one area studied was the uptake normal; in others, average values were much higher. Urinary iodide excretion correlated inversely with these uptakes. The prevalence of clinical goiter also correlated with these data.

In a group of school girls living in Washington, D.C., where the incidence of goiter is very low, the urinary excretion of iodine averaged 123.5 µg. per gm. creatinine (16).

Investigations on the uptake of radioactive iodine in the thyroid gland and the rate of breakdown in the tissues indicate that from 200 to 400 µg. of thyroxin may be manufactured and used daily. Since thyroxin is about two-thirds iodine, approximately 150 to 200 µg. of the mineral would be required daily. It is thought that the body tends to conserve its supply of iodine, reusing about one-third of the mineral which is released when the hormone is broken down. These data agree well with urinary iodine excretion values and support the daily intake of iodine approved by the FNB.

Recommended allowances for iodine have been made. The seventh edition of RDA gives figures for iodine allowances for the different age groups. The amounts increase gradually from 25 µg. daily in early infancy to 120 µg. for the 14- to 16-year-old female and to 150 µg. for the 14- to 18-year-old male. After this the allowances decrease to 80 and 110 µg., respectively, for females and males 55 and older. Iodine needs during pregnancy and lactation are greater. The recommended allowances for all ages may be expressed in terms of energy requirement— approximately 0.5 µg. per 100 kcal.

EFFECTS OF LACK OF DIETARY IODINE

The effects of iodine deficiency have been observed in animals. Goiter may occur in any animal which has a thyroid gland; among farm livestock in certain regions the prevalence of the disease has been of great economic concern. For a time sheep raising in Michigan was seriously crippled and improvement came by the accidental discovery of salt deposits to which the sheep were given access. Iodine was first used intentionally for this purpose by Marine and Lenhart (17) in 1909–10 in Pennsylvania brook trout hatcheries. Pig liver fed to the fish resulted in a goitrous condition, while a diet of sea fish or addition of iodine to the water, in a concentration not greater than 1 mg. per liter, arrested and prevented development of the disease. In the Pacific Northwest, as well as in Wisconsin and other northern states, even though pregnant sows showed no signs of abnormality, many of the young were born dead or died soon after birth; the bodies were hairless, or nearly so, and the necks were thick and pulpy. Hart and Steenbock (18) in 1917 showed this to be the result of iodine deficiency and demonstrated that the addition of 100 mg. of potassium iodide to 100 pounds of the ration used would permit reproduction of normal animals. The thyroid glands of the normal pigs were smaller than those of the diseased animals, and contained iodine, whereas the abnormal glands contained none. As a result of this work addition of iodine to hog rations is now practiced in regions where goiter is known to occur, and the hairless pig malady is no longer prevalent.

Variations exist in susceptibility to goiter. Just as the natural supply of iodine differs according to locality so also does the tendency to develop a goiter. It is well known that simple goiter is more prevalent among women than men and among girls than boys, although in the severest endemic districts both sexes may be so generally affected as to mask the difference. According to Kimball (19), schoolgirls have thyroid enlargement six times as frequently as do schoolboys; for this reason examination for goiter detection among the former is more necessary. In girls the incidence of the disease if left unattended increases steadily up to the 18th year; in boys it reaches its peak at age 12.

Another fact to consider is that this disease is more common at certain times of life, according to Marine (20), particularly during those periods when growth, differentiation, and energy transformation are greatest. During pregnancy special attention to this matter may prevent the disorder in both mother and child; since an excess as well as a lack of iodine is harmful, the physician in charge should assume the responsibility. The breast-fed baby may be treated through the mother. At puberty the incidence of goiter is high and therefore adolescent children should be especially guarded.

Simple goiter does not have extreme effects on the human being but may lead to serious conditions. During pregnancy, fetal life, and adolescence lack of iodine in the diet is manifested in an enlarged thyroid gland, and it is thought that this increase in size is due to the body's effort to compensate for the mineral decrease. The type of cells found in the gland is also different. The change in size and quality of the gland does not seem to have noticeable effects on the person, other than in physical appearance. Another condition which may occur in regions where iodine deficiency continues from generation to generation, as in Switzerland, involves tissue atrophy and decrease in thyroid secretion. This disorder is known as cretinism in the young, myxedema in the adult. In the hypothyroid state the secretion rate of the pituitary growth hormone is lessened; this explains the lack of growth in the cretin. Other symptoms of the disease include a sluggish metabolism, obesity, a thickened connective tissue especially about face, neck, and hands, and a lessening of mental power. It is thought that some types of congenital mental deficiency are due to hypothyroidism and may be corrected by dietary and (or) hormonal treatment. There is slight, if any, effect on the basal metabolic rate in endemic goiter, but in cretinism and myxedema the rate may be very low.

TREATMENT OF THYROID GLAND DISTURBANCES

Simple goiter responds to iodine therapy. After iodine was proved successful in treatment of goiter in fish and farm animals, Kimball and associates (21) undertook the study of goiter in adolescent human beings. With permission, they worked in the public schools in Akron, Ohio, a mildly goitrous district, and, during a period of two and one-half years (1917–19), they examined approximately 10,000 adolescent girls, many of them twice annually. Only girls who had written consent from home to serve as subjects were given treatment of 2 gm. of sodium iodide, administered in 0.2-gm. doses daily for ten consecutive school days, repeated each spring and autumn.

The results of this study indicated that sodium iodide was effective in both prevention and cure of endemic goiter. Of the 1257 normal girls not taking the treatment, 28 per cent developed goiter, while 80 per cent of those having moderately enlarged glands showed improvement with medication. The great success of this experiment resulted in the use of the same treatment in other schools and in industrial plants throughout goitrous regions. In 1918 similar experimental work was instituted in Switzerland, a country which had the largest percentage of endemic goiter of any nation. Today this treatment for goiter is fairly common. When iodine is taken in forms other than food, the careful supervision of a physician or the public health authorities is essential. It also seems well to advocate, especially in goitrous regions, checking the thyroid gland in the periodic physical examination of all children so that curative treatment may be started before the goiter develops to any extent.

Michigan, which was a center of endemic goiter, met the problem by an agreement of the salt manufacturers to add iodine to the extent of 0.02 per cent sodium iodide to their product. The sale of the iodized salt and a well-planned educational campaign were inaugurated in 1924. At that time an extensive survey showed the incidence of goiter in Michigan school children to be 38.6 per cent. This figure was decreased to 9.0 by 1928 and to 1.4 per cent by 1952; this latter figure was secured in a survey of school children in the same Michigan counties where the 1924 study was made.

In Guatemala in 1952 the average prevalence of endemic goiter was 38.5 per cent. In 1962, after 90 per cent of all the salt consumed throughout the country was iodized (one part iodine to 15,000 parts salt), the average prevalence of goiter was 15 per cent, and by 1965 it was further reduced to 5.2 per cent (22).

The importance of the continued use of iodized salt was demonstrated in a study made in Spain (23). In three villages the use of iodized salt over a period of six years brought about an effective regression in goiter in school children. When the administration of iodized salt was stopped for a year the occurrence of goiter increased considerably. The hyperplasia which occurred during the suppression period was significantly greater in girls of ten to 15 years than in those of five to nine.

Several iodine supplements are in use. In the original experiment with Ohio school children sodium iodide was given twice yearly in liquid form. This is not considered a practical procedure for mass prevention or treatment. Neither are tablets or candies which contain iodine. In some localities iodide has been added to the water supply, but this method is not widely used, partly because it does not benefit rural areas, partly because consumption of water by different individuals varies greatly, and partly because it is not economical. Milk and eggs have been iodized by incorporating some form of iodine in the diets of cows and hens but this is not done on a large scale. In two goitrous areas of Australia iodates have been included in bread as a routine procedure. However, a survey (24) showed that the weekly consumption of iodine from iodated bread was much lower than that secured from a tablet containing potassium iodide.

As indicated earlier, salt is generally considered the most acceptable carrier for iodine. At present the level of salt iodization permitted in the United States is 0.5 to 1 part in 10,000. Thus if 10 grams (about 2 teaspoons) of salt are consumed per day, a person would receive from 0.5 to 1.0 mg. iodine, an amount in excess of that needed but not enough to be harmful. Because the iodide may volatilize, a stabilizer such as sodium carbonate sometimes is added. If this is not done the salt offered for sale should be analyzed at intervals by the state health department to be sure the content of iodine is up to standard.

The iodate has been found to be better adapted for fortification than the iodide since it is a more stable compound, especially in areas where moisture and high temperatures prevail. It is not used in salt sold for human consumption in the United States, however; the FDA approves potassium iodide and cuprous iodide, both at a level of 0.01 per cent. Iodates are used as an improver in bread; the amount incorporated is regulated by the FDA. It is thought that these iodine compounds, secured from dairy products and bread, along with iodized salt and natural foods rich in iodine, make the American diet adequate in respect to this mineral.

The other forms of goiter are not amenable to treatment with dietary iodine. Hypothyroidism, the result of an insufficiency of thyroxin, is a pathological condition and is usually treated by the physician with carefully controlled doses of whole thyroid gland or thyroxin. Hyperthyroidism or, as it is sometimes called, exophthalmic goiter, is not nutritional in origin and may not even be primarily a thyroid disease. Symptoms of exophthalmic goiter include bulging eyes, thinness, nervousness, and enlargement of the thyroid gland. A person with this disorder is advised to eliminate iodized products from his diet because they may aggravate the condition in which the basal metabolic rate is already high. Over-exertion and nervous excitement should be avoided and treatment should always be in the hands of a physician.

REFERENCES

1. Fierro-Benitiz, R., *et al.* Endemic Goiter and Endemic Cretinism in the Andean Region. *New Eng. J. Med., 280:*296 (1969).
2. Schaefer, A. E. The National Nutrition Survey. *J. Am. Diet. Ass., 54:*371 (1969).
3. Follis, R. H., Jr. Patterns of Urinary Iodine Excretion in Goitrous and Nongoitrous Areas. *Am. J. Clin. Nutr., 14:*253 (1964).
4. McClendon, J. F., *et al.* Simple Goiter as a Result of Iodine Deficiency. *J. Am. Med. Ass., 80:*600 (1923).
5. Jarvis, M. S., *et al.* Salmon in a Diet for the Prophylaxis of Goiter. *J. Am. Med. Ass., 86:*1339 (1926).
6. Socolow, E. L., *et al.* Possible Goitrogenic Effects of Selected Japanese Foods. *J. Nutr., 83:*20 (1964).
7. Orr, J. B., *et al. Iodine in Nutrition.* Special Report Series, 123. London: Medical Research Council, His Majesty's Stationery Office (1929).
8. Hercus, E. C., *et al.* Iodine Content of Foods, Manures and Animal Products in Relation to the Prophylaxis of Endemic Goiter in New Zealand. *J. Hyg., 26:*49 (1927).
9. Vought, R. L., *et al.* Dietary Sources of Iodine. *Am. J. Clin. Nutr., 14:*186 (1964).
10. Koutras, D. A., *et al.* Dietary Sources of Iodine in Areas With and Without Iodine-Deficiency Goiter. *Am. J. Clin. Nutr., 23:*870 (1970).
11. The Significance of Naturally Occurring Antithyroid Compounds in the Production of Goiter in Man. Borden's Review of Nutrition Research, *21: #*5 Sept.–Oct. 1960.
12. Ekpechi, O. L. Pathogenesis of Endemic Goiter in Eastern Nigeria. *Brit. J. Nutr., 21:*537 (1967).
13. Clark, F. Personal communication.
14. Vought, R. L., *et al.* Iodine Intake and Excretion in Healthy Non-hospitalized Subjects. *Am. J. Clin. Nutr., 14:*124 (1964).
15. North, K. A. K., *et al.* Iodine Intake as Revealed by Urinary Iodide Excretion. *New Zealand Med. J., 65:*512 (1966).
16. Follis, R. H., Jr. *Studies on Iodine Nutrition in Thailand, Washington, D.C., and Jamaica, B.W.I.* Proceedings, Fifth Armed Forces International Nutrition Conference. ICNND (1962).
17. Marine, D., *et al.* Observations and Experiments on the So-called Thyroid Carcinoma of Brook Trout (*Salvelinus Fontinalis*) and Its Relation to Ordinary Goiter. *J. Exptl. Med., 12:*311 (1910).
18. Hart, E. B., *et al.* Thyroid Hyperplasia and the Relation of Iodine to the Hairless Pig Malady. *J. Biol. Chem., 33:*313 (1918).

19. Kimball, O. P. The Prevention of Simple Goiter in Man. *Am. J. Med. Sci., 163:*634 (1922).

20. Marine, D., *et al.* The Pathogenesis and Prevention of Simple or Endemic Goiter. *J. Am. Med. Ass., 104:*2334 (1935).

21. Kimball, O. P. Prevention of Goiter in Michigan and Ohio. *J. Am. Med. Ass., 108:*860 (1937).

22. Béhar, M. Progress and Delays in Combating Goiter in Latin America. *Fed. Proc., 27:*939 (1969).

23. Garcia, F. M., *et al. Prophylaxis with Iodized Salt, Effects of its Suppression in an Endemic Locality.* Proceedings, Fifth Armed Forces International Nutrition Conference. ICNND (1962).

24. Howeler-Coy, J. F. Bread Consumption in Tasmania. *Food & Nutr. Notes & Reviews, 25:*16 (1968).

GENERAL REFERENCE

25. Greer, M. A. Iodine. *In* M. S. Wohl and R. S. Goodhart (eds.), *Modern Nutrition in Health and Disease,* 4th ed. Philadelphia: Lea & Febiger (1968).

Other
Inorganic
Elements

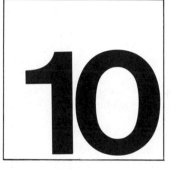

Interest in a number of minerals not discussed in earlier chapters is increasing. These minerals occur in very small amounts and are commonly called "trace elements." Iron and iodine, already discussed, also are included in this category. Elements considered essential for man are chlorine, chromium, cobalt, copper, fluorine, magnesium, manganese, molybdenum, potassium, selenium, sodium, sulfur, and zinc. Other trace elements found in animal tissues are aluminum, arsenic, barium, boron, bromine, cadmium, cesium, lead, lithium, mercury, nickel, rubidium, silicon, silver, strontium, tellurium, tin, titanium, and vanadium. The essentiality of this latter group of minerals is not proven. They occur naturally as salts in foods and water, and they tend to accumulate in body tissues rather than to be excreted.

Several trace elements are thought to be environmental hazards. Mercury, lead, cadmium, and nickel are considered more insidious than pesticides. Cadmium is thought to have a role in developing hypertension.

Chromium

METABOLISM AND FUNCTIONS

These aspects have been studied. The usual daily intake of this trace element in the United States has been estimated to be 30 to 80 μg., of which only a very small per cent is absorbed. Tests with radioactive chromium have shown it at its highest level in the blood of rats one hour after injection (1). Here chromium is bound and transported by siderophilin. The mineral is stored largely in the spleen, kidney, testis, and epididymis; much less is stored in the heart, pancreas, lungs, and brain. Young growing rats retain greater amounts in bones. Chromium has been found in some enzymes and in RNA. Excretion occurs mainly in urine, with minor amounts in the feces. The amount of chromium in the body decreases with age, and it is thought that this may indicate an insufficient dietary intake and be related to the increased incidence of diabetes and degenerative vascular disease found in older people (2).

Chromium deficiency was not recognized until 1959, when it was shown that a retarded glucose tolerance, induced by diet, could be returned to normal by giving rats trivalent chromium; 40 other elements were ineffective as a remedy (3). In other work (4), chromium deficiency has resulted in depressed growth rates, severe glucose intolerance as in diabetes, and incidence of atheromatous lesions in the aorta. It has been found that chromium acts by enhancing the stimulatory effects of insulin. In 1968 it was identified as a cofactor with insulin at the cellular level. Mertz and Roginski (5, 6) believe that this interaction of chromium and insulin is not limited to glucose metabolism but also applies to amino acid metabolism. In rats fed a low protein diet a chromium deficiency resulted in retarded growth and diminished longevity; protein supplementation alone did not improve these conditions. Corneal opaqueness has been noted in rats fed a diet low in both chromium and protein but not in protein alone.

Chromium activates several enzymes involved in the synthesis of fatty acids and cholesterol. It appears to inhibit formation of aortic plaques and its lack may contribute to atherosclerosis. Schroeder's studies (7) on chromium indicate that it may aid in the catabolism or excretion of cholesterol. His studies also suggest that atherosclerotic conditions in human beings may be related to high consumption of refined sugar and grains from which chromium has been removed (8).

STUDIES ON HUMAN BEINGS

Evidence shows that chromium is an essential element for human beings. Most studies on this mineral have been made on rats and mice. However, some have been made on human beings in connection with a diseased state, especially diabetes. Glinsman and associates (9) found that chromium supplementation improved the glucose tolerance in some but not all diabetic patients. Because determining chromium in blood plasma presents technical difficulties Hambidge and co-workers (10) studied the chromium content of the hair of normal and diabetic children. They found significantly low chromium levels in the latter group.

Infants with kwashiorkor also have impaired glucose tolerance. This condition was markedly improved after oral treatment with trivalent chromium, and the fasting blood glucose levels rose from hypoglycemic to normal (11).

No recommended allowance has been set for chromium and little is known about how much is present in the diet. In the study of Type A school lunches (18) the average chromium per lunch was 0.009 to 0.088 mg. This amount was considered marginal.

Copper

OCCURRENCE IN THE BODY

Copper is found in all body tissues; its lack results in a variety of abnormalities. Only about 30 per cent of the copper consumed is absorbed (1). This occurs in the stomach and upper intestine and is favored in an acid medium. From the intestine copper moves into the bloodstream. About 93 per cent of the serum copper is bound tightly to ceruloplasmin and is released from it only when this protein is catabolized. Frieden and co-workers (2) found evidence that ceruloplasmin catalyzes the oxidation of several reducing agents which react with ferric ion. Ceruloplasmin is considered the molecular link in copper and iron metabolism and has been shown to be directly involved in hemoglobin biosynthesis. About 7 per cent of the serum copper is loosely bound to albumin and amino acids, and it is transported to the various body tissues in these forms. Concentrations of copper are high in the brain, liver, heart, and kidney. The liver is the main organ for copper storage. This organ also synthesizes ceruloplasmin and prepares the mineral for biliary excretion. Most of the dietary copper is excreted in the feces, very little in urine.

SYMPTOMS OF LACK

Deficiency is rarely found in man (3). Symptoms of copper deficiency in animals include anemia, skeletal defects, demyelination and degeneration of the nervous system, abnormalities of pigmentation and hair structure, failure to reproduce, and cardiovascular lesions. However, depletion has been noted in some human cases of iron-deficiency anemia, edema, kwashiorkor, sprue, and nephrosis.

FUNCTIONS AND METABOLISM

Functions of copper are known. Several roles of copper involve catalytic action. The mineral helps in hemoglobin formation, probably by releasing iron stores from the liver. It is also essential for activating lipid enzyme systems, particularly those involved in phospholipid synthesis. Copper is a constituent of cytochrome oxidase, an enzyme in the electron transport mechanism from which high-energy phosphate bonds are derived. Copper is found in tyrosinase, an enzyme involved in converting tyrosine into melanin, a black pigment. In animals lack of copper results in loss of hair color; albinism may occur if no copper is present. Copper is necessary in formation of aortic elastin (4); if it is lacking, elastin synthesis is abnormal and aortic rupture may occur.

Several inverse relationships have been found between copper and vitamin A and it is thought that there may be some reciprocal action between the two nutrients, both in metabolism and mode of action (5). As examples, fetal liver contains 5 to 10 per cent more copper than maternal liver, but fetal liver contains only about one-fifth as much vitamin A as does maternal. Also, the copper content of blood plasma is about 10 per cent higher in women than in men, but men's plasma is about 20 per cent higher in vitamin A. In fevers the copper content of the blood is greatly increased, but vitamin A content is decreased. The significance of these contrasts is not understood. Molybdenum and copper interactions are known to exist; the copper-molybdenum complex formed is biologically unavailable (6). As a result of the combination, molybdenum can cause copper deficiency and copper can alleviate molybdenum toxicity.

DIETARY SOURCES AND INTAKES

These have been determined. Among the best food sources of copper are liver, kidney, shellfish, nuts, raisins, and dried legumes (7). Cow's milk contains less copper than human milk. Variations in content of plant foods may be considerable, due to the amount of the mineral in the soil in which the plants are grown. The copper in cooking utensils and piping does not add significant amounts to water or food (8).

Two mg. copper daily are considered sufficient to maintain balance in the adult. In studies on preadolescent girls, daily intakes of 1.3 mg. copper resulted in positive balance (9). Several studies have reported copper intakes which are considered borderline. White (10), who studied the inorganic elements in the weighed diets of high school girls and young women, found the average copper content of the day's meals to be 0.50 ± 0.77 mg., amounts less than those usually recommended. Only four of the 48 composites contained more than 1 mg., and only two of the four had more than 2 mg. per day. In the study of seven- to ten-year-old girls in selected southern states (17), mean daily intakes of 1.180, 1.066, and 1.058 mg. copper resulted in negative balances of 0.028, 0.138, and 0.029 mg., respectively. In Type A school lunches planned to include one-third of the day's nutrient needs a mean of 0.34 mg. copper was found (18). In none of the five regions studied did the average content of copper reach one-third of the 1.3 mg. generally approved. The FNB recommends 0.08 mg. per kg. body weight per day for infants and children. Cordano and associates (11) studied four malnourished infants who were undergoing nutritional rehabilitation. They estimated the daily copper requirement of these rapidly growing infants whose stores were poor to be in the range of 42 to 135 μg. per kg. body weight.

Fluorine

VARIATIONS IN CONTENT OF BODY AND FOODS

The fluoride content of body tissues and foods varies widely. This trace element is present in minute amounts in nearly every human tissue but is found primarily in the skeleton and teeth; the organs contain more fluoride than do other soft tissues. Among the richer food sources of animal origin are gelatin, the organs, seafoods, and infant foods which contain bone meal. Wide deviations in individual foods are found; cow's milk content may vary from 0.09 to 0.32 parts per million (ppm), cheese from 0.16 to 1.31 ppm (1).

In plant foods the fluoride content varies according to environmental conditions; among these are the type of soil, direction and intensity of prevailing winds, and use of fertilizers and sprays which contain fluoride. Green leafy vegetables are especially susceptible to air-borne fluoride; the range of fluoride ion in spinach is 0.1 to 28.3 ppm. Fruits contain little unless sprayed with a fluoride compound; this procedure now is controlled by the FDA to prevent an excess. It has been estimated that an adult may secure 0.5 to 1.0 mg. fluoride daily from his food.

RELATION TO TOOTH DECAY

Fluoride is advocated primarily as a means of controlling tooth decay. Interest in fluoride was aroused when it was found that this element, present naturally in large amounts in the drinking water of certain localities, caused mottled tooth enamel and that this condition could be controlled by limiting the amount of the mineral to about 1.5 ppm. With 1 ppm or less in the water supply, the mottling was controlled but susceptibility to dental caries increased. This effect on tooth decay is evident especially during the time the teeth are forming.

The mechanics of this action is being studied. It has been shown that fluoride combines chemically with hydroxyapatite to form fluorapatite whose crystals are larger and more perfect in form. This in turn results in reduced surface area and solubility. The outer layers of enamel have a higher fluoride content than the inner layers. Also, the fluoride content of the teeth and bones closely parallels the fluoride content of the water supply. These facts probably are related to the resistance of teeth to caries.

Fluoridation of water. Addition of fluoride to the water supply is advocated by public health authorities as a safe, inexpensive, and efficient way to reduce dental caries.

Maximum allowable limits of the fluoride ion in drinking water have been set at 2.4 ppm for cool climates and 1.4 ppm for warm climates where the water intake would be greater. One ppm of sodium fluoride is the amount approved for addition to the water supply. This, plus the amount secured through food, is considered well within the range of safety in fluoride intake. That this amount is not excessive for health has been demonstrated by the absence of mottled enamel. Its positive value has been shown in extensive medical and public health investigations. In communities using fluoridated water a decrease of 50 per cent or more in the incidence of tooth decay has resulted. In a study made in Evanston, Illinois, on more than 26,000 children and covering the period from 1947 to 1961, not only did the amount of tooth decay decline to a great extent but the number of children who were completely free of tooth decay increased markedly (2). A group of 1060 of these children, aged 12, 13, and 14 years, who drank fluoridated water in 1959 was compared with 1701 children of the same ages before the water was fluoridated in 1946. The number of decayed, missing, and filled (DMF) teeth was strikingly less in the 1959 group. Among the 12-year-olds there were about 13 times as many children immune to caries in 1959 as in 1946. Those who benefited most were those who had been exposed to fluoride from prenatal life on. In this study the cost of adding sodium fluoride to the water supply during the 15 years was calculated; it amounted to a little less than 11½ cents per year per person.

Fluoridation of the water supply is by far the most common procedure for supplying this mineral. However, application of a solution of sodium fluoride directly to the teeth may be recommended in areas where the water fluoride content is low. This topical treatment should be started in preschool years and continued at regular intervals throughout the period of tooth formation. During eight years of research in which more than 15,000 children participated, it was demonstrated that a 2 per cent solution of sodium fluoride topically applied reduced new dental decay by 40 per cent.

RELATION OF FLUORIDE TO BONE

Benefits other than caries control have been indicated. There is also evidence that adults profit from the use of fluoride. In 1965 a study was made in five communities in North Dakota where there are both high- and low-fluoride areas (3). Approximately 300 subjects, over 45 years old, from high-fluoride areas (4 to 6 ppm fluoride) and approximately 700 of the same age group from low-fluoride areas (0.15 to 0.3 ppm) were included. X-rays of the lumbar spine were made and graded in terms of relative density. Presence or absence of collapsed vertebrae and calcification of abdominal aortas was also noted. Substantially less osteoporosis in both women and men in the high-fluoride areas was found. In women more than men the incidence of collapsed vertebrae was much lower in the high-fluoride group; the fact that more men had collapsed vertebrae was thought to be due to their heavy labor as farmers. In both sexes the incidence of calcified aortas was much lower in the high-fluoride group. Consumption of milk and cheese was checked and showed no relation to the results.

The favorable effects of fluoride found in North Dakota were not confirmed in a New York check-up made by Korns (4) on adults who had lived for over 20 years in Kingston, with a negligible amount of fluoride in its water, or in Newburgh, with a fluoridated water supply. Even though the effects of fluoridation on dental caries among the children of these two towns had been pronounced, no significant differences were found in prevalence of osteoporosis, collapsed vertebrae, and calcified aortas. In another study (5) made on calcium retention as affected by comparatively small doses of fluoride, the balances were not improved during a 22- to 42-day supplementation period. However, the plasma calcium was lower in most subjects during the fluoride intake.

FLUORIDATION LEGISLATION

Fluoridation of water is a common practice. A survey made in 1969 by the State Dental Directors at the request of the Division of Dental Health of the United States Department of Health, Education, and Welfare gives recent information on fluoridation of water supply systems (6). As of 1969, every state has fluoridated communities. Over 80 million people in 4834 communities received water in which the fluoride concentration was adjusted to the optimal level. An additional 8.4 million people lived in 2624 other communities where the natural water supply contained an adequate amount of fluoride. Thus, in 1970, 56 per cent of the population had access to water whose fluoride content is significant for good dental health. Connecticut was the first state to enact fluoridation legislation and since that time (1965) the total number of people in the state receiving fluoridated water has more than tripled. Other states which have statewide fluoridation laws are Minnesota, Illinois, Delaware, Michigan, South Dakota, and Ohio.

In 1966 the American Institute of Nutrition formally endorsed fluoridation as a safe, effective, and low cost way to improve dental health. The FNB recommends fluoridation of public water supplies where the concentration of fluorine in water is low.

Despite the extensive well-documented evidence in favor of fluoridation, controversy continues. Several contributions in the October, 1969, issue of *The American Journal of Clinical Nutrition* give a variety of opinions (7, 8, 9, 10, 11). The student should become acquainted with these points of view, which show the effects of caution, prejudice, fear, and superstition.

Magnesium

CONTENT OF BODY TISSUES

The amount of magnesium in various body tissues has been studied. Flame photometry and the tracer Mg^{28} have made it possible to obtain considerable accurate information on magnesium in the body. Of the 20 to 25 gm. of the element normally found in the human adult, the skeleton contains from 10 to 12 gm., soft tissues 10 gm. or less, and extracellular fluids about 0.5 gm. Liver and striated muscle have higher concentrations than do other soft tissues. The serum level in a healthy adult is approximately 2 mg. per 100 ml. Bone magnesium is mobilized comparatively slowly and a decrease in dietary magnesium is reflected in a sharp decrease in the serum level. Anast (1) found that the serum levels of magnesium were higher in breast-fed babies than in those fed evaporated milk, as is also true for serum calcium. These higher levels are thought to be related to the greater proportion of phosphorus in cow's milk. Ratios of phosphorus to magnesium were 7.6 to 1 in cow's milk, 4 to 1 in breast milk.

SIGNS OF LACK

Symptoms of magnesium deficiency have been noted in human beings as well as in animals. Experimental work on animals has shown that a diet devoid of magnesium results in marked vasodilation, necrotic changes, hyperirritability, convulsive seizures, and eventually death. On diets marginally deficient in magnesium symptoms were less severe.

Similar symptoms have been observed in man. The resulting disease is like hypocalcemic tetany but shows low serum magnesium levels instead of low calcium levels. In human beings the tetany and low serum levels are associated with alcoholism, diabetes, kwashiorkor, parathyroid disease, and malabsorption syndromes. Surgical patients receiving parenteral feedings and patients receiving diuretic therapy may have symptoms of magnesium deficiency. On the other hand, administration of antacids and cathartics containing magnesium to patients with renal failure may result in hypermagnesia, a condition with severe toxic effects. Pretorius (2) found urinary excretion of the mineral to be low in kwashiorkor. In some cases, negative balance was due to excessive loss of magnesium in the stools, indicating impaired absorption.

The beriberi occurring in this and other Occidental countries frequently is associated with alcoholism. Low serum magnesium concentrations are found in chronic alcoholics and after alcohol ingestion, urinary excretion of the mineral may be increased (3, 4). Zieve and co-workers (5) found, using rats, that magnesium deficiency interfered with the response expected when thiamin was given to a thiamin-deficient animal. Magnesium deficiency also led to some reduction in blood and tissue thiamin levels and to a marked reduction in transketolase activity. This enzyme has been shown to reflect thiamin adequacy.

METABOLIC ROLES

Metabolism of calcium, magnesium, and potassium is related. In subjects tube-fed a diet deficient in magnesium but adequate in calcium, both magnesium and calcium serum levels fell markedly. Potassium levels were also low (6). Following magnesium repletion, calcium levels returned to normal; serum potassium levels also rose. On low intakes of magnesium, high protein, calcium, phosphorus, and vitamin D intakes impede magnesium retention.

Magnesium plays important roles in metabolism. In its common dietary forms this mineral is readily absorbed from the small intestine; this process is favored by an acid medium. Magnesium balance in the body is controlled to a great extent by the kidneys, whose tubules normally reabsorb the mineral as needed.

Magnesium is an essential element in human metabolism; it functions in the work of muscles and nerves, in synthesis of proteins, and in many specific reactions such as glucose utilization, methyl group transfer, and oxidative phosphorylation. This mineral acts in both soft tissues and bones as an activator for many enzymes, particularly for those concerned with the transfer of phosphate from ATP to a phosphate receptor or from a phosphorylated compound to ADP. There is evidence that magnesium is involved in thermoregulation.

Magnesium may have a part in treatment of atherosclerosis. Lipid deposits in the ventrical valves and aortas of rats were prevented by addition of high magnesium levels to an otherwise atherogenic diet, and the lipid deposits formed as a result of feeding the atherogenic diet regressed when magnesium was added. Hellerstein and co-workers (7) found that animals fed moderately low amounts of magnesium often developed calcified lesions in soft tissues. When these animals were fed cholesterol they were more susceptible to atherogenesis. Men who are more susceptible to cardiovascular diseases are also more likely than women to have negative magnesium balances. It has been suggested that one of magnesium's functions is to prevent accumulation of cholesterol in the blood.

DIETARY SOURCES AND INTAKES

The magnesium content of foods and the diet has been studied. An extensive list giving the magnesium content of foods has been compiled in Table 5 of *Composition of Foods,* Agriculture Handbook No. 8. Among foods rich in this mineral (over 100 mg. per 100 gm.) are cocoa and chocolate, nuts, whole grain products, soybeans, dried beans and peas, and beet greens. Those with moderate content (25 to 75 mg. per 100 gm.) include most fish, most green vegetables, bananas, corn, potatoes, dried fruits, and hard cheese. Among the foods relatively poor in magnesium (under 25 mg. per 100 gm.) are refined grain products, eggs, and most fruits, vegetables, meats, and dairy products. Zook and Lehman (8) made spectrographic analyses of 30 fresh fruits. Subtropical fruits such as avocados, bananas, figs, mangoes, papayas, and pineapples were found to have higher magnesium values than citrus fruits and melons.

Cooking, especially boiling, results in magnesium losses. The presence of phytic acid in whole grains interferes with absorption of the mineral.

In the Household Food Consumption Survey conducted in 1965, data were obtained for the magnesium intakes of different age-sex groups

(9). Magnesium consumption averaged 313 and 209 mg. per day for 20-
to 34-year-old males and females, respectively. These intakes were considerably less than those recommended by the FNB. Manolo and co-
workers (10) analyzed 55 hospital diets used in metabolic balance
studies and 30 regular hospital diets of known calorie levels. By a regression analysis of their findings they showed a high correlation between
intake of magnesium and calories. They formulated the following prediction equation:

$$\text{meq}^* \text{ dietary magnesium} = -0.0117 + (0.0099 \times \text{calories}).$$

With this formula these workers have estimated that the average American diet contains about 120 mg. magnesium per 1000 kcal.

White (11) determined, by emission spectroscopy, the amounts of
14 inorganic elements in the weighed diets of 21 college women and
15 high school girls. The average magnesium content of these diets was
85 mg. per 1000 kcal. Only 14.5 per cent of the diets contained 120 mg.
or more per 1000 kcal. Magnesium balances of seven- to ten-year-old
girls were determined in selected southern states (17). In all the studies
reported, mean daily intakes of 121 or more mg. magnesium resulted
in slight positive balances. In the study of nutrient content of Type
A school lunches, an average of 93 mg. was found, whereas the goal
set was 100 mg. Sixty per cent of the 300 schools failed to reach this
goal (18).

RECOMMENDED ALLOWANCES

*The magnesium requirement has been studied and recommended daily
allowances have been set.* Balance studies have been used to determine
the minimal requirement of magnesium. Leichsenring (12), Scoular (13),
and Leverton (14) and their associates found that college women were
in positive balance on 300 mg. magnesium per day.

Seelig (15) summarized and analyzed available data found in 105
balance periods on men and 146 on women, totalling 658 and 781 days,
respectively. On intakes of 4 mg. per kg. per day, negative magnesium
balances were likely to develop in both sexes. There is evidence that
women are in balance on lower intakes than men, but this sex difference
shows up more on low intakes of magnesium. Seelig believes that an
intake of less than 6 mg. per kg. per day is not adequate for equilibrium.

It has been found that the amount of dietary magnesium needed may
depend on other dietary components. High protein, calcium, vitamin D,
phytates, and alcohol tend to impede retention of magnesium or to
increase its requirement, especially when intake is below 6 mg. per kg.
per day. Hunt and Schofield (16), using adult women as subjects,
showed that on a low level of dietary protein (30–48 gm. daily) magne-

---

* One millequivalent (meq) of an ion is equal to atomic weight in mg. divided by
valence.

sium equilibrium or positive balance could be secured on only 178–196 mg. magnesium; this is considerably less than that recommended by the FNB.

The FNB has set 350 mg. per day as the allowance for the adult man, 300 mg. for the adult woman. The RDA for preadolescents and adolescents vary with age. They are 300 to 400 mg. for boys and 300 to 350 mg. for girls. During pregnancy and lactation 450 mg. per day are recommended. For infants and children the allowances are based on the magnesium content of milk. This is about 4 mg. per 100 ml. human milk, 12 mg. per 100 ml. cow's milk.

Manganese

METABOLISM AND FUNCTIONS

The metabolism of manganese has been studied. In the adult human body there are only 10 to 20 mg. of manganese. It is widely distributed, with most of it in the bones, liver, pituitary, pineal, and lactating mammary glands; little in muscle.

Absorption of this mineral from the intestinal tract is rather poor and is adversely affected by large amounts of dietary calcium and phosphorus. Manganese is transported in the plasma, bound to a protein called transmanganin. Conservation of manganese is efficient. Excretion occurs through the intestines, much of it as a choline complex in the bile (1). Urinary losses are very small.

Manganese functions are associated with enzymes. It activates arginase, leucine amino peptidase, bone phosphatase, and enzymes active in oxidative phosphorylation. In animals, deficiency results in retarded growth, lessened reproductive capacity, and nerve disorders; the bones are fragile, deformed, short, and thick (2). In poultry, lack of the mineral results in a bone disorder called perosis. This disease is aggravated by lack of choline in the diet and it is known that manganese and choline are involved in both fat metabolism and skeletal development (3). Manganese has been shown to inactivate pherentasin, a vasoconstrictive compound which is a factor in hypertension (4).

This trace element is considered essential for the human being. Although no deficiency disease has been recognized in man, manganese is considered important for good nutrition. The main dietary sources of manganese are plants, with tea, coffee, blueberries, bran, dry legumes, and nuts being particularly rich. Among the poorer sources are meat, poultry, fish, eggs, dairy products, and the nonleafy vegetables.

No RDA has been set by the FNB. Several investigations have reported on intake. A study by Lang and co-workers (5) showed that a group of men on vegetarian diets containing 7.07 mg. manganese daily retained 0.04 mg. per kg. body weight. Manganese balance was secured on intakes of 3.7 mg. per day in a study by North and co-workers (6) on college women. In White's investigation (7), which included intake only, the manganese content of the diet ranged from less than 0.24 to 1.53 mg. per day.

Coons and Moyer (8), in a metabolic study of preadolescent children, found a daily intake of 2 to 3 mg. per day to be sufficient. In a more recent study on preadolescent girls, Engel and associates (9) estimated that 1.0 mg. per day was required for equilibrium, and they suggested a daily allowance of 1.25 mg. In the study of seven- to ten-year-old girls in selected southern states manganese intakes and output in feces were determined (17). On intakes of approximately 2 to 3 mg. daily manganese was retained. In Type A school lunches the average content of manganese was 0.45 mg., which was not considered a satisfactory amount (18).

Molybdenum

SOURCES AND FUNCTIONS

Traces of molybdenum are found in practically all plant and animal tissues and it is known to be an essential element. Among the food sources of available or enzyme-producing molybdenum, those containing 0.6 ppm dry weight include the legumes, cereal grains, some of the dark green leafy vegetables, and animal organs. Fruits and most root and stem vegetables contain less than 0.1 ppm.

The element is involved in the activity of several flavoproteins and is thought to facilitate the linkage of flavin nucleotide to protein. Xanthine oxidase contains one atom of molybdenum. Body parts containing comparatively large amounts of the element are the liver, kidneys, and bones; it is readily absorbed from the intestinal tract and is excreted mainly in the urine.

DANGERS OF EXCESS STUDIED IN ANIMALS

Molybdenum toxicity has been related to dietary copper and sulfate sulfur (1). In studying molybdenum, more emphasis has been placed on excess intake than on dangers from lack of the mineral. It has been demonstrated in various animal species that a high intake of this mineral promotes copper deficiency and that dietary copper and sulfate ions are related to this disturbance (2). As the molybdenum content of cattle forage increases, more copper is needed to prevent the onset of anemia (3). If molybdenum intake is high and inorganic sulfate is low, however, the copper content of the liver may be increased and anemia prevented. These relationships are complicated and not completely understood. Protein is thought to protect against molybdenum toxicity partly at least because the sulfate formed in the breakdown of body protein causes increased molybdenum excretion.

In rabbits, deformities of the joints at the extremities due to high intakes of molybdenum have been investigated. These abnormalities are not thought to be related directly to the amounts of calcium and phosphorus in the diet or to the deposition of sulfur in the cartilage, in the form of chondroitin sulfate, but to the effect molybdenum has on certain enzyme systems such as the phosphatases.

Practically all the research on molybdenum has been conducted on animals, not on human beings. It is not known whether the relationships discussed above have implications for man.

Studies on molybdenum intake have been conducted. Molybdenum balances were determined in the study of seven- to ten-year-old girls in selected southern states. Mean intakes of 76, 48, and 43 μg. resulted in balances of 5, 11, and 8 μg. Engel (4) has reported storage in six- to ten-year-old girls on intakes of approximately 100 μg. per day. The FNB believes that molybdenum may function nutritionally in man, but there are insufficient data on which to establish a daily allowance.

Sodium, Chlorine, and Potassium

SOURCES AND FUNCTIONS OF THESE MINERALS

These elements have much in common in the body and in food. Sodium, chlorine, and potassium are present in comparatively large amounts in the body—in the 70 kg. adult, about 105 gm. each of sodium and chlorine and 245 gm. of potassium. All three elements are well absorbed. Sodium occurs in greatest concentration in extracellular fluid compartments; potassium almost entirely within the cells; and chlorine in both. Some sodium is found on the surface of bone where it is relatively stable.

Studies have been made on food content and intake. Most of these studies have been made on sodium, some on potassium, few on chlorine. Among natural foods, those from animal sources are higher in sodium than those from plant sources. Relatively high levels of sodium are found in meat, fish, poultry, milk, cheese, and vegetables such as beets, carrots, celery, spinach, chard, and kale. Fruits contain less sodium than vegetables. Zook and associates (1), who analyzed 30 fresh fruits for their mineral content, found that subtropical varieties had the highest sodium and potassium values; considerable variations were found within a producing area. Nuts, grain products, and legumes are low in sodium; shortenings and salad oils contain none. Sodium is found in many prepared products such as baked goods, cereals, and canned foods.

Baking powder, baking soda, some preservatives, artificial sweeteners, and seasoning salts such as monosodium glutamate contain sodium. Some drugs are also available as sodium salts.

The sodium ion content of drinking water in approximately 2100 municipalities in the United States was determined by White and co-workers (2). Water in sections of the Far West and Midwest tended to have higher sodium content than that in other parts of the country. Of all municipalities studied, approximately 40 per cent had levels above 20 mg. sodium ion per liter. These water supplies are considered too high in sodium for use by persons on a low-sodium (500 mg.) diet.

Because ready-to-serve foods may contain considerably more sodium than is listed in a food composition table, Holinger and associates (3) analyzed 69 ready-to-serve foods which appear frequently on sodium-restricted menus. They found considerable variations in amount of sodium, due to methods used in processing, seasonal and geographic fluctuations in sodium content of the soil and of the food fed to animals, and tap water used in cooking.

Usual diets in the United States supply enough sodium, chlorine, and potassium to meet body requirements. No estimates of RDA have been set by the FNB. White (4) determined the amounts of sodium and potassium in the diets of 21 college women and 15 high school girls. In 48 diet composites, analyzed by emission spectroscopy, she found an average of 2.3 gm. sodium and 2.0 gm. potassium daily. In the Type A school lunches fed in 300 schools the sodium and potassium contents averaged 1.466 and 1.190 mg., respectively (18). These amounts are considered within the normal intake range. The seventh edition of *RDA* states that usual adult intakes of sodium and potassium are 100 to 300 meq/day and 50 to 150 meq/day. Expressed in gm. these are 2.3 to 6.9 gm. sodium (equivalent to 6 to 18 gm. sodium chloride) and 1.95 to 5.59 gm. potassium. The daily intake of chlorine is estimated to be 3 to 9 gm.

The daily intake of sodium by the infant fed cow's milk is over three times that of the breast-fed infant. At one year, according to Mayer (5), the average intake of sodium (milk and solid foods) is 6.3 meq per kilogram body weight, as compared with the requirement of one meq per kg. Today many nutritionists advise that salt not be added to baby foods by manufacturers. It is thought that large sodium intakes may be an etiologic factor in hypertension (6).

In functions, sodium, chlorine and potassium are related. With most of the body's sodium located in extracellular fluids, and most of the potassium within the cells, osmosis is made possible and a normal water balance is maintained. The adrenal hormone aldosterone is an important regulator of sodium metabolism. Sodium and potassium are involved in muscle contraction and expansion and in nerve stimulation. Acid-base balance in the blood is regulated to a great extent by the work of these three elements. Chlorine is a constituent of acid in the stomach and aids in the digestive processes. Potassium in the cells is associated with glycolysis, glycogen formation, and protein synthesis and utilization. This mineral is concerned with cellular enzyme function.

METABOLIC PROBLEMS

Under certain conditions the balance of these elements may be upset. Normally when the intakes of sodium and potassium are low, the body conserves its supply by lessening the amounts excreted in the urine. Heat and exercise favor sodium loss in perspiration; salt tablets may be prescribed to prevent excessive loss. Studies made by the Army indicate that people doing sedentary work in hot climates may need approximately 12 gm. of salt daily; for those doing eight hours of hard work, 24 gm. may be required. When more than 4 liters of water are consumed in a day, addition of 1 gm. salt per liter of water is advised.

Diarrhea and regurgitation reduce the body sodium and may upset the balance of sodium and potassium. In such cases and in other extensive fluid losses, intravenous feeding should be used with special consideration of these minerals (7). After severe infection and after surgery, excretion of both potassium and nitrogen in the urine may be expected. Studies made on children suffering from kwashiorkor indicate that depletion of body potassium may be serious (8). When edema occurs, both sodium and water are retained excessively and sodium is restricted as a control measure. Sodium restriction is a generally accepted procedure in hypertension and in many cardiac and renal diseases (9). In severe cases of hypertension, a diet containing only 250 mg. sodium daily may be prescribed. For prevention of edema in cardiac and renal diseases and for edema occurring during pregnancy, sodium intake may be restricted to 1000 mg. daily. It is interesting that in Japan, where salt intake is high (as much as 27 gm. daily in northern Japan and 17 gm. in the southern parts), hypertension is a common disease (10).

For persons on sodium-restricted diets Frank and Mickelsen (11) advocate use of a mixture of sodium- and potassium chloride in place of common salt. Potassium chloride, sometimes used alone, has a bitter, unpleasant flavor, but the mixture of the two salts is palatable. More to the point, it is thought that for a person with hypertension decreasing the Na:K ratio is as important as decreasing the sodium intake.

Sulfur

SOURCES AND FUNCTIONS

Although usually associated with protein needs, sulfur has other functions. The importance of sulfur in relation to protein is due to the sulfur-containing amino acids, methionine, cystine, and cysteine; these were discussed in Chapter 6. Other sulfur-containing nutrients required in the diet are thiamin, coenzyme A, and biotin (see Chapter 12). Compounds containing sulfur include glutathione, lipoic acid, and taurine; pharmacologic agents containing sulfur are sulfa drugs, penicillin, and thiouracil. The sulfur content of foods is not usually included in food composition tables. Among the foods with comparatively large amounts of this mineral are meat, fish, poultry, and eggs, due to their protein content, and certain vegetables, the legumes and members of the Brassica family.

Organic sulfur is better utilized by the body than inorganic, but both are important (1). The availability of the latter is related to the ratio between the two forms. Both contribute to the body's pool of sulfate. Sulfur compounds are important in connective tissue metabolism. Chondroitin sulfates are synthesized in the cartilage; these sulfates are mucopolysaccharides. Lack of dietary sulfate decreases the collagen-forming activity of the fibroblasts (2) in connective tissue.

Although usually considered only as a substitute for methionine, cystine appears to have a function in muscle metabolism which methionine cannot perform; this relates to the prevention of muscular dystrophy in chicks fed a diet deficient in vitamin E (3). The relationship of sulfate to molybdenum was mentioned on page 183.

It is assumed that a person's sulfur requirement is met when the protein intake is adequate. In the United States there is little cause for concern over a lack of this mineral. No RDA for sulfur has been set. In the study on metabolic patterns of seven- to ten-year-old girls in selected southern states 12 subjects were used in assessing sulfur metabolism. On intakes of 237.7 and 270.7 mg. sulfur the balances were 32.5 and 34.3 mg., respectively.

Trace Elements Associated with Vitamins

SELENIUM AND VITAMIN E

Selenium is of interest mainly because it is associated with vitamin E (1). The early concern over selenium resulted from its toxic effects when it occurred at relatively high levels in grains and forage crops eaten by grazing livestock. However, in 1958 Schwarz and Foltz (2) discovered that trace amounts of selenium protected against liver necrosis in rats fed a diet lacking in vitamin E. Since then a variety of animal diseases have been cured with selenium. The mineral occurs in both organic and inorganic forms. It has high potency when combined with cystine and vitamin E; this factor is called Factor 3.

No selenium deficiency disease is known in man. However, children with kwashiorkor who failed to respond to other treatment grew when given selenium supplements (3). Selenium blood levels were lowered in children with kwashiorkor, and it is thought that such children have lower than normal stores of the mineral.

Selenium occurs in very small amounts in the body and in most foods. Selenium and sulfur have much in common and are interchangeable in some plant and micro-organism processes. Selenium is thought to act as a nonspecific antitoxidant (4). Little is known about the site of action and chemical nature. Although selenium and vitamin E are closely related in some of their actions, the two nutrients have some independent functions. The role of the mineral in protein biosynthesis is being investigated.

COBALT

Cobalt is an integral part of vitamin B_{12}. Sheep and cattle raised in Australia and other parts of the world on cobalt-deficient pastures develop a disease once thought to be a simple cobalt lack, now known to be a vitamin B_{12} deficiency. This vitamin contains about 4 per cent cobalt. Bacteria in the rumen of animals synthesize the vitamin when the diet contains enough cobalt and the vitamin is then absorbed. When the fodder is deficient in cobalt the vitamin lack is evident.

In man this synthesis occurs in the colon where absorption is minimal, if any. Therefore, to be of nutritional value to the human being, cobalt must be ingested as the preformed vitamin. The need for cobalt, other than as vitamin B_{12}, is not known. The usual diet supplies from 5 to 8 μg. cobalt; comparatively little is absorbed. In the study of metabolic patterns of seven- to ten-year-old girls in selected southern states daily intakes of 8.6 and 8.0 μg. cobalt resulted in balances of 0.9 and 0.3 μg., respectively. Small amounts are found in the red blood cells and plasma, and some storage takes place in the liver, kidneys, pancreas, and spleen. Excretion is largely in the urine. Because erythropoesis is improved when cobalt is administered in therapeutic doses, the mineral sometimes is used in treatment of some anemias. However, cobalt therapy has produced unpleasant side-effects in some instances and permanent benefit has not always followed treatment.

ZINC

The amount of zinc in the human body is considerably larger than that of most other trace elements. The human body contains about 2 gm. of zinc; comparatively large amounts are found in the liver, voluntary muscle, and bone. The iris, retina, and lens of the eye and the corneal epithelium are high in this mineral, as are the prostate gland and its secretions and spermatozoa. Zinc is found in the teeth, especially in the outer surface of the enamel. The insulin molecule contains about 0.3 per cent zinc.

Human blood contains about 900 μg. of zinc per ml. in plasma, erythrocytes, and leucocytes. The mineral may be bound to protein and often is found associated with enzymes. Under ordinary circumstances, the levels of zinc in the blood are relatively stable. Excretion of zinc occurs largely through the gastrointestinal tract; little is lost in urine.

The functions of zinc and the effects of lack have been investigated. Zinc is a constituent of 15 to 20 enzymes. It is thought that zinc levels in the cells are responsible for formation and regulation of these enzymes (1). The primary site of zinc action is in tissue that has an extremely high turnover rate or where zinc is freely exchangeable. Studies on rats by Reinhold and Kfoury (2) indicate that in zinc depletion the structure of intestinal alkaline phosphatase is modified. Other zinc-containing enzymes have been studied to clarify the mineral's functions (3).

Carbonic anhydrase, present in the erythrocytes and in other parts of the body, aids in carbon dioxide transport. Carboxypeptidase is involved in the breakdown of peptides into amino acids in the intestinal tract. One of the four zinc-containing dehydrogenases oxidizes vitamin A and reduces retinal.

Symptoms of zinc deficiency were first noted in animals. In swine these included growth retardation and a dermatitis called parakeratosis. In rats the hair coat is thin and rough, and growth is very poor. Testicular atrophy is a common symptom in the male rat, as is failure of the reproductive processes in the female (4): few young born to zinc-deficient females live.

Man's need for zinc was not noted until 1961. Clinical signs of zinc deficiency in people living in Iran and Egypt included short stature, marked hypogonadism, hepatosplenomegaly, and anemia (5). Since the diet of these persons consisted primarily of bread made of wheat flour and was negligible in animal protein, they were given supplements of zinc, iron, or animal protein to determine the cause of the trouble. Improvement in sexual characteristics resulted only in the group given zinc. The anemia was found to be due to iron lack, and it responded to iron supplementation. A six-year follow-up (6) on nine of the 13 people originally studied indicated that the abnormalities had disappeared or were much ameliorated in those only on the supplemented diet. In those whose diet remained poor the syndrome continued unabated. This indicated the nutritional origin and reversible nature of the disorder.

In 1969 a pilot experiment on controlled zinc supplementation for 60 malnourished school boys from a rural Iranian area was reported by Ronaghy and associates (7). In all these boys height was below the third percentile of the Iowa growth standard. Three groups were given supplements of placebo, iron, or zinc in capsule form for five months. A seven-month period of no supplementation followed, and then another five months of supplementation. The boys of 12 to 14 years were studied particularly for changes in height, weight, bone development, and sexual maturation. The zinc-supplemented group showed greater progress toward normal for their age, in all respects, than did those receiving placebo or iron. In respect to sexual maturation the increases were statistically highly significant in the zinc group.

Studies have been made of the effects of some nutrients on the availability of zinc (8). The fact that the diet of the Iranians was low in animal protein and high in foods of plant origin, especially grains and legumes, led to studies on protein. Preliminary results of an experiment on chicks indicate that only about 60 per cent of the zinc in cereals and oilseed meals is available for use. The zinc from animal products is known to be utilized more readily than that from plant seeds. It has been suggested that zinc may take part in the pathogenesis of kwashiorkor and marasmus (9). Sandstead (10) found that the serum zinc levels of subjects suffering from kwashiorkor were less than half the normal levels.

A relationship between zinc and calcium is indicated, especially when the diet is based largely on plant seeds. These contain phytate which binds zinc and decreases its availability. When the diet is high in calcium, phytate results in even more zinc-binding.

In the United States there is little danger of zinc lack. This element is widely distributed in foods. Among the better sources are oysters, seafood, liver, wheat germ, and yeast. Green leafy vegetables, fruits, whole grains, meat, and fish are good sources of zinc.

A few studies have been made on intake and output. White (11), who analyzed the diets of high school girls and college women for zinc, found mean daily intakes of 12 mg. for the former, 13.8 mg. for the latter. Coons and Moyer (12) reported intakes of 6.5 to 9.0 mg. zinc per day for preadolescent girls. College women on an average intake of 13.2 mg. zinc per day had a retention of 6.6 mg., and losses of 6.6 mg. in urine and feces. In the study of metabolic patterns of seven- to ten-year-old girls in selected southern states daily intakes of 6.61 mg. or more zinc resulted in positive balances (17). Assuming that seven- to nine-year-old children require 6 mg. zinc daily, the Type A school lunches served in 300 schools were judged adequate. Only five of the samples analyzed had less than 2 mg., one-third of the day's requirement (18).

The FNB considers daily intakes of 10–15 mg. by adults in the United States to be adequate. The usual American diet tends to be low in phytate too, and contains enough animal protein to satisfy the dietary needs for zinc. A strictly vegetarian diet might be inadequate.

REFERENCES

Chromium

1. Hopkins, L. L., Jr. Distribution in the Rat of Physiological Amounts of Injected Chromium[51] (111) with Time. *Am. J. Physiol., 209:*731 (1965).

2. Mertz, W., *et al.* Biological Activity and Fate of Trace Quantities of Intravenous Chromium (111) in the Rat. *Am. J. Physiol., 209:*489 (1965).

3. Schwarz, K., *et al.* Chromium (111) and the Glucose Tolerance Factor. *Arch. Biochem. Biophy., 85:*292 (1959).

4. Schroeder, H. A. Chromium Deficiency in Rats: A Syndrome Simulating Diabetes Mellitus with Retarded Growth. *J. Nutr., 88:*439 (1966).

5. Mertz, W., *et al.* Effects of Chromium (111) Supplementation on Growth and Survival Under Stress in Rats Fed a Low Protein Diet. *J. Nutr., 97:*531 (1969).

6. Roginski, E. E., *et al.* Effects of Chromium (111) Supplementation on Glucose and Amino Acid Metabolism in Rats Fed a Low Protein Diet. *J. Nutr., 97:*525 (1969).

7. Schroeder, H. A. Cadmium, Chromium, and Cardiovascular Disease. *Circul., 35:*570 (1967).

8. Schroeder, H. A. Serum Cholesterol and Glucose Levels in Rats Fed Refined and Less Refined Sugars and Chromium. *J. Nutr., 97:*237 (1969).

9. Glinsman, W. H., *et al.* Plasma Chromium after Glucose Administration. *Sci., 152:*1234 (1966).

10. Hambidge, K. H., *et al.* Concentration of Chromium in the Hair of Normal Children and Children with Juvenile Diabetes Mellitus. *Diabetes, 17:*517 (1968).

11. Hopkins, L. L., Jr., *et al.* Normalization of Impaired Glucose Utilization and Hypoglycemia by Chromium (111) in Malnourished Infants. *Fed. Proc., 25:*303 (1966).

Copper

1. Dowdy, R. P. Copper Metabolism. *Am. J. Clin. Nutr., 22:*887 (1969).

2. Frieden, E. Ceruloplasmin, A Link Between Copper and Iron Metabolism. *Nutr. Revs., 28:*87 (1970).

3. Cartwright, G. E., *et al.* Copper Metabolism in Normal Subjects. *Am. J. Clin. Nutr., 14:*224 (1964).

4. Hill, C. H. A Role of Copper in Elastin Formation. *Nutr. Revs., 27:*99 (1969).

5. Moore, T. Vitamin A and Copper. *Am. J. Clin. Nutr., 22:*1017 (1969).

6. Dowdy, R. P., *et al.* Copper-Molybdenum Interaction in Sheep and Chicks, *J. Nutr., 95:*191; 197 (1968).

7. Hook, L., *et al.* Copper Content of Some Low-Copper Foods. *J. Am. Diet. Ass., 49:*202 (1966).

8. Questions and Answers. Copper Cooking Utensils and Piping. *J. Am. Med. Ass., 200:*426 (1967).

9. Engel, A. W., *et al.* Copper, Manganese, Cobalt and Molybdenum Balance in Preadolescent Girls. *J. Nutr., 92:*197 (1967).

10. White, H. S. Inorganic Elements in Weighed Diets of Girls and Young Women. *J. Am. Diet. Ass., 55:*38 (1969).

11. Cordano, A., *et al.* Copper Deficiency in Infancy. *Pediat., 34:*324 (1964).

Fluorine

1. Waldbott, G. L. Fluoride in Foods. *Am. J. Clin. Nutr., 12:*455 (1963).
2. Hill, I. N., *et al.* Evanston Fluoridation Study: Twelve Years Later. *Dent. Progress, 1:*95 (1961).
3. Bernstein, D. S., *et al.* Prevalence of Osteoporosis in High- and Low-Fluoride Areas of North Dakota. *J. Am. Med. Ass., 198:*499 (1966).
4. Korns, R. F. Relationship of Water Fluoridation to Bone Density in Two New York Towns. *Pub. Health Reports, 84:*815 (1969).
5. Spencer, H., *et al.* Effects of Sodium Fluoride on Calcium Absorption and Balance in Man. *Am. J. Clin. Nutr., 22:*381 (1969).
6. Division of Dental Health, Public Health Service. *Fluoridation Census, 1969.* Washington, D.C.: U.S. Dept. of Health, Education and Welfare (1970).
7. Burgstahler, A. W., *et. al.* Letters to the Editor. *Am. J. Clin. Nutr., 22:*1340 (1969).
8. Rubini, M. E. Fluoridation: The Unpopular Controversy. *Am. J. Clin. Nutr., 22:*1343 (1969).
9. Bronner, F. Fluoridation—Issue or Obsession? *Am. J. Clin. Nutr., 22:*1346 (1969).
10. Sapolsky, H. M. Social Science Views of a Controversy in Science and Politics. *Am. J. Clin. Nutr., 22:*1397 (1969).
11. Waldbott, G. L. Biological Action of Fluoride. *Am. J. Clin. Nutr., 22:*1407 (1969).

Magnesium

1. Anast, C. S. Serum Magnesium Levels in the Newborn. *Pediat., 33:*969 (1964).
2. Pretorius, P. J., *et al.* Magnesium Balance Studies in South African Bantu Children with Kwashiorkor. *Am. J. Clin. Nutr., 13:*331 (1963).
3. Sullivan, J. F., *et al.* Magnesium Metabolism in Alcohol. *Am. J. Clin. Nutr., 13:*297 (1963).
4. McCollister, R. J., *et al.* Urinary Excretion of Magnesium in Man Following the Ingestion of Ethanol. *Am. J. Clin. Nutr., 12:*415 (1963).
5. Zieve, L., *et al.* Effect of Magnesium Deficiency on Growth Response in Thiamine-Deficient Rats. *J. Lab. Clin. Med., 72:*261 (1968).
6. Shils, M. E. Experimental Human Magnesium Depletion. 1. Clinical Observations and Blood Chemistry. *Am. J. Clin. Nutr., 15:*133 (1964).
7. Hellerstein, E. E., *et al.* Studies on the Interrelationships Between Dietary Magnesium, Quality and Quantity of Fat, Hypercholesterolemia, and Lipidosis. *J. Nutr., 71:*339 (1960).
8. Zook, E. G., *et al.* Mineral Composition of Fruits. *J. Am. Diet. Ass., 52:*225 (1968).

9. Agricultural Research Service, USDA, Consumer and Food Economics Research Division. Household Food Consumption Survey, 1965–66.

10. Manalo, R., *et al.* A Simple Method for Estimating Dietary Magnesium. *Am. J. Clin. Nutr., 20:*627 (1967).

11. White, H. S. Inorganic Elements in Weighed Diets of Girls and Young Women. *J. Am. Diet. Ass., 55:*38 (1969).

12. Leichsenring, J. M., *et al.* Magnesium Metabolism in College Women: Observations on the Effect of Calcium and Phosphorus Intake Levels. *J. Nutr., 45:*477 (1951).

13. Scoular, F. I., *et al.* The Calcium, Phosphorus, and Magnesium Balances of Young College Women Consuming Self-Selected Diets. *J. Nutr., 62:*489 (1957).

14. Leverton, R. M., *et al.* Magnesium Requirements of Young Women Receiving Controlled Intakes. *J. Nutr., 74:*33 (1961). .

15. Seelig, M. S. The Requirement of Magnesium by the Normal Adult. *Am. J. Clin. Nutr., 14:*342 (1964).

16. Hunt, S. M., *et al.* Magnesium Balance and Protein Intake Level in the Adult Female. *Am. J. Clin. Nutr., 22:*367 (1969).

Manganese

1. Speckman, E. W., *et al.* Relationships Between Fat and Mineral Metabolism—A Review. *J. Am. Diet. Ass., 51:*517 (1967).

2. Cotzias, G. C. Metabolic Relations of Manganese to Other Minerals. *Fed. Proc., 19:*655 (1960).

3. Tal, E., *et al.* Effect of Manganese on Calcification of Bone. *Biochem. J., 95:*94 (1965).

4. Schroeder, H. A., *et al.* Pressor Substances in Arterial Hypertension. 5. Chemical and Pharmacological Characteristics of Pherentasin. *J. Expl. Med., 102:*319 (1955).

5. Lang, V. M., *et al.* Manganese Metabolism in College Men Consuming Vegetarian Diets. *J. Nutr., 85:*132 (1965).

6. North, B. B., *et al.* Manganese Metabolism in College Women. *J. Nutr., 72:*217 (1960).

7. White, H. S. Inorganic Elements in Weighed Diets of Girls and Young Women. *J. Am. Diet. Ass., 55:*38 (1969).

8. Coons, C. M., *et al.* Minor Minerals and B-Vitamins: Metabolic Patterns in Pre-adolescent Children. *Fed. Proc., 19:*1017 (1960).

9. Engel, A. W., *et al.* Copper, Manganese, Cobalt and Molybdenum Balances in Pre-adolescent Girls. *J. Nutr., 92:*197 (1967).

Molybdenum

1. Miller, R. P., *et al.* Interrelation of Copper, Molybdenum and Sulfate Sulfur in Nutrition. *Fed. Proc., 19:*666 (1960).

2. Arthur, D. Interrelationships of Molybdenum and Copper in the Diet of the Guinea Pig. *J. Nutr., 87:*69 (1965).

3. Dowdy, R. P., *et al.* Copper-Molybdenum Interaction in Sheep and Chicks. *J. Nutr., 95:*191; 197 (1968).

4. Engel, A. W., *et al.* Copper, Manganese, Cobalt and Molybdenum Balances in Pre-adolescent Girls. *J. Nutr., 92:*197 (1967).

Sodium, Chlorine, and Potassium

1. Zook, E. G., *et al.* Mineral Composition of Fresh Fruits. *J. Am. Diet. Ass., 52:*225 (1968).

2. White, J. M., *et al.* Sodium Ion in Drinking Water. 1. Properties, Analysis and Occurrence. *J. Am. Diet. Ass., 50:*32 (1967).

3. Holinger, B. W., *et al.* Analyzed Sodium Values in Foods Ready to Serve. *J. Am. Diet. Ass., 48:*501 (1966).

4. White, H. S. Inorganic Elements in Weighed Diets of Girls and Young Women. *J. Am. Diet. Ass., 55:*38 (1969).

5. Mayer, J. Hypertension, Salt Intake and the Infant. *Postgrad. Med., 45:*229 (1969).

6. Puyau, F. A., *et al.* Infant Feeding Practices 1966. *Am. J. Dis. Childr., 111:*370 (1966).

7. Editorial. Potassium Therapy: A Boon and a Hazard. *J. Am. Med. Ass., 180:*775 (1962).

8. Metcoff, J. Cell Composition and Metabolism in Kwashiorkor. *Med., 45:*365 (1966).

9. Cooper, S. A., *et al.* Sodium Ion in Drinking Water. II. Importance, Problems, and Potential Applications of Sodium-Restricted Therapy. *J. Am. Diet. Ass., 50:*37 (1967).

10. Dahl, L. K. Salt, Fat, and Hypertension: The Japanese Experience. *Nutr. Revs., 18:*97 (1960).

11. Frank, R. L., *et al.* Sodium-Potassium Chloride Mixtures as Table Salt. *Am. J. Clin. Nutr., 22:*464 (1969).

Sulfur

1. Michels, F. G., *et al.* A Comparison of the Utilization of Organic and Inorganic Sulfur by the Rat. *J. Nutr., 87:*217 (1965).

2. Brown, R. G., *et al.* Changes in Collagen Metabolism Caused by Feeding Diets Low in Inorganic Sulfur. *J. Nutr., 87:*229 (1965).

3. Scott, M. L., *et al.* Abstracts of the Fifth International Congress of Nutrition. Washington, D.C., 1960, p. 77.

Selenium

1. Schwarz, K. Role of Vitamin E, Selenium and Related Factors in Experimental Nutritional Liver Disease. *Fed. Proc., 24:*58 (1965).

2. Schwarz, K., *et al.* Factor 3 Activity of Selenium Compounds. *J. Biol. Chem., 233:*245 (1968).

3. Burk, R. F., *et al.* Blood Selenium Levels and *in vitro* Red Blood Cell Uptake of [75]Selenium in Kwashiorkor. *Am. J. Clin. Nutr., 20:*723 (1967).

4. Tappel, A. L. Free-Radical Lipid Peroxidation Damage and Its Inhibition by Vitamin E and Selenium. *Fed. Proc., 24:*73 (1965).

Zinc

1. Leucke, R. W., *et al.* Zinc Deficiency in the Rat: Effect on Serum and Intestinal Alkaline Phosphatase Activity. *J. Nutr., 94:*344 (1968).
2. Reinhold, J. S., *et al.* Zinc-Dependent Enzymes in Zinc-Depleted Rats: Intestinal Alkaline Phosphatase. *Am. J. Clin. Nutr., 22:*1250 (1969).
3. Parisi, A. F., *et al.* Zinc Metalloenzymes: Characteristics and Significance in Biology and Medicine. *Am. J. Clin. Nutr., 22:*1222 (1969).
4. Afgar, J. Effect of Zinc Deficiency on Parturition in the Rat. *Am. J. Physiol., 215:*160 (1968).
5. Prasad, A. G., *et al.* Syndrome of Iron Deficiency Anemia, Hepatosplenomegaly, Hypogonadism, Dwarfism, and Geophagia. *Am. J. Med., 31:*532 (1961).
6. Ronaghy, H., *et al.* A Six-Year Follow-up of Iranian Patients with Dwarfism, Hypogonadism, and Iron-Deficiency Anemia. *Am. J. Clin. Nutr., 21:*709 (1968).
7. Ronaghy, H., *et al.* Controlled Zinc Supplementation for Malnourished School Boys with Zinc: A Pilot Experiment. *Am. J. Clin. Nutr., 22:*1279 (1969).
8. O'Dell, B. L. Effect of Dietary Components upon Zinc Availability. *Am. J. Clin. Nutr., 22:*1315 (1969).
9. Oberleas, D., *et al.* Growth as Affected by Zinc and Protein Nutrition. *Am. J. Clin. Nutr., 22:*1304 (1969).
10. Sandstead, H. H., *et al.* Human Zinc Deficiency, Endocrine Manifestations, and Response to Treatment. *Am. J. Clin. Nutr., 20:*422 (1967).
11. White, H. S. Inorganic Elements in Weighed Diets of Girls and Young Women. *J. Am. Diet. Ass., 55:*38 (1969).
12. Coons, C. M., *et al.* Minor Minerals and B-Vitamins. Metabolism Patterns in Preadolescent Children. *Fed. Proc., 19:*1017 (1960).

GENERAL REFERENCES

17. Moyer, E. Z., *et al. Basic Data on Metabolic Patterns in 7- to 10-Year-Old Girls in Selected Southern States.* Home Econ. Research Rept. 33. ARS, USDA (1967).
18. Murphy, W. W., *et al.,* Regional Variations in Vitamin and Trace Element Content of Type A School Lunches. Proceedings, Fourth Annual Conference on Trace Substances in Environmental Health. University of Missouri (1970).
19. *Present Knowledge in Nutrition,* 3rd ed. New York: Nutrition Foundation (1967).
   Sandstead, H. H., Present Knowledge of the Minerals, p. 117.
   Peden, J. C., Present Knowledge of Copper, p. 129.
   Shaw, J. H., Present Knowledge of Fluoride, p. 130.

Levander, O. A., Present Knowledge of Selenium, p. 138.

Hoekstra, W. G., Present Knowledge of Zinc, p. 141.

Hegsted, D. M., Present Knowledge of Magnesium, p. 152.

20. Ting-Kai Li, *et al.* The Biochemical and Nutritional Role of Trace Elements. *In* M. G. Wohl and R. S. Goodhart (eds.), *Modern Nutrition in Health and Disease,* 4th ed. Philadelphia: Lea and Febiger (1968).

21. Wacker, W. E. C. Magnesium Metabolism. *New Eng. J. Med., 278:*658, 712, 772 (1968).

22. World Health Organization of the United Nations. Fluorides and Human Health. WHO Monograph Series No. 59. Geneva: WHO (1970).

Fat-Soluble Vitamins

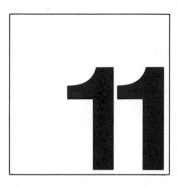

Since 1911 when Casimir Funk first coined the word "vitamine," scientists have been investigating the chemical nature and physiological functions of an increasing number of compounds which may be classified in this category of foodstuffs. According to McCollum, "the vitamins participate as components of catalysts which enable the more inert chemical substances, serving as raw materials for the fabrication of living tissues, to undergo the changes which come under the term metabolism."

Vitamin research is progressing rapidly, in both technical investigations in the biochemical laboratory and practical surveys and studies in clinic and community. For the four fat-soluble vitamins the basic problems of chemical nature and metabolism continue to challenge the researcher. As more is learned it is evident that lack of these vitamins is a problem of practical concern among many persons in both developed and developing countries.

Vitamin A

THE CHEMISTRY AND METABOLISM OF VITAMIN A

Vitamin A exists in various forms. When discovered in 1913, vitamin A was shown to be a fat-soluble substance. Since then chemists have been actively studying its nature. In 1931 it was isolated and its structure determined. Its synthesis was achieved in 1946. By 1949 synthetic vitamin A was on the market. In 1968 the annual requirement for one person cost only five cents.

Vitamin A exists in *trans* and *cis* forms; those predominant in nature have the all-*trans* configuration. Stereoisometric forms with a *cis* configuration are less potent. The various isomers of vitamin A have been studied by means of chromotography and spectrophotometry; some of these isomers react slowly, some fast. Forms containing an extra double bond

197

are designated as vitamin A_2 and are found in greater proportion in fresh-water fish and predatory fish. Vitamin A_1, predominating in salt-water fish and fish of vegetarian habits, occurs as an alcohol ($C_{20}H_{29}OH$) (Figure 11–1). Both forms contain a β-ionine ring and a polyene chain

Figure 11–1
Structural formula of vitamin A_1 (retinol)

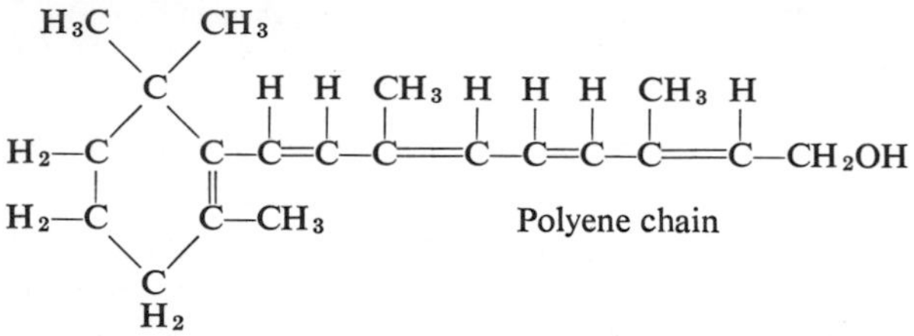

which are considered essential for biological activity. In crystalline form vitamin A is pale yellow.

The vitamin A_1 terms approved for use today are retinol (vitamin A_1 alcohol), retinal (vitamin A_1 aldehyde), and retinoic acid (vitamin A_1 acid). The vitamin A_2 forms have the prefix 3-dehydro. The general term "vitamin A" will be used in this section except in instances where differentiation is necessary.

The carotenoid pigments are related to vitamin A. The relationship of plant carotenoids to vitamin A was shown by Steenbock (1) in 1919. These plant precursors contribute to the vitamin A value of a food and, in a popular manner, frequently are referred to as the vitamin itself, although technically this is incorrect. Of the plant precursors, β-carotene is the most important since it has the highest vitamin A activity and occurs most plentifully in foods. Theoretically, on conversion it could produce two molecules of vitamin A, whereas α- and γ-carotene and cryptoxanthine yield only one molecule. However, in human beings the biologic activity of the carotenes is one-half or less than that of vitamin A, due in part to the extremely variable availability of some of them and the low efficiency of conversion. Beta-carotene is a dark-red crystalline compound (Figure 11–2).

Vitamins A_1 and A_2 and the carotenoid pigments can be distinguished in the spectroscope by their absorption bands. Vitamin A_1 has its absorption maximum at 328 $m\mu$, vitamin A_2 has two distinct bands at 280 and 350 $m\mu$, and the carotenoids which are convertible to vitamin A show distinctive bands in the visible region of the spectrum. These characteristics permit their differentiation in some food materials.

The carotenoid pigments, comparatively stable compounds, are labile on exposure to radiation, especially when in liquid form and when asso-

Figure 11–2
Structural formula of β-carotene

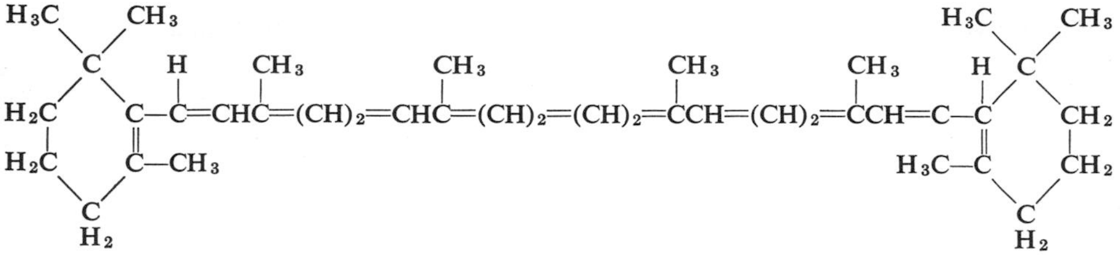

ciated with free radicals or peroxides; films in the solid state are thought to be more stable.

The comparative stability of vitamin A as it is found in foods is a safeguard to health. Because vitamin A and its precursors are soluble in fat and fat solvents and not in water, there is little likelihood of loss by solution in cookery. In spite of the high degree of unsaturation of the molecule, vitamin A is comparatively stable at ordinary cooking temperatures. No doubt this is due to the presence of antioxidants in the food.

Vitamin A is stable to heat, acid, and alkali; loss by oxidation and by exposure to ultraviolet light can be great. When fats become rancid, the vitamin is destroyed. This is thought to be due to formation of peroxide linkages which act as oxidizing agents. Antioxidants are present in many natural oils, but these are removed to a considerable extent by refining processes. To prevent such vitamin A losses, fats and oils should be kept in dark containers in a cold place. Four per cent lecithin or 2 per cent tocopherol may be incorporated commercially to prevent oxidation. Vitamin A esters are more stable than the free alcohol; protein, amino acids, and fatty acids may be used in esterification.

Vitamin A is found in many parts of the body. This vitamin is sometimes referred to as a "complex" because it occurs in the body in the forms of retinol, retinal, and retinoic acid. Leitner, Moore, and Sharman (2) studied the blood levels of vitamin A and carotene in a large group of men and women. They found no sex difference for carotene but higher values for vitamin A in men than women, and an increase in vitamin A in both sexes with age.

Approximately 90 per cent of the vitamin is found in the liver. Some is stored in the kidneys, and with a liberal intake, it may also be found in the lungs, adrenal glands, and fat deposits. In experiments on rats it was found that maximal storage of vitamin A occurred in the animal's body at maturity and when there had been a liberal intake of the factor throughout the growth period. In the retina retinal combines with the protein opsin to form the pigment rhodopsin; the amount here represents only about 0.1 per cent of the total body vitamin A.

The carotenes and various forms of vitamin A are metabolized in preparation for use by the body (3, 4). The carotenes present in food are cleaved in the intestinal mucosa by dioxygenase, an enzyme which requires molecular oxygen. In the cleavage, retinal is formed which is then reduced to retinol. Vitamin A is present in food mainly as its palmitate ester, which is hydrolyzed to retinol in the lumen of the small intestine by an enzyme of the pancreatic juice. Bile salts are necessary for activation of this enzyme and for formation of a micelle suitable for absorption. In the intestinal mucosa most of the retinol is re-esterified, incorporated into the chylomicra, and transported by the lymph to the liver and adipose tissues. Small amounts of retinol may be oxidized to retinal and then to retinoic acid, which may be converted to glucuronides and absorbed through the portal circulation. It is now thought that some retinol, retinal, and retinoic acid may be absorbed as such through the portal route.

A specific protein is necessary for retinol transport. This protein, reported by Goodman (5), has a molecular weight of about 21,000 and binds one mole of retinol per mole of protein. In this form retinol is carried to the liver and to the various tissues. Retinol is stored in ester form within the liver. Retinoic acid is not stored but most of it, as a glucuronide, is taken up by bile. Some of the retinol and retinoic acid in the liver may be decarboxylated and it is thought that the products formed may retain some biological activity. Vitamin A metabolites are excreted largely from the bile into the feces; small amounts are excreted in urine.

THE FUNCTIONS OF VITAMIN A

The part played by vitamin A in vision is well known. The retina of the eye has two kinds of light receptors. The cones in the center contain the pigment iodopsin or visual violet and are associated with bright light or photopic vision. The remainder of the retina has cones and rods, the proportion of the rods increasing as the periphery is reached. The photoreceptor substance in the rods is called rhodopsin or visual purple and is associated with scotopic or dim light vision. Both 11-*cis*-retinal and 11-*cis*-3-dehydro retinal combine with opsin in the human eye to form rhodopsin. This action takes place in the dark. The pigment breaks down in the presence of light and is rebuilt in the dark. Some vitamin A is used in the reaction and, unless there is a sufficient supply in the diet or in the body, rod vision is impaired and night blindness results. A person's light threshold, which may be related to vitamin A metabolism, can be measured. It has been demonstrated that retinoic acid has no visual function. If it is fed instead of retinol or retinal, blindness ensues.

Growth and reproduction are affected by various forms of vitamin A. The relationship of vitamin A to growth was the first function studied by Osborne and Mendel at Yale, McCollum and Davis at Wisconsin, and

Sherman and his associates at Columbia (6). The latter group conducted a good deal of research on various phases of this relationship. In their studies rats received a diet containing an adequate amount of vitamin A until they reached specified ages. The animals were then placed in four groups, one of which was given a diet which had no vitamin A; the other three groups received a diet supplemented with varying amounts of cod liver oil. Growth and the length of time the rats survived depended on two variables. First was the age at which depletion of vitamin A began. With a longer preliminary period which permitted greater body storage the rats were able to prolong the time during which growth and survival could continue. Second was the amount of vitamin A the animals received. Survival time was related to this variable also. The rats receiving the largest cod liver oil supplement lived the longest. The relationship between growth and survival has been demonstrated in other studies.

Today it is known that retinol promotes growth and that a diet lacking retinol prevents reproduction in rats. In the male, spermatogenesis stops; in the female, fetal resorption results. When retinoic acid is fed in place of retinol, the rat grows normally and mated females conceive. However, their fetuses invariably resorb. Thompson and co-workers (7) investigated the relationship of the chemical structure of vitamin A to the early development of the chick embryo. Baby chicks fed retinoic acid grew well. The hens produced eggs, and fertility was high after artificial insemination, but the eggs from hens fed retinoic acid always failed to hatch. The abnormalities occurring in these eggs were found to be due to the hens' failure to transfer retinoic acid to their eggs. The embryo became deficient in vitamin A and died. These studies indicate a specific role of retinol in the embryo's development.

Optimal storage of vitamin A in the liver is important since normal development of fetal tissue may be affected adversely by a prenatal diet low in the factor. When the food of pregnant rats was deficient in vitamin A, Warkany and co-workers (8) found that the young at birth had congenital malformations; these defects occurred in both skeletal and soft tissues. Parts frequently affected included the tibia, mandible, ribs, eyes, and cardiovascular system. It also has been shown that the offspring of cows fed a diet low in vitamin A developed eye abnormalities and paralysis.

However, it is known that man has a comparatively short organogenetic period, the time when most malformations are determined. The first trimester of pregnancy is considered the critical period and lack of vitamin A then may cause miscarriage. A specific relationship between dietary lack and congenital malformations in human beings has not been demonstrated and, according to Warkany, is difficult to prove.

Specific functions of vitamin A are related to various body tissues. Vitamin A is thought to play a fundamental role at the cellular level and to maintain the mucopolysaccharide structure of the cell. It influences several enzyme systems and for a time it was thought to serve as a co-enzyme in these reactions but this is not now considered probable. The vitamin causes release of a proteolytic enzyme from intracellular particles called lysosomes, which are similar in size to mitochondria. This release stimulates secretion of mucus by the epithelia. The tracts and organs of the body are lined with epithelial cells which protect and keep healthy the various parts. Studies made on the eyes, certain glands, and the respiratory and genitourinary tracts indicate that when vitamin A is lacking these cells change form, becoming stratified and keratinized, and the cilia normally present in the tracts are lost.

In the young of a species the eyes may be the first body part to be affected by lack of vitamin A. Biomicroscopic examination will show ocular lesions, a condition known as xerosis conjunctivae. This is the early stage of a condition which is later recognized as xerophthalmia.

In older animals the lungs frequently are affected. A correlation between the amount of vitamin A in the diet and the prevalence of tuberculosis has been noted in human beings. Sinus trouble and kidney and bladder disorders may also arise as a result of epithelium abnormalities during avitaminosis A.*

Lucy, Luscombe, and Dingle (9) investigated the effects of retinol and retinoic acid on the structure of cell membranes. Their work indicates that retinol may have a major function as a stabilizing effect on structural integrity and normal permeability of cell membranes and membranes of subcellular particles.

In studying the possible relationship of vitamin A to infection Bieri (10) used germfree rats. He found that conventional rats on a vitamin A-free diet died rapidly as compared with germfree rats on the same diet. He believes that this survival difference is due to bacterial infection. However, most of the germfree rats on a vitamin A-free diet had urinary bladder stones; many had hemorrhagic lung areas and respiratory failure related to extensive keratinization of epithelial tissue. These symptoms indicate that vitamin A has a primary anti-infection function.

Studies on human beings have shown that during acute infection both the serum levels of vitamin A and the reserves of the factor in the liver decrease. This has been demonstrated in patients with rheumatic fever, pneumonia, abscesses, tonsillitis, and other febrile diseases. It is thought that these decreases may indicate increased need for vitamin A by other tissues during an infection, or possibly increased destruction of the vitamin.

It has been shown that retinol and retinoic acid take part in corticosterone synthesis. Production of cortical steroids is depressed on vitamin

* The term "avitaminosis" is used to indicate a condition or state caused by the lack of a vitamin.

A-deficient diets. When the factor is added, normal formation is renewed.

Teeth, bones, and the nervous system may be affected by lack of vitamin A. Because changes in body weight are easily assessed in rat experiments, the requirement for vitamin A has been associated specifically with gain in weight. However, it is known that hard tissues and the nervous system also are affected. Vitamin A is important in tooth formation. Like other epithelia, the enamel-forming cells are affected by lack of vitamin A; instead of an even protective layer of enamel, fissures will be present and the teeth will tend to decay. Also the odontoblasts which form dentine are atrophied when there is a shortage of the vitamin.

Bone development may be slowed if vitamin A is lacking during the rapid-growth period. According to Wolbach (11), the multiplication of cartilage cells is retarded. He also states that if the brain and spinal cord grow too fast for the stunted skull and spinal column, injury of brain and nerves may occur and paralysis result. Irving and Richards (12) showed that the various types of body tissue require different amounts of the vitamin for normal development and that tissue sensitivity to the lack differs with age. Obviously, a liberal supply of this vitamin, especially during prenatal life and childhood, is important.

Vitamin A reacts with macromolecules. Olson (4) has discussed the possible interactions of vitamin A with protein, lipids, and nucleic acid in relation to fundamental functions. Vitamin A and the carotenoids occur naturally, bound to lipoproteins. The importance of the protein opsin in vision has been explained. It is thought that vitamin A and protein may serve as enzymes, as repressors, or as membrane transport carriers. With lipids Olson suggests that vitamin A may have a role in membrane function. Interrelationships between vitamin A and nucleic acid are not known, but Olson suggests that vitamin A may function with DNA or RNA in processes of differentiation and growth through interaction with the genetic apparatus.

METHODS OF DETERMINING VITAMIN A VALUES OF FOODS

Vitamin A values are expressed in terms of international units and of micrograms. In 1934, when only impure preparations of vitamin A were obtainable, the Health Organization of The League of Nations defined the vitamin A activity of pure β-carotene in terms of international units (IU) of vitamin A. In 1949, the Sub-Committee on Fat-Soluble Vitamins of the WHO set further equivalents. Today, in accord with current, more specific terminology, the following standards are used: one IU of β carotene (0.6 μg. all-*trans* β-carotene) is equivalent to one IU of vitamin A (0.3 μg. all-*trans* vitamin A alcohol (retinol) or 0.344 μg. all-*trans* vitamin A acetate (retinyl acetate) in the rate. It is thought that the same potency relationships apply to human beings. For practical purposes it is generally assumed that two IU of carotene are equivalent to one IU of vitamin A. But other factors of 3 or 4 carotene to one vitamin A are sometimes used to compensate for the lower availability of carotenes from different foods. Pharmaceutical companies in the United States have established a reference standard for the vitamin A potency of their products. The United States Pharmacopoeia Reference Standard contains vitamin A acetate dissolved in cottonseed oil in amount to make one USP unit identical with one IU. Therefore the two terms may be used interchangeably.

The bioassay method of determining vitamin A value of a food was the first to be used. The first measurements of vitamin A value were stated in terms of rat growth. This biological method is still used in some laboratories even though animal studies are exacting. With this method it is possible to have a controlled situation in which one variable at a time can be studied, to conduct an experiment on a sufficiently large number of animals to give reliability to results, to complete the problem in a comparatively short period of time, to observe the onset of disease, its development and course from day to day, and, by autopsy, to detect the effects of lack of vitamin on all parts of the body. Procedures used in bioassays of vitamin A have been standardized so they include in one test not only growth of the animal but also storage of the vitamin in the liver and the degree of vaginal keratinization.

Chemical and spectrometric methods are preferred today. Because the bioassay is time consuming, more objective methods have been sought. The specificity of the absorption bands of vitamin A_1 and A_2 and of the carotenoids forms the basis of the spectrometric method of determining vitamin A values of foods. In a chemical test developed by Carr and Price a comparatively stable blue color is secured when antimony trichloride is added to vitamin A. The color can be measured in a tintometer or in terms of its absorption bands. When the blue color, measured photometrically, is compared with the intensity of the absorption band at 328 $m\mu$, good agreement is reached. A factor has been determined which may be used to convert the "blue value" into IU of vitamin A. Many improvements in technique have been made since these objective methods were first set up. Chromatography is being used to eliminate nonspecific substances. The photoelectric colorimeter prevents errors in measuring results. Micromethods permit the use of very small samples.

Certain problems arise in determining and expressing the values. The biological activity of dehydroretinol is about 40 per cent of that of retinol, as indicated in rat growth tests (13). In areas where fresh-water fish is the main source of vitamin A this fact should be considered. Measurement of vitamin A values of foods which contain the carotenoid pigments is complicated. Many of the carotenoids in yellow- and red-pigmented foods are not physiologically available. Therefore, if total carotenoids are determined by physical methods, the vitamin A value is greatly over-estimated. If β-carotene only is determined, the figure is low because it does not include cryptoxanthin and other biologically active carotenes. In addition, in some foods the total carotenoid pigments increase con-siderably with advancing maturity or during storage. Thus, vitamin A values for foods have to be estimated using the data available. Table 11–1 gives data on the estimated distribution of retinol, carotene, and other carotenoids in a variety of foods. More precise figures for vitamin A values of foods cannot be stated until specific analytical methods are

Table 11–1

Estimated Distribution of Sources of Vitamin A Activity (as IU)
*in Various Foods**

Source	From retinol[†]	β-carotene	Other carotenoids
Animal origin			
Meat and meat organs	90	10	
Poultry	70	30	
Fish and shellfish	90	10	
Eggs	70	30	
Milk and milk products	70	30	
Animal or fish oil	90	10	
Plant origin			
Cereals			
Maize, yellow		40	60
Others		50	50
Legumes and seeds		50	50
Vegetables			
Green vegetables		75	25
Deep yellow (carrots, sweet potatoes—			
deep orange type, etc.)		85	15
Sweet potatoes—pale type		50	50
Other vegetables		50	50
Fruits			
Deep yellow (apricot, sapote, etc.)		85	15
Other fruits		75	25
Vegetable oils			
Red palm oil		65	35
Other vegetable or seed oils		50	50

* From INCAP/ICNND, *Food composition tables for use in Latin America* (1961).
† Including that derived from retinyl esters.

developed for determining each carotenoid and further study given to the behavior of each one during maturing and storing. In Agriculture Handbook No. 8, most of the vitamin A values are based on physical and chemical determinations of total carotenoids or of individual carotenes and of the biologically active pigment cryptoxanthin.

THE VITAMIN A VALUE OF FOODS

Plant foods contain only the precursor forms. Orange-yellow and green parts of plants are known to be superior to other parts in their vitamin A value. Hubbard squash, the more intense-colored sweet potatoes, yellow turnips, and yellow peaches are superior to the paler varieties of the same families; the orange butternut squash contains considerably more of the carotenes than the Hubbard squash.

Plant parts which contain chlorophyll are so rich in the yellow pigments that it is thought the green pigment may play a role in formation of the carotenes. The bright green, thinner leaves have more carotenes than the pale, thicker ones. The vitamin A value of other green vegetables such as asparagus, broccoli, string beans, and peppers also may be judged by their color. Cereal products and legumes are relatively poor sources of the precursors of vitamin A. Yellow corn owes only about half its pigmentation to the carotenes. Occasionally the yellow color is masked by still another pigment; for example, tomatoes and prunes are considered good sources of the precursor. Among the fruits, apricots, yellow peaches, cantaloupes, and persimmons are excellent sources. Red palm oil, produced extensively in parts of Africa and the Far East, is a very rich source of carotene. In areas where animal sources of vitamin A are limited the use of this oil should be encouraged (14).

Animal foods may contain both vitamin A and its precursors. As stated previously, the body can convert the carotenes into vitamin A. Both the hen and the cow are efficient in this respect, the hen probably more so, but in neither is the conversion complete. Since carotene in concentrated form is orange-yellow, whereas vitamin A in concentrated form is only slightly yellow, the color of the animal food does not necessarily indicate its vitamin A value. Fish liver oils, which are by far the most potent source of this factor, contain only vitamin A and are very pale. The egg yolk from a hen fed cod liver oil, although light in color, will be rich in vitamin A.

The amount of vitamin A in milk and eggs varies with the diet of the animal. Summer milk, butter, and eggs tend to contain more carotene than do the winter products. However, properly cured alfalfa, dried grass, and corn silage produce milk of nearly as great a potency.

Halibut and codfish derive their vitamin A from eating smaller fish which, in turn, have consumed carotene-containing marine plants. Since most of the vitamin is stored in the liver, fish liver oils are a superior source of vitamin A. The livers of animals and fowl are excellent sources: in order of vitamin A content are lamb, beef, chicken, calf, and pork. Muscle meats contain negligible amounts, but some seafood such as swordfish, mackerel, salmon, and oysters are good sources. The meat of whale, a mammal, ranks high.

The original value of foods is not greatly changed by food processing. The comparative stability of vitamin A and carotene to heat and their insolubility in water make for good retention, in general, during the processes through which foods pass from production to service at the table. Recommendations to the farmer include selection of superior varieties, fertilization of poor soil, and harvesting while the plant is young, since these steps favor optimal carotene content. Purchase of fresh, unwilted vegetables, green rather than bleached, and their storage in a cool, moist compartment are practices the homemaker should follow to retain the full quota of carotene in the plant. Fats and oils, because of their tendency to become rancid, require a cold dark storage place. Pasteurized, irradiated, and evaporated milks may be bought without fear that vitamin A was destroyed when the milk was processed.

Experimental work indicates that ordinary methods of cooking meat, fish, and vegetables decrease the vitamin A value little, if at all. Likewise in canning and in freezing there is little or no loss. In dehydration there may be a serious depreciation, especially if the process is prolonged at a high temperature and if oxidation occurs. Sulfur dioxide used in drying fruits conserves the vitamin A value, while sun-drying is destructive.

Fortified foods and concentrates are on the market. Fortification of margarine with vitamin A has been approved on an optional basis by the FDA as a means of making vitamin A available at low cost. The Administration has set a minimum of 9000 IU of vitamin A per pound but most margarines contain 15,000 or more units, thus making this product the approximate equivalent of butter, for which the year-round average is also 15,000 IU per pound. Margarine is considered an ideal carrier of vitamin A. Usually tocopherol and an emulsifying agent such as lecithin are added to margarine; tocopherol serves as an antioxidant and lecithin improves fat absorption in the body. In addition, fluid skim, or nonfat, milk is now often fortified with vitamin A.

Many concentrates of vitamin A are available, both in combination with vitamin D and as multivitamin preparations of fat-soluble and water-soluble factors. Today it is realized that there is danger of toxic effects from vitamin A excess. If large doses of vitamin A (20 to 30 times the RDA) are taken for long periods of time symptoms of toxicity are manifest. Carotene in large amounts accumulates in the body and a yellow skin is the only evident sign of excess. On the other hand, excessive amounts of vitamin A are indicated by anorexia, hyperirritability, skin lesions, bone decalcification, and increased intracranial pressure. Infants and children are more apt to receive excessive amounts of vitamin A than adults. For an infant of three to six months a daily dose of 18,500 IU of a water-dispersed vitamin A-D preparation taken for one to three months is considered to be toxic. Authorities recommend that persons administering vitamin A concentrate should be cautioned about its high potency and the importance of acurate dosage.

MEANS OF DETERMINING THE VITAMIN A STATUS
OF A HUMAN BEING

Studies are made on the blood. The general methods for determining vitamin A and carotene values in foods are used with blood plasma, but some adaptations are necessary. A method found to be superior to the Carr-Price technique uses trifluoroacetic acid (TFA) as the chromogen in place of antimony trichloride; in the presence of moisture the latter produces turbidity and has film-forming properties. Both macro- and micromethods using TFA have been perfected for use with blood serum. Physical methods also are employed.

The carotenoid content of the blood of a healthy adult eating an ordinary diet ranges from 80 to 120 μg. per 100 ml.; the level for serum vitamin A is between 100 and 300 IU per 100 ml., or approximately 30 to 90 μg. This is thought to be a better criterion than the carotene level because it reflects the intake of both the preformed vitamin and the precursors and includes the vitamin A the body has made from the ingested carotenoids. Levels have been shown to be affected by such factors as type of diet, completeness of absorption, storage in the liver, and lipid concentration of the serum, as well as by certain diseases.

Interpretation of data on the vitamin A and carotenoid concentrations in the serum is complicated. The problem is still more confused by the fact that the vitamin A serum level may not be lowered appreciably until the diet lacks the factor for months, whereas the carotene value drops rapidly when the food intake of vitamin A and carotenoids is low. A study of the blood is useful in determining whether the day-to-day intake of vitamin A is low or excessive.

Absorption of vitamin A and of carotene has been investigated. When a measured amount of vitamin A is given and blood levels are determined before and at set intervals after the test dose, the rate of absorption may be studied. Such a procedure is valuable in certain diseases where absorption may be poor or delayed.

Another way of studying absorption involves a quantitative analysis of vitamin A and carotene in the feces, since neither carotene nor vitamin A is excreted in the urine in the normal person. Therefore quantitative measurement of vitamin A and its precursor in the feces, on ingestion of known amounts of these factors, may show variations in degree of absorption, hence the comparative values of various sources in meeting the body's requirement. Small losses may occur through the skin and there may be some destruction in the intestines, but until more is known about these problems the data must be interpreted cautiously.

The degree of absorption explains, to a large extent at least, why dietary carotene is not the equivalent of vitamin A in promoting health and why certain food sources are better than others. Studies on absorption have proved that mineral oil retards absorption of both carotene and vitamin A, more the former than the latter; the presence of fat and cooking of vegetables increase the absorption of carotene.

The excretion of vitamin A has not been applied to any extent as a technique in surveys of groups of people. It is useful in explaining an individual's poor vitamin A nutriture when he seems to be consuming an adequate amount of the factor.

The eye's ability to adjust to a change in light intensity may measure vitamin A nutriture. The part vitamin A plays in vision has been discussed. It is known that the speed with which the eye adjusts to a change in light intensity depends on the amount of vitamin A in the system; thus the ability of a person to adjust to a change from dark to light, or vice versa, is used to determine both state of vitamin A health and body requirement.

Adaptometers have been designed to measure the dark adaptation of a person under different conditions. This equipment may be used to determine the amount of vitamin A necessary to prevent night blindness, as a criterion of minimal requirement.

Some workers question the test's reliability since administration of vitamin A does not always improve a poor visual acuity and since the threshold value seems to have no direct relationship to the vitamin A value of blood plasma. An explanation of why so few cases of night blindness have been found in recent surveys is that the threshold value is lowered only when the vitamin A intake is extremely low. Also it is thought that factors other than vitamin A impair dark adaptation. If avitaminosis A is to be judged by this method, a serial study of the individual is advised to overcome deviations from test to test and from errors in measurement.

Certain physical signs are associated with poor vitamin A status. Clinical findings such as dryness and scaling of the skin, follicular keratosis, xerophthalmia, and xerosis conjunctivae may be observed during a physical examination. These skin and ocular lesions are evident macroscopically in certain advanced cases of vitamin A lack. In some research studies correlation has been found between one or more of these symptoms and the serum levels of carotene or vitamin A. By means of a slit lamp which permitted a biomicroscopic investigation of the eye Kruse (15) found evidence of specific lesions at an early stage of vitamin A deficiency. When he studied 143 persons in a low income group he found that 45 per cent of them had gross ocular lesions, and another 54 per cent had microscopic lesions, both types characteristic of avitaminosis A.

A critical evaluation of vitamin A nutriture may include several methods of study. Several research investigations have been reported in which more than one means of evaluating vitamin A status have been used. One reported in 1949 by the Vitamin A Subcommittee of the Accessory Food Factors Committee of the (British) Medical Research Council (16) was based on blood studies, dark adaptation, and excretion as well as on clinical examination. Twenty-three conscientious objectors, 19 to 34 years old, served as volunteer subjects for periods of from six and one-half to 25 months; seven were positive controls, 16 ate a diet practically free of vitamin A or carotene but otherwise adequate. The first effect of lack of the vitamin was noted within three months when the carotenoid content of the blood had dropped from an average of about 150 IU per 100 ml. of plasma to about 40 IU. Only in eight months was a decrement in vitamin A plasma level evident and then in only ten of the experimental subjects. On the deficient diet the dark adaptation levels deteriorated gradually, slightly in 13 of the 16 subjects, markedly in the other three, and then in ten, 12, and 20 months, respectively. Fecal analysis of the carotenoids was used in connection with carotene utilization. Dryness of the skin, eye discomfort, and deterioration of hearing were the most commonly observed clinical symptoms. The investigators expected to ascertain requirement after depletion, but only the three subjects who were recognized as being completely depleted could be used as criteria of the effectiveness of varying amounts of vitamin A and carotene. For these three, 1300 IU of vitamin A daily was considered the minimal protective dose; 2500 IU was set as the amount which would cover the varying needs of individual healthy males, 20 to 30 years old, and allow a safety margin.

For carotene the minimal protective dose was thought to be indicated by that part of the intake not excreted in the feces. This amount differed, not only with the source of carotene (carotene in oil, in margarine, in carrots, cabbage, and spinach), but also with individuals, and with the same individual at different times. To cover these variations and provide a safety factor, a daily intake of 7500 IU of carotene was recommended. This British investigation disclosed that vitamin A deficiency in adult human beings is not induced easily or quickly and that the best criteria for judging depletion are the level of plasma carotenoids and the rate of dark adaptation.

RECOMMENDATIONS FOR VITAMIN A IN THE DAILY DIET

A liberal intake is advised. The RDA for reference man and woman set by the FNB is 5000 IU of vitamin A daily. In the United States it is assumed that about half of this will come from the carotenoids. Since a margin of safety is included in this allowance, further adjustments for variations which may exist in the proportions of carotenoids in a specific diet are not thought needed. The RDA for infants is based on the amount of vitamin A consumed in human milk; this is approximately 1500 IU in a day. Since little knowledge is available on the needs during childhood and adolescence, the FNB uses interpolated estimates based on body weight and growth needs. These allowances range from 2000 IU vitamin A for the child of one to two years, to 4500 IU for the ten- to 12-year-old. The main sources of vitamin A in the diet of infant and child are the supplement given almost without exception in the first few years, eggs, green leafy and yellow vegetables, and milk. From 14 years on the adult allowance is recommended.

Six thousand IU of vitamin A daily during the last two trimesters of pregnancy and 8000 IU daily during lactation are recommended by the FNB. These amounts are indicated by the demands of the rapidly growing fetus and infant on the maternal organism, as well as by the greater needs of the woman herself. The extra milk and vegetables and the vitamin A concentrate advocated throughout the reproduction period should care for the extra requirement.

The Joint FAO/WHO Expert Group (13) recommends a daily intake of 2500 IU of preformed vitamin A. This recommendation assumes that the availability of β-carotene is one-third that of vitamin A, the efficiency of conversion is only one-half that available, and, consequently, the utilization efficiency of carotene is only one-sixth that of vitamin A. Therefore, in areas of the world where the vitamin A intake is derived from both preformed vitamin and carotene the recommended intake for the vitamin should be adjusted upward.

Physiological variations in the use of vitamin A and carotene affect the need. Brief reference has already been made to some of the factors affecting absorption and storage of vitamin A and carotene. It is known that carotenes of various foods have different utilization values. Callison and Orent-Keiles (17) found that to maintain normal dark adaptation human beings needed only 62 per cent as much β-carotene from cooked garden peas as from the pure carotene in oil, 82 per cent as much from cooked spinach, and 143 per cent more from cooked carrots. In a study on rats about two-thirds of the carotene in cooked kale, and about one-third of the pigment in cooked carrots was utilized.

In jaundice, cirrhosis of the liver, infectious hepatitis, and obstruction of the bile duct, conditions in which bile is lacking, a considerable amount of the vitamin and its precursors may not be assimilated. In such cases bile may be given as a supplement, or vitamin A may be administered parenterally. However, oral administration of vitamin A is thought to be more effective in producing storage in the liver than is either subcutaneous or intramuscular injection. Therefore, an aqueous dispersion of vitamin A may be prescribed. It has been found that the vitamin is absorbed more rapidly and completely when given in this form than when it is dissolved in oil. Dietary fat is needed for absorption of carotene and vitamin A but its deteriorating effect on utilization is not significant unless rancid oils are present.

Vitamin E, which has antioxidant properties, when given simultaneously seems to protect vitamin A and carotene against oxidation in the intestinal tract and to increase storage of vitamin A in the liver. Ames (18) has demonstrated that either oral or intramuscular administration of vitamin E along with vitamin A increased the storage of vitamin A in the liver by three to six times. It also has been found that cattle are less able to synthesize ascorbic acid when vitamin A is lacking, and that vitamin A preservation is enhanced by added ascorbic acid.

The relationship of protein to vitamin A absorption and transport in the blood has been mentioned. From a practical standpoint the supply of protein is very important for vitamin A nutriture. Children with kwashiorkor are likely to have low levels of vitamin A in the serum and it is thought that dietary vitamin A may not reach the liver. Arroyave (19) has shown that if protein malnutrition is treated by protein supplements alone the clinical manifestations of vitamin A deficiency may suddenly become evident.

Utilization of vitamin A is retarded in several diseases. In hypothyroidism, clinical evidence of vitamin A deficiency may be associated with high levels of carotene in the blood. It is possible that thyroxin aids in conversion of carotene to vitamin A. Another theory is that abnormal thyroid metabolism affects intestinal absorption. Other diseases in which the relationship is not clear are cirrhosis of the liver, nephrosis, hydrocephalus, and pernicious anemia.

VITAMIN A VALUES IN THE DIET

In many countries lack of vitamin A in the food supply is a serious problem (20). Table 11–2 gives average daily intakes of calories, protein, and vitamin A value in ten countries. In parts of the South and in East Asia and other developing countries hypovitaminosis A is common (14). This is evident mostly in infants and young children.

A report by Olson (3) describes the problems in Thailand and presents a plan for correction. He found that the diets of those who live in rural villages lacked vitamin A, primarily because of age-old customs, lack of contact with provincial health officials, and poor availability of foods containing the vitamin. This was particularly true of children in the postweaning, preschool period. Olson suggested a plan involving a series of rather large protective doses of vitamin A to be given to children age one to six in regions where a high incidence of deficiency of this vitamin exists. The plan is based on the facts that only a small amount, about 5–7 μg. per kg. body weight, is required daily; a relatively large amount of vitamin A can be stored in the liver and other body organs; and vitamin A is avidly conserved when liver stores become low.

Studies conducted in Hyderabad (21) have shown the amount of

Table 11–2

*Average Daily Intake of Calories, Protein, and Vitamin A Activity in Sample Populations in 10 Countries**

	Calories	Protein gm	Vitamin A value, IU	Source vegetable, % of vitamin A
Thailand	1,821	49	1,781	84
Burma	2,501	54	1,150	60
East Pakistan	2,251	57	1,590	90
Jordan	2,182	70	3,125	75
Lebanon	2,173	70	4,000	75
Nigeria	2,143	49	7,542	Red palm oil
Ethiopia	2,512	65	2,901	
Trinidad and Tobago (Negroes)	1,912	62	2,660	
Chile	2,801	81	2,315	
Uruguay	2,562	91	2,774	66

* Courtesy of Patwardhan and *American Journal of Clinical Nutrition* 22:1108 (1969).

water-dispersible retinyl acetate which may be administered in a single large dose to afford maximal protection without being toxic. Under a plan approved by the Nutrition Division of the Thai Ministry of Public Health, all young children in selected villages in Thailand will receive a large annual or semiannual injection of water-dispersible retinyl acetate. These children will be followed over a four- to five-year period. The expectation is that the incidence of eye disease and blindness will be greatly reduced. It also is hoped that the rate of general infection will decline and that the children's weights, heights, and brain size will be significantly improved.

The food supply in the United States contains liberal amounts of foods high in vitamin A value. The survey (22) made of households in the United States in the spring of 1965 indicates that 74 per cent of the diets contained as much or more vitamin A value than the RDA; 16 per cent, two-thirds or more; and 10 per cent, below two-thirds. This last group included more women than men. When the vitamin A value of the diet was calculated in terms of percentage of total food the following distribution was found: milk, cream, and cheese, 12.5 per cent; meat, poultry, and fish, 15.7 per cent (of this 11.5 per cent came from liver); eggs, legumes, soups, and mixtures, 8.4 per cent; vegetables, 42.5 per cent; fruit, 7.3 per cent; grains, 1.4 per cent; fats and oils, 11.0 per cent; and sugars and miscellaneous, 1.1 per cent. Figure 11–3 shows how the food sources varied in three selected time periods. Since 1909–1913 use of green and yellow vegetables and margarine has markedly increased, while that of sweet potatoes and butter has declined.

Table 11–3 indicates that it is possible to obtain a liberal amount of vitamin A even at a low income level. In this low-cost dietary the large percentage of vitamin A was supplied by the meat, fish, egg group; this was due to the use of one pound of liver in the week's menus. Without the liver the vitamin A needs would not have been met. Carrots, broccoli, and sweet potatoes furnished more than one-fourth of the total. If all the milk had been whole its contribution would have been much greater.

Over the past few years use of skim milk and margarine has increased. These substitutes are fortified with vitamin A to balance the losses which might occur from replacement of whole milk and butter in the dietary. Practically all the margarines on the market and some of the fluid skim and dry skim milks have this vitamin added.

Blood studies indicate that many (but not all) people in the United States have satisfactory vitamin A nutriture. In the blood analyses reported in *Nutritional Status U.S.A.* (23), concentration of vitamin A in the serum was generally fair to good. The vitamin A and carotene levels in the blood of New York children and of children and adults in eight

Figure 11–3

Sources of vitamin A value in the American diet. (From Consumer and Food Economics Research Division, Publ. 62–20. Washington, D.C.: ARS, USDA, [1969].)

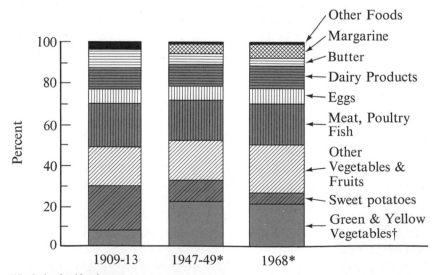

*Includes fortification.
†1968 data preliminary.

Table 11–3

Distribution of Vitamin A Values in the Low-Cost Dietary for a Family of Four*

Food Groups	Animal Sources IU	Animal Sources %[1]	Plant Sources IU	Plant Sources %[1]	All Sources IU	All Sources %[1]
Milk, cheese	15742	4.3			15742	4.3
Meat, fish, eggs	213438	57.9			213438	57.9
Dark-green and deep-yellow vegetables			96255	26.1	96255	26.1
Citrus fruit, tomatoes			8401	2.3	8401	2.3
Legumes, potatoes, other fruits and vegetables			15410	4.2	15410	4.2
Grain products					0	0.0
Margarine, oil	500	0.0	18750	5.2	19250	5.2
Sugar, sweets					0	0.0
Total for week	229680	62.2	138816	37.8	368496	100.0
Total for day	32811		19831		52642	
Recommended allowance for day[2]					18000	

* For description of family see Chapter 6, page 113.

[1] Expressed to one decimal.

[2] Recommended Dietary Allowances, Seventh Revised Edition. Washington, D.C.: FNB, NAS-NRC Publ. 1694 (1968).

western states were within the range of serum vitamin A expected in healthy persons (30–90 μg. per 100 ml.). In general, the figures for vitamin A closely paralleled those for carotene. Here it may be recalled that the carotene levels reflect the recent and current intake of sources of carotene, whereas the serum vitamin A level is considered a more reliable means of judging vitamin A nutriture.

In the first phase of the NNS (24) the preliminary findings appear to indicate a greater degree of vitamin A deficiency in the United States than was previously thought. In a group of 50 pre-school children in South Carolina, High (25) found 15 with less than 20 μg. per 100 ml. serum, and four of the 15 had levels under 10 μg. per 100 ml. None of the 50 had levels considered high.

Vitamin D

THE NATURE OF VITAMIN D AND ITS PRECURSORS

Vitamin D and its precursors belong to the sterol family. The prevalence of rickets through the centuries may be assumed by observing outward symptoms of the disorder in infants portrayed in paintings of the Madonna and Child. It has been estimated that in 1915 in the United States 50 to 75 per cent of all formula-fed infants suffered from rickets. It was not until 1918 that this disease was associated with the lack of a specific substance—vitamin D. Today, rickets still occurs (1), partly because infants tend to grow at a faster rate than in former times and consequently have greater need for the vitamin.

Much is known about the chemistry of vitamin D. Among the many sterols which have vitamin D activity, only two are considered of practical importance. One is formed from the animal precursor, 7-dehydrocholesterol; the other, from the plant precursor, ergosterol. Both are activated by exposure to ultraviolet light; the former, when activated, is called vitamin D_3, or cholecalciferol; the latter, D_2, ergocalciferol or viosterol. Their formulas are quite similar. However, in the side chain vitamin D_3 ($C_{27}H_{44}O$) lacks a double bond and has one less methyl group than vitamin D_2 ($C_{28}H_{44}O$) (Figure 11–4). Pure vitamins D are white, odorless crystals.

Figure 11–4
Structural formulas of vitamin D

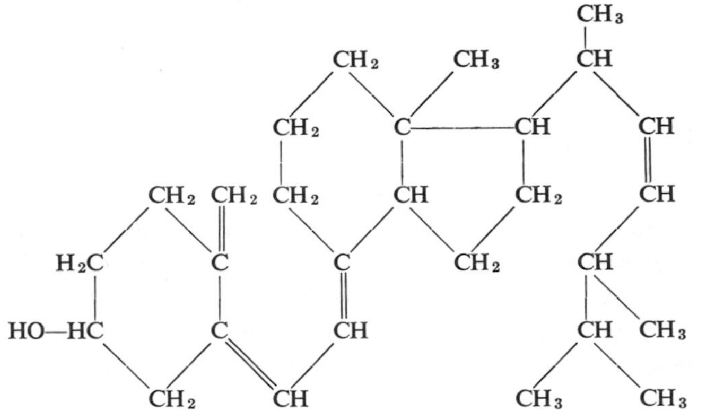

Vitamin D_2 (Calciferol; Viosterol; Activated Ergosterol; Ergocalciferol)

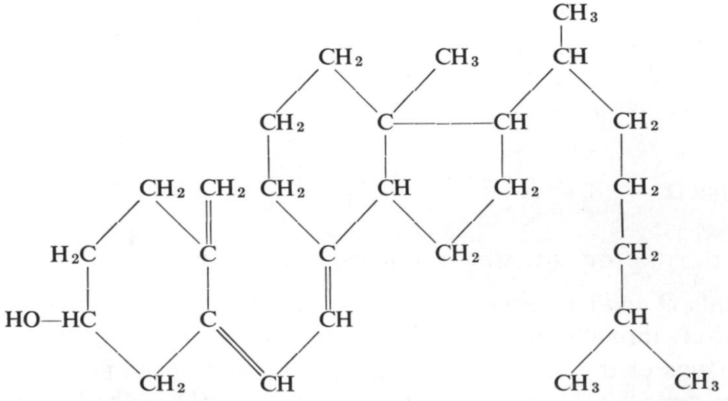

Vitamin D_3 (Activated 7-Dehydrocholesterol; Cholecalciferol)

Vitamin D is more stable than vitamin A. Like vitamin A, vitamin D is fat-soluble and for a time the two were thought to be a single entity. Their differentiation was proved by the greater lability of vitamin A in the presence of oxygen. Vitamin D is comparatively stable to both heat and oxidation, as well as to acid and alkali. Some destruction of the factor occurs if the fat which serves as its carrier becomes rancid. Vitamin D_3 is more stable than vitamin D_2; esters of both forms are remarkably stable if kept away from light. Excessive irradiation of the precursors may result in formation of toxisterol and suprasterol, slightly toxic compounds which show no antirachitic potency.

The precursors may be activated by ultraviolet rays. Certain wave lengths of the spectrum, coming in contact with 7-dehydrocholesterol in the skin and in animal foods, change it into vitamin D_3 (2). Ergocalciferol also is activated by the same wave lengths.

The sun as a source of ultraviolet rays is not constant or dependable. Its antirachitic effectiveness varies with altitude, latitude, time of day, clouds, fog, smoke, and dust in the air. The quality and intensity of the rays are more important than their duration. At high altitudes the ultraviolet intensity is great. Only when the sun's altitude is above 35° are the ultraviolet rays strong enough to be curative. This means that radiation at noon is more effective than that during early morning and late afternoon hours, and it is more effective in summer than in winter. During several winter months the rays which reach the earth in the northern states are not of much value. Children living in tropical countries get more benefit from the sun's potent rays than do those living in cooler regions, and statistics prove that rickets is correspondingly less common there.

Pigmentation is a factor in the absorption of ultraviolet rays (3). The more pigment there is in the skin, the less the amount of vitamin D produced in the body by irradiation. A dark-skinned person may profit by this protection if he lives in the tropics, but not if he resides in the temperate zone. Reflected light from the sun retains its antirachitic properties, although the protection provided by reflected light may not be as great as that from direct sunshine. In cloudy countries such as England skyshine may be the chief source of ultraviolet rays. Large cities tend to have little solar radiation, direct or indirect, partly due to smoke and dust which may filter out about half of the potent rays, partly due to tall buildings.

People who are indoors all day do not secure their quota of ultraviolet rays, even though they may sit in the sunshine and feel its warmth. This is because ordinary window glass cuts off all light of wave lengths as short as 310 to 320 mμ. Quartz glass permits the active rays to penetrate, but it may be too expensive for home use. Several window-glass substitutes of more moderate cost are now available. They allow some protection from rickets, and tests have been made which show their comparative light transmissions. However, the advisability of the special glasses for home use is questioned, since a few minutes a day in direct sunshine usually is feasible.

Ultraviolet rays from artificial sources may be used to activate the precursors of vitamin D. Because of the irregularity and uncertainty of the sun's rays and because of screening materials such as smoke, fog, windowpanes, and clothing, it is often considered advisable to use an artificial source of ultraviolet light. Mercury vapor quartz and carbon arc lamps are used in hospitals, clinics, and homes. Since the rays from these lamps are much more powerful than those from the sun and vary depending on the type of lamp and distance, their use may be dangerous, and special care must be taken to regulate the dosage. Too long or too close an exposure may burn the body seriously; the eyes are especially sensitive. Ordinarily the first treatments are very short, a half-minute each on front and back. The time is gradually increased to a half-hour or more. In all cases these lamps should be controlled by an intelligent, trained person, with careful consideration of the individual and his reaction.

THE METABOLISM AND FUNCTIONS OF VITAMIN D

Studies employing radioactive vitamin D indicate the processes through which the vitamin is metabolized. It is known that calcium is actively transported through the intestinal wall and that this transport is minimal in animals lacking vitamin D. Research involving radioactive vitamin D conducted by DeLuca and co-workers (4) indicates that the vitamin induces the formation or elaboration of a protein, α_2-globulin, in the intestinal mucosa. This protein carries vitamin D to the liver, where the vitamin is converted to 25-hydroxycholecalciferol (25-HCC). Antirachitic assays in rats and chicks have demonstrated that 25-HCC is metabolically active and that it is more potent than cholecalciferol.

From the liver 25-HCC is carried to bone and intestine. In nuclear membranes, according to DeLuca (5), it probably unmasks a specific DNA, which in turn makes RNA. The resultant enzyme actively enhances calcium and phosphorus in the plasma which causes normal bone mineralization.

It is also known that parathyroid hormone stimulates vitamin D action by inducing mobilization of calcium and phosphate in old or deep bone. This elevates plasma calcium and phosphorus which brings about normal bone mineralization. This hormone may also aid intestinal transport of vitamin D.

Other studies show how vitamin D acts to promote good nutrition. Vitamin D favors utilization of phosphorus. By raising the renal threshold for phosphate excretion, the vitamin permits an increased rate of reabsorption by the renal tubules, which results in a more normal blood phosphorus level. Alkaline phophatase changes organic to inorganic phosphorus in bone. The increase in this enzyme noted early in rickets is thought to be related to an increased need for osteoblasts to recalcify the weak bones. On treatment of the rachitic infant with vitamin D, the level of the enzyme returns gradually to normal.

Phytase, an enzyme present in the intestines, hydrolyzes dietary phytates, thus increasing the availability of the phosphorus (6). Vitamin D has been found to increase the activity of phytase and the bone ash content of rats fed a rachitogenic diet. The relationships of the vitamin to citrate and sulfur metabolism also are being investigated. All these studies on vitamin D's mode of action indicate that various factors are active in bone metabolism, but their significance is not fully understood at this time.

It is believed that the functions of vitamin D are more far reaching than the absorption of calcium and phosphorus from the gastrointestinal tract, the accretion and resorption of these minerals in the bone, and the effect of the renal handling of the minerals. Vitamin D has been found to increase both the volume and acidity of gastric secretions. Growth of soft tissue is accelerated by vitamin D; Steenbock and Herting (7) demonstrated this in a rat experiment in which the diet was low in calcium but otherwise adequate. When the antirachitic factor was administered, the level of rat growth was greater than when extra calcium was used as the supplement. These workers believed that this increased growth is only one indication of the vitamin's general effect on organic tissue metabolism.

Vitamin D prevents and cures rickets. This disease, often evident in a mild form among infants, involves a faulty calcification of growing bones and is related to a deficiency of either or both calcium and phosphorus in the blood. Lack of vitamin D or of ultraviolet light exaggerates this condition, and one or both are included, along with a liberal supply of the two minerals, in treatment of the disorder.

Among the symptoms to be observed in a clinical examination of a rachitic child are misshapen bones, enlargement of the ends of the long bones and at rib junctions, delayed closing of the fontanelle, and slow eruption of the teeth. The musculature may be affected, causing protrusion of the abdomen. Rickets often is associated with rapid growth of muscle tissue. This may explain low phosphorus rickets, the form most commonly observed.

Tetany accompanies the low calcium type, which may be associated with parathyroid disturbance. Osteomalacia, a rickets-like disorder common among women in the Orient, is related to their inadequate diet, lack of direct sunshine, and frequency of pregnancies; calcium, phosphorus, and vitamin D are used in its treatment.

Another form of the disorder is known as vitamin D-resistant or refractory rickets. Bone deformities and blood conditions are similar to those found in vitamin D-deficiency rickets. However, an ordinary dosage of the vitamin has no curative effect. The condition occurs both in infancy and throughout childhood and adult life. Since the outward signs of rickets do not appear until the disease is well developed, two blood chemistry tests are used in diagnosis of the disease: first, the calcium and phosphorus content of the blood; second, the alkaline phosphatase in the serum. Normally the infant's blood contains approximately 10 mg. of calcium and 5 mg. of phosphorus per 100 ml., and in health throughout the growth period this ration of 2:1 stays quite constant. A low phosphorus serum indicates the most common form of rickets; on treatment with usual doses of vitamin D a rise in this mineral can be expected in about ten days. The alkaline phosphatase technique was developed by Bodansky in 1933 and levels are expressed in terms of Bodansky units. Bessey and co-workers (8) have developed a micromethod for determining the amount of the enzyme in the serum. The normal level of the phosphatase in the serum is between 3 and 12 units per 100 ml. up to 12 years, 3 to 5 units in adults. In mild rickets, the level may be 20 to 30 units; in severe cases, as high as 60 units. With this microtechnique it is thought that the alkaline phosphatase test may serve as a sensitive and reliable tool in nutrition surveys, as well as a means of diagnosis in individuals. Another method of studying rickets involves a study of the bones by x-ray. However, rickets cannot be recognized in the x-ray film until the disease is well advanced, so this technique is used less in detection than in following the course of treatment. The bone density indicates its degree of calcification. Too, the ends of the long bones of a rachitic child, as seen in x-rays, are concave, with frayed edges. With usual doses of vitamin D, deposition of calcium salts may be noted in about 21 days.

Vitamin D aids in dentition. Jeans and Stearns (9) studied the relation of the amount of vitamin D consumed to the time of tooth eruption, linear growth, and mineral retention in infants. Their results indicate that an intake of 300 to 400 IU daily is more conducive to good dentition and growth than is a smaller amount or a massive dose.

Eruption of the temporary teeth may be delayed during rickets, and their order of appearance is often deranged. Frequently a rachitic child may have two or less teeth at the first birthday; these will eventually erupt and their enamel probably will be normal. However, the permanent teeth which are forming in the jaw during this time may show thinning, pitting, or grooving of the enamel, defects which will be evident as a definite line across the teeth. The defective area tends to decay more easily. The beneficial effect of vitamin D on tooth formation may be expected only when calcium and phosphorus intakes are satisfactory. Eliot and co-workers (10) in studies on 450 children found that enamel hypoplasia and tooth decay were common among those who had a history of rickets.

THE SOURCES OF VITAMIN D

Several tests may be used to determine the vitamin D potency of a product. Chemical tests for measuring quantitatively the amount of vitamin D in a food have been proposed. Photometric methods may give reliable data when the vitamin is in a simple solution. A microbiological assay for vitamins D_2 and D_3 has been developed, based on reactions of *Lactobacillus casei,* and this technique may be used in the future in place of the line test, long the accepted procedure for measuring vitamin D values. Since bone is the tissue most commonly associated with vitamin D, it has been used in a special technique, devised by McCollum and associates (11), for testing a food's antirachitic potency. This procedure is based on the marked reducing action of newly deposited bone on silver salts; the narrow and continuous line across the distal ends of the radii and ulnae of the normal rat indicates the presence of calcium and hence normal bone.

A biological procedure employing radioactive phosphorus has been perfected by Numerof and co-workers (12). It gives results similar to those of the line test. In addition, it is more objective in nature and its results are not affected by such complications as weight gain and variations in food consumption.

The potency of a food may be expressed in terms of IU, USP units, or micrograms. In 1949 the Subcommittee on Fat-Soluble Vitamins of the WHO (13) set a new standard of reference for vitamin D for international use. One international unit is the equivalent of 0.025 mg. of pure crystalline vitamin D_3. The standard used previously was based on irradiated ergosterol. One USP unit is equal to one IU.

Few natural foods are good sources of vitamin D. Of the foods included in the normal diet, only eggs, liver, and a few fish are considered significant sources. The amount of vitamin D present in eggs and liver depends largely on the amount of the vitamin in the food of the hen or animal. Salmon, sardines, herring, tuna, and fish roe are good sources of vitamin D. Milk and butter contain some; muscle meats, fruits, vegetables, and cereal products contain mere traces, if any. In general, it can be assumed that the food commonly eaten cannot be counted on to supply the body's need unless the milk has been fortified with vitamin D.

Rich sources of vitamin D are on the market. Cod liver oil, long considered the best and cheapest source of the vitamin, is required by the United States Pharmacopoeia to contain at least 85 units per gm. and many brands have two or three times this amount. Thus one teaspoon of cod liver oil, 4 gm., supplies from 340 to 1000 units of vitamin D. The use of this oil in infant feeding has decreased, partly because of its odor and flavor, which often are more distasteful to the adult who administers it than to the child, and partly because other potent products are now sold at the same price level. Viosterol, the plant form of vitamin D_2, is one of these. According to the United States Pharmacopoeia, this must be standardized to contain 10,000 IU of vitamin D per gm., or 200 to 222 IU per drop. It is tasteless and can be administered directly. The vitamin may be incorporated in an oil base or in propylene glycol, in which form it mixes easily with milk or other foods.

Fish oils such as percomorph and halibut liver oil are considerably richer than cod liver oil in both the D and A vitamins and are diluted with a less potent oil so that the dose may be easily measured. By law, all these oils must be diluted to be uniform in vitamin D potency and equivalent to that supplied by viosterol in oil. Since many preparations containing vitamin D, with or without other vitamins and minerals, are available, it is of the utmost importance that the information on the label be read and the dosage adjusted to give the amount of vitamin the physician prescribes.

A number of foods are fortified with vitamin D. Milk has been approved by both the Council on Foods of the American Medical Association and the FDA as a carrier of vitamin D. Today a high proportion of all fluid milk and practically all evaporated and nonfat dry milk is fortified with this factor. The common way to fortify is to add a measured amount of vitamin D concentrate prior to pasteurization, homogenization, evaporation, or drying. The particular effectiveness of vitamin D in milk is thought to be due partly to its combination and dispersion with lactalbumin, and partly to the presence of calcium and phosphorus in the milk. Since this product can be purchased at little if any added cost and the antirachitic factor can be easily incorporated, it is believed that vitamin D milk may well be the accepted source of the vitamin in the diets of older children and adults, and especially of pregnant and lactating women.

Some cereals, breads, milk flavorings, fruit juices, and margarines are fortified with vitamin D. When considered in relation to the amount per serving, the amounts secured seem small; however, when added to that received from milk and other supplementary sources, the total amount of vitamin D in the diet may be excessive.

THE AMOUNT OF VITAMIN D THE BODY NEEDS

Vitamin D is needed throughout the growth period. Since this factor can be acquired both by ingestion and by exposure to ultraviolet rays, dietary needs will vary; a lack will occur only when both sources are inadequate. The FNB recommends a daily intake of 400 IU of vitamin D throughout the growth period. It is thought that maximal retention of calcium by healthy infants is probable when from 300 to 400 units of vitamin D are taken, provided the calcium consumption at the same time is adequate; larger amounts of the vitamin have not been shown to be associated with greater calcium retention or better dentition. In some normal full-term infants as little as 100 IU per day have prevented rickets.

The premature infant is sometimes given a larger daily supply since he is growing fast and his exposure to sunlight is delayed. Because the infant's ability to utilize fats is apt to be poor, a water-miscible preparation of vitamin D may be used. Provided the premature baby has an adequate intake of calcium it is thought that he will thrive on 400 IU vitamin D per day.

Throughout the growth period the child continues to need vitamin D. Studies on children, two to 14 years of age, have shown that rickets may continue to puberty, although the frequency and severity diminish as the child grows older. The adolescent boy and girl are advised to take as much vitamin D as does the infant, along with a liberal supply of milk. The type of vitamin D, whether from a plant or an animal precursor, is not a matter of concern in child nutrition since both are equally well utilized.

During reproduction there is a demand for vitamin D. Since vitamin D is necessary for normal development and growth, it is to be expected that some source should be included in the diets of the pregnant and lactating woman. Vitamin D mobilizes calcium and phosphorus for building fetal bones and teeth; without it the baby at birth may have a predisposition to rickets, and this tendency may be further exaggerated during lactation owing to the lack of vitamin D in the mother's milk. Throughout the reproductive period 400 IU daily are recommended.

The importance of normal bone growth throughout life is especially evident at the time of childbirth. The small, malformed pelvic arch resulting from childhood rickets may so increase the danger of delivery to both mother and infant that a Caesarean operation is necessary.

The normal adult's need for vitamin D is minimal. The healthy adult leading a normal life has a minimal requirement for this vitamin. His rate of loss of calcium and phosphorus from the skeleton is thought to be less rapid than that of the growing organism; also, summer sunshine may so help in the storage of the factor in the liver that the year's needs may be taken care of in a few weeks' time. The FNB states that ordinarily adult needs for vitamin D are met by exposure to the sun and by the amount of the vitamin secured in the normal diet.

Many physicians and nutritionists consider it wise to prescribe vitamin D throughout the winter months; year-round supplements may be advisable for those who are confined indoors or who work the night shift or whose clothes shield them completely from the sun's direct rays. The vitamin is also advised for the aged and patients recovering from fractures and bone operations.

Hypervitaminosis is a serious condition. High levels of vitamin D are toxic. Excessive amounts may cause high levels of calcium and phosphorus in the blood and excessive excretion of calcium in the urine;

calcification of soft tissues and of the walls of blood vessels and kidney tubules result. The abnormalities cause a condition known as the idiopathic hypercalcemia syndrome.

In 1950 the Committee on Nutrition of the British Medical Association recommended 800 IU of vitamin D daily for children up to two years, and British welfare foods (cod liver oil and "national" dried milk) and proprietary infant foods were prescribed accordingly. In 1957 fortification reduction, to supply 400 IU vitamin D per day, was followed by an almost complete disappearance of hypercalcemia but by no apparent increase in the incidence of rickets (14).

Until recently it was thought that there was a large margin between the amount of vitamin D recommended and a toxic dose, an amount considered to be 1000 to 3000 IU per kg. body weight per day. However, in some cases of infantile hypercalcemia the intakes of vitamin D have been found to be much less than these amounts. Therefore, the FNB now recommends that the amount of vitamin D given an infant should not appreciably exceed 400 IU per day. The Board also approves limiting the intake to this amount for older children and adults.

The amount recommended includes the total secured through a vitamin supplement, milk, and other foods in the diet. That received from food sources should be determined before deciding on the need for a supplement. Even in pregnancy and lactation a quart of vitamin D milk daily may be expected to supply the needed amount.

Vitamin E

THE CHEMISTRY AND OCCURRENCE OF VITAMIN E

The chemical nature of vitamin E is significant. Vitamin E was discovered in 1922 by Evans and Bishop (1), at which time it was shown to be essential for normal reproduction in the rat. It was isolated from wheat germ, identified as an alcohol, and named vitamin E. Later it received the name "tocopherol," derived from Greek words meaning "offspring" and "to bear." Four naturally occurring tocopherols are known. Three of these, β-, γ-, δ-, have relatively low biological potency and are usually disregarded in nutritional evaluations. Occasionally data on total tocopherol are found but the alpha form is the one most often determined (Figure 11–5). One IU of vitamin E is the equivalent of 1 mg. of synthetic dl-α-tocopherol acetate. The naturally occurring form, d-α-tocopherol acetate is equal to 1.36 IU per mg.; the free alcohol, dl-α-tocopherol, 1.1 IU, and d-α-tocopherol, 1.49 IU.

Vitamin E is unstable in the presence of oxygen. Other factors which lessen its biological potency are ultraviolet light, alkali, and lead and iron salts; heat catalyzes these effects. The primary value of this vitamin is its action as an antioxidant; this is thought to be due to the presence of an

Figure 11–5
Structural formula of vitamin E (α-tocopherol)

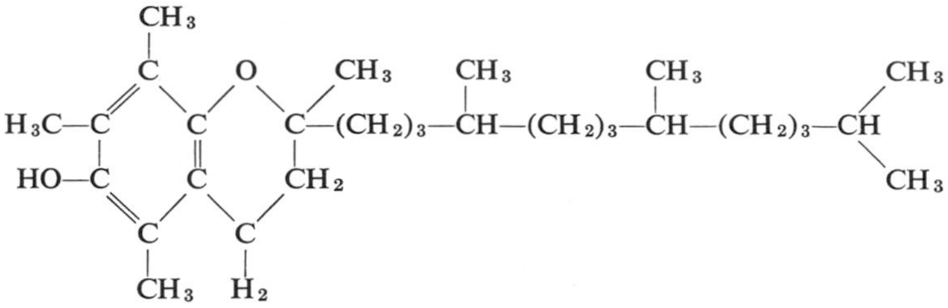

$$CH_3$$
$$|$$
$$C$$
$$H_3C-C \quad O \quad CH_3 \quad CH_3 \quad CH_3 \quad CH_3$$
$$| \quad | \quad | \quad |$$
$$H_3C-C \quad C \quad C-(CH_2)_3-CH-(CH_2)_3-CH-(CH_2)_3-CH$$
$$HO-C \quad C \quad CH_2 \quad CH_3$$
$$C \quad C$$
$$| \quad |$$
$$CH_3 \quad H_2$$

easily oxidized phenol group on the aromatic ring. Tocopherols are found in one or more forms wherever fat occurs in nature and cause an increase in the fat's stability. The vitamin may be used commercially to prevent flavor changes due to rancidity. Ascorbic acid also may be incorporated into commercial fat mixtures since it increases the antioxidant power of the tocopherols. Vitamin E hinders oxidative destruction of vitamin A, carotene, and fat.

Vitamin E is found in both plant and animal foods. Chemical, physical, and biological assays are used to measure vitamin E values. Paper chromatography is now being used to a great extent as a means of assay.

The richest natural sources of the factor are some of the plant oils (2); there is a wide range of values—from 2 μg. per gm. total tocopherol in coconut oil to 1896 μg. per gm. in wheat germ oil. Of the oils commonly used as food, cottonseed oil is considered a superior source. Margarine, which is made largely of plant oils, is considered a good source of vitamin E; when oils are hydrogenated in the manufacture of some margarines and shortenings, the tocopherol content is not thought to be lessened.

Fruits and vegetables do not supply large amounts of vitamin E (3). Whole grains contain more vitamin E than do the refined products; if flour is bleached with chlorine dioxide it contains little or no tocopherol. Meats, fish, and poultry contribute from low to moderate amounts of this vitamin, fish being a better source. Although animal products do not contain as much tocopherol as plants the relative amount of α- to total tocopherol in animal foods is high. The vitamin E content of milk and milk products has been studied because these foods are important in infant feeding. Herting and Drury (4) have reported that human milk contains an average of 1.14 mg. α-tocopherol per quart, homogenized cow's milk contains about 0.21 mg. per quart in early spring and about 1.06 mg. per quart in midfall. Evaporated, condensed, and nonfat dry milk when reconstituted for use supply about 0.66, 1.29, and 0.02 mg. per quart, respectively. No loss of the vitamin results from pasteurization of milk and other foods show only slight losses from ordinary cooking processes.

Since foods high in fat are among the best sources of α-tocopherol Bunnell and associates (5) analyzed foods which were cooked in vegetable oils. Little loss was noted on cooking but the loss of α-tocopherol was great in foods which were frozen and stored after cooking. This is due to oxidation, even at low temperatures. These investigators suggested that vegetable oils to be used in pre-freezing processes should be fortified with α-tocopherol acetate, which is stable to heat and oxidation.

Body tissues contain varying amounts of tocopherol. Comparatively little is known about absorption and metabolism of this vitamin. No active metabolite has been found in studies using labelled α-tocopherol, and no specific enzyme involved in its metabolism has been detected (6).

From the intestine vitamin E passes into the lymph and is carried to the liver where some is stored. The amount stored appears to be in linear relation to the amount in the diet but this relationship may not hold when very large amounts are eaten. Tocopherol is also stored in fatty tissues, in the blood, some glands, and other internal organs. The amount of α-tocopherol in the plasma was determined by Herting and Drury (7) in two groups of subjects. In those living in Pittsburgh, Pa., the plasma contained 358 ± 21 μg. per cent; those living in Rochester, N.Y., had 507 ± 32 μg. per cent. These results, based on α-tocopherol only, are lower than figures found previously when the method used included all forms of tocopherol.

THE ESSENTIAL NATURE OF VITAMIN E

Experimental studies have shown the many-sided nature of vitamin E. Rats were used in the earliest experiments which showed the relationship of vitamin E to normal reproduction. Since then, several disorders have been related to a deficiency of vitamin E in many different animals and under a variety of conditions (8). These are associated with hematopoetic, muscular, vascular, central nervous, and reproductive systems. A wide variety of symptoms occur in different species of animals; among these are creatinuria, low hemoglobin values, erythrocyte hemolysis, and accumulation of ceroid pigments in tissues. The last-mentioned is thought to be due to oxidative changes in unsaturated fatty acids.

The body of a mature animal which has appreciable stores of vitamin E will be depleted very slowly when the vitamin is withheld. The young animal, with relatively small stores, is more quickly affected. Malabsorption syndromes lead to acute symptoms; the signs of marginal lack may be obscured by the effects of other dietary deficiencies. Poor reproduction and muscular dystrophy have been successfully treated with vitamin E therapy in animals; neither disorder responds to such treatment in human beings.

Anemia is common in the vitamin E-depleted Rhesus monkey (9). Bone marrow RNA and DNA were found to be greatly increased in the deficient monkey. On treatment with α-tocopherol the animals responded with reticulocytosis and blood regeneration.

Some investigators believe that vitamin E plays a role in intracellular respiration. They have studied the mitochondria, where respiration takes place, and other cell granules rich in many enzymes and trace elements. The fat-splitting enzymes free unsaturated fatty acids which then inhibit cell respiration. If present, tocopherol will stop this respiratory decline.

The presence of selenium in the enzymes is thought to be significant. In 1957 this trace element was identified in Factor 3, a compound which also contains vitamin E and cystine. Schwarz (10) has stated that these three substances, together or separately, may explain the different forms of disease which are associated with vitamin E deficiency.

A structural similarity exists between ubiquinone (also called coenzyme Q) and vitamin E (11). Some workers believe that members of the coenzyme Q group of compounds have a primary role in explaining the activities. A decreased amount of ubiquinone in the tissues has been found during a lack of vitamin E. Also it is known that coenzyme Q can cure vitamin E-deficient animals. The theory has been advanced that such substances as vitamin E, other antioxidants, and selenium, and a diet low in polyunsaturated fatty acids, may prevent coenzyme Q from oxidative destruction. Other authorities believe the biochemical relationship between vitamin E and coenzyme Q is not very direct.

In man certain beneficial effects of vitamin E have been observed. Despite its failure to benefit the two disorders mentioned in the preceding paragraph, α-tocopherol administered to the human being has brought about some favorable effects. These include a decrease in creatinuria in patients with cystic fibrosis and xanthomatous biliary cirrhosis, and a decrease in creatinuria and an increase in reticulocyte formation in children with protein-calorie malnutrition and macrocytic anemia. Both erythrocyte survival and reticulocyte levels were related to dietary tocopherol in a study made by Horwitt, Century, and Zeman (12). To determine the change in life span of the red blood cells the following technique was employed: blood was removed from each of four subjects, labeled with radioactive Cr^{51}, and reinjected into the same subject's blood stream. An isotope-counting mechanism was used to measure the survival time of these reinjected erythrocytes. After a tocopherol depletion period of 72 to 76 months, there was a small but significant decrease in the Cr^{51} erythrocyte life span. When three of Horwitt's tocopherol-depleted subjects were given a daily supplement of 300 mg. of tocopherol, there was a significant increase in reticulocyte level. These favorable effects on the blood indicate that vitamin E is a hematopoetic agent in man as well as in animals.

Analysis of tocopherol in the blood and the peroxide hemolysis test are two means of evaluating vitamin E nutriture. The latter, devised by Rose and György (13) in 1952, was used first on animals and later on human beings; it measures the increase in rate of erythrocyte hemolysis as affected by a deficiency of vitamin E, and the improvement on therapy.

Horwitt and his associates demonstrated the antioxidant action of vitamin E in their long-time investigations in the Elgin State Hospital, referred to in Chapter 1. The subjects were 38 male patients. One group received a diet considered adequate in all respects except that it was low in tocopherol (approximately 3 mg. daily). The diet contained 55 gm. fat daily, of which 30 gm. was lard that had been stripped—a process involving heat to remove much of the tocopherol. Another group received the same diet plus a supplement of 15 mg. α-tocopherol acetate daily. Still others were given an *ad libitum* hospital diet. After two and one-half years on this regime, the first group of subjects showed positive reactions to the hemolysis test and the plasma tocopherol averaged only about 0.5 mg. per 100 ml.—approximately one-half the level noted at the beginning of the experiment. At this time corn oil, stripped to remove much of the tocopherol, was substituted for the lard; the level of plasma tocopherol decreased still more in the next nine months to 0.4 mg. per 100 ml. Later, as the stripped corn oil in the diet was doubled to 60 gm., replacing more of the lard, levels of 0.1 and 0.2 mg. per 100 ml. were recorded. Figure 11–6 shows the effect of increasing the amount of PUFA, as secured in the corn oil diets, on both the plasma tocopherol and the peroxide hemolysis. Horwitt observed that the fatty acid content of the erythrocytes and depot fat remained high longer than did the to-

Figure 11–6

Changes in plasma tocopherol and peroxide hemolysis on a single representative subject. (*From Horwitt, in* Vitamins and Hormones, 20:547 [*1962*]. © *The Academic Press. Reprinted by permission of The Academic Press.*)

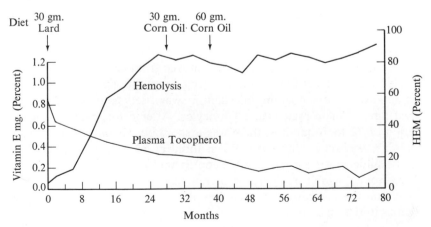

copherol levels, thus destroying the natural relationship between PUFA and tocopherol and increasing the severity of the deficiency. Horwitt attributes the different types of symptoms of vitamin E lack to the varying concentrations of PUFA and tocopherol in the different tissues as well as to the level of intake of fatty acids and tocopherol (14). Another factor involved was the elapsed time on the diet.

In the infant and child a lack of vitamin E may result in an anemia. Hemolytic anemia is a condition in which the normal resistance of the erythrocytes to rupture by oxidizing agents is markedly reduced. During pregnancy placental transfer of vitamin E is negligible. Therefore at birth little of the vitamin has been stored in the newborn's body, and serum tocopherol levels are low. The bottle-fed baby acquires little vitamin E from cow's milk, and anemia is likely to develop. This condition is exaggerated in a premature infant. Oski and Barnes (15) showed that premature infants with hemolytic anemia respond to vitamin E supplements with increases in plasma tocopherol levels, decreases in erythrocyte hemolysis, return to normal hemoglobin levels, and decreases in reticulocyte count.

Because it has been shown that the need for vitamin E is related to PUFA in the diet much work on infants has centered on this phase of the problem. Both full-term and premature babies have developed symptoms of vitamin E lack when the diet was high in PUFA and low in vitamin E (E/PUFA ratio of 0.19). Barness (16) reported that anemia in premature infants is preventable if their diet contains 1.5 per cent protein, 50 per cent unsaturated fat, and about 4 mg. vitamin E per quart of formula.

A possible relationship between vitamin E and protein has been indicated in studies of young children who have kwashiorkor. Majaj and co-workers (17), working with infants who suffered from protein-calorie malnutrition, found a macrocytic anemia to be very prevalent. This did not respond to treatment with iron, vitamin C, or vitamin B_{12}, but administration of tocopherol brought a rapid increase in reticulocytes and an improvement in hemoglobin. Herting (20) has suggested that the kwashiorkor syndrome may contribute to the vitamin E lack through decreased absorption or low levels of serum protein which transports the vitamin.

INTAKE AND RECOMMENDED ALLOWANCE OF VITAMIN E

Dietary surveys indicate the amount of vitamin E eaten. Few studies have been made on the consumption of vitamin E. Harris and Embree (18) estimated the probable intake of vitamin E in the American diet. Using data on foods available to the average consumer in 1960 they calculated that the daily diet supplied 14.9 mg. of d-α-tocopherol and 24.2 gm. of PUFA. The ratio E/PUFA was 6.16. Based on the statement that 93 to 96 per cent of normal persons in the United States have serum tocopherol levels above the deficiency level of 0.5 mg./100 ml., Harris and Embree believe that the usual intake of 15 mg. vitamin E per day is sufficient. They state that an E/PUFA ratio above 0.6 will protect, below 0.6 may result in depletion.

Bunnell and associates (5) calculated the α-tocopherol contents of eight typical breakfast, lunch, and dinner menus. They found wide ranges in the vitamin E content of the meals: in breakfasts, 0.59 to 3.68 mg.; in lunches, 0.44 to 5.37 mg.; in dinners, 1.61 to 6.38 mg. The daily totals ranged from 2.6 to 15.4 mg. α-tocopherol, with an overall average of 7.4 mg. The FNB states that about 64 per cent of the α-tocopherol included in the usual American diet comes from salad oils, shortening, and margarine, about 11 per cent from fruits and vegetables, and about 7 per cent from grain products.

The recommended allowance takes into consideration the amount and type of fat consumed. As the total amount of fat and PUFA increases the requirement for vitamin E increases. Assuming that the fat consumption in the United States is liberal (about 40 per cent of the total calories) and the PUFA is high (over 35 gm. per day), the FNB recommends 30 IU daily of vitamin E. If PUFA intake was under 7 gm. per day the RDA for vitamin E would be only about 10 IU.

The vitamin E requirement is not related to calorie intake or directly to body weight; it appears to be related to body weight in kg. to the three-quarter power (kg.$^{0.75}$). This is designated as physiologic or metabolic size. This parameter does not include needs for growth. Studies on vitamin E requirements of 11 species of animals of very different sizes indicated that their requirements were related to body weight to the 0.73 power, a figure close to that suggested for man. The allowances listed in the RDA (Table A–3 in the Appendix) were determined by multiplying body weight in kg.$^{0.75}$ by 1.25. Table A–2 in the Appendix gives body weights in kilograms (kg.) and kg.$^{3/4}$

No danger from large intakes of vitamin E have been detected. Even at daily intakes of 800 IU per kg. body weight over a period of five months no toxic symptoms were noted.

Vitamin K

THE CHEMISTRY AND PHYSIOLOGY OF VITAMIN K

Natural and synthetic forms of the vitamin are known. In 1929 Dam and co-workers (1) of the University of Copenhagen described a hemorrhagic disease of chicken, associated with a delayed blood-clotting time. In 1935 they reported the presence of a fat-soluble, antihemorrhagic substance in foods which they called the "Koagulations-vitamin." Since then numerous compounds which have vitamin K activity have been isolated and synthesized, and their chemical and physiological properties have been investigated. Several laboratory tests, including radioactivity, have been used in these studies. The products are derivatives of 2-methyl-1, 4-naphthoquinone. There are two natural forms of vitamin K. K_1, which contains a phytyl group, was first isolated from alfalfa and is found especially in green leafy vegetables. K_2, representing a series of compounds with varying lengths of side chains, contains the difarnosyl group; it was originally secured from putrefied fish meal (Figure 11–7).

Figure 11–7
Structural formulas of the K vitamins

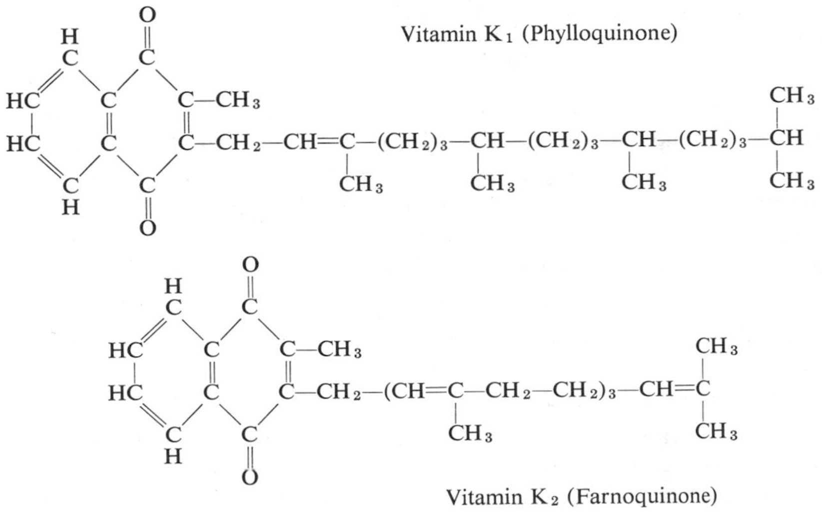

Vitamin K_1 (Phylloquinone)

Vitamin K_2 (Farnoquinone)

An International Committee (2) has adopted the terms "phylloquinone" (K_1), "menaquinone" (MK_n) in which *n* is the number of isoprene units in the side chain, and "menadione." The latter term, as used by the International Committee, is a synthesized yellow crystalline powder, devoid of the phytyl side chain (Figure 11–8).

The compounds are heat-stable and are destroyed by irradiation. While the natural K vitamins are fat-soluble, some of the synthetic compounds are water-soluble, in which state they are well adapted for therapeutic use. Vitamin K_1 is preferred over menadione for use as a supplement since excessive doses of menadione may produce toxic symptoms such as increased breakdown of red blood cells and inhibition of glucoronide formation.

Early in the study of the anti-hemorrhagic vitamin an association was made with coumarin anticoagulants, one of which was found in improperly cured clover hay. When cattle were fed this hay they suffered from

Figure 11–8

Structural formula of menadione

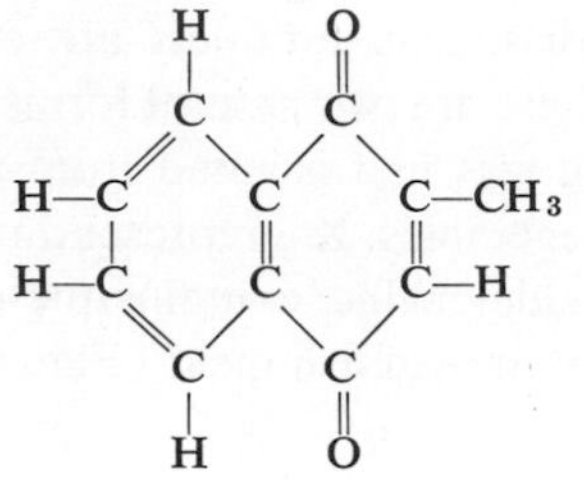

severe bleeding. One of these coumarin derivatives, wayfarin, is being used in investigations on the effectiveness of vitamin K as a blood coagulant (3).

Both exogenous and endogenous vitamin K are used by the body. Dietary sources of vitamin K are absorbed in the small intestine where fats are absorbed (4). Bile salts are necessary for effective absorption. The vitamin passes into the lacteals, through the thoracic duct, and into the liver. Here it functions in synthesis of the proteins, prothrombin (factor II), proconvertin factor (factor VII), plasma thromboplastin component (PTC, factor IX), and the Stewart factor (factor X) (5). All these are necessary for blood clotting. The mechanism of this synthesis is not known but it is believed that vitamin K is not incorporated in the prothrombin molecule.

Vitamin K is synthesized by bacteria in the intestinal tract. This may supply considerable of the vitamin K adult needs. In the newborn baby the intestinal flora do not yet function to synthesize the vitamin and so hemorrhaging may occur (6). Excretion of vitamin K is largely through the feces. In the rat coprophagy (consumption of feces) has been shown to supply the animal with all the vitamin it requires.

THE BODY'S NEED FOR VITAMIN K

Vitamin K is necessary for normal coagulation of the blood. Early experiments on young chicks fed a low-fat diet resulted in bleeding and death; treatment with vitamin K prevented the hemorrhaging. This disorder was found to be associated with a lack of prothrombin in the blood. Use of the vitamin was extended to treatment of obstructive jaundice in man and hemorrhage in the newborn; in both these conditions the bleeding was associated with a deficiency in the blood-clotting mechanism. The factors involved in coagulation are low in the blood of the newborn and decrease still more during the first week of life. In the following weeks their concentrations return spontaneously toward adult levels.

In some mammalian tissue and in bacteria vitamin K has been shown to function in electron transport and oxidative phosphorylation. It probably serves as a prosthetic group in essential enzyme systems in liver cells. It is not thought to act through messenger RNA (5).

The need for vitamin K has been related to other nutrients and hormones. The relationships of vitamin K to other compounds are complex. Doisy (7) demonstrated that vitamin A, even at low intake levels, markedly decreased the plasma prothrombin level in the absence of vitamin K. The mechanism of the interrelationship of vitamins A and K is not understood, but it appears that prothrombin levels vary inversely with the amount of dietary vitamin A. It has been suggested that vitamin E may have a deleterious effect on vitamin K similar to that of vitamin A. This may be because vitamin E as an antioxidant preserves vitamin A, which then serves as an antagonist for vitamin K. Matschiner and Doisy (8) showed that the effects of vitamin K deficiency on blood coagulation were less in rats when a deficiency of protein occurred simultaneously.

It is known that the male animal is more subject to hemorrhage than the female. Mellette and Leone (9) found that administration of male hormones (androgens) intensifies hemorrhages. Administration of female hormones (estrogens) ameliorates the bleeding caused by lack of vitamin K (10). The vitamin K requirements of rat, chick, and monkey are increased by addition of sulfonamides or antibiotics. This probably is the result of decreased intestinal synthesis of the vitamin.

THE REQUIREMENT FOR VITAMIN K

No daily allowance for this vitamin has been set. Observations made on human adults indicate that a deficiency of vitamin K is uncommon. This favorable condition is assumed to be due both to synthesis by intestinal microorganisms and to a sufficiency in the diet.

The vitamin is widely distributed in natural foods; animal products are poorer sources than plants; hog liver is the richest known animal source. Cow's milk and human milk contain 60 and 15 μg. per liter, respectively. Green leaves such as spinach and kale are excellent sources; cauliflower and cabbage are also good sources. Cereals, roots, and fruits contain small amounts.

Frick and co-workers (11) used antibiotics in a study of ten elderly subjects who were maintained entirely on intravenous feedings, which consisted of a solution of glucose, minerals, and water-soluble vitamins. Seven subjects who received antibiotics as well as the nutrient solution had no lowering of the clotting factors II, VII, and X. The three who received only the nutrient solution had no lowering of the clotting factors. Next, four of the seven who had developed vitamin K deficiency were studied to find the minimum amount of vitamin K required daily to permit a sustained elevation of clotting time for 24 hours. This was found to be approximately 0.03 µg. vitamin K per kg. body weight. This amount elevated clotting time to about 30 per cent of normal levels.

Zieve and Solomon (3) used wayfarin in a study of vitamin K requirement. They measured the response in blood clotting time of six adult human volunteers to a single dose of the anticoagulant. No record of the diet was kept. The individual effect varied considerably in both magnitude and duration of response. Varying sized doses of vitamin K were then injected intravenously and the effects on clotting time noted. When 2.5 or 5.0 mg. vitamin K was given 48 hours after 40 mg. wayfarin, the clotting time of three subjects returned to normal in six hours. Such a study is very complicated because of individual variations in synthesis and absorption of vitamin K, hormone activity, and diet and other exogenous factors.

Special consideration should be given to the needs of the·newborn. Danger of hemorrhage in the baby at birth is great, due to low values of the coagulation factors. Sutherland and co-workers (12) studied 3338 full-term newborn infants to ascertain the qualitative and quantitative need for vitamin K. At birth these babies were given either a placebo, or 5 mg., or 100 µg. of menadione sodium bisulfite. Hypothrombinemic bleeding was noted only in breast-fed babies given the placebo. To prevent bleeding, 100 µg. of the vitamin K compound was found to be as effective as 5 mg.

The vitamin is usually administered as a water-miscible form in a single oral dose: sometimes it is given parenterally or intramuscularly. It is especially important to give vitamin K when there is increased susceptibility to hemorrhage due to prematurity or anoxia (oxygen shortage), and when the mother has received anticoagulant therapy.

The greater susceptibility of breast-fed infants to hemorrhage is explained by the vitamin K content of milks. Human milk has 15 µg. vitamin K per liter, while cow's milk contains 60 µg. per liter.

At one time the vitamin was customarily given to the mother four to 24 hours before delivery. However, the Committee on Nutrition of the American Academy of Pediatrics (13) does not advocate this practice. If large amounts of water-soluble vitamin K are given to the mother, they may be harmful to the infant; smaller amounts are apt to be ineffective in preventing hemorrhage. Harmful effects have included hyperbilirubinemia, mild hemolytic anemia, and kernicterus; these conditions are more noticeable in premature than in full-term infants.

PROBLEMS

1. Calculate the IU of vitamin A in the food intake records used in Problem 1, Chapter 2. Determine the average number of units in your daily diet. How does the figure compare with the standard given? If it is low, make suggestions to correct the deficiency.

2. A college girl trying to economize ate the following:

		kcal
Breakfast	Coffee, 1 cup black	0
	Sugar, 1 teaspoon	13
	Bread, whole wheat, 2 slices	130
	Margarine, 2 pats	70
	Jam, 1 tablespoon	55
Dinner	Boiled ham, 1 slice	135
	Mashed potato, ½ cup	93
	Boiled cabbage, ¾ cup	23
	Pickles, 2 small	40
	Applesauce, ½ cup	115
Supper	Bread, white enriched, 2 slices	140
	Peanut butter, 2 tablespoons	190
	Butterscotch pie, 1 sector	350
	Cola-type beverage, 12 ounces	145
11 P.M.	Milk chocolate, 1 ounce	145
	Total	1644

Calculate the units of vitamin A she obtained. Suggest a menu which will meet the standards set in the food check sheet and supply her with 2000 calories and 5000 IU of vitamin A. Keep the cost as low as possible.

REFERENCES

Vitamin A

1. Steenbock, H. White Corn vs. Yellow Corn and a Probable Relation Between the Fat-Soluble Vitamin and Yellow Plant Pigments. *Sci.,* *50:*352 (1919).

2. Leitner, Z. A., *et al.* Vitamin A and Vitamin E in Human Blood. I. Levels of Vitamin A and Carotenoids in British Men and Women, 1948–57. *Brit. J. Nutr., 14:*157 (1960).

3. Olson, J. A. Metabolism and Function of Vitamin A. *Fed. Proc., 28:*1670 (1969).

4. Olson, J. A. Some Aspects of Vitamin A Metabolism. *In* R. S. Harris, I. G. Wool, and J. L. Loraine (eds.), *Vitamins and Hormones. 26:*1. New York: Academic Press (1968).

5. Goodman, D. S. Retinol Transport in Human Plasma. *Am. J. Clin. Nutr., 22:*911 (1969).

6. Sherman, H. L. *et al.* A Quantitative Study of the Storage of Vitamin A. *J. Biol. Chem., 68:*69 (1926).

7. Thompson, J. N., *et al.* Vitamin A in Development of the Embryo. *Am. J. Clin. Nutr., 22:*1063 (1969).

8. Warkany, J. Congenital Malformations Induced by Maternal Dietary Deficiency. *Nutr. Revs., 13:*289 (1955).

9. Lucy, J. A., *et al.* Studies on the Mode of Action of Excess of Vitamin A. 8. Mitochondrial Swelling. *Biochem. J., 89:*419 (1963).

10. Bieri, J. G., *et al.* Survival of Germfree Rats without Vitamin A. *Sci., 163:*574 (1969).

11. Wolbach, S. B. Vitamin A Deficiency and Excess in Relation to Skeletal Growth. *J. Bone and Joint Surg., 29:*171 (1947).

12. Irving, J. T., *et al.* The Protective Action of Vitamin A upon Various Tissues in the Avitaminotic Rat and the Sensitivity of These Tissues to Vitamin A Deficiency. *Brit. J. Nutr., 10:*7 (1956).

13. Joint FAO/WHO Expert Group. *Requirements of Vitamin A, Thiamin, Riboflavin and Niacin.* Tech. Report Series 362. WHO, Rome (1967).

14. Lian, O. K., *et al.* Red Palm Oil in the Prevention of Vitamin A Deficiency. A Trial in Preschool Children in Indonesia. *Am. J. Clin. Nutr., 20:*1267 (1967).

15. Kruse, H. D. The Ocular Manifestations of Avitaminosis A with Special Considerations of the Detection of Early Changes by Biomicroscopy. *Milbank Mem. Fund Quart., 19:*207 (1942).

16. Hume, E. M., *et al. Vitamin A Requirement of Human Adults: An Experimental Study of Vitamin Deprivation in Man.* London: Medical Research Council (1949).

17. Callison, E. C., *et al.* Availability of Carotene from Carrots and Further Observations on Human Requirements for Vitamin A and Carotene. *J. Nutr., 34:*153 (1947).

18. Ames, S. R. Factors Affecting Absorption, Transport and Storage of Vitamin A. *Am. J. Clin. Nutr., 22:*934 (1969).

19. Arroyave, G. Interrelations Between Protein and Vitamin A and Metabolism. *Am. J. Clin. Nutr., 22:*1119 (1969).

20. Patwardhan, V. N. Hypovitaminosis A and Epidemiology of Xerophthalmia. *Am. J. Clin. Nutr., 22:*1106 (1969).

21. György, P. Protein-Calorie and Vitamin A Malnutrition in Southeast Asia. *Fed. Proc., 27:*949 (1968).

22. Agricultural Research Service, USDA, Consumer and Food Economics Research Division. Household Food Consumption Survey, 1965–66. Report 6.

23. Morgan, A. F. (ed.), *Nutritional Status U.S.A.* Berkeley: Calif. Agr. Expt. Sta. Bull. 769 (1959).

24. Schaefer, A. E. The National Nutrition Survey, *J. Am. Diet. Ass., 54:*371 (1969).

25. High, E. G. Some Aspects of Nutritional Vitamin A Levels in Preschool Children of Beauport County, S.C. *Am. J. Clin. Nutr., 22:*1128 (1969).

GENERAL REFERENCES

26. Goodhart, R. S. Vitamin A. *In* M. G. Wohl and R. S. Goodhart (eds.), *Modern Nutrition in Health and Disease,* 4th ed. Philadelphia: Lea and Febiger (1968).

27. Roels, O. A. Present Knowledge of Vitamin A. *In Present Knowledge in Nutrition,* 3rd ed. New York: Nutrition Foundation (1967).

Vitamin D

1. Weick, M. T. A History of Rickets in the United States. *Am. J. Clin. Nutr., 20:*1234 (1967).
2. Blunt, K., *et al. Ultra Violet Light and Vitamin D in Nutrition.* Chicago: University of Chicago Press (1930).
3. Loomis, W. F. Skin-Pigment Regulation of Vitamin D Biosynthesis in Man. *Sci., 157:*9 (1967).
4. DeLuca, H. F. Recent Advances in the Metabolism and Function of Vitamin D. *Fed. Proc., 28:*1678 (1969).
5. DeLuca, H. F. Mechanism of Action and Fate of Vitamin D. *In* R. S. Harris, I. G. Wool, and J. L. Loraine (eds.), *Vitamins and Hormones, 25:*315, New York: Academic Press (1967).
6. Roberts, A. H., *et al.* Effect of Phytate and Other Dietary Factors on Intestinal Phytase and Bone Calcification in the Rat. *Brit. J. Nutr., 15:*457 (1961).
7. Steenbock, H., *et al.* Vitamin D and Growth. *J. Nutr., 57:*449 (1955).
8. Bessey, O. A., *et al.* A Method for the Rapid Determination of Alkaline Phosphatase with Five Cubic Millimeters of Serum. *J. Biol. Chem., 164:*321 (1946).
9. Jeans, P. C., *et al.* Effect of Vitamin D on Linear Growth in Infancy. *J. Pediat., 13:*730 (1938).
10. Eliot, M. M., *et al.* A Study of the Teeth of a Group of School Children Previously Examined for Rickets. *Am. J. Dis. Childr., 48:*713 (1934).
11. McCollum, E. V., *et al.* Studies on Experimental Rickets. XVI. A Delicate Biological Test for Calcium-Depositing Substances. *J. Biol. Chem., 51:*41 (1922).
12. Numerof, P., *et al.* The Use of Radioactive Phosphorus in the Assay of Vitamin D. *J. Nutr., 55:*13 (1955).
13. WHO Subcommittee on Fat-Soluble Vitamins. *Chronicle of World Health Organization, 3:*147 (1949).
14. Panel on Recommended Allowances of Nutrients. *Recommended Intakes of Nutrients for the United Kingdom.* Report No. 120. London: Dept of Health and Social Security (1969).

GENERAL REFERENCES

15. Forbes, G. B. Present Knowledge of Vitamin D. *In Present Knowledge in Nutrition,* 3rd ed. New York: Nutrition Foundation (1967).
16. Goodhart, R. E. Vitamin D. *In* M. G. Wohl and R. S. Goodhart (eds.), *Modern Nutrition in Health and Disease,* 4th ed. Philadelphia: Lea and Febiger (1968).

Vitamin E

1. Evans, H. M. The Pioneer History of Vitamin E. *In* R. S. Harris and I. G. Wool (eds.), *Vitamins and Hormones, 20:*379. New York: Academic Press (1962).

2. Herting, D. C., *et al.* Vitamin E Content of Vegetable Oils and Fats. *J. Nutr., 81:*335 (1963).

3. Booth, V. H., *et al.* Tocopherol Contents of Vegetables and Fruits. *Brit. J. Nutr., 17:*575 (1963).

4. Herting, D. C., *et al.* Vitamin E Content of Milk, Milk Products, and Simulated Milks: Relevance to Infant Nutrition. *Am. J. Clin. Nutr., 22:*147 (1967).

5. Bunnell, R. H., *et al.* α-Tocopherol Content of Foods. *Am. J. Clin. Nutr., 17:*1 (1965).

6. Draper, H. H., *et al.* Metabolism and Function of Vitamin E. *Fed. Proc., 28:*1690 (1969).

7. Herting, D. C., *et al.* Plasma Tocopherol Levels in Man. *Am. J. Clin. Nutr., 17:*351 (1965).

8. Century, B., *et al.* Biological Availability of Various Forms of Vitamin E with Respect to Different Indices of Deficiency. *Fed Proc., 24:*906 (1965).

9. Fitch, C. D. The Red Blood Cell in the Vitamin E-Deficient Monkey. *Am. J. Clin. Nutr., 21:*51 (1968).

10. Schwarz, K. Factor 3, Selenium, and Vitamin E. *Nutr. Revs., 18:*193 (1960).

11. Symposium of Interrelationships Among Vitamin E, Coenzyme Q, and Selenium. *Fed. Proc., 24:*55 (1965).

12. Horwitt, M. K., *et al.* Erythrocyte Survival Time and Reticulocyte Levels after Tocopherol Depletion in Man. *Am. J. Clin. Nutr., 12:*99 (1963).

13. Rose, C. S., *et al.* Specificity of Hemolytic Reaction in Vitamin E-Deficient Erythrocytes. *Am. J. Physiol., 168:*414 (1952).

14. Horwitt, M. K. Interrelations Between Vitamin E and Polyunsaturated Fatty Acids in Adult Man. *In* R. S. Harris and I. G. Wool (eds.), *Vitamins and Hormones, 20:*541. New York: Academic Press (1962).

15. Oski, F. A., *et al.* Hemolytic Anemia in Vitamin E Deficiency. *Am. J. Clin. Nutr., 21:*45 (1968).

16. Barness, L. A. Tocopherol-Responsive Anemia in Premature Infants. *In* R. S. Harris, I. G. Wool, and J. L. Loraine (eds.), *Vitamins and Hormones, 26:*70. New York: Academic Press (1968).

17. Majaj, A. S., *et al.* Vitamin E-Responsive Megaloblastic Anemia in Infants with Protein-Calorie Malnutrition. *Am. J. Clin. Nutr., 12:*374 (1963).

18. Harris, P. L., *et al.* Quantitative Consideration of the Effect of Polyunsaturated Fatty Acid Content of the Diet upon the Requirements for Vitamin E. *Am. J. Clin. Nutr., 13:*385 (1963).

GENERAL REFERENCES

19. Gordon, H. H., and Nitowsky, H. M. Vitamin E. *In* M. G. Wohl and R. S. Goodhart (eds.), *Modern Nutrition in Health and Disease,* 4th ed. Philadelphia: Lea and Febiger (1968).

20. Herting, D. C. Perspective on Vitamin E. *Am. J. Clin. Nutr., 19:*210 (1966).

21. Horwitt, M. K. Lipids, α-Tocopherol and Erythrocyte Hemolysis. *In* R. S. Harris, I. G. Wool, and J. L. Loraine (eds.), *Vitamins and Hormones, 26:*487. New York: Academic Press (1968).

22. Roels, O. A. Present Knowledge of Vitamin E. *In Present Knowledge in Nutrition,* 3rd ed. New York: Nutrition Foundation (1967).

Vitamin K

1. Dam, H., *et al.* Isolation of Vitamin K in Highly Purified Form. *Helvetica Chimica Acta, 22:*310 (1939).

2. International Union of Pure and Applied Chemistry-International Union of Biochemistry, Commission of Biochemical Nomenclature, Tentative Rules. Nomenclature of Quinones with Isoprenoid Sidechains. *Biochim. Biophys. Acta, 107:*5 (1965).

3. Zieve, S. D., *et al.* Variation in the Response of Human Beings to Vitamin K. *J. Lab. Clin. Med., 73:*103 (1969).

4. Udall, J. A. Human Sources and Absorption of Vitamin K in Relation to Anticoagulation Stability. *J. Am. Med. Ass., 194:*127 (1965).

5. Suttie, J. W. Control of Clotting Factor Biosynthesis by Vitamin K. *Fed. Proc., 28:*1696 (1969).

6. Aballi, A. J., *et al.* Coagulation Studies in the Newborn Period. III. Hemorrhagic Diseases of the Newborn. *Am. J. Dis. Childr., 97:*524 (1959).

7. Doisy, E. A. Nutritional Hypoprothrombinemia and Metabolism of Vitamin K. *Fed. Proc., 20:*989 (1961).

8. Matschiner, J. T., *et al.* The Effect of Dietary Protein in the Development of Vitamin K Deficiency in the Rat. *J. Nutr., 86:*93 (1965).

9. Mellette, S. J., *et al.* Influence of Age, Sex, Strain of Rat, and Fat-Soluble Vitamins on Hemorrhagic Syndromes in Rats Fed Irradiated Beef. *Fed. Proc., 19:*1045 (1960).

10. Rama Roa, P. B., *et al.* Relationship of Estrogen and Vitamin K. *Proc. Soc. Expl. Biol. Med., 112:*393 (1963).

11. Frick, P. G., *et al.* Dose Response and Minimal Daily Requirement for Vitamin K in Man. *J. Appl. Physiol., 25:*387 (1967).

12. Sutherland, J. M., *et al.* Hemorrhagic Disease of the Newborn—Breast Feeding as a Necessary Factor in the Pathogenesis. *Am. J. Dis. Childr., 113:*524 (1967).

13. American Academy of Pediatrics, Committee on Nutrition. Vitamin K Compounds and the Water-Soluble Analogues. *Pediat., 28:*51 (1961).

GENERAL REFERENCES

14. Goodhart, R. S. Vitamin K. *In* M. G. Wohl and R. S. Goodhart (eds.), *Modern Nutrition in Health and Disease,* 4th ed. Philadelphia: Lea and Febiger (1968).

15. Olson, R. E. Present Knowledge of Vitamin K. In *Present Knowledge in Nutrition,* 3rd ed. New York: The Nutrition Foundation (1967).

Water-Soluble Vitamins

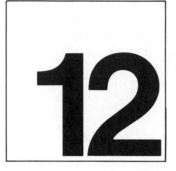

At approximately the same time that the first fat-soluble factor was discovered, a water-soluble substance essential for growth was also found. Later it became clear that this was not a single entity but was composed of many distinct factors, and that some foods contained a water-soluble constituent separate from fat-soluble A and water-soluble B. Today many vitamins more or less soluble in water have been identified and synthesized. However, much still needs to be learned about their chemistry, biochemical and physiological functions, and sources as well as human requirements for them.

In this chapter ascorbic acid, also known as vitamin C, and three members of the vitamin B complex—thiamin, riboflavin, and niacin— are discussed in detail. Significant facts about vitamin B_6, biotin, pantothenic acid, folic acid, and vitamin B_{12} are presented, and brief mention is made of *para*-aminobenzoic acid, choline, and inositol. Actually, when considering the B vitamins, it must be remembered that the various factors usually occur simultaneously in foods and that a disease syndrome resulting from lack of only one member of the B complex seldom occurs.

Ascorbic Acid (Vitamin C)

THE CHEMISTRY OF ASCORBIC ACID

The vitamin was discovered through a search for an antiscorbutic substance. A cure for scurvy was known long before its relationship to ascorbic acid was suspected. As early as 1493 scurvy was reported as a scourge of the sea, prevalence of the disease depending largely on the length of time the crew was on the ship without reprovisioning with fresh foods. When Magellan circumnavigated the globe in 1522, the majority of his men were stricken with scurvy. Cartier, in his journal kept on a 1535 voyage to Newfoundland, described the symptoms of the dread disease. He told how his captain secured from the Indians branches of a tree (spruce) whose growing tips, when brewed, were a miraculous cure. An infusion made of rose hips has been used as a dietary supplement in Russian nurseries and preschools. This source of ascorbic acid is now thought to be both impractical and uneconomical.

In 1928 hexuronic acid, isolated from orange juice, cabbage juice, and ox adrenal glands, was found to be identical with vitamin C, an antiscorbutic material obtained from lemon juice. By 1933 the structure of the vitamin had been determined and it had been synthesized. It is now available in tablet form at very low cost.

Much is known about the chemistry of ascorbic acid. This vitamin is readily soluble in water, is odorless, and in pure form occurs as white crystals. It is insoluble in fat and fat solvents. Its formula is $C_6H_8O_6$; it closely resembles glucose in structure but contains an acid lactone and a dienol group (Figure 12–1). To the latter group it owes its strong re-

Figure 12–1
Structural formulas of ascorbic acid

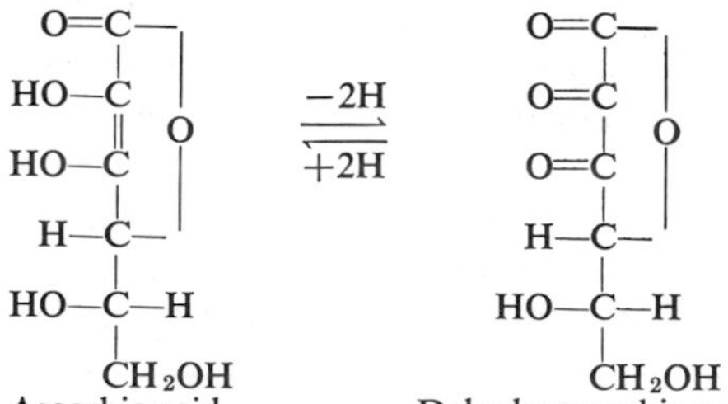

L-Ascorbic acid   Dehydroascorbic acid

ducing action. The L-isomer is the physiologically active form. It is rapidly oxidized by the cytochrome oxidases and some other tissue catalysts to dehydroascorbic acid; in this form it is also biologically active. Dehydroascorbic acid may be reversibly reduced to ascorbic acid by di- and tri-phosphopyridine nucleotides and related enzyme systems in the presence of sulfhydryl compounds such as cysteine and glutathione. Or if the pH of the medium is above 4, dehydroascorbic acid may be further and irreversibly reduced to 2,3-diketogulonic acid and finally to oxalic acid and L-threonic acid. In some analyses of foods, diketogulonic acid has been included as ascorbic acid but it has no ascorbic acid potency. An acid medium and buffer substances tend to protect the factor from oxidation; heat in the presence of air, alkali, and catalysts such as copper and iron speed the breakdown. Erythorbic acid, a compound which differs from L-ascorbic acid only in its space configuration around the fifth carbon atom, has little or no antiscorbutic activity.

Glucoascorbic acid is known to be an antagonist to the vitamin. The rat, normally able to synthesize a sufficiency of the vitamin, will develop scurvy when fed glucoascorbic acid. It is not known whether this analogue of ascorbic acid is an antivitamin or whether it hinders synthesis by intestinal bacteria.

Except for guinea pigs, fruit bats, and the primates, animals can convert D-glucose to L-ascorbic acid; failure of synthesis has been identified as a lack of the enzyme L-gulono-lactone oxidase.

Tests for ascorbic acid are based on its chemical reactions. The reducing property of the factor is the basis of chemical tests used to measure quantitatively the vitamin value of a sample. In a commonly used technique, 2,6-dichloro-phenol-indophenol is decolorized by ascorbic acid; measurement of the amount of reagent reduced is made either by titration or, preferably, by means of a spectrophotometer or a photometric colorimeter. The dinitrophenylhydrazine method has been adapted for use in nutrition surveys and requires very small samples of blood serum. Values for this vitamin are reported most frequently on reduced ascorbic acid, the form in which most of the factor occurs in fresh foods. Dehydroascorbic acid, the oxidized form, is found in significant amounts in processed or stored foods. Since few investigators have reported both these forms, or total ascorbic acid, the data in tables of nutritive value may give lower than actual amounts. However, higher than actual figures may be secured by analysis in the presence of interfering substances which react like the vitamin chemically but not physiologically; such substances are apt to be found in high-carbohydrate foods which have been heated or stored under unfavorable conditions.

THE ROLES PLAYED BY ASCORBIC ACID IN THE BODY

This factor is found in many parts of the body. Since ascorbic acid is water-soluble, it is readily absorbed from the gastrointestinal tract into the blood stream. Studies using radioactive ascorbic acid show that it is rapidly taken from the serum and transported to the adrenal glands, kidneys, and liver. Transfer to such tissues as the eyes, muscles, testes, and brain is more gradual. Tissues which have higher metabolic activity contain the highest concentrations of this vitamin. The rate of transfer has nothing to do with the amounts present in the various body parts. Observations indicate that the ascorbic acid content of tissues tends to decrease with age and that excretion is greater in the older person.

The oxidized form of the vitamin crosses cellular barriers more readily than does reduced ascorbic acid and is thought to be the form which penetrates the erythrocytes, brain, and placenta. Comparatively little of the vitamin, probably about 1 gm., is stored in the body.

The major part of the intake is excreted within a few hours after ingestion. The kidneys are the main excretory organ. Abt and co-workers

(1) demonstrated that the respiratory tract is also an elimination pathway. The amount excreted varies with the amount of intake and the degree to which the body tissues are saturated.

The only metabolic end products of ascorbic acid are ascorbic acid, dehydroascorbic acid, and oxalate. Baker and associates (2) studied three healthy men whose ascorbic acid intakes were about 100 mg. per day. Their ascorbic acid pool was 2 to 3 gm. and the turnover half-time was about 20 days.

Ascorbic acid performs several functions. It serves as a co-factor or a coenzyme in several metabolic systems. It takes part in hydroxylation of proline to hydroxyproline, in the synthesis of collagen, hydroxylation of tryptophan to 5-hydroxytryptophan, conversion of 3, 4-dihydroxy-phenylethylamine to norepinephrine, and hydroxylation of p-hydroxy-phenylpyruvate to homogentisic acid in the metabolic pathway of tyrosine. Other systems in which ascorbic acid participates are the hydrolysis of alkyl mono-thioglycosides and the regulation of the respiratory cycle in mitochondria and microsomes. Ascorbic acid is involved in reduction and release of the ferric ion from transferrin, a plasma protein, and its incorporation into tissue ferritin; in this transfer ATP is necessary (3).

It has been shown that ascorbic acid lowers the blood cholesterol content of patients with atherosclerosis and a deficiency of this vitamin has been suggested as a contributing factor in development of this disorder. But it has also been demonstrated in experimental animals that a deficiency of ascorbic acid may result in atherosclerosis without an accompanying increase in blood cholesterol and deposition of lipids in the tissues. This indicates that ascorbic acid does not have a specific relationship to cholesterol metabolism. Shaffer (4) suggests that the vitamin lack, by disturbing the integrity of intercellular tissues, provides a medium which favors deposition of cholesterol and plaques.

There is a high concentration of ascorbic acid in the adrenal cortex. This gland tends to hypertrophy in scurvy, as well as in conditions of stress such as exposure to cold, x-ray, and thermal shock; injections of large doses of the vitamin prevent this. There must be a close relationship between the metabolism of ascorbic acid and corticosteroid hormone synthesis.

During a deficiency of ascorbic acid, wound healing is retarded and defective; it has been found that collagen synthesis also is very poor (5). Shortly after surgical incision, content of ascorbic acid at the wound site is high. A plasma concentration of 0.4 to 1.0 mg. of ascorbic acid per 100 ml. of serum is associated with tissue saturation and with normal wound healing.

The role of ascorbic acid in infection is mentioned frequently. Low blood ascorbic acid values have been reported in infectious diseases such as tuberculosis, diphtheria, rheumatic fever, and pneumonia. It is not known whether this lack is due to increased demand by the diseased tissues or to accelerated losses; direct action of the vitamin on the harmful bacteria has been suggested. Contrary to popular belief there is no experimental evidence that vitamin C has a deterring effect on the incidence, duration, or severity of the common cold. Walker and co-workers (6) conducted both *in vitro* and *in vivo* experiments on this subject, the latter in both animals and human beings. Objective means were used in determining the results. In one part of the investigation, 91 human volunteers were used. They ate an *ad libitum* mixed diet containing fresh fruits and cooked vegetables. All subjects were inoculated with viruses known to be frequent causes of colds. For three days prior to the inoculations and for six days after, 47 subjects received 1 gm. ascorbic acid three times a day and 44 subjects received placebo tablets. No evidence was noted of a general prophylactic effect of ascorbic acid, nor was there any difference in the number or severity of colds in the two groups.

Scurvy results from a deficiency of ascorbic acid. When this vitamin is lacking, abnormalities are found in supporting or intercellular tissues of cartilage, dentine, and bone matrix, the collagen of fibrous tissues, and nonepithelial cement substances. These play important parts in the structure and functioning of bones and teeth, capillaries, muscle, and glandular organs. In scurvy, failure to maintain normal collagen is the primary cause of most of the obvious physical changes. The scientific relationship between ascorbic acid and collagen has been understood only recently. Collagen is unique in that it contains much hydroxyproline, whereas other proteins contain proline (7). Feeding hydroxyproline does not result directly in collagen formation. First, proline is built into a protein unit by cellular ribosomes. Then an enzyme, collagen protein hydroxylase, catalyzes the action in which ascorbic acid and oxygen are essential to adding a hydroxyl group to carbon-4 of the proline.

Lack of ascorbic acid results in abnormalities in the supporting tissues evidenced by hemorrhage, soft swollen gums, teeth with resorbed porotic dentine, malformed and weak bones, anemia, and degeneration of muscle fibers, including those of the heart. Beading of the ribs at the costochrondal junctions is evident and may be confused with that seen in rickets. Fractures are apt to occur near the ends of the long bones which are swollen and brittle and in which new trabeculae do not form at a normal rate. X-ray examination shows a very characteristic transverse band of increased density, called the "white line of scurvy." This is caused by accumulation of calcified matrix which under normal circumstances would be removed. The epiphyses show a "halo" appearance, also due to the abnormal calcium deposition. These deficiency symptoms are evident to a greater or lesser degree in scurvy. Latent scurvy, more prevalent especially among low-income groups and accompanying certain diseases, is evidenced by lassitude, fleeting pains, especially at the joints, bleeding gums, and internal hemorrhages resulting in black-and-blue spots.

The positive effect of ascorbic acid on mineral retention is thought to relate to its favorable influence on the intercellular structure of bone matrix, cartilage, and teeth; in a similar way the ascorbic acid in the nonepithelial cement substances of the capillaries prevents bleeding.

Greater body growth in the guinea pig has been associated with higher intakes of ascorbic acid. Evans and Hughes (8) have shown that this is due to a metabolic effect on tissue formation rather than to food consumption.

FOODS WHICH SUPPLY ASCORBIC ACID

Plant sources are superior to animal sources in ascorbic acid. The chemical assays referred to earlier are being used more than the bioassay in determination of ascorbic acid values. When the latter technique is used, the guinea pig is the test animal, and on an ascorbic acid-free diet a young guinea pig develops scurvy in from two to three weeks. The technique used in the preventive method involves growth and the conditions of bones and blood on autopsy. Ascorbic acid values are expressed in terms of milligrams.

Citrus fruits and strawberries are excellent plant sources of the factor; other good sources include tomatoes, green peppers, and cantaloupes, the more acid berries such as gooseberries and currants, and the more actively growing parts of the edible plant such as the leaves. Animal sources are as a whole poor; liver is superior to muscle tissue, and raw fresh milk from a cow fed green grass may contain considerable ascorbic acid. However, when the liver is cooked and the milk pasteurized or allowed to stand, a large proportion of the original amount has been destroyed. The importance of the care given to milk between time of milking and delivery to the home was shown by Holmes (9) in a study of 126 samples of commercial retail milk. Milk sold in stores averaged 3.8 mg. of ascorbic acid per liter; that delivered to the home, 6.3 mg. Exposure to light is also an important factor in retention or loss of the vitamin. This loss on standing may also be expected in vegetables and non-acid fruits.

The ascorbic acid content of plant foods is known to vary greatly with such factors as variety, climate, amount of sunshine, soil, and degree of maturity. Agronomists are studying these problems, and many state experiment stations make recommendations to farmers on selection of seed, growing conditions, harvesting, and marketing.

Various parts of the plant differ in vitamin content. In a study of the turnip, values of ascorbic acid, thiamin, riboflavin, and carotene were determined in the blade and midrib of the leaf and in the root; for all vitamins tested the leaf blade was found to be the best source, the root the poorest. Sixty-six per cent of the total ascorbic acid was in the blade; only 9 per cent in the root.

Ascorbic acid loss may be expected because of its instability. The chemical properties of ascorbic acid related to its loss or retention were given earlier. These should be kept in mind during the selection, storage, and preparation of food to obtain maximal amounts of the vitamin.

Practices carried on at the market and in the home before the food is prepared for eating play a large part in its vitamin value. When selecting fresh fruits and vegetables, it is wise to patronize stores which use modern methods of storing and exhibiting; a cold temperature for storage is better than room temperature although not all foods are equally affected. Cabbage, tomatoes, and green peppers when kept for 48 hours in air at room temperature retained respectively 94, 88, and 85 per cent of their original ascorbic acid—more than did kale (64 per cent), carrots (56 per cent), beets (75 per cent), and peas (67 per cent). It has been found that vegetables stored in crushed ice retained a greater percentage of ascorbic acid than did those kept on ice or in the refrigerator. Broccoli stored for two days in crushed ice had no ascorbic acid loss. Stored in the refrigerator, retention was 92 per cent; on top of ice, 91 per cent; when left at room temperature, 56 per cent. Some large produce markets use crushed ice in their open display cases.

It is important to choose young fresh produce; a wilted item is seldom a bargain. When the food is brought into the home, it should, with a few exceptions, be kept in a cold place until used—preferably a short storage time for maximal ascorbic acid content. In preparation use a sharp knife and avoid crushing, grinding, or bruising. More ascorbic acid will be secured from oranges or grapefruit which are halved, sliced, or sectioned than from those which are juiced. Juice squeezed the night before it is drunk should be kept cold and covered, with as little space as possible between the juice and the cover. If the food is to be cooked, a minimal cooking time and a comparatively small amount of water should be used.

Noble (10) studied the effect of overcooking on eight commonly used vegetables. The methods used included cooking in boiling water and in a pressure saucepan at 15 lb. pressure. Mean ascorbic acid retention decreased significantly as cooking time increased, in both methods of cookery, but the quantitative decrease was small. The amounts of the vitamin dissolved in the cooking waters did not increase with longer cooking but much more was lost in boiling than in the pressure saucepan —38 and 7 per cent, respectively. Regardless of the method used, approximately 15 per cent of the ascorbic acid present in the uncooked vegetable was not present in either the cooked vegetable or the cooking water. Apparently, this ascorbic acid had been changed to a biologically inactive substance.

Experiments have been conducted to compare retention of the factor in microwave and conventional cooking of vegetables. Eheart and Gott (11) tested frozen spinach, broccoli, peas, and fresh potatoes cooked by these two methods and found that only in spinach was a significantly greater amount of the vitamin retained by the electronic method.

Although cooking time can be reduced by using soda in vegetable cookery, the practice is not recommended. Soda increases the alkalinity of the cooking medium and thus contributes to ascorbic acid loss.

Quick freezing conserves ascorbic acid to a higher degree than other methods of preserving. There has been considerable research on quick-freezing methods for retention of ascorbic acid. Recommendations include: (1) use produce harvested in the prime of condition and ripeness; (2) permit the shortest possible time to elapse between harvesting and placing the packaged product in the freezer; (3) blanch with steam or boiling water for only the shortest time necessary to inactivate the enzymes which otherwise would destroy the factor; and (4) freeze at 0°F. and store at this temperature or lower. This degree of coldness retained all the ascorbic acid content of peas for a one-year period, whereas 10°F. resulted in a 50 per cent loss; in strawberries and snap beans there was a 33 per cent loss at 0°F. in a year, but at 10°F. the berries lost 65 per cent, and the beans, 80 per cent of their ascorbic acid. It seems probable that the open-freezer compartment, common in many supermarkets today, is not conducive to maximal retention of this vitamin.

Orange juice, when concentrated and frozen by modern acceptable methods and stored at the freezing point, retains much of its original ascorbic acid. Lopez, Krehl, and Good (12) studied the stability of ascorbic acid under conditions of controlled time and temperature, in fresh, canned, frozen, and synthetic orange juices and in an ascorbic acid solution. The products were prepared as for the table, with distilled water if dilution was necessary. A remarkable stability of the vitamin was found in all products even when stored at room temperature for as long as eight days. These researchers concluded that ascorbic acid in citrus fruits and related products is highly stable under appropriate storage conditions (in covered glass or plastic containers) and in the absence of undue exposure to air or added metallic ions. Even vigorous boiling for ten minutes in a glass container, with distilled water, caused only partial loss.

Canning, when done by modern methods which guard against oxidation, causes less loss of ascorbic acid than used to occur with old methods, the amount depending on such factors as the oxidation potential of the food itself and the blanching and processing time and temperature. De-aeration and protection from metal ion contamination are approved practices. A commercially canned product may be superior to the freshly cooked one because the canned food may have been fresher and better in quality before canning and because it was heated in vacuum—a process the homemaker does not use. Addition of 150 mg. of ascorbic acid in tablet form to a pint of home-canned tomato juice will raise its ascorbic acid content to the level of orange juice, even after the product has been stored for six months.

Although modern methods of dehydration tend to result in less destruction of ascorbic acid than did older ones, this process does not conserve ascorbic acid as well as freezing or canning. Sulfite used to retain natural color favors retention of the vitamin. In experiments performed on reconstituted dehydrated potatoes and fresh mashed potatoes (13), the former retained only about one-half as much of the vitamin as did the latter; the longer the dehydrated potatoes were stored before use, the greater was the loss. It has been suggested that when dehydrated potatoes are used as a primary source of this vitamin, they should be fortified with ascorbic acid.

THE AMOUNT OF ASCORBIC ACID RECOMMENDED

Several procedures are used to determine whether the body's needs are met. Among the methods of estimating the status of ascorbic acid nutriture are measurements of the factor in the blood, both plasma and white blood cells (referred to as buffy coat), excretion in the urine, and the size of the body pool. In the latter method C^{14} isotopes are used (2). Such determinations are necessary because clinical manifestations of scurvy do not appear for a considerable time when the intake is low. In blood tests microchemical methods which utilize small amounts of blood are frequently employed, usually after a short period of fasting. Some research workers favor use of white cell measurements because this level is the last to be depleted and the first to become saturated when therapy is given. Plasma levels reflect more closely the present intake; white cell levels, the body stores. The white blood cell-blood platelet ascorbic acid concentration sometimes is recommended in assessing body store since it reaches a minimum almost simultaneously with the onset of scurvy (14). Table 12–1 gives guidelines for use in relating serum ascorbic acid levels to intakes of ascorbic acid.

Urine studies of ascorbic acid are made to determine saturation of body tissues, more being excreted when the intake becomes excessive

Table 12–1

*Serum Ascorbic Acid Levels and Intakes**

Serum Ascorbic Acid mg/100 ml	Ascorbic Acid Intake mg
<0.1	<10
<0.2	10–29
0.2–0.5	30–70
0.6–1.4	≥70

* From W. N. Pearson, in M. G. Wohl and R. S. Goodhart, (eds.), *Modern Nutrition in Health and Disease,* 4th ed. Philadelphia: Lea & Febiger, (1968).

or when the plasma threshold is reached. To judge ascorbic acid status, a large test dose is fed and the amount appearing in the urine within 24 hours is measured; an excretion of 50 per cent of the dose is considered indicative of an adequate supply of ascorbic acid in the diet. Some workers use a shorter period of time and base adequacy of diet on excretion in four hours of 40 per cent or more of the test dose. Others determine the time required for excretion of half the test dose and relate this to tissue saturation; still others use a fasting level. Because individual personal variations must be expected and because the determination techniques may be subject to error, results of both urinary and blood tests must be interpreted with caution.

Another test, used by some workers, is based on the fact that the capillary walls are fragile and that internal hemorrhages occur when the diet does not contain sufficient ascorbic acid to make normal intercellular tissue. The capillary resistance test measures the number of petechiae in a given area on the arm when a positive or a negative pressure is applied. However, it is known that factors other than diet affect the fragility of the walls; also, mild cases of scurvy are not detected by this technique. For these reasons the test is not generally accepted.

The FNB recommends a liberal intake of ascorbic acid. The amount of ascorbic acid actually utilized by healthy men has been measured by use of C^{14} isotopes in studies of body pools. Mean utilization was 21.5 mg. per day, with a standard deviation of 8.1 mg. The FNB recommends more to provide for individual variability and to compensate for possible losses in food. Beyond age 12 the recommended allowance has been calculated, on the basis of metabolic body size, as 2.5 mg. per kg. body weight to the three-fourths power. For the average American man this amounts to 60 mg. ascorbic acid, for the woman, 55 mg.

In the United Kingdom recommended intakes of ascorbic acid are much lower. The basis of the United Kingdom allowance is an amount sufficient to prevent signs of deficiency, with some margin to allow for individual variation and for stress (15). This is stated as 30 mg. per day for both men and women.

At certain times increased ascorbic acid intake is desirable. During growth the requirement of ascorbic acid is greater. Studies have been made on the blood and urine of groups of children and on individual cases to ascertain the intake of ascorbic acid associated with tissue saturation; for the young infant, standards have been set by determining the ascorbic acid content of the amount of human milk consumed daily. The allowances for infants and children recommended by the FNB are from 35 to 40 mg. daily, depending on age and sex. During adolescence both sexes should have 45 to 55 mg. ascorbic acid daily. The greater amount recommended during pregnancy and lactation, 60 mg. daily, relates to the drainage of maternal tissue by the fetus and nursing infant.

Large doses of ascorbic acid have not been shown to have beneficial effects on physical and psychomotor performance of men, or on their ability to work in hot environments. A cold climate increases excretion of the vitamin in urine but taking more does not hasten adaptation to the cold. It is thought that larger than usual amounts of ascorbic acid are needed in such disorders as rheumatic fever, arthritis, hyperthyroidism, and pernicious anemia, and in the treatment of wounds, ulcers, and severe burns. Crandon (16), who has investigated blood ascorbic acid levels in surgical patients, states that major surgery causes an average decrease of 17 to 20 per cent in plasma and buffy coat levels. He recommends 100 to 300 mg. of the vitamin per day as a means of preventing wound dehiscence. Some physicians have used ascorbic acid therapy successfully in the control of hay fever and bronchial asthma. Since doses of 1 to 2 gm. daily over prolonged periods have shown no harmful effects, this factor is considered nontoxic.

THE ASCORBIC ACID CONTENT OF THE AMERICAN DIET

The diet is likely to be low in ascorbic acid. Today the diet contains much more of this vitamin than it did in 1900, but it still tends to be lacking in this factor. In 50 weighed dietary studies made in 1900 by Atwater and his associates, ascorbic acid content was estimated at 69 mg. per person per day; no corrections were made for losses in cooking. In 1957–59 the average ascorbic acid available for civilian consumption was estimated to be 105 mg. and in 1970, 108 mg. (43). The peak was reached in the mid-forties when many home gardeners had victory gardens. In 1900 almost half the vitamin was secured from potatoes and sweet potatoes (45); in 1970, only one-fifth. In 1970, 94 per cent of the total ascorbic acid in the diet came from fruits and vegetables; of this, citrus fruits supplied 22 per cent. The practice of adding ascorbic acid to foods such as fruit juices and drinks increases the amount of ascorbic acid available.

Many studies have been reported in *Nutritional Status U.S.A.* (48) on the intakes of ascorbic acid by boys and girls, men and women, living in different sections of the country. The number of cases represented is large: 2800 boys, 3200 girls, 1047 men, and 2684 women. As a group the boys and men met their allowances well. Girls from 12 to 16 years and women from 30 to 45 and over 70 tended to consume less.

In a Louisiana study half of the eight- to 11-year old children had blood ascorbic acid values of 0.6 mg. per cent or less. In general, blood levels are an indication of long-range dietary customs, but food intake as shown in seven-day diet records like these studies reflects current, and perhaps only temporary, food consumption.

Five North Central states cooperated in a study of 568 women, aged 20 to 80. Data on basal excretion of vitamin C and on excretion after a

400 mg. load dose were secured on 135 of the subjects; when the average daily intake exceeded 1.1 mg. per kg. of body weight there was a nearly linear relation between intake and excretion. Also on this level of intake blood values tended to be above 0.8 mg. per cent. An ascorbic acid intake of 1.1 mg. per kg. of body weight was considered satisfactory. There were frequent instances of lower consumption among the women studied.

Studies were made in California of 525 men and women over 50 years of age who lived in their own homes. Their self-selected diets contained adequate mean amounts of ascorbic acid of 99 mg. for the men and 86 mg. for the women; their blood levels averaged 0.83 and 1.07 mg. per cent, respectively. More men than women had low levels. Dodds (17) has suggested that there is a sex difference in blood levels of ascorbic acid. Using existing data on almost 5000 individuals, male and female, on equivalent ascorbic acid intakes, she found that for ages four to 12 there was little difference between the sexes in blood response to intake, but that from 13 years on the males showed lower blood levels than females. This indicates hormonal interrelationships in ascorbic acid metabolism.

Biochemical tests and clinical examinations were included in the National Nutrition Survey conducted by the Nutrition Program of the Public Health Service. It was found that 12 to 16 per cent of all age groups had serum ascorbic acid levels below 0.2 mg. per 100 ml. (18).

A liberal daily intake of ascorbic acid is important. Table 12–2 gives data which indicate that the FNB standards for ascorbic acid can be met

Table 12–2

*Distribution of Ascorbic Acid in the Low-Cost Dietary for a Family of Four***

Food Groups	Ascorbic Acid mg.	Ascorbic Acid per cent[1]
Milk, cheese	130	3.2
Meat, fish, eggs, legumes	151	3.8
Dark-green and deep-yellow vegetables	544	13.5
Citrus fruit, tomatoes	1211	30.1
Potatoes	730	18.1
Other fruits and vegetables	1263	31.3
Grain products	0	0.0
Fats, oils	0	0.0
Sugar, sweets	0	0.0
Total for week	4029	100.0
Total for day	576	
Recommended allowance for day[2]	195	

* For description of family, See Chapter 6, p. 113.
1 Expressed to one decimal.
2 Recommended Dietary Allowances, Seventh Revised Edition. Washington, D.C.: FNB, NAS-NRC Publ. 1694 (1968).

even on a limited food budget. In this low-cost plan, citrus fruits and tomatoes, more limited in use than in many menus, furnish 30 per cent of the ascorbic acid intake, other fruits and vegetables supply 45 per cent, and potatoes, 18 per cent.

An adequate ascorbic acid supply is considered important for several reasons. Because this vitamin is unstable it seems probable that people actually get a good deal less ascorbic acid into their systems than might be expected from the data recorded in printed tables. Long shipments, exposure to the warm dry atmosphere of a market, poor storage conditions in the home, and careless cooking methods considerably decrease the ascorbic acid content of the diet. Variations in the individual's utilization of ascorbic acid may be expected; common infections and mechanical injuries may result in lack of saturation of body tissues and excessive elimination. Thus an intake which might seem sufficient under ordinary circumstances may actually be dangerously low. Sherman (19) states that scientific evidence, although fragmentary and inconclusive, nevertheless seems to indicate that consistently high daily intake of ascorbic acid will defer the aging process. Since there are many arguments for a liberal intake and no known harmful effects from it, the optimal dietary should include plenty of foods rich in ascorbic acid.

Thiamin (vitamin B_1)

THE CHEMISTRY OF THIAMIN

The search for a cure for beriberi led to the isolation and synthesis of thiamin. In the latter part of the nineteenth century Eijkman, a Dutch physician working in a military hospital in Java, reported that feeding rice polishings to fowl prevented a disease similar to beriberi in man. Eijkman thought that a toxic substance in polished rice, probably formed from the large amounts of carbohydrate, caused the disease, which he termed "polyneuritis," and that the toxin was neutralized by an antitoxin contained in the rice polishings. Later his associate, Grijins, suggested that beriberi was a deficiency disease and that rice polishings contained an unknown nutrient. Thereafter, many scientists sought to isolate the substance. Among them were Casimir Funk, who suggested the word "vitamin," and McCollum and Davis, who referred to the beriberi-curative substance as water-soluble B. Finally, in 1926 Jansen and Donath isolated the factor and in 1936, after years of dedicated research, Williams and Cline (1, 2) synthesized thiamin. Today, it is available on the market in pure form, usually as thiamin hydrochloride $C_{12}H_{18}N_4OSCl_2$ (Figure 12–2), or the mononitrate. Biological activity is associated with the pyrimidine and thiazole nuclei found in it. It is a white substance with the odor of yeast and a salty nutlike flavor. Frequently thiamin is referred to as vitamin B_1. Jansen named it *aneurin* when it was isolated because of its specific action on the nervous system, but this name has

Figure 12–2

Structural formula of thiamin hydrochloride

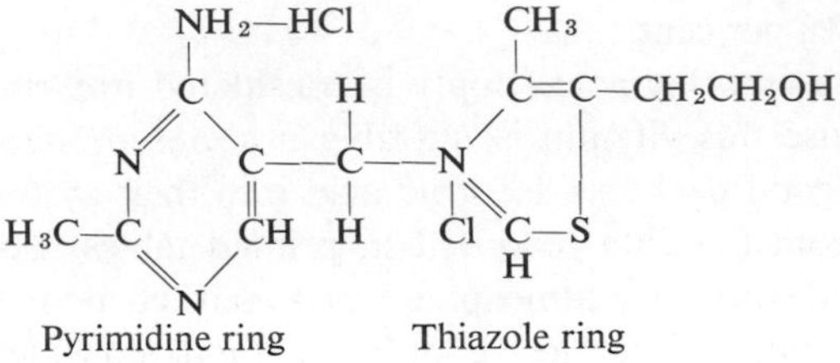

Pyrimidine ring   Thiazole ring

gone out of general use since it is now known that the vitamin acts in biological processes involving a variety of tissues.

Derivatives of thiamin—allithiamin and dithiopropylthiamin—have been prepared. These compounds are absorbed faster than thiamin itself and thus produce high levels of blood and urine thiamin and of liver cocarboxylase with greater rapidity (3, 4).

Several antithiamins have been synthesized in the laboratory but are not known to occur in nature. Neopyrithiamin and oxythiamin both produce symptoms comparable to those caused by a lack of thiamin in the diet. A heat-labile enzyme found in certain seafoods and a heat-stable compound of unknown identity occurring in bracken ferns and some other plants destroy thiamin. Bacteria which secrete thiaminases have been detected in the intestinal tracts of patients with thiaminase disease.

Its properties are of significance in food preparation. Because thiamin is soluble in water considerable loss occurs in the preparation and cooking of foods. Soaking vegetables and fruits during the processes of washing and freshening, cooking in an excess of water, long cooking, and discarding the water in which foods have been cooked or canned are practices which should be avoided.

Thiamin is comparatively stable to heat and oxidation in the dry form and in solution when the pH is less than 5. Sterilization in an acid medium for 30 minutes at 120°C. permits the vitamin to be well retained. At a pH of 7 or more, boiling or even storing at room temperature causes rapid loss, the vitamin being hydrolyzed into its pyrimidine and thiazole rings. Addition of baking soda to cooking water may result in almost total loss of the vitamin.

THE FUNCTIONS OF THIAMIN

Specific symptoms are observed in cases of thiamin deficiency. Beriberi, a specific polyneuritis originally associated with vitamin B lack, is a disorder of the nerves and may result in paralysis of the legs and in heart failure. This disease, thought to be due to a multiple deficiency, is not common in the United States. However, thiamin-deficiency syndromes are found in alcoholics. Such conditions have been attributed to poor dietary habits, low thiamin intakes, and liver damage, resulting in decreased activation of thiamin to thiamin pyrophosphate and reduced hepatic thiamin storage (4). Recent research suggests that impaired thiamin absorption is the major cause of thiamin deficiency in alcoholics (5). As more is known of the signs of a mild deficiency in thiamin, it seems evident that proper provision for this vitamin must be a matter of practical concern in this country. Williams and his collaborators (6) fed a diet deficient in the factor to a group of human beings for almost three months. Specific symptoms, evident early, were fatigue, lassitude, and loss of interest in food. Subjects also showed depressed mental states, dizziness, backache, insomnia, loss of weight, muscle atony, lowered blood pressure, and bradycardia. Capacity for muscular work fell progressively as the period lengthened. Other workers have found thiamin to prevent fatigue of the central nervous system, including the brain.

In the Orient beriberi is prevalent. The poor economic condition of the people, their preference for a highly polished rice, and the tendency to eat raw sea food explain the high incidence of the disorder in such countries as China, Japan, and the Philippines. Nutrition surveys made on the armed forces of the Philippines by the ICNND (7) indicate that deficiency of thiamin is common among these people. Forty-one per cent of the cases studied had an abnormally low urinary excretion of the vitamin.

Thiamin is especially involved in carbohydrate metabolism. The vitamin is found in the body both in the free form and combined with phosphate as the coenzyme thiamin pyrophosphate. The coenzyme known as cocarboxylasc combines with magnesium and specific proteins to form active enzymes, the carboxylases, which function in cell respiration, being capable of reversible oxidation and reduction. Thus thiamin aids in the complete breakdown of carbohydrates into carbon dioxide and acetaldehyde, releasing energy for the body to use. The coenzyme cocarboxylase acts with diphosphopyridine nucleotide (a nicotinic acid-containing compound), coenzyme A (a pantothenic acid-containing compound), and lipoic acid to bring about the breakdown of pyruvic acid, one of the intermediate products in carbohydrate metabolism, to acetyl coenzyme A. The B-vitamins, riboflavin and vitamin B_6 are involved in these reactions also. Thiamin pyrophosphate is necessary, also, in other enzyme systems in carbohydrate metabolism. Therefore, when thiamin is lacking or deficient, pyruvic acid and other intermediate compounds accumulate in the tissues. These products are presumed to produce the deficiency symptoms. In any event, accumulation of these metabolites is a biochemical abnormality related to inadequate thiamin intake. It has been suggested, too, that cocarboxylase is necessary as a coenzyme in reactions leading to the production of ribose, the pentose sugar needed for the formation of DNA and RNA. In addition, evidence is accumulating from studies with rats that link thiamin with protein catabolism. High tissue levels of glyoxylic acid have been found in thiamin-deficient animals. It has been suggested (8) that the increase in glyoxylic acid, formed in the breakdown of the amino acid glycine, may be responsible for some of the symptoms of thiamin deficiency not explainable by the known changes in carbohydrate metabolism.

In animal experiments several substances have been found to have a sparing action on thiamin (9, 10). The list includes protein, sorbitol, ascorbic acid, and penicillin. Explanations given for the sparing action include interrelated effects on growth and metabolic processes, on synthesis of thiamin in the intestines, and on suppression of growth of thiaminase-secreting bacteria. The significance of these thiamin sparers for the human being is not considered great. Fat frequently is called a "thiamin sparer." It has been found that when fat calories replace carbohydrate calories less thiamin is required, but the reduction is small (11).

Specific functions of thiamin are known. It seems probable that catalytic action of thiamin in carbohydrate metabolism is the explanation of several of the functions associated with this factor. A poor appetite, one of the earliest symptoms of lack, is known to be directly related to thiamin deficiency. The quantity of food eaten may be increased as the result of the addition of thiamin only. This increased intake may in turn promote growth. Experimental work on infants and children indicates that an amount of the vitamin greater than is ordinarily received promotes more consistent growth and a more stable appetite. In thiamin lack, loss of appetite or anorexia, as this condition is technically termed, may be accompanied by nausea and vomiting. The peak of the pyruvate level in the blood coincides with that of the nausea. This and the intermittent nature of the anorexia suggest that the cause is chemical rather than a nervous stimulus.

It is believed that thiamin functions in maintaining normal muscle tonus, especially in the digestive system and in the heart. The poor intestinal motility commonly associated with constipation may be, in part, the result of thiamin lack. In clinical cases of athiaminosis constipation usually is present. The cardiovascular system is frequently involved resulting in reduced capacity of the heart muscles to work. The lowered rate of heart beat, as measured on the electrocardiograph, is the basis of a test for determining the thiamin value of a food.

This factor has been called the "morale" vitamin because of its relation to a healthy nervous system and its effect on mental attitude. As stated earlier, the neuritis accompanying beriberi involves paralysis of the lower extremities. With a less serious lack of the antineuritic factor, early in the deficiency, certain symptoms of nerve disturbance such as irritability, forgetfulness, confusion, and fear occur. It is thought that a short period of vitamin therapy may alleviate these signs of neurasthenia. Horwitt and co-workers (12) studied the psychological effects of lack of thiamin on psychiatric patients in an institution over several years. The subjects received varying amounts of thiamin in an otherwise adequate diet. The men were tested for various deficiency effects. Among the mental conditions noted when the daily diet approximated 0.4 mg. of thiamin were loss of inhibitory emotional control, paranoid trends, manic or depressive features, and confusion. A study by Brozek (13) on healthy young men investigated the impact of a thiamin-free diet. After a long period of partial restriction and during a period of 15 to 27 days on the thiamin-free regime, tests showed neurasthenia, marked emotional upset, lowering of pressure-pain threshold, general weakness, extreme anorexia, pronounced incoordination of the legs, and hyperpyruvinemia. No effect was noted on intelligence. When generous thiamin supplements were administered, most of the above conditions returned to normal promptly, but signs of peripheral neuropathy lingered for some time.

Effort has been made to relate thiamin intake to learning capacity in animals and children. Such a relationship probably does not exist. In one experiment (14), the improvement noted in children who were given supplementary doses of 2 mg. thiamin daily was credited to better utilization of food and to lessened fatigue rather than to a direct effect of the vitamin on learning capacity.

THE SOURCES OF THIAMIN

There are several methods for determining the thiamin content of a food. Chemical techniques for securing data on thiamin values are based either on the fluorescence of the product formed by the vitamin's oxidation into thiochrome or on the color intensity of thiamin when combined with a diazotized amine. Paper chromotography and paper electrophoresis permit separate measurements of the vitamin and its phosphorylated esters.

Bioassays using the rat, chicken, or pigeon have been used. However, because these methods are time-consuming and may require expensive apparatus, they have been superseded by methods using molds, bacteria, yeasts, and protozoa. The reproducibility of results, low cost, and short time required for such studies make them especially useful.

Thiamin is found in both animal and plant materials. This factor is widely distributed in common food materials but, with few exceptions, in only small amounts. Among the foods classed as excellent (0.45 mg. or more thiamin per 100 gm.) are dried legumes, pork, some organ meats, rolled oats and whole wheat flour and cereals, and most nuts. In the good group (0.3 to 0.44 mg. per 100 gm.) are whole corn meal and brown rice, enriched flour and some enriched cereals, dried milk, dried egg yolks, dried whole eggs, and green peas. Fair sources (0.09 to 0.29 mg. per

100 gm.) include eggs, particularly the yolks, peanut butter, many vegetables, most dried fruits, and some fish and meat. Most fruits, some vegetables, chicken, milk, and the nonenriched white breadstuffs contain very little thiamin, but when eaten in liberal amounts they may furnish a significant part of the daily requirement. Brewer's yeast and wheat germ are very rich sources of thiamin, containing 15.61 mg. and 2.01 mg. per 100 gm. respectively. However, since they are eaten in only small amounts and by relatively few people, they cannot be considered important sources of thiamin in the average dietary.

Methods used in producing, processing, and preparing food may alter the thiamin content. Pork is considered one of the best of the foods in thiamin, yet it is known that considerable variation exists in samples. Research has proven that the amount of thiamin in the hog's diet is reflected in the flesh; a practical suggestion is to supplement the animal's food with thiamin-rich sources, such as dried yeast or peanut skins.

The relationship of such conditions as soil fertility, temperature, and light to thiamin content of plant foods has been investigated. There are indications that certain environmental factors are more favorable than others, and to certain plants more than others. Light and moisture, a temperature adjusted to the most desirable rate of growth, and such chemicals as phosphorus, nitrates, and boron have been shown in research studies to increase thiamin value of the tested foods. Genetic variations in hens have been shown to affect thiamin utilization by the fowl and the thiamin content of eggs. Howes and Hutt (15) found that eggs from White Leghorn hens contained 43 to 66 per cent more thiamin than eggs from breeds such as Plymouth Rocks and Rhode Island Reds.

The properties referred to earlier in this section explain many thiamin losses noted when a food is cooked. In general it may be said that loss of thiamin may be expected owing to solution in water, to heat, and to an alkaline medium. Research (16) has shown that adding soda markedly increases destruction of the factor in vegetable cookery and in baking some quick breads.

Thiamin retention in meats has been studied extensively. Experiments on roast lamb have shown that from 56 to 75 per cent of the thiamin present in the raw meat was retained, whether the meat was cooked electronically or in conventional ovens (17, 18). The variations in the results reported were due either to differences in cooking time or to the final internal temperature of the meat. Thiamin retention in beef and pork, roasted and pan or oven broiled, has been found to average about 70 per cent. The effect of cooking on the vitamin retention in variety meats has been studied by Noble (19). She found the average retention of thiamin in braised and simmered sweetbreads averaged 60 per cent; that in beef kidney, 41 per cent; and that in beef, veal, and pork hearts, approximately 29 per cent. In addition, it has been reported that the drippings, or cooking juices, from meat contain appreciable amounts of thiamin; their use is recommended. Braising and simmering meat result in greater losses of thiamin than does roasting, but some of the vitamin is retained in the braising and simmering liquids. Since thiamin destruction continues throughout the heat processing of meats, the lowest temperatures and the shortest times consistent with other requirements should be used for maximum thiamin retention (20, 21). Freeze-drying of chicken has been reported to result in little loss of thiamin, whereas pork has been shown to lose about one-third of the initial thiamin when subjected to similar processing (22, 23). Irradiation of freeze-dehydrated meats, up to as much as 4.5 megrads*, has resulted in no significant loss of thiamin (24). Storage of canned meats for one year at room temperature results in losses of 30 to 40 per cent of the initial thiamin, but none appears to be lost from freeze-dried products stored for comparable lengths of time. Studies on thiamin content of frozen meats and their cookery indicate that little of the vitamin is lost in the freezing process, and that immediate cooking in the frozen state tends to conserve it.

Studies made on milk products indicate only slight differences in thiamin content of milk with variations in the cow's ration and only insignificant loss on dehydration. Some decrease was noted during pasteurization by the hold process; this is done at a temperature of not less than 142°F. for 30 minutes. The thiamin content of cheeses varies depending on the type and processing procedure. Hard cheeses and cream cheese generally contain little since most of the vitamin is dissolved and removed in the whey. Cottage cheese compares favorably with milk in thiamin content. The studies by Morgan and co-workers (25) demonstrated that the sulfuring process used in dehydration of fruits causes a loss in thiamin. The sulfite dip used to prevent discoloration of pared white potatoes, however, results in no appreciable loss of the vitamin (26). In bread baking there is not more than a 15 per cent thiamin loss and often much less; a 10 per cent decrease from that in the dough is thought to be a liberal estimate of loss.

Rice which has been soaked and parboiled before milling is available in many parts of the world and is marketed in the United States under the trade name "converted" rice. It looks like white rice but contains 0.2 mg. of thiamin per 100 gm. in contrast to 0.07 mg. in the refined product. The parboiling process redistributes the water-soluble nutrients within the grain, going from the outer layers toward the inner, and also causes part of the germ to adhere to the endosperm. In general, modern practices in food processing are directed toward retention of thiamin as well as of all other nutrients.

---

* 4.5 megrads equals 4,500,000 rads. A rad is the absorption of 100 ergs of radiation per gram of tissue.

Enriched cereal products make an important contribution to the dietary. In their natural state the grains are a good source of thiamin, but much of the nutrient is removed in the milling and refining process. Since cereal products occupy so large a part of the dietary of many people, they have been approved for fortification by the Council on Foods and Nutrition of the American Medical Association. In setting the standards for the allowances, restoration of the thiamin in these refined products to the original levels in the whole grains has been the general policy. The actual value adopted was that in oatmeal, the cereal having the highest thiamin content of all of the whole grain cereals. Various manufacturers of refined cereal products have used this standard in their enrichment programs.

The name given to the enriched products and the recommended amounts of the materials to be added (not only thiamin but also niacin, iron, and riboflavin) were decided on by nutrition experts including the FNB, the Council on Foods and Nutrition of the American Medical Association, government nutrition authorities, and representatives of milling and baking industries (27). Early in 1941 the FDA defined enriched flour as that to which the approved amounts of the four supplements had been added. Up to July, 1943, riboflavin addition was deferred. The quantities of thiamin, niacin, riboflavin, and iron found in whole wheat and brown rice and in unenriched and enriched wheat flour, macaroni, corn meal, and rice are given in Table 12–3. Many bakers use enriched

Table 12–3

Vitamin and Iron Content of Some Grain Products*

EXPRESSED IN MG. PER POUND AS PURCHASED

Product	Thiamin	Riboflavin	Niacin	Iron
	mg.	mg.	mg.	mg.
Wheat Flour				
Whole	2.49	0.54	19.7	15.0
All-purpose, unenriched	0.28	0.21	4.1	3.6
All-purpose, enriched[1]	2.00	1.20	16.0	13.0
Macaroni, dry				
Unenriched	0.42	0.29	7.7	5.9
Enriched[1]	4.00	1.70	27.0	13.0
Cornmeal, dry				
Bolted, nearly whole grain	1.36	0.36	8.6	8.2
Degermed, unenriched	0.64	0.23	4.5	5.0
Degermed, enriched[1]	2.00	1.20	16.0	13.0
Rice, dry				
Brown	1.52	0.24	21.4	7.3
White, unenriched	0.32	0.12	7.2	3.6
White, enriched[1]	2.00	1.20[2]	16.0	13.0

* Compiled from *Composition of Foods—raw, processed, prepared.* Agriculture Handbook No. 8, Agricultural Research Service, United States Department of Agriculture, Revised 1963.
1 Minimal Level of Enrichment, Food, Drug, and Cosmetic Act.
2 Enrichment of rice with riboflavin optional pending further study and federal hearings.

flour, and others use wheat germ to fortify bread. Some authorities prefer adding a natural product such as dried milk or soy bean meal to the flour. They believe that the quality of the protein is likely to be very poor in low-cost diets and hence should receive as much consideration as the B vitamins.

There is some question on the amounts of vitamins which should be added in enrichment. Westerman and associates (28) showed that adding greater amounts of thiamin and riboflavin than are now used, plus pyridoxine, choline, and calcium pantothenate, results in even greater growth in rats than was evident when the approved enriched flour was fed at a level of 40 to 50 per cent of the diet.

Federal standards for enriched rice became effective in 1958 for all the nutrients except riboflavin. The requirement for this vitamin has not been set because the yellow pigment of riboflavin discolors the product; this may be objectionable to some individuals and thus limit its use. One method used to enrich rice involves coating the polished grain with a highly concentrated solution of thiamin, niacin, and iron (29). This product is called a premix; when one part of it is added to 200 parts of polished rice, the thiamin content of the mixture is approximately equal to that of unmilled rice. This product was manufactured in the United States and shipped to the Philippines where it was mixed with native rice and used in a beriberi-prevention program. Before this program was begun a clinical survey was conducted (October, 1947, to February, 1948), and it was found that an average of 12.76 per cent of the population of Bataan Province had either beriberi or one or more symptoms of the disease (30). After furnishing the enriched rice in an experimental area for approximately two years another survey showed a decrease in incidence of the disorder from 12.76 per cent to 1.55 per cent. In 1950 an increase in hemoglobin level was observed. The continued low urinary riboflavin was considered evidence that the decrease in beriberi incidence was related to use of the premix rather than to improvement in the diet as a whole. It points to the need for enrichment of rice with riboflavin as well as with thiamin, niacin, and iron. This study indicates a comparatively simple and successful way to eliminate beriberi in Oriental countries.

Enrichment of rice is required by law in South Carolina, and much of the rice available elsewhere in the United States is enriched. Further, all rice distributed in the national school lunch program must be enriched according to a 1962 federal law. Because the nutrients added to the premix are not always rinse resistant, the FDA requires that the label on packaged enriched rice carry the statement, "To retain vitamins do not rinse before or drain after cooking." If the label does not carry such a statement, or if cooking directions are given that require washing or draining, the nutrients must be present in such a quantity or form that 85 per cent of the minimum standards for enriched rice is retained after cooking (31).

Corn and macaroni enrichments have been approved, and definitions and standards have been issued in the Federal Register (27). Most of the degerminated corn meal and grits sold in the southeastern states now is enriched. This should help prevent recurrence of pellagra in states where corn is consumed in large quantities. However, in rural areas corn is still ground at country mills and hence is not enriched.

In Newfoundland, improvement in the health of the people has been largely associated with enrichment of flour, through a law enforced by the government. Two surveys, one before the law went into effect, the other four years after, show the results of the change in diet. Levels of thiamin in the urine were low in 1944; in 1948 they were satisfactory. Benefits from the other enrichment nutrients were also observed (32, 33).

THE NEED FOR THIAMIN

Several methods are used to determine how much of this factor the body requires. Both urine and blood tests are performed in the study of thiamin metabolism. In the urine, measurement may be made during fasting or during a period of time following oral or parenteral administration of a test dose of the vitamin. The amount of thiamin excreted in the urine diminishes rapidly as the intake decreases, and it approaches zero when the intake is about 0.07 mg. per day. On the other hand, when large doses of thiamin are given, particularly by intravenous injection, much of it spills over into the urine because the kidneys have no threshold for retaining it. Therefore, the reliability of "saturation tests" for assessing thiamin nutriture in individuals is questioned, although such tests are still considered useful in nutrition status studies of population groups. Keys and associates (34) advise that, when the diet is very low in thiamin, nutritional status is best determined by a yeast fermentation method which measures the amount of pyramine in the urine.

In blood studies determination of thiamin levels is considered less significant in evaluating nutritional status than the measurement of pyruvic and lactic acid levels. In a normal person there is a definite ratio of these two acids in the blood, but during thiamin deficiency the balance is upset and an excess of pyruvic acid is found. Therefore, the ratio of the two acids is considered to be more important than the amount of either acid present, especially that of pyruvic acid. Horwitt and co-workers (35) have formulated a carbohydrate metabolic index, called CMI, which under the specifications of their test may be used to diagnose early and mild degrees of thiamin lack. Analysis of blood for glucose, lactic acid, and pyruvic acid is done following a measured metabolic load which consists of ingested glucose and mild exercise. Their formula

is $\text{CMI} = \dfrac{L - \dfrac{G}{10} + 15P - \dfrac{G}{10}}{2}$, in which G, L, and P are levels of the three substances in mg. per 100 ml. of blood. Healthy subjects have been found to have an index below 15; thiamin-deficient subjects, an index over 15.

Brin (36) has reported a specific relationship between thiamin nutrition and transketolase activity in the enzyme or cellular level. Thiamin pyrophosphate is known to be necessary for activating transketolase, an enzyme involved in the oxidation of glucose in all cells except skeletal cells. Since large amounts of transketolase occur in erythrocytes of well-nourished individuals, Brin has suggested use of the erythrocyte for evaluation of thiamin adequacy. Such an assay measures the erythrocyte-transketolase activity. It appears to be sufficiently sensitive to demonstrate a biochemical defect before the appearance of clinical signs and thus reveal marginal deficiency states. Baker and associates (37) developed a method for assaying thiamin levels in biologic fluids and tissues using protozoa. They report that the technique yields reproducible results and accurately reflects thiamin status in both man and animals. More recently, the excretion of thiamin metabolites in the urine has been used as an indication of the utilization of thiamin (38). These methods should prove to be of value in clinics as well as in research and in nutritional status surveys.

The amount of thiamin needed is related to energy metabolism. The thiamin requirement is based on the calorie intake; as the intake increases, however, the proportion of thiamin required decreases. On the basis of much evidence the minimal thiamin requirement for the adult is believed to approximate 0.33 mg. per 1000 kcal per day.

The 1968 revision of the RDA lists 0.5 mg. thiamin per 1000 kcal per day as the amount required to maintain satisfactory thiamin nuriture. Further, an intake of no less than 1 mg. per day is recommended for older adults even when the intake is less than 2000 kcal per day. The need for thiamin is known to vary with the individual and the relationship between thiamin intake and excretion per 1000 kcal is debatable. Therefore, the recommended allowances for all age groups are based on 0.5 mg. of thiamin per 1000 kcal. Much still has to be learned about the thiamin-sparing action of certain nutrients and other substances, and about such factors in foods as thiamin stabilizers and thiaminases which favor or hinder thiamin potency.

The FNB recommends the same allowance in relation to calories, for infants, children, and adolescents. The requirement for thiamin during pregnancy is thought to be increased. Studies have shown decreased excretions during pregnancy which appear to indicate greater need during this period. Consequently, an additional allowance of 0.1 mg. per day is recommended for the pregnant woman. The allowance during lactation is 0.5 mg. per day above that for the nonlactating woman. This is based on a thiamin need of 0.5 mg. per 1000 kcal; the recommended calorie intake for lactating women is 1000 kcal daily above that recommended for nonpregnant, nonlactating women.

The body sometimes requires more thiamin. The vitamin need may be expected to be greater in diseases in which energy metabolism is increased. These include fever, especially of long duration, and hyperthyroidism. In gastrointestinal disturbances a greater amount of thiamin is often recommended. In constipation more of the vitamin is advised because of its effect in stimulating peristalsis. On the other hand, in diarrhea of long standing the system does not assimilate what it needs. Manifestations of thiamin deficiency are apt to appear in the polyneuropathies occuring in beriberi, pellagra, alcoholism, and diabetes, and in these disorders favorable response may be expected with thiamin therapy. Cardiac patients often improve when given thiamin. The vitamin may be used successfully in treating neurasthenia but therapy is valid only when there is a thiamin deficiency. It is thought that alcohol may require thiamin for its metabolism.

If a large amount of thiamin is prescribed, it should be given parenterally since excessive amounts are not completely utilized when taken by mouth. Experiments performed on human subjects indicate that a 5 mg. dose is the maximum for complete absorption. Some of the vitamin is normally excreted in the feces; some is destroyed in the colon. Intolerance to thiamin is rare. No ill effects have been observed in patients who received daily injections of up to 500 mg. for periods of as long as a month.

THIAMIN IN THE DIET

Even though the food supply in the United States provides sufficient amounts of thiamin, the diets of many people are not adequate in this respect. From 1935 to 1939, the amount of thiamin available in the United States averaged 1.47 mg. per capita per day (39). In 1970 the food supply for civilian consumption was estimated to provide 1.84 mg. per person per day. This increase was due largely to the grain enrichment program and to the increased meat consumption.

The studies on the thiamin content of the diets of large groups of adults and children in many areas of the country, reported in *Nutritional Status U.S.A.* (48), indicate that the intake of this vitamin met or was above the recommended dietary allowances except for women over age 65. These data are in contrast to those reported from the 1965 nationwide Food Consumption Survey. In the latter study, thiamin intakes were found to be 5 to 15 per cent below the recommended allowances for all age groups of females and for boys of 12 to 14 years. Other age groups of males, infants, and children met or exceeded the recommended allowance by up to 15 per cent.

Changes in food practices and public health nutrition education programs have had an effect. Reduced consumption of bread and cereals, and increased use of lean meats, have been due partly to health education programs concerned with obesity and coronary artery disease, and to the high level of the economy in the United States. A study of Table 12–4 will indicate the difficulty of meeting the recommended allowances for thiamin if grain products are eliminated from the diet. The inclusion of two slices of bread, whole wheat or enriched, or one slice of such bread and one serving of enriched cereal, will supply approximately 15 per cent of the day's quota of thiamin. Further, if foods from the meat, fish, egg, and legume groups are limited, the thiamin intake may not meet the recommended level.

The figures for available nutrients compiled by the USDA are based on the assumption that the food supply is evenly distributed among individuals. No deduction is made for loss or waste of food in households, or for destruction or loss of nutrients during food preparation. Thus, although the amount of thiamin available in the food supply appears to

Table 12–4

Distribution of Thiamin, Riboflavin, and Niacin Equivalent in the Low-Cost Dietary for a Family of Four*

Food Groups	Thiamin		Riboflavin		Niacin Equivalent[2]	
	mg.	%[1]	mg.	%[1]	mg.	%[1]
Milk, cheese	4.59	9.4	25.70	36.8	157.5	14.6
Meat, fish, eggs, legumes	14.71	30.0	25.67	36.7	548.1	50.9
Dark-green and deep-yellow vegetables	1.10	2.2	1.33	1.9	15.8	1.5
Citrus fruit, tomatoes	2.26	4.6	0.82	1.2	14.2	1.3
Potatoes, other fruits and vegetables	7.39	15.1	4.89	7.0	100.3	9.3
Grain products	18.85	38.5	11.06	15.8	237.4	22.1
Fats, oil	0.04	0.1	0.07	0.1	0.0	0.0
Sugars, sweets	0.03	0.1	0.35	0.5	3.1	0.3
Total for week	48.97	100	69.89	100	1076.4	100
Total for day	7.00		9.98		153.9	
Recommended allowance for day[3]	4.7		5.6		61.0	

* For description of family, See Chapter 6, p. 113.
1 Expressed to one decimal.
2 In the case of a few foods, tryptophan data were not available and data on preformed niacin were used.
3 Recommended Dietary Allowances, Seventh Revised Edition. Washington, D.C.: FNB, NAS-NRC Publ. 1694 (1968).

be adequate to meet the recommended dietary allowances, this may not always be so in practice.

The bread enrichment program is largely responsible for the increased thiamin content of the diet in the United States. The thiamin content of the average diet in 1942 was about 0.8 mg. per 2500 calories. This figure, below the recommended daily allowance, represents the situation in this country prior to the advent of enriched flour and bread.

According to estimates of the United States food supply made by the USDA, the quantities of thiamin consumed decreased gradually from 1909 to the mid-thirties, due largely to the decreasing consumption of grain products. The rise noted after 1937 is credited to greater supplies of meat, poultry, and fish, and by 1943, to the enrichment of white bread and flour. In 1968 and 1969 enrichment of grains added over 30 per cent more thiamin to the food supply of the nation than if enrichment had not been in effect.

Riboflavin

THE CHEMISTRY OF RIBOFLAVIN

Riboflavin is a thermostable fraction of the B complex. The concept of several B vitamins was formed gradually as a result of biological and chemical studies. Numerous investigators found that when yeast was autoclaved the beriberi-preventive factor—that is, thiamin—was destroyed, but a growth-promoting factor remained. This unknown substance was termed "vitamin G" by research workers in the United States and "vitamin B_2" by British scientists. At first it was thought to be a single entity; later it was found that the heat-stable fraction of vitamin B was composed of several factors.

In 1932 Warburg and Christian reported isolation of a substance from yeast which they found was involved in oxidative processes, serving as a hydrogen carrier. This factor, first termed the "yellow enzyme" and later the "Warburg enzyme," was yellow in water solution, exhibited a green fluorescence, and was a flavoprotein. Other investigators reported isolation of similar yellow-fluorescent pigments from a variety of animal and plant products. Finally, in 1933, riboflavin was isolated and the fluorescent materials from foods such as eggs, milk, and liver which had been called ovoflavin, lactoflavin, and heptoflavin were established as identical with one another. In 1935, the vitamin was synthesized almost simultaneously by Kuhn and associates and Karrer and others in Germany. In 1937, on the recommendation of the Council of Pharmacy and Chemistry of the American Medical Association, the name "riboflavin" was adopted since the factor contains the pigment flavus and the pentose sugar D-ribose and is nitrogenous in nature. Its formula is $C_{17}H_{20}N_4O_6$

(Figure 12–3), and in pure form it exists as fine orange-yellow crystals which are practically ordorless and bitter-tasting. In water solutions riboflavin shows a characteristic yellow-green fluorescence.

Figure 12–3
Structural formula of riboflavin

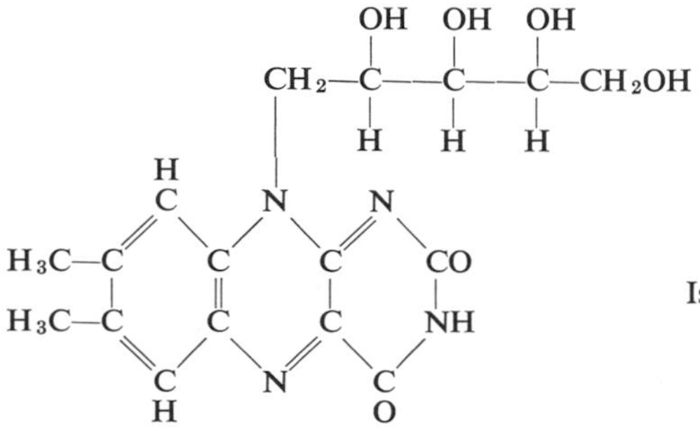

Other chemical properties of riboflavin are important. It is known to be stable to oxidizing agents and to heat, decomposing at 275°C. It is much less soluble in water than thiamin but, like thiamin, it is stable to acid and labile to alkali. In dry form riboflavin is not much affected by diffused light, but as a liquid it is destroyed rapidly on exposure to either visible or ultraviolet rays; alkali and a high temperature speed destruction. In a study (1) made in Montreal a two-hour exposure of milk in quart bottles to sunshine at a temperature of 63 to 68°F. resulted in a loss of 54 to 68 per cent of the factor. Opacity of foods is thought to prevent much loss from exposure during cooking.

THE FUNCTIONS OF RIBOFLAVIN

Like thiamin, riboflavin is involved in cell respiration. The vitamin exists in free form in certain foods and is excreted in this form in urine and feces. In tissues where respiration is taking place, riboflavin occurs in combination with phosphoric acid as flavin mononucleotide (FMN), and with phosphoric acid and adenine as flavin adenine dinucleotide (FAD). These, combined with specific proteins, make up a number of different flavoprotein enzyme systems in which the riboflavin-containing nucleotides are the coenzymes. These flavoprotein enzymes, of which at least 30 are now known, function in oxidative processes in living cells. They play a major role with thiamin- and niacin-containing enzymes in a long chain of oxidation-reduction reactions by which hydrogen is released and finally combines with oxygen to form water. Thus riboflavin functions in the metabolism of amino acids, fatty acids, and carbohydrates. In addition, riboflavin is necessary for conversion of tryptophan to niacin, is thought to be a component of the retinal pigment of the eye, and appears to be involved in adrenocortical function. Katagiri and associates (2) suggested a nonrespiratory function of riboflavin, that of serving as a glycosyl carrier in the synthesis of polysaccharides. They reported isolation of glycosyl-, galactosyl-, and fructosyl-riboflavin in studies using microorganisms, the three hexose sugars being linked to the ribose of riboflavin. Further study with animals and higher plants is needed to determine whether riboflavin actually plays an important role in the synthesis of polysaccharides.

Lack of riboflavin affects growth, the skin, eyes, and nerves. One of the first symptoms of riboflavin deficiency is growth failure: this effect led to isolation of the vitamin. In animals maintained on riboflavin-deficient diets, ocular changes, including conjunctivitis and cataract formation, lesions of the lips and oral cavity, dermatitis, digestive disturbances, anemia, and nerve degeneration occur. In severe deficiencies sudden collapse and death result.

The first controlled studies of riboflavin deficiency in human beings were made in 1939 by Sebrell and Butler (3). Eighteen women in good general condition, except for mental disorders, were put on a restricted diet known to be adequate in all respects except riboflavin, of which there was very little, and niacin, which was somewhat low. Cheilosis, seen as lesions of the lips, fissures in the angles of the mouth, and seborrheic accumulations around the nose resulted, even when a supplement of niacin was given. On administration of riboflavin the mouth and nose conditions disappeared.

A very early sign of riboflavin deficiency occurs in the eyes and involves invasion of the cornea by the capillaries (4). Burning and watering of the eyes, dimness of vision, and photophobia are common symptoms. In extreme cases there may be complete opacity of the cornea. Vascularization of the cornea occurs in both vitamin A and protein deficiencies, and there is some evidence that lack of these nutrients may produce a conditioned or secondary deficiency of riboflavin in the cornea. Glossitis and dermatitis about the scrotum have been reported also. The glossitis of riboflavin deficiency is quite similar to that of pellagra and pernicious anemia except that the tongue is magenta in color in contrast to the scarlet-red color observed in niacin deficiency and pernicious anemia. However, these conditions are not specific evidence of lack of riboflavin, although they may be produced by this deficiency. In such cases they are relieved promptly by riboflavin therapy. Horwitt and co-workers (5) reported no unusual vascularization of the cornea in subjects maintained for several months on a diet low in riboflavin, although scrotal dermatitis was observed. The appearance of specific lesions in the human being varies with the individual, and their absence cannot be used as an indication that the diet contains an adequate amount of riboflavin.

Anemia has been reported in riboflavin-deficient animals of several species. Some investigators now believe that this anemia may have been due to deficiencies of other nutrients such as folic acid and vitamin B_{12} rather than riboflavin (6). However, Lane and co-workers (7) have shown that riboflavin is involved in red blood cell formation in man. In their studies they used the riboflavin antagonist, galactoflavin, in a semi-synthetic riboflavin-free diet in order to produce an acute riboflavin deficiency. In addition to the usual signs of riboflavin deficiency, an anemia appeared. This and all the other symptoms responded rapidly to riboflavin therapy.

A severe riboflavin deficiency disease in human beings has not been identified. The vitamin authority R. R. Williams (8) does not include ariboflavinosis among the classical deficiency diseases, since no human deaths have been known to result from a lack of this vitamin. It has been suggested that acute uniform manifestations of riboflavin deficiency seldom are observed because of the absorption from the intestinal tract of riboflavin synthesized by the intestinal bacterial flora.

THE SOURCES OF RIBOFLAVIN

The riboflavin values of foods may be studied in several ways. Assays are based on physiochemical properties of the vitamin and include colorimetric, fluorometric, polarigraphic, enzymatic, and microbiological methods. Rat-growth assays also have been used. In determining the riboflavin content of foods, fluorometric and microbiological methods are preferred now to the early cumbersome and expensive biologic assays with laboratory animals (9). The color of the active principle may be determined by colorimetric means. Its fluorescence in blue or ultraviolet light may be measured fluorometrically, or it may be converted into lumiflavin, which may be determined either colorimetrically or fluorometrically. These methods require a preliminary acid or enzymatic digestion to release riboflavin from its combined forms. Discrepancies in the values stated for riboflavin content of foods occur because in some cases the release of bound riboflavin is not complete.

Riboflavin is found in many of the foods which supply thiamin. Like thiamin, riboflavin is widely distributed in both plant and animal tissues. Richest of all the foods are the glandular organs; muscles of animals and fish are a good source and so, also, are milk, both whole and skim, eggs, and cheese. Best among the plant foods are the actively growing leaves. Legumes, including peanuts, are also good sources. Fruits, roots, tubers, and grain products are only fair sources. The use of enriched flour and dry milk in breadmaking is recommended since they are rich in riboflavin. This supplementation is especially important when meat is expensive. The fact that enrichment of rice with riboflavin is not required by federal law was discussed in the preceding section on thiamin.

The amount of riboflavin in the diet has been shown by experiments to influence the content of the hen's egg, the tissue and the organs of the chicken, and the muscle of pork. In the latter study an optimal consumption beyond which there was no further storage was found. Other investigators (10) have reported genetic variations in the utilization of riboflavin by hens. Significantly more riboflavin has been found in the eggs of some White Leghorn hens than in those of New Hampshires. In another study only small amounts of the vitamin were found in the eggs of other White Leghorns.

There are several antagonists of riboflavin. In these another compound is substituted for ribose in the molecule. Galactoflavin, for example, contains galactose in place of ribose. Little is known about the presence of these compounds in natural foods.

Losses of riboflavin in food preparation and processing are comparatively small. Despite the fact that riboflavin is heat-stable, some loss is to be expected in cookery. This results partly from solution and partly as a result of the medium in which the food is cooked; alkali and light, factors favoring its loss, may be present. In general, when cooked in liquid form, precautions taken to conserve thiamin will also protect riboflavin.

It has been reported that less than 5 per cent of the riboflavin content of enriched farina is destroyed by home cookery methods. In the blanching processes used prior to canning or freezing certain foods, losses of from 5 to 20 per cent of the factor have been found; relatively little further loss occurs in the subsequent stages of canning or freezing. Noble and associates (11, 12) have reported several studies on vitamin retention of meats cooked by varying methods. They found average riboflavin retentions of from 70 to 92 per cent in meat after roasting, braising, or broiling, with an additional 2 to 20 per cent contained in the drippings. Riboflavin retention was similar when the meat was roasted electronically or in conventional ovens. When variety meats were cooked by either braising or simmering, veal, beef, lamb, and pork hearts retained, on the average, 75 per cent of the riboflavin; sweetbreads, 65 per cent; and beef kidneys, 55 per cent (13).

Dehydration and freeze-drying processes apparently have little effect on the riboflavin content of food. Only marginal losses have been noted in foods stored for periods of as long as ten months after such processing. Pasteurization, drying, and evaporation of milk result in relatively small losses of riboflavin. The use of paper cartons and amber-colored bottles for fluid milk prevents destruction of riboflavin by light.

THE NEED FOR RIBOFLAVIN

Blood and urine are studied to assess riboflavin nutriture. Riboflavin is found in several components of the blood, the plasma, red blood cells and white blood cells, and in several forms: as free riboflavin, as FAD, and as FMN. Investigations have been made to ascertain which component and which form are most closely related to dietary intake of the vitamin. Bessey, Horwitt, and Love (14) in a long-time study on human beings found that the riboflavin content of the red blood cells is a sensitive and practical indicator of riboflavin nutriture but that free riboflavin in the plasma or in the white blood cells, or FAD, or FMN was not a reliable measure. In the red blood cells a level of 20 μg. of riboflavin per 100 ml. of blood is thought to indicate an adequate diet, one which contains from 1.5 to 2.2 mg. of riboflavin per day. A red blood cell level below 15 μg, of riboflavin was associated with a sub-optimal intake.

Urinary excretion of riboflavin varies with the amount of the vitamin consumed and may be investigated with or without administration of a test dose. The rate of excretion also varies during a 24-hour period, being less at night than during the day (15). Therefore, when urinalysis without a test dose is used to assess the riboflavin status of the body, it is recommended that a 24-hour urine specimen be obtained. If this is not possible, a 6-hour fasting specimen may be used. If neither procedure is practical, a random sample may be used and excretion of the vitamin related to the creatinine excretion (16). Since the creatinine content of the urine tends to be constant throughout a 24-hour period, excretion of riboflavin per gram of creatinine has been found to be a fairly reliable indicator of the true excretion rate of the vitamin. Such a relationship is thought to exist also for thiamin and niacin. When test doses of riboflavin are administered, either orally or parenterally, the amount of the vitamin passed in the urine during the following four hours is determined. In general, low return levels are indicative of a deficiency of the vitamin. However, since saturation of tissues takes place only gradually after riboflavin depletion, studies employing test doses should be relatively long.

In a study on adult men (17) it was shown that tissue reserves of the vitamin could not be maintained when less than 1.1 mg. was ingested daily. It is believed that a loss of less than 10 per cent of the intake indicates an inadequate amount of the factor in the diet. This loss was found when the amount of riboflavin in the daily diet was between 0.55 and 1.1 mg. At and above an intake of 1.6 mg., more than 25 per cent was excreted in the urine. This investigation indicates that an intake of 1.1 to 1.6 mg. of riboflavin daily is adequate. Similar studies (18) performed on healthy young women showed that 1.0 to 1.5 mg. of riboflavin daily met their tissue requirements.

Urinary excretions of riboflavin were determined on 30 subjects in the study mentioned in Chapter 1 of the metabolic response of young women to a standardized diet. The mean daily intake was approximately 0.9 mg. of riboflavin, which is only 60 per cent of the recommended allowance. Only three subjects excreted over 25 per cent of the intake, an indication that the level of riboflavin in the standardized diet was too low to maintain the subjects in adequate riboflavin nutriture.

In the nutrition surveys conducted by the ICNND (19) riboflavin nutriture was assessed by determining the ratio of riboflavin to creatinine excreted in random samples of urine. Excretions of less than 80 μg. of riboflavin per gm. of creatinine per day were considered indicative of riboflavin deficiency and have been found with intakes of less than 1.1 mg. of riboflavin per day.

A liberal daily allowance of riboflavin is recommended. The requirement for riboflavin has been computed both from calorie intake and from protein requirement. Bro-Rasmussen (20), in 1958, thoroughly reviewed the literature on the riboflavin requirements of both man and animals and concluded that the requirement is related to oxygen consumption, and therefore to energy expenditure. In his survey of the studies on man he found that when the diet contained less than 0.25 to 0.27 mg. of ribo-flavin per 1000 kcal signs of deficiency occurred. The minimal require-ment to prevent clinical signs of deficiency is assumed to be about 0.3 mg. per 1000 kcal for adults, and between 0.4 and 0.5 mg. per day for infants and young children. The critical point of urinary excretion of this vitamin is an indication of tissue saturation, provided the subject is in nitrogen balance. It may be noted that 0.5 to 0.6 mg. of riboflavin per 1000 kcal is sufficient for tissue saturation in the adult, 0.4 to 0.7 mg. per 1000 kcal for the child. These investigations indicate that, while riboflavin requirement increases in proportion to energy requirement, the riboflavin requirement per 100 gm. of protein falls as the protein require-ment increases.

More recent studies of the quantitative human riboflavin requirements have indicated that need is related to body size, metabolic rate, and rate of growth (21, 22). Accordingly, the 1968 RDA for riboflavin were calculated on the basis of metabolic body size. The 1963 riboflavin al-lowances were related to calorie intake. In 1958, they were calculated from the protein allowances, using a factor of 0.025 mg. of riboflavin per gm. of protein. It is interesting to note that, in actuality, the recommended allowances for riboflavin do not differ to any extent whether they are based on metabolic body size, calorie intake, or the protein allowance. This is so because these three factors are interrelated.

Horwitt (23) has suggested that the riboflavin requirements be re-turned to a protein base because it has been found in growth studies that the amounts of riboflavin and protein in the diet are proportionately limiting. He believes that relating the riboflavin and protein allowances would simplify calculation of the needs of individuals who are growing faster than the average, of pregnant and lactating women, and of those who need more protein and riboflavin for tissue repair as a result of sur-gery or burns.

The 1968 RDA for riboflavin are calculated on the basis that adults require 0.07 mg. and infants 0.1 mg. per kg.$^{0.75}$ (17, 24, 25). Since there are insufficient data on the riboflavin requirements of children aged ten to 14 years, an arbitrary age-group adjustment was made (26). The allowances for children ten to 12 and 12 to 14 years old are calculated on riboflavin needs of 0.09 and 0.08 mg. per kg.$^{0.75}$, respectively, in order to meet the increased needs for growth.

The allowance during pregnancy is 1.8 mg. per day. This was computed from the factor 0.07 mg. per kcal$^{0.75}$ plus approximately 0.3 mg. of riboflavin daily to meet the increased needs brought about by the growth of the fetus and accessory tissues (27, 28).

Human milk supplies on the average 40 μg. of riboflavin per 100 ml. and the mean daily excretion during an average lactation period of six months is 850 ml., which amounts to 0.34 mg. of the vitamin (29). Since the utilization of riboflavin for milk production is about 70 per cent, an additional daily intake of 0.5 mg. above that calculated on the basis of 0.07 mg. per kg.$^{0.75}$ is recommended—a total of 2.0 mg. per day during lactation (30). The breast-fed infant apparently receives adequate amounts of riboflavin.

Several factors influence the riboflavin requirement. Other nutrients in the diet as well as external factors may be concerned in riboflavin metabolism. The relationship between riboflavin and protein has been mentioned. Protein seems to be necessary for retention of the factor. During dieting, which is extreme enough to induce a negative nitrogen balance, riboflavin will be lost from the body. Patients convalescing from surgery when nitrogen loss is great also have a high urinary excretion of riboflavin. In addition, marked increases in urinary excretion of riboflavin have been observed in human subjects during one- to seven-day fasts (31), in acute (but not in chronic) starvation, in diabetes mellitus, and after taking antibiotics.

Certain carbohydrates such as dextrin and starch have a greater sparing action on riboflavin than do the more soluble carbohydrates; here the slower breakdown and absorption favor synthesis of the factor in the intestines. A high-fat diet is thought to increase the riboflavin requirement since it furnishes an unfavorable medium for bacterial growth. Since a lack of one of the B-complex factors may upset the vitamin balance and result in manifestations of other deficiencies, use of B-complex mixtures is advocated in treating vitamin deficiency diseases. In pellagra this practice is always followed.

A relationship between folic acid and synthesis of riboflavin has been demonstrated in bacteria and it is suggested that folic acid may possibly be substituted partially for riboflavin in mammals (32). In stress, when the need for adrenal hormones is increased, riboflavin has been found to be especially important. The theory has been propounded that riboflavin is required either for synthesis of these hormones or as an aid in their elaboration.

The coefficient of digestibility of a food may affect the biological availability of riboflavin. Everson and co-workers (33) studied the digestibility of ice cream, green peas, almonds, and soy beans, all rich in riboflavin. The almost complete digestibility of ice cream and the less complete digestibility of the other three foods indicate that their values to the body may be quite different than those shown by chemical analysis. Among the disorders which may affect absorption and metabolism of riboflavin are diarrhea, vomiting, ulcers, infection, and hyperthyroidism. As a therapeutic measure oral administration of 5 mg. of riboflavin three times a day has been recommended. Occasionally as much as 30 mg. daily may be needed. Sometimes when a person fails to respond to treatment by mouth a parenteral injection is advised.

RIBOFLAVIN IN THE DIET

Intake of riboflavin is closely associated with consumption of protein-rich foods. Since 1966 there has been a slight decrease in riboflavin in the national food supply due to lower consumption of fluid whole milk (43). There were 2.26 mg. of riboflavin available per capita per day in 1970 compared to 2.28 mg. in 1957–59. Meats provided approximately 26 per cent of the riboflavin in the food supply in 1970, and dairy products, excluding butter, 42 per cent.

Despite the fact that consumption of grain products has dropped almost 50 per cent since the early 1900's, the level of riboflavin they furnished has been maintained as a result of enrichment. In 1969 they furnished 14 per cent of the riboflavin in the food supply. In Israel enrichment of flour has been found to provide from 33 to 41 per cent of the riboflavin intake of pregnant women in the lower income groups (34).

Riboflavin needs are not always met. Despite the increased availability in the United States of foods rich in riboflavin, some diets tend to be short of this vitamin. In the studies reported in *Nutritional Status U.S.A.* (48) the average intake of riboflavin for all age groups except women over 65 tended to meet or exceed the recommended allowances. However, deficiencies in riboflavin intake were noted, particularly in the diets of girls and women in the Northwest and north central states and in West Virginia. Symptoms of mild riboflavin deficiencies have been reported among a group of 15- and 16-year-old boys and girls in the state of Washington. Although the dietary intake of riboflavin of these adolescents could be described as adequate, laboratory findings indicated that their riboflavin nutriture was only poor to fair.

Reports of the nutrition surveys conducted by ICNND on population groups in other countries indicate that riboflavin deficiencies exist in many areas of the world, although clinical diagnosis of ariboflavinosis has not always been made.

In the low-cost dietary given in Table 12–4 the total riboflavin content is over the recommended allowance. Meat, fish, eggs, and legumes supply 36.7 per cent of the total riboflavin; milk and cheese, 36.8 per cent. The importance of the whole grain and enriched products in this dietary is evident, since grain products provide 15.8 per cent of the total riboflavin. Nonfat milk solids are an excellent and inexpensive source of riboflavin and their use should be encouraged, particularly in low-cost diets.

Nicotinic Acid (Niacin)

THE CHEMISTRY OF NIACIN

Research on the heat-stable fraction of vitamin B led to identification of niacin as the pellagra-preventing factor. In 1725 the Spanish physician Casal described a disease, *mal de la rosa,* which was prevalent among peasants. Later in the eighteenth century the Italian physician Frapoli named the disease "pellagra," a term derived from the Italian *pelle agra,* meaning "rough skin." For years the disease was believed to be due to a toxic or infectious substance in spoiled corn. In the United States in the early part of the twentieth century it was endemic in many southern states, and the mortality rate was high.

In pellagra the skin, gastrointestinal tract, and central nervous system are affected. The most obvious symptom is a bilateral dermatitis, red in color, which burns and itches. The mucous membranes of the mouth, stomach, and intestines also are affected. A classical symptom is the dermatitis outlining the neck which has often been referred to as "Casal's collar." Loss of appetite is common and in advanced cases diarrhea is noted. Early nervous symptoms include depression, dizziness, and insomnia; later dementia occurs. Pellagra has been known as the disease of the "four D's"—dermatitis, diarrhea, dementia, and death. At times reference is made to only "three D's," the final D, death, being omitted. Effects on two or three parts of the body may be noted simultaneously, but sometimes the oral, gastrointestinal, skin, or nervous symptoms may occur singly. This complicates diagnosis. Sunlight aggravates the skin condition and patients are advised to avoid direct sunshine.

About 1915 Goldberger of the USPHS in a series of studies on convicts proved that the disorder was caused not by infection but by a dietary deficiency. He also showed that "black tongue" in dogs is the analogue of pellagra in man. In 1926 this scientist subjected yeast to the high temperature of an autoclave, thus destroying thiamin. He observed that the heat-treated yeast contained a factor which prevented or cured the pellagra-like condition in rats. He termed this heat-stable material the "P-P factor." Elvehjem and coworkers (1) reported the cure of canine "black tongue" with nicotinic acid or nicotinamide, substances identified as the pellagra-preventive factor described by Goldberger.

Nicotinic acid and its chemistry have been known to organic chemists since Huber isolated it from nicotine in 1867. The name niacin was suggested by Cowgill to avoid confusion with the nicotine of tobacco. He coined this word from the first two letters of the words *ni*cotinic and *ac*id and the last two of vitam*in*. The terms, "niacin" and "niacinamide," were adopted by the American Medical Association, the American Institute of Nutrition, and the FNB. However, in many countries nicotinic acid and nicotinamide continued to be the accepted names. In 1966 the Commission on Nomenclature of Biological Chemistry of the International Union of Pure and Applied Chemistry (IUPAC) (2) ruled that the correct designations of the vitamin be nicotinic acid and nicotinamide. At the same time they changed thiamine to thiamin, pyridoxine to pyrodoxol, and ruled that the vitamin B_6 group be designated pyridoxine. In the United States the custom currently prevailing is to use "niacin" as a generic term for both nicotinic acid and nicotinamide. This practice will be followed in this section.

Tryptophan is a precursor of niacin. Goldberger's experiments indicated that the large amount of corn in the diet was a causative factor in pellagra. At one time he considered the possibility that pellagra was due to an amino acid deficiency but later concluded that the disease was the result of a lack of an unknown dietary factor. About the same time, investigators in Egypt suggested that pellagra was caused by a deficiency of an essential amino acid, probably tryptophan. Since the diets of pellagrans usually included a large amount of corn, it was thought generally, following the isolation of niacin, that the low content of this vitamin in corn caused the disorder. When the niacin values of Goldberger's diets were calculated, however, it was found that the corn ration contained more niacin than the milk diet used in prevention of pellagra.

In the meantime, work by Krehl and co-workers (3) showed that in rats tryptophan could be substituted for niacin in certain proportions, and Perlzweig and associates (4) reported that the human being could convert the amino acid into the vitamin. Today it is known that tryptophan is a precursor of niacin, and it appears that thiamin, riboflavin, and vitamin B_6 are essential for this conversion.

In the long-time study at the Elgin institution, referred to in Chapter 1, Horwitt and associates (5) determined the quantitative relationship of niacin and tryptophan for the human being. While some men ate only the basal diet, low in both niacin and tryptophan, others received this diet plus varying amounts of the two nutrients. By comparing the totals ingested with the niacin metabolites excreted in the urine these investigators were able to formulate a ratio of 60 mg. of tryptophan to 1 mg. of niacin as equivalents. They state that this relationship is not inflexible but believe it is necessary to assume a ratio in studying niacin metabolism problems.

Goldsmith (6) at the same time was investigating the niacin requirements of women. Her work confirmed the ratio recommended by Horwitt. The term "niacin equivalent," referring to the tryptophan-niacin relationship, was introduced in 1955.

It appears from recent studies on the biosynthesis of niacin from tryptophan that an amino acid imbalance in the diet may have an adverse effect on the conversion of tryptophan to niacin. Belavady and associates (7) reported that excesses of leucine result in reduced production of niacin from tryptophan. Pearson (8) found that high levels of threonine had a similar effect. These observations on the importance of amino acid balance may be another explanation for the early belief that ingestion of large amounts of corn might be the cause of pellagra and for incidence of the disease in areas where people subsist on low quality protein diets. Horwitt (9) has suggested that it may be more nearly correct to think of pellagra as a result of a tryptophan deficiency rather than of a niacin deficiency. In any event, niacin needs must be considered in relation to the amount of tryptophan in the diet.

Niacin is a stable compound. Niacin is the β-carboxylic acid of pyridine and has the formula $C_6H_5O_2N$. It was first isolated in 1912, from yeast by Funk and from rice bran by Suzuki, during their efforts to secure the antiberiberi factor. It also has been synthesized. It is available in both acid and amide form (Figures 12–4 and 12–5). In the human body nicotinic acid is easily converted to nicotinamide. The vitamin occurs in plant tissues in the acid form and in animal tissues as the amide. Since nicotinic

Figure 12–4
Structural formula of nicotinic acid

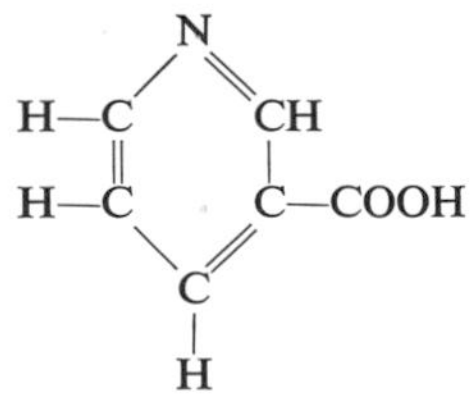

Figure 12–5
Structural formula of nicotinamide

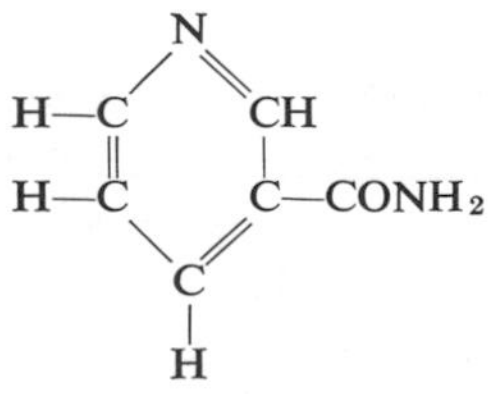

acid is a mild vasodilator and may cause flushing of the face, an increase in skin temperature, and momentary hypotension and dizziness, nicotinamide is preferred in therapeutic preparations. The amide is much more soluble in water than the acid form, but neither is affected by acid or alkali. Both are stable in air to light and to heat, even at autoclaving temperatures.

THE FUNCTIONS OF NIACIN

Niacin functions in glycolysis and tissue respiration. In the body niacinamide is a component of two important coenzymes, nicotinamide adenine dinucleotide (NAD) and nicotinamide adenine dinucleotide phosphate (NADP). NAD is a compound composed of nicotinamide, adenine, two molecules of d-ribose, and two of phosphoric acid. NADP is similar in structure except that it contains three molecules of phosphoric acid. Formerly NAD was referred to as diphosphopyridine nucleotide (DPN), and NADP, as triphosphopyridine nucleotide (TPN).

These coenzymes function in many important enzyme systems which are necessary for cell respiration. They are involved in utilization of protein, fat, and carbohydrate. Along with flavoproteins they act as hydrogen acceptors and donors in a series of oxidation-reduction reactions concerned with the release of energy from the body, and with riboflavin and other members of the vitamin B complex, in oxidation of glucose and synthesis of fatty acids. When niacin is lacking there is a reduced amount of these coenzymes in the tissues, and deviations from the expected amounts of the metabolites of both niacin and tryptophan occur in the urine. In man the main urinary products are N^1-methylnicotinamide (NMN) and its pyridone, with either the 2 or 6 carbon in the pyridine ring having an oxygen attached to it. Smaller amounts of quinolinic acid are found also. This compound is one of the intermediary products formed in tryptophan metabolism. Its excretion level in the urine is a measure of the extent of tryptophan utilization in the body.

Niacin has other functions. This factor is thought to have a specific effect on growth. Certain microorganisms have been shown to require niacin in order to grow. However, in the rat and some other animals intestinal synthesis by bacteria has complicated study of this function. Sure and co-workers (10) were able to produce niacin deficiency in the rat by incorporating sulfathalidine in the diet. This sulfa drug prevented bacterial synthesis of niacin and thus growth was retarded; resumption of growth was obtained by feeding niacin.

Macrocytic anemia occurs in niacin deficiency in dogs, pigs, and some other animals, but it has not been found to result from a lack of this vitamin in man. The anemia occurring in pellagra appears to be due to a deficiency of the vitamin folacin. There have been reports that nicotinic acid, but not nicotinamide, reduces the levels of cholesterol, β-lipoproteins, and triglycerides in the blood. However, large doses of nicotinic acid have been used to accomplish this and undesirable side effects from administration of the vitamin have been observed. Niacin is known to be involved in the conversion of vitamin A to retinal but the exact mechanism of action is not known (11, 12, 13).

SOURCES OF NIACIN

Determination of the preformed niacin in a food is based on chemical and microbiological methods. Bioassay is not used in measuring the niacin values of foods because many animals can synthesize the vitamin in the intestinal tract and then absorb and utilize considerable amounts of it. Dogs are satisfactory subjects, but experiments with them are expensive and time-consuming and assays have not been put on a quantitative basis. Chemical assay methods have been modified and improved so that the free acid can be measured and interfering substances removed. Microbiological techniques measure the free acid following its release from the food sample by enzyme, acid, or alkali treatment and are based on growth of an organism such as *Lactobacillus arabinosus* or *Shigella paradysenteriae*.

Niacin is found in both animal and plant tissue. The factor is widely distributed in foods. Yeast is the richest source, and frequently dried brewer's or Torula yeast are incorporated in recipes used in pellagra regions. Meat and poultry are rich sources, the organs being superior to the muscle tissue. Salt water fish is on the whole richer in niacin than fresh water fish and ranks along with meat in value. Milk and eggs are poor sources of the preformed vitamin, but since they are excellent sources of tryptophan, they contribute considerable niacin to the diet. Fruits and vegetables vary in niacin content. Nuts and legumes are better sources than are the leaves, stems, and roots of plants. Even though whole cereals contain appreciable amounts of niacin, they are considered poor sources because the vitamin occurs in "bound" form that becomes available only on alkaline hydrolysis. Treating corn with alkali or heat makes the vitamin more available. However, alkali releases more niacin than heat does and in a shorter time (14). This may be one explanation of the low incidence of pellagra in Central-American countries where the custom is to cook corn in lime and serve it as tortillas (15). During milling, from 80 to 90 per cent of the niacin of cereals is removed. Enrichment of grain products adds considerable niacin to refined flours and breakfast foods. Niacin is retained to a great extent in the process of making "converted" rice.

Niacin is the most stable of the B-complex vitamins, but because it is water-soluble some may be lost in cooking water and in meat drippings. Freezing, dehydration, canning, and food storage result in little destruction of the vitamin. In a study (16) of niacin content of potatoes stored for six months at 40°F. only small niacin losses were observed.

Niacin equivalents have been estimated. Both the tryptophan and niacin contents of a food are significant when nutritive value is to be considered. Within the past few decades many foods have been analyzed for tryptophan and thus niacin equivalents for them can be estimated. In such calculations it is assumed that 60 mg. of tryptophan are equal to 1 mg. of niacin. Most tables of nutritive values of foods include figures for preformed niacin rather than for niacin equivalents, as does the food value table in the Appendix of this book. Table 12–5 gives niacin equiv-

Table 12–5

Niacin Equivalents in Foods*

EXPRESSED AS RAW, EDIBLE PORTION†

Food	Weight gm.	Approximate Measure	Trypto- phan mg.	Niacin mg.	Niacin Equiva- lent mg.
Almonds	142	1 cup	250	5.0	9.2
Asparagus	113	4 spears	31	1.7	2.2
Avocados	108	½(3″ × 4¼″ × ¼″ diam.)	15	1.7	2.0
Bacon, broiled or fried crisp	16	2 slices	15	0.8	1.1
Bananas, A.P.	150	1 medium (6″ × ½″)	27	1.1	1.5
Barley, pearled	203	1 cup	325	6.3	11.7
Beans, lima, dried	100	½ cup	195	1.9	5.2
Beans, lima, fresh	100	½ cup	97	1.4	3.0
Beans, navy, dried, raw	95	½ cup	189	2.3	5.4
Beans, navy, canned	261	1 cup	149	1.5	4.0
Beans, snap, green	100	⅔ cup	33	0.5	1.1
Beef, chuck	100	1 piece (2″ × 2″ × 1½″)	217	4.5	8.1
Beef, hamburger	100	1 patty (approx. ¼ lb.)	187	4.3	7.4
Beef, rib roast	100	1 piece (5″ × 2½″ × ¼″)	203	3.6	8.3
Beef, round	100	1 piece (2¼″ × 2″ × 1″)	228	4.8	8.6
Beef, sirloin	100	1 piece (4″ × 3″ × ¾″)	202	4.1	7.5
Beef, chipped	100	5–6 thin slices (4″ × 5″)	401	3.8	10.5
Beets	100	¾ cup	14	0.4	0.6
Beet greens	100	2¼ cups, packed	24	0.4	0.8
Bluefish	100	1 piece (3″ × 3″ × 1″)	203	1.9	5.3
Bologna	114	4 slices (4″ × ⅟₁₀″)	147	3.0	5.4
Bran flakes (40%)	30	⅔ cup	36	1.9	2.5
Bran breakfast cereal (all bran)	30	½ cup	59	5.3	6.3
Bread, white, enriched	23	1 slice (½″ thick)	21	0.6	1.0

Niacin Equivalents in Foods* (continued)

Food	Weight gm.	Approximate Measure	Trypto- phan mg.	Niacin mg.	Niacin Equiva- lent mg.
Bread, white, unenriched	23	1 slice (½" thick)	21	0.3	0.7
Broccoli	100	2 stalks (5")	37	0.9	1.5
Brussel sprouts	100	7 medium (1½" diam.)	44	0.9	1.6
Buttermilk	244	1 cup	93	0.2	1.8
Cabbage	100	1 cup, shredded	11	0.3	0.5
Cantaloupe, A.P.	385	½ melon (5" diam.)	4	1.2	1.3
Carrots	50	1 (5½" × 1")	5	0.3	3.1
Cashew nuts	100	¾ cup	471	1.8	9.7
Cauliflower	100	1 cup, flower buds	33	0.7	1.3
Celery	40	1 stalk (8" × 1½")	5	0.1	0.2
Celery	100	1 cup diced	12	0.3	0.5
Chard, Swiss, leaves and stalks	100	2½ cups, packed	14	0.5	0.7
Cheese, cheddar	17	1" cube	58	Trace	1.0
Cheese, cottage	225	1 cup	403	0.2	6.9
Cheese, cream	15	1 tablespoon	12	Trace	0.2
Chicken, broiler or fryer	142	1 leg, boned	355	7.5	13.4
Chicken, hen	113	3 slices (4" × 2½" × ¼")	293	11.4	16.3
Cod, fresh	100	1 piece (4" × 1½" × 1")	164	2.2	4.9
Cod, dried	100	1 piece (4" × 2¼" × ½")	811	10.9	24.4
Collards, leaves	100	2 cups, packed	55	1.7	2.6
Corn, sweet, canned	256	1 cup	31	2.3	2.8
Cornflakes (added nutrients)	28	1 cup	15	0.8	1.0
Cornmeal, whole	118	1 cup	66	2.4	2.8
Cornmeal, degermed, enriched	100	⅔ cup	48	3.5	4.3
Cornmeal, degermed, unenriched	100	⅔ cup	48	1.0	1.8
Cucumbers	50	6 slices (⅛" thick)	3	0.1	0.2
Dates	89	½ cup	54	2.0	2.9
Eggs, whole	50	1 medium	106	Trace	1.8
Farina, enriched	169	1 cup	210	5.9	9.4
Farina, unenriched	169	1 cup	210	1.2	4.7
Flour, rye, light	80	1 cup, sifted	85	0.5	1.9
Flour, wheat, whole	120	1 cup, sifted	197	5.2	8.5
Flour, wheat, all purpose, enriched	110	1 cup, sifted	142	3.9	6.2

Niacin Equivalents in Foods* (continued)

Food	Weight gm.	Approximate Measure	Trypto-phan mg.	Niacin mg.	Niacin Equiva-lent mg.
Flour, wheat, all purpose, unenriched	110	1 cup, sifted	142	1.1	3.8
Flour, buck-wheat, light	98	1 cup, sifted	88	0.4	1.9
Flour, soybean, full fat	72	1 cup, stirred	390	1.5	8.0
Frankfurters, cooked	51	1 (5¼″ × 1″ diam.)	61	1.4	2.4
Gelatin	10	1 tablespoon	1	0	0
Grapefruit, A.P.	285	½ medium	3	0.2	0.3
Haddock	100	1 piece (4″ × 1¾″ × ¾″)	181	3.0	6.0
Halibut	100	1 piece (4″ × 1¾″ × ¾″)	185	8.3	10.4
Ham, smoked, medium fat	100	1 slice (4½″ × 4½″ × ¼″)	162	4.1	6.8
Ham, boiled	100	2 slices (4½″ × 4½″ × ⅛″)	219	2.6	6.3
Heart, beef	100	1 piece (2″ × 3″ × ½″)	219	7.5	11.2
Kale	100	2 cups, packed	42	2.1	2.8
Lamb, medium fat, rib chop	100	1 medium chop	193	3.8	7.0
Lamb, medium fat, leg roast	100	1 slice (4½″ × 5″ × ¼″)	233	4.9	8.8
Lentils, dry, split	100	½ cup	216	2.0	5.6
Lettuce, headed	50	2 large leaves	6	1.5	1.6
Liver, beef	100	2 slices (3″ × 2¼″ × ½″)	296	13.6	18.5
Liver, calf	100	2 slices (3″ × 2¼″ × ½″)	286	11.4	16.2
Liver, chicken	100	3–4 livers	332	10.8	16.3
Macaroni, enriched	100	⅔ cup	150	6.0	8.5
Macaroni, unenriched	100	⅔ cup	150	1.7	4.2
Mackerel	100	1 piece (2″ × 3″ × 1″)	186	8.2	11.3
Milk, whole	244	1 cup	120	0.2	2.2
Milk, skim	246	1 cup	121	0.3	2.3
Milk, evaporated	252	1 cup	249	0.5	5.7
Milk, condensed	306	1 cup	349	0.6	6.4
Milk, dried, whole	128	1 cup	466	0.9	8.7
Milk, dried, skim	120	1 cup	602	1.1	11.1
Mushrooms	100	1½ cups	6	4.2	4.3
Mustard greens	100	2¼ cups, packed	37	0.8	3.2
Noodles, egg, enriched	73	1 cup (1½″ strips)	97	4.4	7.0
Oatmeal	80	1 cup	146	0.8	3.2
Okra	100	10 pods	18	1.0	1.3
Onions, mature	110	1 (2½″ diam.)	23	0.2	0.6
Oranges, A.P.	215	1 medium (3″ diam.)	6	0.9	1.0

Niacin Equivalents in Foods* (continued)

Food	Weight	Approximate Measure	Trypto-phan	Niacin	Niacin Equiva-lent
	gm.		mg.	mg.	mg.
Orange juice	246	1 cup	7	1.0	1.1
Peanuts	144	1 cup	490	23.6	31.8
Peanut butter	16	1 tablespoon	53	2.4	3.3
Peas, green	100	¾ cup	56	2.9	3.8
Peas, dry, split	200	1 cup	518	6.0	14.6
Pecans	108	1 cup	149	0.9	3.4
Peppers, green, A.P.	76	1 medium	7	0.4	0.5
Pineapple	140	1 cup, diced	7	0.3	0.4
Pork loin	100	1 medium chop (½" thick)	213	4.2	7.8
Pork sausage	100	5 small links	92	2.3	4.8
Potatoes	100	1 medium (2½" diam.)	21	1.5	1.9
Radishes, A.P.	40	4 small	2	0.1	0.2
Rice, brown	208	1 cup	168	9.8	13.6
Rice, white, enriched	191	1 cup	157	6.7	9.3
Rice, white, unenriched	191	1 cup	157	3.1	5.7
Rice, puffed (added nutrients)	14	1 cup	6	0.6	0.7
Salmon	100	1 piece (3" × 4" × ¾")	173	7.2	10.1
Salmon, canned	100	½ cup, flaked	200	7.3	10.6
Spaghetti, enriched	94	1 cup (2" pieces)	141	5.6	7.6
Spinach	100	2 cups, packed	37	0.6	1.2
Squash, summer	100	1 medium	5	1.0	1.1
Sweet potatoes	200	1 medium	62	1.2	2.2
Tangerines, A.P.	114	1 medium (2½" diam.)	6	0.1	0.2
Tomatoes	150	1 medium (2" × 2½")	14	1.0	1.2
Tongue, beef, medium fat	100	5 slices	197	5.0	8.3
Turnip greens	100	2¼ cups, packed	45	0.8	1.6
Veal, medium fat, cutlet	100	1 piece (4" × 2½" × ½")	256	6.5	10.8
Veal, medium fat, stew meat	100	4 pieces (2½" × 1" × 1")	240	6.3	10.3
Walnuts, English	100	1 cup, halves	175	0.9	3.8
Wheat germ	68	1 cup	180	2.9	5.9
Wheat, shredded	28	1 large biscuit	24	1.2	1.6

* Data concerning tryptophan are from *Amino Acid Content of Foods,* by M. L. Orr and B. K. Watt. Home Economics Research Report No. 4, United States Department of Agriculture, 1957. Data on niacin are from *Composition of Foods—raw, processed, prepared.* Agriculture Handbook No. 8, Agricultural Research Service, United States Department of Agriculture, Revised 1963.

† A few of the foods are listed as A.P. or as canned or cooked, and are so indicated.

alent data for 123 foods. However, there is a need for tryptophan over and above that used to form niacin. Rose (17) estimated this to be about 500 mg. per day. Consequently it has been suggested that a deduction of 500 mg. of tryptophan be made when the niacin equivalent values of a dietary are computed. On this basis the USDA estimates that the niacin equivalent value of the nation's food supply is about 50 per cent higher than the figure for the content of preformed niacin.

THE NEED FOR NIACIN

Biochemical tests for assessing niacin nutriture are complicated and less satisfactory than those for thiamin and riboflavin. One reason for this is the conversion of tryptophan to niacin in the body; another is the multiplicity of end products of niacin metabolism excreted in the urine. Studies evaluating niacin nutritive status indicate that both niacin and tryptophan intakes must be determined. The vitamin occurs in blood mainly as NAD, and on low niacin intakes concentration of this coenzyme varies according to the amount of tryptophan available for synthesis to niacin. From the reports of the few studies that have been made on blood, it appears that much more information is needed before NAD levels can be used in evaluating niacin nutrition.

Urinary excretion studies are commonly used for judging niacin nutritional status. The metabolites of niacin usually measured are NMN and 2-pyridone. Both Horwitt and Goldsmith and associates (5, 6, 18, 19) have reported the relationship of these urinary metabolites to the tryptophan-niacin ratio. They found that when large amounts of the two nutrients are eaten, excretion of 2-pyridone is greater in proportion to that of NMN. In pellagra, however, NMN is excreted long after that of 2-pyridone ceases. These variations complicate the findings in niacin nutriture studies. Another complication may arise when studies are made after giving large doses of niacin. It seems probable that under these circumstances part of the metabolite is a detoxication product rather than a normal one. Horwitt concludes that a deficiency level is necessary in a study designed to estimate human requirements of niacin.

In the ICNND nutrition surveys of population groups, determinations were made of the excretion of NMN per gm. of creatinine. Excretions of less than 1.6 mg. of NMN per gm. of creatinine were considered indicative of niacin deficiency and have been found on daily intakes of less than 10 mg. of preformed niacin. DeLange and Joubert (20) suggested that the ratio of 2-pyridone per gm. of creatinine to NMN per gm. of creatinine excreted in the urine be used to evaluate niacin status in nutrition surveys. From the results of their studies it appears that ratios of 1.3 to 4 indicate tissue saturation, and that anything below the ratio of 1.0 is evidence of niacin inadequacy.

The amount of niacin recommended is stated in terms of niacin equivalents. The niacin requirement is related to caloric intake and is influenced by the amount and kind of dietary protein available. On the basis of the findings from well-controlled studies in which both niacin and tryptophan were considered, the minimum requirement for niacin (including that formed from tryptophan) to prevent pellagra is believed to average 4.4 mg. niacin equivalents per 1000 kcal per day, with an absolute minimum need of 9 mg. niacin equivalents per day for adults on caloric intakes of less than 2000 kcal. A 50 per cent margin of safety above the minimum requirement has been added to allow for variations in individual needs as well as for differences in conversion of the precursor into the vitamin. The niacin allowance, expressed in niacin equivalents, recommended in 1968 by the FNB for all age groups is 6.6 mg. per 1000 kcal. Human milk contains approximately 0.17 mg. of niacin and 22 mg. of tryptophan per 1000 ml. which amount to about 8 niacin equivalents per 1000 kcal. The recommended allowance for infants, based on Holt's studies (21) and on the amount of niacin equivalent estimated to be in human milk, were set in 1968 at 5 to 8 niacin equivalents daily. Six niacin equivalents derived from tryptophan appear to meet the daily requirement for infants fed a purified diet devoid of niacin. Although there is an increased conversion of tryptophan to niacin during pregnancy (22), an additional 2 mg. niacin equivalent per day is recommended for pregnant women because of increased calorie intake. During lactation the recommendation is for an additional 7 mg. of niacin equivalent daily. This amount approximates the niacin equivalent of the quantity of human milk that furnishes 1000 kcal.

Under certain conditions a larger intake of niacin is deemed wise. When pellagra is suspected niacin and tryptophan intake should be increased. Spies and associates (23) list three groups of people who should be watched for pellagra symptoms: first, the indigent and those with poor food habits and idiosyncrasies; second, people with organic disease such as tuberculosis, gastrointestinal disorders, nephritis, diabetes, influenza, and typhoid fever; and third, chronic alcoholics. A fourth group might include people with mental or nervous disorders.

In prevention and treatment of these conditions associated with pellagra physician and nutritionist have a task of education as well as of feeding. An adequate well-cooked diet is more beneficial than is a vitamin tablet, but occasionally a supplement of wheat germ, brewer's yeast, liver extract, or niacinamide is prescribed.

In recent years isonicotinic acid hydrazide (INH) has been used successfully in treatment of tuberculosis. This compound is related structurally to both niacin and vitamin B_6. It is known to act as an antimetabolite against vitamin B_6 and may be an antagonist of niacin also. It has been suggested that the intake of niacin as well as that of vitamin B_6 be increased during treatment with INH.

NIACIN IN THE DIET

The food supply furnishes liberal amounts of niacin and proteins which contain tryptophan. The niacin available for civilian consumption in the food supply in the United States in 1970 was 22.6 mg. per person per day (43) compared to 20.6 in 1957–59. This change is due largely to the increased availability and consumption of poultry. Enriched grain products may add considerable to niacin intakes, but full advantage of this source is not achieved when use of bread and cereals is reduced. The USDA reports that plenty of tryptophan is available.

The need for niacin may not always be met unless sufficient tryptophan is included in the diet. In the nutrition surveys reported in *Nutritional Status U.S.A.* (48) deficiencies of preformed niacin intakes were observed in some of the groups studied. However, when the data obtained were recalculated on the basis of 1 per cent tryptophan for dietary protein, the niacin equivalent of the diets was found to be adequate. The FNB estimates that the average diet in the United States furnishes from 500 to 1000 mg. or more of tryptophan daily and from 8 to 17 mg. of preformed niacin, which amounts to a total of from 16 to 33 mg. of niacin equivalents.

Table 12–6 gives an estimate of the niacin equivalent content of the low-cost diet for the family of four. A few of the foods, mostly the fruits, sweets, and fats, were not calculated in niacin equivalents because data on their tryptophan content were not available. Data on preformed niacin were used for these foods. Of the estimated total of 1076.4 mg. of niacin equivalent in the week's dietary, 54 per cent was preformed niacin and 46 per cent was calculated as the maximum potential contribution of niacin from tryptophan. If the need for tryptophan over and above that used for niacin synthesis is considered and an allowance of 500 mg. per day made for each member of the family, approximately 31 per cent of the total niacin equivalent value of the dietary would be contributed through conversion of tryptophan to niacin. It is interesting to note the shift in importance of the "milk, cheese" food group when data on niacin equivalents replaced that on preformed niacin. Milk and cheese, which contain only small amounts of preformed niacin, contribute much tryptophan.

The theoretical probability that the American diet is adequate in niacin equivalents is supported by the knowledge that pellagra is practically nonexistent in the United States today. Pellagra and subclinical niacin deficiencies do occur in many areas of the world where the food supply is limited and diets are low in tryptophan as well as in niacin.

Table 12–6

*A Comparison of the Nutritive Value of the Low-Cost Dietary for A Family of Four When Niacin Equivalent and Preformed Niacin Data Were Used**

Food Groups	Niacin Equivalent[2]		Preformed Niacin	
	mg.	%[1]	mg.	%[1]
Milk, cheese	157.5	14.6	26.5	4.6
Meat, fish, eggs, legumes	548.1	50.9	303.0	52.2
Dark-green and deep-yellow vegetables	15.8	1.5	8.7	1.4
Citrus fruits, tomatoes	14.2	1.3	12.3	2.1
Potatoes, other fruits and vegetables	100.3	9.3	82.7	14.3
Grain products	237.4	22.1	143.6	24.9
Fats, oils	0.0	0.0	0.0	0.0
Sugars, sweets	3.1	0.3	3.1	0.5
Total for week	1076.4	100	579.9	100.
Total for day	153.9		82.8	
Adjusted for day[3]	120.6			
Recommended allowance for day[4]	61.0			

* For description of family, See Chapter 6, p. 113.
1 Expressed to one decimal.
2 In the case of a few foods, tryptophan data were not available.
3 Calculated from total tryptophan less 500 mg. per person per day.
4 Recommended Dietary Allowances, Seventh Revised Edition. Washington, D.C.: FNB, NAS-NRC Publ. 1694 (1968).

Vitamin B$_6$ (Pyridoxine)

THE CHEMISTRY AND SOURCES OF VITAMIN B$_6$

There are three naturally occurring vitamin B$_6$ compounds. In 1934 György observed that a substance found in yeast was effective in treatment and cure of a well-marked dermatitis in rats which was similar to the human disease acrodynia. This new factor was first called "adermine" or "vitamin B$_6$." Later, following its isolation in 1938 and synthesis in 1939, György proposed the name "pyridoxine" for the vitamin since it is a derivative of pyridine and contains several methoxy groups. Pyridoxol has the empirical formula $C_8H_{11}O_3N$ and is a white crystalline powder, odorless, and slightly bitter in taste (Figure 12–6). It is readily soluble in water, fairly stable to heat, acid, and alkali, but it is destroyed by ultraviolet light and oxidation. When vitamin B$_6$ is administered therapeutically it is usually in the form of pyridoxol hydrochloride.

Figure 12–6

Structural formulas of vitamin B_6 group

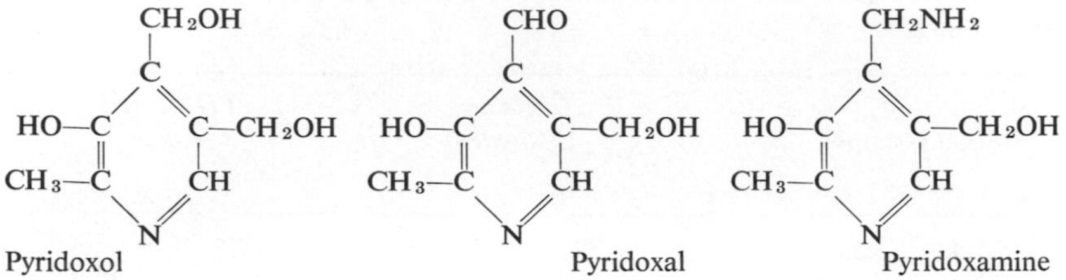

Pyridoxol   Pyridoxal   Pyridoxamine

    The original factor is now known to be one in a group of three related compounds, pyridoxol, pyridoxal, and pyridoxamine, the latter two being derived from pyridoxol by partial oxidation and by amination, respectively. The terms "pyridoxine" and "vitamin B_6" have been used as group names for the three forms of the complex. In the United States the current practice is to use "vitamin B_6" as the group name. This terminology conforms with that used by the United States National Agricultural Library, not with that recommended by the IUPAC.

Several methods are used to ascertain the vitamin B_6 content of foods. Distribution of the three natural forms of the factor has been determined by microbiologic, chromatographic, fluorometric, and enzymatic procedures. Bioassay, with rats or chicks, has been used to ascertain comparative values of total vitamin B_6 (1, 2). However, the results from these different methods do not always agree because of difficulties in analysis due partly to the presence of interfering substances. Although precise methods for determining the vitamin B_6 content of foods have not been established, the most reliable results appear to be obtained when the three forms of the vitamin are first separated by chromatographic procedure and then the vitamin content of each fraction determined by microbiological assay. The total vitamin B_6 content is obtained from the summation of the values for the three separated components. It is known that vitamin B_6 is widely distributed in foods and that few can be classed as poor sources.

    In animal tissues and yeast the vitamin occurs largely in its pyridoxal and pyridoxamine forms. In plants all three members of the group are found, but pyridoxol appears to predominate (3). The best sources of vitamin B_6 are muscle and organ meats, fish, whole-grain cereals, legumes, peanuts, molasses, yeast, bananas, and some vegetables including corn, cabbage, and yams (4, 5). In milling wheat flour, over one-half the original vitamin B_6 content has been reported to be lost (6). Foods that contain vitamin B_6 as pyridoxal or as pyridoxamine tend to lose more of their vitamin B_6 activity as a result of the commonly used methods of processing and storage than those that contain pyridoxol. In a study on the effect of cooking on vitamin B_6 content of beef, Meyer and co-workers (7) reported retentions of 72 per cent after oven-roasting and 49 per cent after oven-braising, with retentions in the drip averaging 16 per cent and 34 per cent, respectively. Richardson and associates (8) have found that freeze-dehydration and subsequent storage have no adverse effects on the vitamin B_6 content of meat and chicken. Studies (9) on vitamin retention in several varieties of potatoes have demonstrated that storage for as long as six months at 40°F. results in no loss of vitamin B_6.

FUNCTIONS OF VITAMIN B_6

Vitamin B_6 has several important metabolic roles. The vitamin is active metabolically in its phosphorylated forms, mainly as pyridoxal-5-phosphate (PLP). However, in some reactions pyridoxamine-5-phosphate (PMP) has been found to be active. In these forms it functions as the coenzyme in several enzyme systems, most of which are concerned with protein metabolism. It serves as the coenzyme for the enzymes that remove carboxyl groups from amino acids (decarboxylases), transfer amino groups from one compound to another (transaminases), remove amino groups from certain amino acids (deaminases or dehydrases), remove sulfhydryl groups from some sulfur-containing amino acids (desulfurases), and enhance utilization of D-amino acids by converting them to the L-form (racemases). The transamination reactions are thought to involve interconversion of pyridoxal phosphate and pyridoxamine phosphate. Pyridoxal phosphate is essential for conversion of tryptophan to niacin, and when vitamin B_6 is lacking, abnormal metabolites of tryptophan are excreted in the urine. Measurement of the excretion of these, especially that of xanthurenic acid, is used as a basis for studying vitamin B_6 deficiency. It is thought that the vitamin B_6 coenzymes are involved in nearly all reactions concerned with the synthesis and catabolism of amino acids.

Vitamin B_6 is thought to take part in fat metabolism, but the exact functions have not been explained. It may be involved in the metabolism of PUFA and in the lengthening of the fatty acid chain (10, 11). The skin lesions observed in deficiencies produced by the use of deoxypyridoxine, a vitamin B_6 antagonist, have responded to large doses of linolenic acid or to administration of 5 mg. of any one of the three members of the vitamin B_6 group (12). There is evidence also that a relationship exists between the vitamin and cholesterol metabolism and that vitamin B_6 may be involved in the control of atherosclerosis.

The vitamin has an important role in carbohydrate metabolism. As PLP, it has been found to be an essential part of the enzyme, glycogen phosphorylase, which brings about the conversion of glucose to glucose-1-phosphate (13). It has been estimated that over 50 per cent of the vitamin B_6 stored in the body is in this enzyme (14).

Vitamin B_6 assists in energy transformation in brain and nerve tissues and therefore is important in the functioning of the central nervous system. When the factor is lacking, convulsive seizures result in both experimental animals and human infants. Tower (15) studied the part played by the coenzyme in the brain and associated the epileptiform seizures with a deficiency of the vitamin. It has been demonstrated (16) that vitamin B_6 is necessary for formation of serotonin, a product formed in the decarboxylation of tryptophan, which is involved in central nervous system metabolism. Symptoms of lack of the vitamin are thought to be due to failure of the conversion of glutamic acid to γ-aminobutyric acid, a substance necessary for oxygen metabolism in the brain (17). Vitamin B_6 deficiency has been reported (18, 19) to cause increased urinary excretion of oxalates, and thus a lack of the vitamin may result in the formation of renal calculi. In addition, it appears from the findings of experimental studies that the vitamin is involved in antibody formation, messenger RNA synthesis, nucleic acid and folic acid metabolism, and adrenocortical, pituitary, and thyroid functions (20, 21). In studies on humans (22) vitamin B_6 has proved to be effective in the treatment of iron-resistant anemias, and supplemental vitamin B_6 during pregnancy seems to provide some protection against dental caries (23). It has been reported from studies with animals that vitamin B_6 deficiency interferes with the absorption of L-amino acids, iron, and vitamin B_{12}. The vitamin is a nutrient of great metabolic importance both biochemically and physiologically.

The human being uses all three forms of vitamin B_6. Pyridoxol, pyridoxal, and pyridoxamine are interchangeable in human metabolic processes and have equal vitamin activity. Pyridoxal is absorbed more completely and rapidly than the other two members of the group.

Microorganisms in the intestinal tract are known to synthesize vitamin B_6. However, since oral administration of streptomycin and of neomycin has resulted in no reduction in the amounts of vitamin B_6 and 4-pyridoxic acid excreted in the urine, it is considered doubtful that any of this potential source of the vitamin is absorbed and utilized. Small amounts of pyridoxal and of pyridoxamine are excreted normally in the urine; the total excretion of these factors varies between 0.2 and 0.3 mg. per 24 hours. Almost no pyridoxol is found in the urine. The chief excretory product of vitamin B_6 metabolism is 4-pyridoxic acid, which is biologically inactive. However, accurate measurement of this compound is difficult because interfering substances present may give erroneously high values.

The vitamin B_6 content of human blood has been reported to vary considerably in adults. Levels in infants under 18 months of age tend to be more than three times higher than those observed in adults.

THE NEED FOR VITAMIN B₆

Several laboratory tests are used in vitamin B_6 studies. The most widely used method for determining vitamin B_6 status is measurement of xanthurenic acid in a 24-hour urine specimen following oral administration of tryptophan. Normally, the excretion ranges from 0 to 50 mg. Amounts of from 200 to 500 mg. of xanthurenic acid are indicative of vitamin B_6 deficiency. However, comparison of results from different studies is difficult because of the amount and form (DL- or L-) of tryptophan given, and the analytical methods used are not always the same. Standardization of the tryptophan load test, therefore, has been suggested (24). Two gm. of L-tryptophan have been recommended for studies with adults and 50 mg. per kg. for studies with infants. Another test is based on the relationship of vitamin B_6 to alanine metabolism. When a deficiency occurs, the blood urea levels remain abnormally high 12 hours after administration of a test dose of 30 gm. of alanine. Both blood and urine levels of vitamin B_6 may be measured by microbiologic assay. Results from these analyses are not very accurate because the amounts of the vitamin present are so low.

Whole blood and serum transaminase activities have been tried as tests to assess vitamin B_6 nutriture (25). However, since blood transaminase levels of vitamin B_6 increase markedly after administration of the vitamin in both well-nourished and malnourished individuals, these assays are not effective in determining vitamin B_6 deficiency.

The urinary excretion of 4-pyridoxic acid may be determined by either photofluorometric or chromatographic procedures (26). The photofluorometric method is simpler than the chromatographic and may have value for clinical studies in which test doses of pyridoxine hydrochloride are administered.

Clinical signs of vitamin B_6 deficiency have been observed. It is difficult to create a dietary deficiency of the vitamin in human beings because vitamin B_6 is so widely distributed in foods. In experimental work, a vitamin B_6 antagonist has been used. In such a study Vilter was able to develop a deficiency state using deoxypyridoxine (27). The symptoms noted were a seborrheic dermatitis observed first about the eyes, in the naso-labial folds, and around the mouth. Later the lesions spread to other parts of the body. Loss of weight, muscular weakness, irritability, and mental depression were noted commonly, as were susceptibility to infection and lymphopenia. When a test dose of tryptophan was administered, large amounts of xanthurenic acid were excreted in the urine. Administration of as little as 5 mg. of pyridoxol, pyridoxal, or pyridoxamine promptly relieved all the abnormalities observed.

Vitamin B_6 deficiency syndromes have occurred in infants maintained inadvertently on vitamin B_6-deficient diets. In the early 1950's widespread occurrences of hyperirritability, twitchings, and convulsive seizures were reported among infants fed a commercial canned liquid-milk formula (28). The similarity of the convulsive seizures to those observed in vitamin B_6-deficient rats suggested that the disturbances might be due to a lack of vitamin B_6. Intramuscular administration of pyridoxine hydrochloride relieved the symptoms within five minutes. It was found later that the formula's natural vitamin B_6 content had been destroyed in the sterilization process. Since then the manufacturer has added a thermostabile form of vitamin B_6 to the product.

The human requirement for vitamin B_6 has been established. Sufficient data on the need for vitamin B_6 have become available so the FNB could include specific recommendations for it in the 1968 edition of the RDA. On the basis of a variety of studies (29, 30) on vitamin B_6 nutriture, the allowance has been set at 2 mg. per day for adults. This allowance is planned to provide a reasonable margin of safety and for daily intakes of 100 gm. or more of protein. Since there is evidence (16) that marginal or low intakes of vitamin B_6 may have detrimental effects on physical and mental growth and development, the allowance for children is 0.5 to 1.2 mg. daily from ages two to ten years. The FNB states that sufficient information is not available to make a definite statement on the vitamin B_6 requirements of adolescents. The allowances for adolescents are in the range of 1.4 to 2.0 mg. daily.

The average diet in the United States has been reported to contain 2 mg. of vitamin B_6 daily (31). The FDA found that 16- to 19-year-old boys ingesting a high-calorie, moderate-cost diet obtain 2.2 to 2.9 mg. of vitamin B_6 daily (32). It would appear, therefore, that, because of the widespread distribution of the vitamin in foods, it is not likely to be deficient in the diet and, under ordinary conditions, the RDA can be met. However, preliminary data from the 1965 Nationwide Food Consumption Survey (40) indicate that adolescent males tended to meet the allowance, but that adolescent females did not.

During infancy the protein-vitamin B_6 relationship is critical. Under normal circumstances the breast-fed infant receives sufficient vitamin B_6. The metabolic requirements of the bottle-fed infant will be satisfied if the formula contains 0.015 mg. of the vitamin per gm. of protein or 0.04 mg. per 100 kcal. According to the FNB, the needs during pregnancy and lactation will be met by an intake of 0.5 mg. per day above that recommended for the nonpregnant, nonlactating female (23). Therefore, the allowances for these periods are 2.5 mg. per day. Although there is some evidence that the need for vitamin B_6 increases in the elderly, no additional allowance is suggested for this age group.

Several factors may influence the amount of vitamin B_6 required. When the diet is high in protein, low in essential fatty acids, or low in other members of the vitamin B complex, the requirement for the vitamin may be increased. When the functions of vitamin B_6 are recalled, it can be understood readily why a high protein diet may increase the body's need for the vitamin.

An inborn error of metabolism in which there is an abnormally high requirement for the vitamin has been described (33). The convulsive seizures in infants with this disorder have been controlled by administration of 2 mg. of vitamin B_6 daily. This metabolic defect apparently increases the vitamin B_6 requirement for normal brain metabolism.

During pregnancy alterations in vitamin B_6 and in tryptophan metabolism have been reported (34). Some pregnant women excrete excessively large amounts of xanthurenic acid following a test load of tryptophan. Such abnormalities have been relieved quickly by administration of small amounts of pyridoxol. In other studies abnormal responses to administration of alanine have been reported in pregnant women. Blood urea nitrogen levels were found to remain high for more than 12 hours after the alanine test dose was given (35). Normal responses to the alanine load tests were observed in the same women following daily vitamin B_6 supplements. It is not known that these findings actually indicate an increased need for vitamin B_6 during pregnancy, particularly since the excretion pattern of the various metabolites of tryptophan has been found to differ in many respects from that observed in vitamin B_6 deficiency. However, the increased need of the pregnant woman for protein and calories indicates the advisability of including liberal amounts of vitamin B_6 in the daily diet.

Patients with hypochromic anemia, but whose serum and bone marrow iron levels are high, respond to pyridoxol in daily doses of 10 mg. or more. It is thought that such conditions involve a metabolic block, probably in porphyrin formation, which increases the requirement for vitamin B_6.

Isonicotinic acid hydrazide (INH), commonly used in the treatment of tuberculosis, hydralazine, an anti-hypertensive drug, and penicillamine, a metabolite of penicillin, have been found to interfere with certain activities of pyridoxal phosphate, causing convulsions in animals and a peripheral neuritis in human beings. These symptoms can be prevented by daily administration of vitamin B_6. In human beings, therapeutic doses of as much as 50 to 100 mg. appear to be required.

Folic Acid (Folacin, Pteroylglutamic Acid)

CHEMISTRY AND SOURCES OF FOLIC ACID

The terms "folic acid" or "folacin" are used to designate a group of closely related substances. Isolation of folic acid in 1945, and its synthesis in 1946, ended years of research to find the factor important in the prevention and control of certain types of anemias, and necessary for the growth of microorganisms and many species of animals. It soon became apparent that the various growth-promoting and anemia-preventing substances reported in the literature, including vitamin M, vitamin U, vitamin B_c, and the *Lactobacillus casei* factor, were either folic acid or conjugates of it.

Folic acid is a compound that contains the pteridine group and one molecule each of glutamic acid and *para*-aminobenzoic acid (Figure 12–7). Its empirical formula is $C_{19}H_{19}N_7O_6$. Sometimes it is referred

Figure 12–7
Structural formula of folic acid

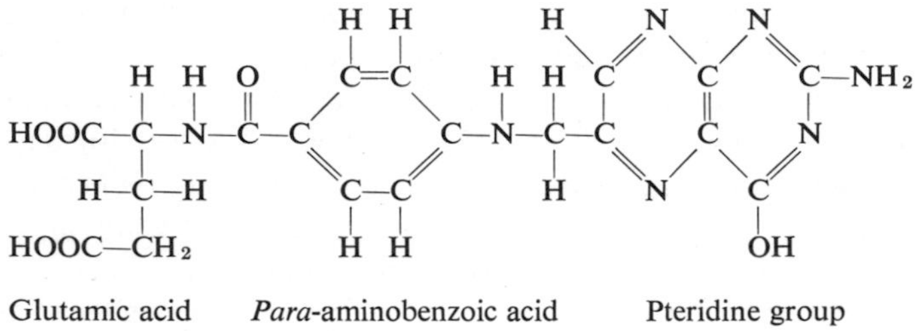

Glutamic acid   *Para*-aminobenzoic acid   Pteridine group

to by its chemical name, pteroylglutamic acid. It is a yellow crystalline substance, slightly soluble in water, relatively unstable to heat, and labile to acid and to sunlight when in solution.

The vitamin occurs in foods of animal and plant origin, some of it in the free form but usually as folic acid conjugates in which it is combined with two or six additional molecules of glutamic acid. A derivative of folic acid, folinic acid, often called the citrovorum factor, leucovorum, or N^5-formyltetrahydrofolic acid, also occurs in foods usually conjugated with additional glutamic acid molecules (Figure 12–8).

Figure 12–8
Structural formula of folinic acid (citrovorum factor, N^5-formyltetra-hydrofolic acid)

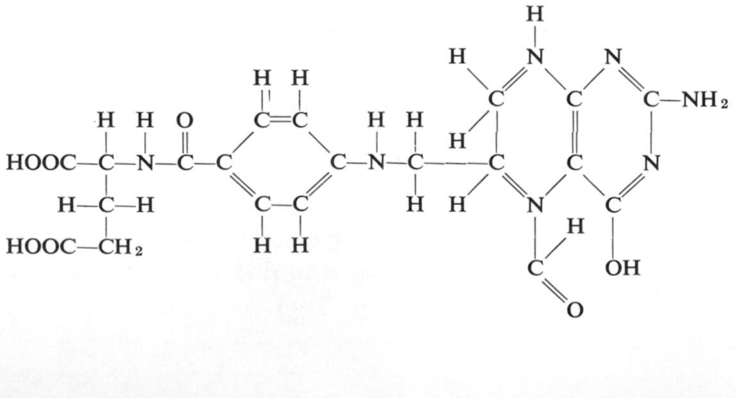

Many foods have been analyzed for folic acid content (1). Although bioassays with the monkey, rat, or chick and spectophometric techniques have been used in the determination of folic acid in foods, microbiological assay is the most commonly used method. In this procedure the vitamin is released from its bound forms by enzymatic hydrolysis prior to assay for total folic acid content with *Lactobacillus casei* or *Streptococcus faecalis*. In recent years chromatographic fractionation has been used to determine the pteroylglutamate components of individual foods (2, 3, 4). Liver and dark-green leafy vegetables (4) are the richest sources. Other green vegetables, kidney, legumes, nuts, and whole grains are good sources. Most other foods contain varying small amounts of the vitamin.

Studies made on eggs have shown that approximately nine-tenths of the folic acid is in the yolk. The amount (5) the hen deposited in the egg was increased by addition of vitamin B_{12} to the hen's ration. The commercial process of "converting" rice results in considerable increase in the concentration of folic acid over that in polished rice. Ordinary cooking procedures and dehydration processes have been reported to cause, on the average, 50 per cent destruction of the vitamin. Similar losses have been found to occur during the vegetable storage.

THE BIOLOGICAL SIGNIFICANCE AND NEED FOR FOLIC ACID

Folic acid is involved in many biochemical processes. The exact mechanisms by which folic acid acts have not been determined. However, it is known that folic acid is changed in the body into biologically active forms by a process of reduction, which is facilitated by niacin and ascorbic acid and with the addition of formyl, hydroxymethyl, methyl, or formimine groups (6). These substances are tetrahydrofolic acids (TFA) and serve as coenzymes in the transfer of single carbon units important in the metabolism of many body compounds. The folic acid coenzymes act in formation of purines and pyrimidines that are used in making nucleoproteins, methylation of homocysteine to form methionine, conversion of glycine to serine, formation of porphyrin compounds necessary for hemoglobin, and synthesis of choline and other compounds of the labile methyl group (7, 8). Vitamin B_{12} appears to be involved in the activity of the folic acid coenzymes in many of these metabolic processes (9, 10). Folic acid has been shown to take part in the metabolism of the amino acids tyrosine, tryptophan, and histidine.

This factor is required for normal hematopoiesis. Lack of folic acid results in macrocytic anemia with megaloblastic arrest of the maturation of red blood cells due to an inadequate supply of nucleoproteins. This condition may occur in infancy, during pregnancy, in persons on exceedingly poor diets, and during a primary liver disease. It has been suggested that in some instances megaloblastic anemia is due to an unknown metabolic defect in the production of the folic acid coenzymes. Patients with pernicious anemia may respond to treatment with folic acid, but only in respect to remission of the blood condition. Since its use in amounts in excess of 0.1 mg. per day may prevent the blood changes symptomatic of pernicious anemia while the neurological changes of the disease progress, federal law prohibits sale without prescription of vitamin preparations recommending doses of more than 0.1 mg. of folic acid per day.

The metabolism of folic acid by the human being is being investigated. Both folic acid and folinic acid are used by the body when taken orally or administered parenterally. However, naturally occurring conjugates of folic acid must be reduced to the monoglutamate form to be absorbed. In cases of nontropical sprue it has been found that oral administration of pteroyldiglutamic acid or of sodium pteroyltriglutamic acid is more effective than folic acid (11). The extent to which the vitamin is absorbed from food sources is not known. Antagonists of folic acid occur in nature and limit the availability of the vitamin to the body (12). One of these, aminopterin, is used frequently to develop a deficiency in the human being.

Synthesis of both folic acid and folinic acid may occur through the action of microorganisms in the intestinal tract. This was demonstrated in an experiment on germ-free rats. Biotin was shown to be necessary for the synthesis. Folic acid and folinic acid are found in the urine. The amount excreted following a test dose is used to indicate nutritional status. In a study of sprue patients 1.2 per cent of the test dose was excreted in the urine. In control subjects and in sprue patients who had been treated with folic acid, 26 and 24 per cent, respectively, were excreted. Folic acid nutritional status may be determined also by administering a test dose of histidine and measuring the urinary excretion of formiminoglutamic acid, an intermediate in the metabolism of histidine (13). In subjects with folic acid deficiency large amounts of formiminoglutamic acid are excreted, the formimino group having been attached to glutamic acid in the absence of sufficient TFA (14).

The utilization of folacin has been shown to be adversely affected by a deficiency of iron. In studies on iron-deficient animals and adults with iron-deficiency anemia, abnormally high urinary excretions of formiminoglutamic acid have been reported. It has been suggested that the functional defect in folacin utilization in iron deficiency states is due to a reduction in the activity of the enzyme formimino-transferase (15). Utilization and functions of folic acid have been reported to be impaired when protein malnutrition exists (16, 17).

The urinary excretion of citrovorum factor in healthy men after administration of folic acid or citrovorum factor with and without ascorbic acid supplements has been studied. On an ordinary diet the average amounts of folic acid and citrovorum factor per ml. of urine were 5 to 10 mμg. and 1 mμg., respectively. Excretion of the citrovorum factor was increased from two to three times when ascorbic acid was given in combination with the test dose of folic acid, indicating that ascorbic acid plays a role in the biosynthesis of folinic acid.

In a study (18) on the megaloblastic anemia of infancy, 25 per cent of the infants were scorbutic and about 50 per cent showed a suboptimal intake of ascorbic acid. It has been found that this anemia can be prevented by administering ascorbic acid, but, once having developed, it responds to treatment only with folic acid or folinic acid. This disease of infancy has disappeared almost entirely, since ascorbic acid supplements are included in the proprietary foods fed to babies. Adults with scurvy who were fed test doses of folic acid excreted much less citrovorum factor than did normal subjects (19). When the scorbutic patients were fed ascorbic acid with folic acid, the return to normal citrovorum factor excretion was delayed, showing a metabolic derangement. Vilter and associates (20) reported the occurrence of megaloblastic anemia resulting from combined folic acid and ascorbic acid deficiencies in persons with scurvy and in infants maintained on unsupplemented milk diets.

Deficiency of folic acid in man has been found with increasing frequency. The deficiency may be caused by inadequate dietary intake, impaired absorption, excessive body tissue demands, or metabolic derangements. It has been estimated that about 20 per cent of all cases of megaloblastic anemia are due to dietary lack of folic acid. The anemia, glossitis, and diarrhea resulting from the deficiency respond promptly to therapeutic doses of 5 to 10 mg. of folic acid daily.

In mice and in man, leukemia can be controlled to some extent by use of folic acid antagonists which reduce the number of white blood cells produced, but cure has not been possible. There is some evidence from studies on experimental animals that antagonists of folic acid may inhibit the growth of tumors.

Allowances for dietary folic acid have been recommended. The FNB has recommended a daily allowance of 0.4 mg. of folacin daily for both males and females age ten and over. Since present knowledge of the availability of the various forms of folic acid in foods is limited (21), the allowances are based on dietary sources as determined by *Lactobacillus casei* assay. The FNB suggests that intakes of less than one-fourth of the recommended allowances may be effective if pure forms of folic acid are used. Studies on babies have shown that they require approximately 0.005 to 0.02 mg. (22) per day. Because of the frequent occurrence of megaloblastic anemia in infants which responds to folic acid therapy, the allowance for infants has been set at 0.05 to 0.2 mg. per day. The recommended intakes during pregnancy and lactation are 0.8 mg. and 0.5 mg. daily to take care of the increased demands on folacin stores and prevent development of megaloblastic anemia (23).

It has been reported that a balanced diet in the United States contains as much as 0.6 mg. of total folacin activity when measured by *Lactobacillus casei* assay. Therefore, during pregnancy, folacin-rich foods should be stressed in the diet in order to meet the fetal and maternal needs and to prevent development of megaloblastic anemia.

Vitamin B_{12} (Cobalamin)

CHEMISTRY AND SOURCES OF VITAMIN B_{12}

Studies on control and treatment of pernicious anemia led to discovery of vitamin B_{12}. In 1948, after years of research, a red crystalline material was isolated from liver and proved to be active in treatment of pernicious anemia. It was named vitamin B_{12} and was found to contain about 4 per cent cobalt as well as some phosphorus and nitrogen, but no sulfur. Since then several closely related compounds have been identified. The generic name of cobalamin has been given to this group of substances because they contain cobalt. Vitamin B_{12}, which has the cyano group in the molecule, is called cyanocobalamin. Chemical analysis has shown that the vitamin has the empirical formula $C_{63}H_{90}O_{14}N_{14}PCo$. Its structure has been elucidated and is extremely complex (Figure 12–9).

Cyanocobalamin is freely soluble in water and stable to boiling temperature in neutral solution, but autoclaving causes some destruction. It is labile to strong acids, alkali, and light, and loses its potency to some extent in the presence of oxidizing and reducing agents. Hydroxocobalamin, which contains the hydroxy group in place of the cyano group, has biological activity equal to that of cyanocobalamin. Both substances are available commercially in plentiful supply.

Microbiological tests are used for determining the vitamin B_{12} content of foods. The microorganism most widely used to determine vitamin B_{12} in foods is *Lactobacillus leichmanni*. It has been found that vitamin B_{12} occurs bound to protein in foods of animal origin. There is very little, if any, of the vitamin in plant foods. Vitamin B_{12} is synthesized by many bacteria and by microorganisms in the rumen of herbivorous animals. The original source of the vitamin in the animal kingdom is thought to result from such microbiological synthesis. Some is formed by bacteria in the human intestinal tract, but it appears that little, if any, of this is absorbed and available for use. Man apparently is dependent on a preformed source of vitamin B_{12} in foods.

Liver and kidney are the richest sources of vitamin B_{12} (1). Muscle meats, eggs, fish, milk, and cheese also supply good amounts (2, 3).

THE FUNCTIONS OF VITAMIN B_{12}

Vitamin B_{12} plays many important biological roles. The vitamin functions as a coenzyme and at least five different forms have been identified. These are termed "cobamide coenzymes." Conversion of the vitamin to

Figure 12–9
Structural formula of vitamin B$_{12}$.

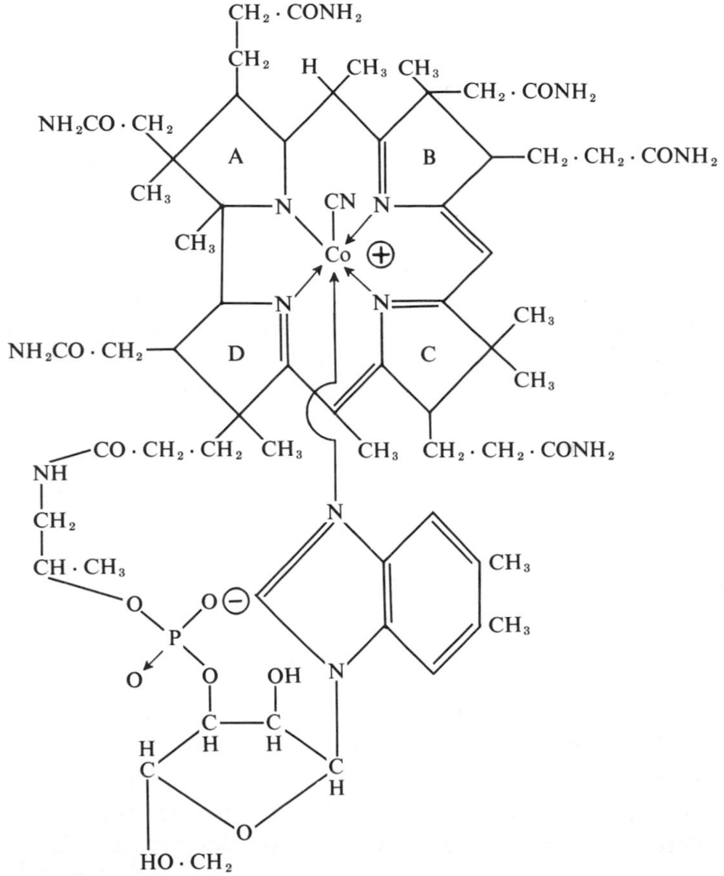

the coenzyme requires many nutrients, including riboflavin, nicotinic acid, and magnesium.

Vitamin B$_{12}$ has many important functions in metabolic processes, but the mechanism of action of the cobamide coenzymes is not fully understood. It is known that like folic acid, vitamin B$_{12}$ in coenzyme form is concerned with metabolism of purines and pyrimidines in the synthesis of nucleoproteins, and therefore is essential for normal blood cell formation. Vitamin B$_{12}$ is necessary also for normal metabolism of nervous tissue. A review of the literature on the role of vitamin B$_{12}$ by Vilter (4) indicates that the vitamin is involved in protein, fat, and carbohydrate metabolism. It appears that cobamide coenzyme is concerned with the biosynthesis of amino acids rather than with protein synthesis (5). It may be important also in thyroid function and ascorbic acid metabolism (6). In animals vitamin B$_{12}$ has been found to be a growth-stimulator.

However, no convincing evidence has been found for a growth role in human beings (7).

In man a deficiency of cobalamin results in pernicious anemia characterized by megaloblastic anemia and subacute combined degeneration of the spinal cord. The anemia of vitamin B_{12} deficiency appears to be due to an inability of the bone marrow cells to form DNA brought about by disturbances in folic acid metabolism. Apparently, vitamin B_{12} is necessary for activation of folic acid coenzymes required for DNA synthesis.

Experimental evidence indicates that cobalamin is involved in the transfer of single carbon intermediates, particularly in transmethylation processes such as synthesis of choline from methionine, serine from glycine, and methionine from homocysteine. It appears also that the vitamin serves as a coenzyme in propionic and methylmalonic acid metabolism (8), in biosynthesis of methyl groups, and in reduction reactions such as conversion of disulfide to the sulfhydryl group.

Studies on pernicious anemia have demonstrated that vitamin B_{12} is the extrinsic factor. Control of this disease was first brought about by feeding liver, later liver extract, and still later beef muscle and normal gastric juice. These findings led Castle and his associates to conclude that two factors were involved, one endogenous, the other exogenous. The endogenous substance called the intrinsic factor (IF) is a mucoprotein found in normal gastric juice and in an extract of hog mucosa. It appears to be necessary for absorption of vitamin B_{12} from the intestinal tract (9, 10). The IF apparently binds vitamin B_{12}, forming the B_{12}-IF complex. Then, in a reaction catalyzed by calcium, B_{12}-IF is attached to the ileum wall through which the vitamin is absorbed. In the absorptive process it is thought that the IF is either removed or altered since none is found in lymph or blood plasma. The intrinsic factor has been shown by means of radioactive cobalt-vitamin B_{12} tracer tests to increase absorption of the vitamin in individuals who have pernicious anemia. The endogenous substance was found to be vitamin B_{12}. In pernicious anemia patients, the blood serum levels and urinary excretion of the vitamin are low, but both may be increased on administration of a test dose of cobalamin (11). Normal blood serum levels of free and bound vitamin B_{12} range from 200 to 300 μg. per ml. In pernicious anemia, serum levels average only about one-tenth of the normal level. Since after a test dose both healthy persons and individuals with this disease tend to excrete the vitamin in comparable amounts, urinary excretion cannot be used as an index in metabolism experiments. However, tracer tests with radioactive cobalt-vitamin B_{12} are effective in studying the disease.

In treating pernicious anemia vitamin B_{12} is the therapeutic agent to be used. Full hematopoietic and clinical responses have been observed following oral administration of 1 to 5 mg. of IF with 5 to 10 μg. of vitamin B$_{12}$. Cooperative studies (12, 13, 14) have shown that daily oral doses of 300 μg. of cyanocobalamin without IF are effective in treating pernicious anemia. Apparently the mass action of such large oral doses results in absorption of approximately 1 per cent of the vitamin which is as available and utilizable as that absorbed with IF. However, it is thought generally that the parenteral administration of vitamin B$_{12}$ is more effective than when it is given orally. Daily doses of 10 to 15 μg. are usually prescribed until all symptoms are relieved and blood values have become normal. Thereafter, maintenance doses of 15 to 30 μg. may be given at intervals as infrequently as every three to four weeks. Sometimes both vitamin B$_{12}$ and folic acid are used in this treatment. Folic acid cannot be used alone since, although it may benefit the hematological condition, it is not effective in controlling the neurological complications of the disease and even may hasten degeneration of the spinal cord.

THE NEED FOR VITAMIN B$_{12}$

Sufficient data are available so that recommended allowances have been established. In studies (15) with normal persons using a radioactive form of the vitamin it has been shown that more than 70 per cent of a 0.5 μg. dose is absorbed and that absorption decreases as the amount of vitamin B$_{12}$ administered increases, with 30 per cent or less of a 5 μg. dose being absorbed. Total daily excretion of vitamin B$_{12}$ has been estimated at about 1.3 μg. per day (16). Heyssel and co-workers (17) reported that vitamin B$_{12}$ from food sources is as well absorbed as crystalline vitamin B$_{12}$. On the basis of these and other investigations the FNB recommends a daily intake of 5 μg. for adults. The allowance for infants during the first year ranges from 1 to 2 μg. per day. This is gradually increased until age eight to ten when the recommended intake reaches 5 μg. During pregnancy (18, 19) serum vitamin B$_{12}$ levels tend to fall gradually. Although this may be due to hemodilution, there is evidence of excessive vitamin B$_{12}$ demand by the fetus (20). A significant increase in absorption of an orally administered test dose of vitamin B$_{12}$ by the pregnant woman has been demonstrated (21). The recommended allowance for pregnant women, therefore, is increased to 8 μg. daily; for lactation, it is 6 μg. daily. The level of vitamin B$_{12}$ in the blood has been found to decrease with age (22). Since absorption may be poor and hypoacidity frequently occurs in older persons, the allowance for those over 55 has been set at 6 μg. per day. Sometimes the administration of IF and crystalline vitamin B$_{12}$ is recommended for elderly persons.

In a study of high-cost, low-cost, and poor diets Mangay Chung and associates (23) found the daily average vitamin B$_{12}$ contents were 31, 16, and 2.7 μg. respectively. Tentative data from the 1965 Nationwide

Food Consumption Survey indicate that the daily intake of vitamin B_{12} of all age groups studied, except women 75 years or over, exceeded 5 μg. Judging from these data, it would appear that average diets in the United States should meet the recommended allowances.

Other conditions may affect the need for vitamin B_{12}. Experimental work (24) has shown that deficiency of pyridoxine in the diet decreases the blood level and the absorption of cobalamin and that increased storage of the vitamin in the liver and kidneys occurs when intakes of riboflavin and folic acid are not limited. Vitamin B_{12} is given frequently with folic acid in treatment of both sprue and nutritional macrocytic anemia (25).

Decreased absorption of vitamin B_{12} may occur in persons with blind intestinal loops or pouches, small bowel diverticula, sprue and other malabsorption syndromes, and in those infested with fish tapeworm. Since these conditions involve deficiencies of folic acid and other essential nutrients, multiple-vitamin therapy should be effective. It is thought that the beneficial hematological influence of antibiotics, sometimes noted, may result from their eliminating certain intestinal bacteria which, if remaining, would have inhibited normal absorption of the factor. In stress conditions such as infections, a cold temperature, and hyperthyroidism there may be an increased demand for cobalamin.

Vitamin B_{12} therapy is usually necessary following total gastrectomy and ileum resection and may be required after subtotal gastrectomy or pernicious anemia may result. Removal of the IF-secreting parts of the stomach or the absorbing surfaces of the small intestine are responsible for the conditioned vitamin B_{12} deficiency.

Vegetarian diets containing no foods of animal origin are practically devoid of cobalamin, and persons living on such diets have been reported (26, 27) to require supplementary sources of the vitamin to prevent development of the neurological manifestations of vitamin B_{12} deficiency. Anemia occurs only rarely among strict vegetarians.

Pantothenic Acid

CHEMISTRY AND SOURCES OF PANTOTHENIC ACID

Studies on the nutrients necessary for the growth of yeast resulted in isolation and synthesis of pantothenic acid. In 1933 R. J. Williams reported the presence in a variety of plant and animal tissues of an acidic substance which was a specific growth stimulator for yeast. Because of its widespread distribution, he named the factor "pantothenic acid," a word derived from the Greek meaning "from everywhere." Concurrently, investigators in other laboratories were attempting to isolate an "antidermatitis factor" for chicks, a "liver filtrate factor" for rats, and a "growth factor" for lactic acid bacteria. The isolation of pantothenic acid in 1939, and its synthesis in 1940, proved it to be identical with these factors.

Pantothenic acid is fairly stable in neutral solutions, but it is destroyed by acid and alkali, and by prolonged dry heat. Its formula is $C_9H_{17}O_5N$ (Figure 12–10). The calcium salt of the vitamin is the form in which it is used generally. Calcium pantothenate is odorless and slightly bitter in taste. Pantothenic acid in pure form is a pale yellow viscous oil.

Figure 12–10
Structural formula of pantothenic acid

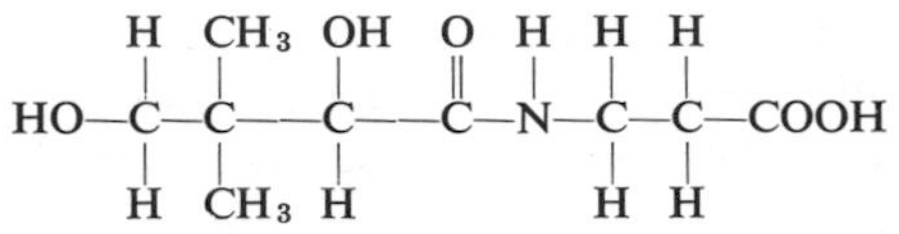

The pantothenic acid content of foods may be determined by microbiologic or rat assay. The most commonly used method is microbiological, using *Lactobacillus plantarium*. Since the vitamin occurs in bound as well as free forms in foods, the bound form must be released by enzymatic digestion before assay with microorganisms. Zook and associates (1) have developed an enzymatic-microbiological method for determination of both free and bound pantothenic acid, the results of which are in general agreement with those obtained by rat assay.

Among the best sources of the vitamin are liver and other organ meats, egg yolk, salmon, legumes, peanuts, mushrooms, broccoli, kale, avocados, and dried brewer's and Torula yeast. Lean muscle meats, poultry, whole grain products, and most nuts are good sources. Milk and cheese contain about half as much pantothenic acid as do muscle meats. Most fruits and vegetables are fair sources of the vitamin.

Ordinary cooking processes appear to result in only negligible losses of pantothenic acid (2). Heat-dried beef has been found to lose 30 per cent of its original pantothenic acid (3). The milling of whole wheat results in loss of about one-half the vitamin.

THE BIOLOGICAL SIGNIFICANCE AND NEED FOR PANTOTHENIC ACID

Pantothenic acid is vital in metabolic processes. It has been shown that pantothenic acid is an essential constituent of CoA. This bound form of pantothenic acid is heat stabile. Pantothenic acid first combines with β-mercaptoethylamine (a sulfur-containing compound) to form pantetheine or the *L-bulgaricus factor*. This unites with phosphate, ribose, and an adenine molecule to form CoA. However, the structure of this large molecule is still tentative.

CoA aids in acetyl transfer. Thus it is involved in many metabolic processes which include carbohydrates, fats, and proteins. It functions in acetylation of choline and of *para*-aminobenzoic acid, and in formation of porphyrins (4). It is concerned in synthesis of cholesterol, steroids, and fatty acids (5). Lessened activity of the adrenal glands in secreting adrenocortical hormones is associated with pantothenic acid deficiency (6). CoA has been shown to function also in the synthesis of arachidonic acid from linoleic acid, and of aminolevulinic acid which is a precursor of heme, important in hemoglobin formation. The coenzyme appears to be necessary for maintenance of normal blood sugar levels and for antibody formation (7).

Symptoms of a lack of the vitamin have been found in many animals. These include dermatitis, graying of feathers, and degeneration of the spinal cord in chicks; achromatricia or graying of the hair, failure of growth, inability to acetylate *para*-aminobenzoic acid, and necrosis of the adrenal glands in rats; and hypoglycemia, fatty degeneration of the liver, and gastrointestinal disturbances in dogs. These and other signs demonstrate the vitamin's fundamental enzymatic role.

A diet high in protein has a sparing effect on the pantothenic acid requirement. In a study on rats (8), methionine was found to be as effective as protein; it is thought that a sulfur-containing amino acid such as methionine may improve utilization of pantothenic acid for synthesis of CoA. Ascorbic acid also takes part in pantothenic acid metabolism in some animals. Addition of small amounts of ascorbic acid to diets lacking pantothenic acid has been shown to prevent symptoms of pantothenic acid deficiency in rats. However, Pudelkewitz and Roderuck (9), found that large amounts of ascorbic acid were not beneficial in pantothenic acid deficiencies in guinea pigs.

The metabolism of pantothenic acid in human beings is being investigated. Since pantothenic acid occurs commonly in foods, under usual dietary circumstances a deficiency is seldom seen. Bean and co-workers (10) induced a deficiency of the vitamin in man by administering the pantothenic acid antagonist, *omega*-methyl-pantothenic acid. The results of their extensive studies indicate that pantothenic acid deficiency causes fatigue, weakness, headache, nausea, emotional instability, dizziness, impaired motor coordination, muscle cramps, and changes in heart function, including fluctuations in heart beat and blood pressure. Biochemical tests showed impaired ability of acetylation, increased sensitivity to insulin resulting in low blood sugar levels, poor adrenal functioning, decreased gastric secretions, and impaired immune body formation. Water imbalance and abnormal electrolyte control were noted also. All the adverse effects were reversed when the antagonist was discontinued and pantothenic acid was administered.

Deficiency of pantothenic acid has been associated with the "burning feet syndrome" which occurred in the Philippines and Japan among prisoners during World War II. Malnourished people in India have shown a similar condition which is thought to be due to lack of pantothenic acid. Ralli (11) has reported that administration of calcium pantothenate in large doses improves the ability of well-nourished human subjects to withstand stress conditions.

CoA does not circulate in the blood but is found in other body tissues. The liver, adrenal glands, kidneys, brain, and heart have the highest concentrations. Apparently, the coenzyme is synthesized from pantothenic acid intracellularly whenever it is needed. Free pantothenic acid is found in the blood, particularly in the plasma, and it is excreted in the urine. Considerable variation in blood levels and urinary excretion of the vitamin has been observed in normal subjects. Blood levels have been found to range from 3 to 32 μg. per 100 ml. and urinary excretion from 2 to 7 mg. daily (12).

A relationship between riboflavin and pantothenic acid metabolism has been reported by Spies and co-workers (13). They found low blood levels of pantothenic acid in patients with pellagra, beriberi, and ariboflavinosis. When calcium pantothenate was administered parenterally a rise in the blood level of riboflavin as well as of pantothenic acid resulted.

This factor is considered an essential nutrient for the human being. Although the amount of the vitamin required by the human being is not known, R. J. Williams (14) has estimated that a typical 2500-calorie diet which includes foods from both animal and plant sources provides about 10 mg. of pantothenic acid per day. Other reports (15) indicate that the usual diets consumed by adults in the United States furnish about 10 to 15 mg. of pantothenic acid daily with a range of from 6 to 20 mg. Studies (16) on the dietary intakes of children age seven to nine years have shown that when the other recommended allowances are met the diets provide about 4 to 5 mg. of pantothenic acid. On the basis of these figures and of urinary excretions of from 2 to 7 mg. daily, the FNB suggests that a daily intake of 5 to 10 mg. per day should satisfy human requirements. Obtaining enough of the vitamin during pregnancy and lactation is important, but there is no evidence to suggest that the requirement should be increased during these periods.

Although pantothenic acid has been shown to prevent graying of hair and feathers in animals and fowl, clinical evidence has not corroborated the early reports that it is an anti-gray hair factor for human beings.

Biotin

CHEMISTRY AND SOURCES OF BIOTIN

Biotin has been isolated and synthesized. The discovery of bios, a growth-promoting substance for yeast known since 1901, and the search for the factor in raw egg white which was reported in 1916 to be toxic for rats, led to isolation of biotin in 1936. It was established then that biotin was identical with vitamin H (the anti-egg white injury factor), Bios II, and coenzyme R. These were some of the names suggested for the factor as the search for its identification progressed. In 1942 biotin was synthesized by du Vigneaud. The free compound has the formula $C_{10}H_{16}O_3N_2S$ (Figure 12–11) and is a colorless compound. It is readily soluble in hot

Figure 12–11
Structural formula of biotin

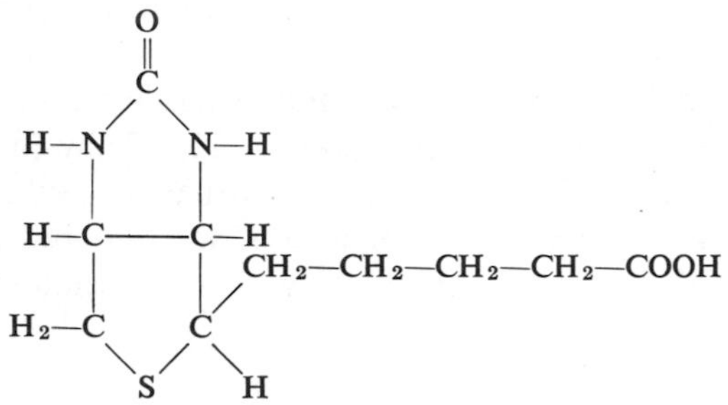

water, but only sparingly so in cold water, stable to heat, and inactivated by oxidizing agents, alkalis, and strong acids.

The biotin content of foods may be determined either microbiologically or by bioassay. The vitamin occurs in natural products principally in a bound form and is a biotin-protein complex. The microbiological techniques used to determine quantitatively the biotin in foods and body tissues therefore involve a preliminary acid or enzymatic hydrolysis. Assays on chicks and rats measure equally well both the bound and free forms as they occur in natural products. In such assays growth is measured under controlled conditions and is the basis for data on the biotin content of food. Liver, kidney, milk, egg yolk, and yeast are among the richest sources of the vitamin. Legumes, nuts, chocolate, fish, and some fruits and vegetables are good sources. Muscle meats, and corn and wheat products contain only small amounts.

THE FUNCTIONS AND NEED FOR BIOTIN

The mode of action of the vitamin is being studied in order to establish biochemical mechanisms. Microorganisms, rats, mice, and guinea pigs are used in efforts to determine the metabolic processes for which biotin is required. It is known that the vitamin is an essential part of a coenzyme which is involved in carbon dioxide fixation and in deamination and decarboxylation processes (1). It has been demonstrated (2) that biotin aids in the synthesis of saturated fatty acids, a mechanism which is thought to involve the carboxylation of acetyl CoA. Biotin has been found necessary also in conversion of ornithine into citrulline, an important step in urea formation, for protein synthesis, oxidative phosphorylation, and carbohydrate metabolism. The factor is required for purine metabolism (3), and, in the presence of carbon dioxide, for conversion of pyruvate to oxalacetate and then to aspartate. It is closely related to folic acid (4), pantothenic acid, and vitamin B_{12} in metabolic processes. It has been suggested that these three nutrients participate in one-carbon metabolism.

Signs of biotin deficiency have been observed. In experimental animals when biotin is not available, certain manifestations are evident. The rat (5) will show spectacled eye symptoms and alopecia or loss of hair. Later, paralysis, spasticity, myocardial necrosis, and death ensue. Pantothenic acid deficiency in mice has been cured more quickly when biotin was fed with pantothenic acid than when pantothenic acid was fed alone. Also, biotin aided in the restoration of hair and hair color.

Symptoms of biotin deficiency do not occur in human beings under ordinary circumstances. This is to be expected because the vitamin is widely distributed in foods and considerable quantities are made available to the body through biosynthesis by intestinal bacteria. Oppel (6) found in a study of healthy adults that the daily excretion of biotin in urine and feces exceeded the intake by three to six times, thus showing the significance of biosynthesis of the factor.

It is known that a protein called avidin in raw egg white combines with biotin to form a compound which cannot be absorbed from the intestinal tract and therefore is excreted in the feces. In addition, the biotin synthesized in the intestines may be lost if enough raw egg white is ingested (7).

Sydenstricker and associates (8) produced a biotin deficiency in man by feeding volunteers a diet containing a minimal amount of the vitamin plus raw egg white equal to at least 30 per cent of the total calories. Adequate amounts of synthetic vitamins, iron, and calcium were supplied. Symptoms, evident in about seven weeks, included dermatitis, a grayish pallor of skin and mucous membranes, a diminution of hemoglobin and erythrocytes, and a striking rise in serum cholesterol. Depression, muscle pains, and anorexia appeared. Excretion of biotin in the urine was much below that of a person on a normal diet. When 150 or more mg. of biotin were injected daily, the symptoms became less evident. The ashy pallor disappeared in four days, serum cholesterol was reduced, and urinary excretion of biotin increased.

The requirement of biotin for the human being has not been determined. The FNB does not make a specific recommendation for biotin but suggests a daily intake of from 150 to 300 μg., a range that should be secured easily in the average American diet. Studies by Sydenstricker and co-workers (8) have shown that deficiency symptoms in man do not occur when the intake of biotin is 150 µg. or more per day.

The biotin requirement may be increased during administration of some sulfa compounds and certain antibiotics. It has been found that large and prolonged doses of sulfasuxadine, sulfathalidine, streptomycin or terramycin can cause almost complete cessation of intestinal synthesis of biotin. Consideration of a possible biotin deficiency from continued use of these drugs appears to be necessary.

It is considered highly unlikely that the usual diet contains enough avidin from raw egg white to produce a biotin deficiency. Clinical cases of biotin deficiency have been described in individuals who have included large amounts of raw eggs in their diets. It should be borne in mind that the avidin in egg white is destroyed by cooking, and thus the usual dietary includes little of the biotin-interfering substance.

The results of studies on biotin metabolism indicate that it is a nutrient necessary for utilization of fat, protein, and carbohydrate. Although it is required probably in only micro-amounts, it is presumed to be essential for man.

Other Nutrient Factors

THE VITAMIN STATUS OF PARA-AMINOBENZOIC ACID, CHOLINE, AND INOSITOL

These three factors have been classified as members of the B complex. However, there is some question now whether they are actually vitamins. The fact that *para*-aminobenzoic acid (PABA) is a unit in the structure of folic acid may be a reason for its tentative status as a vitamin. At one time PABA was classified as a vitamin. It is no longer considered such for human beings, since it is now known to be a component of pteroylglutamic acid. Further, it is not a necessary constituent in the human dietary. PABA is essential, however, for organisms that are able to synthesize pteroylglutamic acid. In synthetic diets choline and inositol are needed in large amounts compared to the requirements for the known vitamins; both substances are synthesized in the body under ordinary circumstances, and their action as coenzymes in metabolic processes has not been demonstrated (Figure 12–12). Therefore, it has been suggested that choline and inositol be classified as essential nutrients, rather than as vitamins for fowl and certain species of bacteria and animals. Whether they are essential dietary constituents for man is unknown.

The biological significance and need for the three substances have not been established. It has been shown that PABA is a growth-promoting factor for many bacteria and for chicks. There is evidence also that it

, *et al.* Vitamin Retention in Meat Cooked Electronically. *J. Am.*
*s., 41:*217 (1962).

. Thiamine and Riboflavin Retention in Cooked Variety Meats.
*iet. Ass., 56:*225 (1970).

gh, C. H., *et al.* Thiamine Retention in Meats after Various Heat
nt. *J. Am. Diet. Ass., 40:*35 (1962).

A. M., *et al.* Microwave and Conventional Cooking of Meat.
*iet. Ass., 45:*139 (1964).

E., *et al.* Thiamine Retention in Freeze-Dehydrated Irradiated
*od Tech., 16:*107 (1962).

). M., *et al.* Effect of Freeze-Drying on Thiamine, Riboflavin,
in Content of Chicken Muscle. *Food Tech., 17:*111 (1963).

J. The Bioassay of Thiamine in Beef Exposed to Gamma Radia-
*Jutr., 62:*107 (1957).

A. F., *et al.* The Vitamin Content of Sultanina Grapes and
*J. Nutr., 9:*369 (1935).

i, S. R., *et al.* Effects of Sulphiting on Potatoes. *J. Am. Diet.*
214 (1962).

tates Food and Drug Administration. Definitions and Standards
y: Cereal Products and Related Products; Enriched Cornmeals.
*ister, 27:*618; Code of Fed. Regulat. Title 21, part 15, Sec. 15.513

an, B. D., *et al.* Improving the Nutritive Value of Flour. I. The
Supplementing Enriched Flour with Other B-Complex Vita-
*Nutr., 33:*301 (1947); II. Further Studies on the Effect of Sup-
ng Enriched Flour with B-Complex Vitamins and Some Ob-
s on the Use of 80 Per Cent Extraction Flour. *J. Nutr., 36:*187

. J., *et al.* Enrichment of Rice with Riboflavin. *Food Tech.,*
1962).

H. B., *et al.* Nutrition Resurvey in Bataan, Philippines, 1950.
*46:*239 (1952).

er, E. N. Cooking Enriched Rice. *J. Am. Diet. Ass., 42:*139

Survey of Nutrition in Newfoundland. *Can. Med. Ass. J., 52:*227

Resurvey of Nutrition in Newfoundland, 1948. *Can. Med. Ass.*
2 (1949).

. *et al.* The Performance of Normal Young Men on Controlled
Intakes. *J. Nutr., 26:*399 (1943).

M. K., *et al.* The Determination of Early Thiamine-Deficient
Estimation of Blood Lactic and Pyruvic Acids after Glucose
ration. *J. Nutr., 37:*411 (1949).

Erythrocyte as a Biopsy Tissue for Functional Evaluation of
Adequacy. *J. Am. Med. Ass., 187:*762 (1964).

., *et al.* A Method for Assaying Thiamine Status in Man and
*Am. J. Clin. Nutr., 14:*197 (1964).

Figure 12–12

Structural formulas of para-*aminobenzoic acid, choline, and inositol*

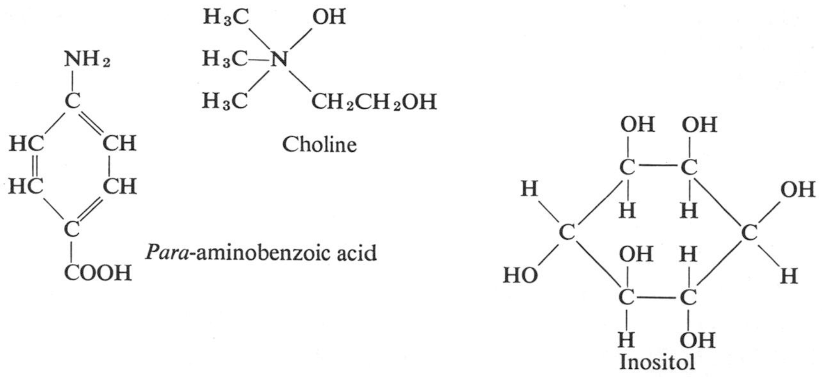

prevents the graying of fur in black rats and mice. The only indication
that it may play a role in human metabolism is that oral administration
of PABA has been shown to reduce mortality in several types of ricket-
tsial infections, including Rocky Mountain spotted fever. However,
aureomycin and similar antibiotics now appear to be more effective than
PABA in treatment of these diseases.

Both choline and inositol are constituents of phospholipids and act as
lipotropic agents. Experimental evidence indicates that choline serves as
a methyl group donor and inositol as a methyl group acceptor in biochemical reactions. The exact mechanisms are not fully understood, but
it is thought that dietary choline is oxidized to betaine before use in
transmethylation reactions. It appears that methionine, folic acid, and
vitamin B_{12} also are involved in the synthesis, transfer, and utilization of
methyl groups.

Choline and inositol are found rather widely distributed in foods, and
it is assumed that lack of them is unlikely in the usual dietary.

PROBLEMS

1. Calculate the milligrams of ascorbic acid, thiamin, riboflavin, niacin equivalents, vitamins B_6 and B_{12}, and pantothenic acid in the food intake records used in Problem 1, Chapter 2. Carry decimals to one place.

2. Calculate the milligrams of thiamin, ascorbic acid, riboflavin, niacin equivalents, vitamins B_6 and B_{12}, and pantothenic acid supplied by average
   servings of representative foods.

3. Plan a week's menus for an orphanage in which most of the children are
   underweight and have finicky appetites. The diet in the past is known to
   be low in thiamin, but supplies sufficient calories and adequate protein.
   Write a letter to the director, a woman untrained in nutrition, and explain
   the reasons for the new diet.

4. A woman living in a southern mountain area has been eating a subcalorie diet composed of corn meal, 500 calories; salt pork, 500 calories; potatoes, 300 calories; and molasses, 300 calories. Her fuel needs are 2200 calories. Plan a low-cost pellagra-preventing diet. Calculate the cost of this diet according to local prices.

5. Plan two days' low-cost menus for a ten-year-old child which will furnish 40 mg. of ascorbic acid per day.

REFERENCES

Ascorbic Acid

1. Abt, A. F., *et al.* Vitamin C Requirements of Man Reexamined. *Am. J. Clin. Nutr.,* *12:*21 (1963).

2. Baker, E. M., *et al.* Ascorbic Acid Metabolism in Man. *Am. J. Clin. Nutr.,* *19:*371 (1966).

3. Mazur, A. Role of Ascorbic Acid in the Incorporation of Plasma Iron into Ferritin. *Ann. N.Y. Acad. Sci.,* *92:*225 (1961).

4. Schaffer, C. F. Ascorbic Acid and Atherosclerosis. *Am. J. Clin. Nutr.,* *23:*27 (1970).

5. American Medical Association, Council on Foods and Nutrition. Vitamin C and the Healing of Wounds. *J. Am. Med. Ass.,* *184:*307 (1963).

6. Walker, G. H., *et al.* Trial of Ascorbic Acid in Prevention of Colds. *Brit. Med. J.,* *i:*603 (1967).

7. Udenfriend, S. Formation of Hydroxyproline in Collagen. *Sci.,* *152:*1335 (1966).

8. Evans, J. R., *et al.* The Growth-Maintaining Activity of Ascorbic Acid. *Brit. J. Nutr.,* *17:*251 (1963).

9. Holmes, A. D. Store vs. Delivered Milk as a Source of Reduced Ascorbic Acid. *J. Am. Diet. Ass.,* *27:*578 (1951).

10. Noble, I. Ascorbic Acid and Color of Vegetables: Effect of Length of Cooking. *J. Am. Diet. Ass.,* *50:*304 (1967).

11. Eheart, M. S., *et al.* Conventional and Microwave Cooking of Vegetables. *J. Am. Diet. Ass.,* *44:*116 (1964).

12. Lopez, A., *et al.* Influence of Time and Temperature on Ascorbic Acid Stability. *J. Am. Diet. Ass.,* *50:*308 (1967).

13. Bring, S. V., *et al.* Total Ascorbic Acid in Potatoes. *J. Am. Diet. Ass.,* *45:*149 (1964).

14. Pearson, W. N. Blood and Urinary Vitamin Levels as Potential Indices of Body Stores. *Am. J. Clin. Nutr.,* *20:*514 (1967).

15. Panel on Recommended Allowances of Nutrients. *Recommended Intakes of Nutrients for the United Kingdom.* Rept. No. 120. London: Dept. of Health and Social Security (1969).

16. Crandon, J. H., *et al.* Ascorbic Acid Economy in Surgical Patients. *Ann. N.Y. Acad. Sci.,* *92:*246 (1961).

17. Dodds, M. L. Sex as a Factor in Blood Levels of Ascorbic Acid. *J. Am. Diet. Ass.,* *54:*32 (1969).

18. Schaefer, A. E. The National Nutrition S (1969).

19. Sherman, H. C. *The Nutritional Improv* lumbia University Press (1950).

Thiamin

1. Williams, R. R., *et al.* Synthesis of Vi *58:*1504 (1936).

2. Wurst, H. M. The History of Thiamine (1962).

3. Review. Physiological Properties of Dif *18:*181 (1960).

4. Latham, M. C. Present Knowledge of T *in Nutrition,* 3rd ed. New York: Nutrit

5. Tomasulo, P. A., *et al.* Impairment of T ism. *Am. J. Clin. Nutr.,* *21:*1341 (1968).

6. Williams, R. D., *et al.* Induced Thiami Requirement of Man: Further Observat (1942).

7. Berry, F. B., *et al.* Nutrition Surveys in of the Interdepartmental Committee on *Am. J. Clin. Nutr.,* *6:*342 (1958).

8. Liang, C. C. Tissue Breakdown and Gly *J.,* *83:*101 (1963).

9. Binet, L., *et al.* Contribution à l'étude de la Vitamine B$_1$ (thiamine). *Nutr. A*

10. Washmann, B. S., *et al.* The Influence upon Growth and Liver Thiamine of Stock Rats Fed a Thiamine-Deficient D

11. Jones, J. H. A Striking Difference in Fat on Deficiencies Produced by Oxythi *78:*353 (1962).

12. Horwitt, M. K., *et al.* *Investigations Complex Vitamins.* National Research D.C. (1948).

13. Brozek, J. Psychological Effects of Th tion in Normal Young Men. *Am. J. Clin*

14. Daum, K., *et al.* Influence of Various Physiologic Response. VII. Thiamine tions. *J. Am. Diet. Ass.,* *25:*398 (1949).

15. Hutt, F. B. Nutrition and the Genes in *19:*225 (1961).

16. Johnston, C. H., *et al.* The Effect of C Bicarbonate on the Thiamine, Riboflavi Peas. *J. Nutr.,* *26:*227 (1943).

17. Noble, I. Thiamine and Riboflavin Re *Diet. Ass.,* *45:*447 (1964).

18. Noble, *Diet. A*

19. Noble, *J. Am.*

20. Lushbo Treatm

21. Kylen, *J. Am.*

22. Karmas Pork. *F*

23. Rowe, and Ni

24. Day, E. tion. *J.*

25. Morgan Raisins.

26. Mudam *Ass., 40*

27. United of Iden Fed. Re (1962)

28. Wester Effect mins. *J.* plement servatio (1948).

29. Lease, *16:*146

30. Burch, *J. Nutr.*

31. Todhun (1963)

32. Medica (1945).

33. Medica *J., 60:3*

34. Keys, A Thiamin

35. Horwitt States b Adminis

36. Brin, M Thiamin

37. Baker, Animals

38. Ariaey-Nejad, M. R., *et al.* Thiamine Metabolism in Man. *Am. J. Clin. Nutr., 23:*764 (1970).

39. Stitt, K. R. Nutritive Values of Diets Today and Fifty Years Ago. *Nutr. Revs., 21:*257 (1963).

Riboflavin

1. Williams, R. R., *et al.* Destruction of Riboflavin by Light. *Sci., 96:*22 (1942).

2. Review. Non-respiratory Function of Riboflavin. *Nutr. Revs., 20:*95 (1962).

3. Sebrell, W. H., *et al.* Riboflavin Deficiency in Man. *Pub. Health Repts., 54:*2121 (1939).

4. Sydenstricker, V. P., *et al.* The Ocular Manifestations of Ariboflavinosis. *J. Am. Med Ass., 114:*2437 (1940).

5. Horwitt, M. K., *et al.* Effects of Dietary Depletion of Riboflavin. *J. Nutr., 39:*357 (1949).

6. Mickelson, O. Present Knowledge of Riboflavin. *In Present Knowledge in Nutrition,* 3rd ed. New York: Nutrition Foundation (1967).

7. Lane, M., *et al.* The Anemia of Human Riboflavin Deficiency. *Blood, 25:*632 (1965).

8. Williams, R. R. Can We Eradicate the Classical Deficiency Diseases? *J. Am. Diet. Ass., 36:*34 (1960).

9. Watt, B. K., *et al.* Composition of Foods—raw, processed, prepared. USDA., Agr. Handbook No. 8 (revised 1963).

10. Review. Genetic Differences in Riboflavin Utilization. *Nutr. Revs., 22:*273 (1964).

11. Noble, I., *et al.* Vitamin Retention in Meat Cooked Electronically. *J. Am. Diet. Ass., 41:*217 (1962).

12. Noble, I. Thiamine and Riboflavin Retention in Braised Meat. *J. Am. Diet. Ass., 47:*205 (1965).

13. Noble, I. Thiamine and Riboflavin Retention in Cooked Variety Meats. *J. Am. Diet. Ass., 55:*225 (1970).

14. Bessey, O. A., *et al.* Dietary Deprivation of Riboflavin and Blood Riboflavin Levels in Man. *J. Nutr., 58:*367 (1956).

15. Tucker, R. G., *et al.* The Influence of Sleep, Work, Diuresis, Heat, Acute Starvation, Thiamine Intake, and Bed Rest on Human Riboflavin Excretion. *J. Nutr., 72:*251 (1960).

16. Pearson, W. N. Biochemical Appraisal of the Vitamin Nutritional Status in Man. *J. Am. Med. Ass., 180:*49 (1962).

17. Horwitt, M. K., *et al.* Correlation of Urinary Excretion of Riboflavin with Dietary Intake and Symptoms of Ariboflavinosis. *J. Nutr., 41:*247 (1950).

18. Davis, M. V., *et al.* Riboflavin Excretions of Young Women on Diets Containing Varying Levels of the B Vitamins. *J. Nutr., 32:*143 (1946).

19. Interdepartmental Committee on Nutrition for National Defense. *Manual for Nutrition Surveys,* 2nd ed. Washington, D.C. (1964).

20. Bro-Rasmussen, F. The Riboflavin Requirement of Animals and Man and Associated Metabolic Circumstances. *Nutr. Abstr. Revs., 28:*369 (1958).

21. Leverton, R. M., *et al.* The Metabolic Response of Young Women to a Standardized Diet. *Home Econ. Res. Rept. No. 16,* Washington, D.C.: USDA (1962).

22. Technical Committee of the Southern Regional Research Project (S-28). Metabolic Patterns in Preadolescent Children. *Southern Cooperative Series, Bull. No. 64.* Blacksburg: Virginia Agr. Expt. Sta. (1959).

23. Horwitt, M. K. Nutritional Requirements of Man, with Special Reference to Riboflavin. *Am. J. Clin. Nutr., 18:*458 (1966).

24. Snyderman, S. E., *et al.* The Minimum Riboflavin Requirement of the Infant. *J. Nutr., 39:*219 (1949).

25. Stearns, G., *et al.* Excretion of Thiamine and Riboflavin by Children. *Am. J. Dis. Childr., 95:*185 (1958).

26. Donald, E. A., *et al.* Nutritional Status of Selected Adolescent Children. V. Riboflavin and Niacin Nutrition Assessed by Serum Level and Subclinical Symptoms in Relation to Dietary Intake. *Am. J. Clin. Nutr., 10:*68 (1962).

27. Oldham, H., *et al.* Thiamine and Riboflavin Intakes and Excretion During Pregnancy. *J. Nutr., 41:*231 (1950).

28. National Academy of Sciences-National Research Council, Food and Nutrition Board. *Maternal Nutrition and Child Health.* Bull. 123 (1950) (reprinted 1957).

29. National Academy of Sciences-National Research Council, Food and Nutrition Board. *Composition of Milks.* Publ. 254 (1953).

30. World Health Organization. *Nutrition in Pregnancy and Lactation.* Tech. Rept. Ser. No. 302 (1965).

31. Windmueller, H. G., *et al.* Elevated Riboflavin Levels in Urine of Fasting Human Subjects. *Am. J. Clin. Nutr., 15:*73 (1964).

32. Clapper, W. E., *et al.* Relation of Folic Acid and Concentration of Medium to Riboflavin Metabolism of *Streptococcus faecalis. J. Bact., 76:*48 (1958).

33. Everson, G. *et al.* Biological Availability of Certain Foods as Sources of Riboflavin. *J. Nutr., 46:*45 (1952).

34. Pozanski, R., *et al.* Value of Flour Enrichment to Pregnant Israeli Women. *J. Am. Diet. Ass., 40:*120 (1962).

Nicotinic Acid

1. Elvehjem, C. A. Relation of Nicotinic Acid to Pellagra. *Physiol. Revs., 20:*249 (1940).

2. Commission on Nomenclature, International Union of Pure and Applied Chemistry. Tentative Rules. *J. Biol. Chem., 241:*2987 (1966).

3. Krehl, W. A., *et al.* Factors Affecting the Dietary Niacin and Tryptophan Requirement of the Growing Rat. *J. Nutr., 31:*85 (1946).

4. Perlzweig, W. A., *et al.* A Study in Nicotinic Acid Deficiency in Man. *J. Am. Med. Ass., 118:*28 (1942).

5. Horwitt, M. K., *et al.* Tryptophan-Niacin Relationships in Man. *J. Nutr., 60,* Supp. *1:*3 (1956).

6. Goldsmith, G. A. Niacin-Tryptophan Relationships in Man and Niacin Requirements. *Am. J. Clin. Nutr., 6:*479 (1958).

7. Belavady, W. N., *et al.* The Effect of Oral Administration of Leucine on the Metabolism of Tryptophan. *Biochem. J., 87:*652 (1963).

8. Pearson, W. N., *et al.* Amino Acid Imbalance and the Excretion of Tryptophan Metabolites in the Rat. Proc. 6th. Internat'l Congress of Nutr. Edinburgh and London: E. & S. Livingston, Ltd. (1964). pg. 482.

9. Horwitt, M. K. Niacin-Tryptophan Requirements of Man. *J. Am. Diet. Ass., 34:*914 (1958).

10. Sure, B., *et al.* The Specific Effect of Niacin on Growth. *J. Nutr., 46:*55 (1952).

11. Mickelson, O. Present Knowledge of Niacin. *In Present Knowledge in Nutrition,* 3rd. ed. New York: Nutrition Foundation (1967).

12. Emerson, G. A. Recent Research in the B Vitamins. *J. Am. Diet. Ass., 36:*220 (1960).

13. Goldsmith, G. A. Niacin Antipellagra Factor, Hypocholesterolemic Agent. Model of Nutrition Research Yesterday and Today. *J. Am. Med. Ass., 194:*167 (1965).

14. Harper, A. E., *et al.* Effect of Alkali Treatment on the Availability of Niacin and Amino Acids in Maize. *J. Nutr., 66:*163 (1958).

15. Squibb, R. L., *et al.* A Comparison of the Effect of Raw Corn and Tortillas (Lime-Treated Corn) with Niacin, Tryptophan, or Beans on the Growth and Muscle Niacin in Rats. *J. Nutr., 67:*351 (1959).

16. Page, E., *et al.* Vitamin B$_6$ and Niacin in Potatoes. *J. Am. Diet. Ass., 42:*42 (1963).

17. Rose, W. C., *et al.* The Amino Acid Requirements of Man. XV. The Valine Requirement; Summary and Final Observations. *J. Biol. Chem., 217:*987 (1955).

18. Goldsmith, G. A., *et al.* Efficiency of Tryptophan as a Niacin Precursor in Man. *J. Nutr., 73:*172 (1961).

19. Moyer, E. Z., *et al.* Metabolic Patterns in Preadolescent Children. VII. Intake of Niacin and Tryptophan and Excretion of Niacin and Tryptophan Metabolites. *J. Nutr., 79:*423 (1963).

20. deLange, D. J., *et al.* Assessment of Nicotinic Acid Status of Population Groups. *Am. J. Clin. Nutr., 15:*169 (1964).

21. Holt, L. E. The Adolescence of Nutrition. *Arch. Dis. Childr., 31:*427 (1956).

22. Wertz, A. W., *et al.* Tryptophan-Niacin Relationships in Pregnancy. *J. Nutr., 64:*339 (1958).

23. Spies, T. D., *et al.* Pellagra, Beriberi, and Riboflavin Deficiency in Human Beings. *J. Am. Med. Ass., 113:*931 (1939).

Vitamin B₆

1. Toepfer, E. W., *et al.* Estimation of Vitamin B₆ in Foods. In R. S. Harris, I. G. Wool, and J. L. Loraine (eds.), *Vitamins Hormones, 22:*825, New York: Academic Press (1964).

2. Storvick, C. A., *et al.* Estimation of Vitamin B₆ in Biological Material. In R. S. Harris, I. G. Wool, and J. L. Loraine (eds.), *Vitamins Hormones, 22:*833 (1964).

3. Rabinowitz, J. C., *et al.* Distribution of Pyridoxal, Pyridoxamine, and Pyridoxine in Some Natural Products. *J. Biol. Chem., 176:*1157 (1948).

4. Polansky, M. M., *et al.* Vitamin B₆ Components in Fruits and Nuts. *J. Am. Diet. Ass., 48:*109 (1966).

5. Polansky, M. M., *et al.* Vitamin B₆ Components in Fresh and Dried Vegetables. *J. Am. Diet. Ass., 54:*118 (1969).

6. Polansky, M. M., *et al.* Nutrient Composition of Selected Wheat and Wheat Products. IV. Vitamin B₆ Components. *Cereal Chem., 46:*664 (1969).

7. Meyer, B. H., *et al.* Pantothenic Acid and Vitamin B₆ in Beef. *J. Am. Diet. Ass., 54:*122 (1969).

8. Richardson, L. R., *et al.* Comparative Vitamin B₆ Activity of Frozen, Irradiated, and Heat-Processed Foods. *J. Nutr., 73:*363 (1961).

9. Page, E., *et al.* Vitamin B₆ and Niacin in Potatoes. *J. Am. Diet. Ass., 42:*42 (1963).

10. Wakil, S. J., Jr. Mechanism of Fatty Acid Synthesis. *J. Lipid Res., 2:*1 (1961).

11. Witten, P. W., *et al.* Polyethanoic Acid Metabolism. VI. Effects of Pyridoxine on Essential Fatty Acid Conversion. *Arch. Biochem. Biophys., 41:*266 (1952).

12. Mueller, J. F., *et al.* Effect of Desoxypryidoxine Induced Vitamin B₆ Deficiency on Polyunsaturated Fatty Acid Metabolism in Human Beings. *Am. J. Clin. Nutr., 12:*358 (1963).

13. Krebs, E. G., *et al.* Phosphorylase and Related Enzymes of Glucose Metabolism. In R. S. Harris, I. G. Wool, and J. L. Loraine, (eds.), *Vitamins Hormones, 22:*399, New York: Academic Press (1964).

14. Baranowski, T., *et al.* The Isolation of Pyridoxal-5-Phosphate from Crystalline Muscle Phosphate. *Biochem. Biophys. Acta, 25:*16 (1957).

15. Tower, D. B. Pyridoxine and Cerebral Activity. *Nutr. Revs., 16:*161 (1958).

16. Coursin, D. B. Relationship of Nutrition to Central Nervous System Development and Function. Overview. *Fed. Proc., 26:*134 (1967).

17. Roberts, E. Some Thoughts about the γ-Amino-butyric Acid System in Nervous Tissue. *Nutr. Revs., 21:*161 (1963).

18. Faber, S. R., *et al.* The Effects of Induced Pyridoxine and Pantothenic Acid Deficiency on Excretions of Oxalic Acid and Xanthurenic Acid in Urine. *Am. J. Clin. Nutr., 12:*406 (1963).

19. Gershoff, S. N. Vitamin B₆ and Oxalate Metabolism. In R. S. Harris, I. G. Wool, and J. L. Loraine (eds.), *Vitamins Hormones, 22:*281, New York: Academic Press (1964).

20. Axelrod, A. E., *et al.* Vitamin B_6 and Immunological Phenomena. In R. S. Harris, I. G. Wool, and J. L. Loraine (eds.), *Vitamins Hormones, 22:*591, New York: Academic Press (1964).

21. Hodges, R. E., *et al.* Factors Affecting Human Antibody Response. IV. Pyridoxine Deficiency. *Am. J. Clin. Nutr., 11:*180 (1962).

22. Hines, J. D., *et al.* Pyridoxine-Responsive Anemia. *Am. J. Clin. Nutr., 14:*137 (1964).

23. Hillman, R. W., *et al.* Pyridoxine Supplementation During Pregnancy. Clinical and Laboratory Observations. *Am. J. Clin. Nutr., 12:*427 (1963).

24. Coursin, D. B. Recommendations for Standardization of the Tryptophan Lead Test. *Am. J. Clin. Nutr., 14:*56 (1964).

25. Raica, N., *et al.* Blood Cell Transaminase Activity in Human Vitamin B_6 Deficiency. *Am. J. Clin. Nutr., 15:*67 (1964).

26. Linkswiler, H., *et al.* Urinary and Fecal Elimination of B_6 and 4-Pyridoxic Acid on Three Levels of Intake. *J. Nutr., 41:*523 (1950).

27. Vilter, R. W., *et al.* The Effect of Vitamin B_6 Deficiency Induced by Desoxypyridoxine in Human Beings. *J. Lab. Clin. Med., 42:*335 (1953).

28. Bessey, O. A., *et al.* Intake of Vitamin B_6 and Infantile Convulsions: A First Approximation of Requirements of Pyridoxine in Infants. *Ped., 20:*33 (1957).

29. Baker, E. M., *et al.* Vitamin B_6 Requirement for Adult Men. *Am. J. Clin. Nutr., 15:*59 (1964).

30. Sauberlich, H. E. Human Requirement for Vitamin B_6. In R. S. Harris, I. G. Wool, and J. L. Loraine (eds.), *Vitamins Hormones, 22:*807, New York: Academic Press (1964).

31. Borsook, H. Relation of Vitamin B_6 Requirement to Amount of Diet (Man). In R. S. Harris, I. G. Wool, and J. L. Loraine (eds.), *Vitamins Hormones, 22:*855, New York: Academic Press (1964).

32. Food and Drug Administration. Total Diet Study: A. Strontium-90 and Cesium-137 Content. B. Nutrient Content. C. Pesticide Content. *J. Am. Off. Agr. Chem., 46:*749 (1963).

33. Hunt, A. D. Abnormally High Pyridoxine Requirement. *Am. J. Clin. Nutr., 5:*561 (1957).

34. Brown, R. R., *et al.* The Effect of Vitamin Supplementation on the Urinary Excretion of Tryptophan Metabolites in Pregnant Women. *J. Clin. Invest., 40:*617 (1961).

35. McGanity, W. J., *et al.* An Effect of Pyridoxine on Blood Urea in Human Subjects. *J. Biol. Chem., 178:*511 (1949).

Folic Acid

1. Toepfer, W. W., *et al. Folic Acid Content of Foods.* USDA, Agr. Handbook No. 29 (1951).

2. Butterworth, C. E., Jr., *et al.* The Pteroylglutamate Components of American Diets as Determined by Chromatographic Fractionation. *J. Clin. Inves., 42:*1929 (1963).

3. Butterworth, C. E., Jr. Annotation. The Availability of Food Folate. *Brit. J. Hematol., 14:*339 (1968).

4. Hurdle, A. D. F., *et al.* A Method for Measuring Folate in Food and Its Application to a Hospital Diet. *Am. J. Clin. Nutr., 21:*1202 (1968).

5. Welch, B. E., *et al.* The Relation of Vitamin B$_{12}$ to Egg Yolk Storage of Folic Acid. *J. Nutr., 54:*601 (1954).

6. Stokstad, E. L. R., *et al.* Folic Acid Metabolism. *Physiol. Revs., 47:*85 (1968).

7. Bleiler, R. E., *et al.* Metabolism of Folic Acid and Citrovorum Factor by Human Beings. *J. Nutr., 56:*163 (1955).

8. Greenberg, G. R. Role of Folic Acid Derivatives in Purine Biosynthesis. *Fed. Proc., 13,* No. *3:*745 (1954).

9. Alperin, J. B. Effect of Vitamin B$_{12}$ Therapy in a Patient with Folic Acid Deficiency. *Am. J. Clin. Nutr., 15:*117 (1964).

10. Luhby, A. L., *et al.* Folic Acid Deficiency in Man and Its Interrelationship with Vitamin B$_{12}$ Metabolism. *Adv. Metab. Disord., 1:*263 (1964).

11. Baker, H., *et al.* Mechanisms of Folic Acid Deficiency in Non-Tropical Sprue. *J. Am. Med. Ass., 187:*119 (1964).

12. Berlin, N. I., *et al.* Folic Acid Antagonists. *Ann. Intern. Med., 59:*931 (1963).

13. Mikhlin, S. Y. A. Effect of Folic Acid Deficiency (Caused by Aminopterin) on Enzymatic Secretion of the Main Digestive Glands. *Fed. Proc., 22,* No. 5, Part II (Translation Supplement): T918 (1963).

14. Luhby, A. L., *et al.* Urinary Excretion of Formiminoglutamic Acid. *Am. J. Clin. Nutr., 7:*397 (1959).

15. Vitale, J. J. Present Knowledge of Folacin. *In Present Knowledge in Nutrition,* 3rd. ed. New York: Nutrition Foundation (1967).

16. Spector, I., *et al.* Observations on Urocanic Acid and Formiminoglutamic Acid in Infants with Protein Malnutrition. *Am. J. Clin. Nutr., 18:*426 (1966).

17. Ghitis, J., *et al.* Malabsorption in the Tropics. 2. Tropical Sprue Versus Protein Malnutrition: Vitamin B$_{12}$ and Folic Acid Studies. *Am. J. Clin. Nutr., 20:*1206 (1967).

18. Ivak, G., *et al.* The Effect of Small Doses of Folic Acid in Nutritional Megaloblastic Anemia. *Am. J. Clin. Nutr., 13:*369 (1963).

19. Review. Folacin and Megaloblastic Anemia. *Nutr. Revs., 22:*3 (1964).

20. Vilter, R. W., *et al.* Interrelationships of Vitamin B$_{12}$, Folic Acid, and Ascorbic Acid in the Megaloblastic Anemias. *Am. J. Clin. Nutr. 12:*130 (1963).

21. Review. Folacin Activity in United States Diets. *Nutr. Revs., 22:*142 (1964).

22. Velez, H., *et al.* Cali-Harvard Nutrition Project. I. Megaloblastic Anemia in Kwashiorkor. *Am. J. Clin. Nutr., 12:*54 (1963).

23. Alperin, J. B., *et al.* Studies of Folic Acid Requirements in Megaloblastic Anemia of Pregnancy. *Arch. Intern. Med., 117:*681 (1966).

Vitamin B$_{12}$

1. Scheid, H. E. *et al.* Vitamin B$_{12}$ Content of Organ Meats. *J. Nutr., 53:*419 (1954).

2. Denton, C. A., *et al.* Effect of Injecting and Feeding Vitamin B_{12} to Hens on Content of the Vitamin in the Egg and Blood. *J. Nutr., 54:*571 (1954).

3. Hartmann, A. M., *et al.* Vitamin B_{12} Content of Milk and Milk Products as Determined by Rat Assay. *J. Nutr., 59:*77 (1956).

4. Vilter, R. W. Vitamin B_{12}. *In* M. G. Wohl and R. S. Goodhart (eds.), *Modern Nutrition in Health and Disease,* 4th ed., Philadelphia: Lea & Febiger (1968).

5. Arnstein, H. R. U., *et al.* An Effect of Vitamin B_{12} on the Biosynthesis of Certain Amino Acids by *O Chromonas Malhamnesis. Biochem. Biophys. Acta, 36:*286 (1959).

6. Vilter, R. W., *et al.* Interrelationships of Vitamin B_{12}, Folic Acid and Ascorbic Acid in Megaloblastic Anemia. *Am. J. Clin. Nutr., 12:*130 (1963).

7. Scrimshaw, N. S., *et al.* Growth and Development of Central American Children. II. The Effect of Oral Administration of Vitamin B_{12} to Rural Children of Preschool and School Age. *Am. J. Clin. Nutr., 7:*180 (1959).

8. Barness, L. A. Vitamin B_{12} Deficiency with Emphasis on Methylmalonic Acid as a Diagnostic Aid. *Am. J. Clin. Nutr., 20:*573 (1967).

9. Wilson, H. T. Intrinsic Factor and Vitamin B_{12} Absorption—A Problem in Cell Physiology. *Nutr. Revs., 23:*33 (1965).

10. Chow, B. F., *et al.* Factors Affecting the Absorption of Vitamin B_{12}. *Am. J. Clin. Nutr., 6:*386 (1958).

11. Sullivan, L. W., *et al.* Delineation of Minimal Daily Requirements and Relative Potency of Vitamin B_{12} Analogues Using Minimal Dosage Therapeutic Trials. *Am. J. Clin. Nutr., 10:*354 (1962).

12. Brody, E. A., *et al.* Treatment of Pernicious Anemia by Oral Administration of Vitamin B_{12} Without Intrinsic Factor. *New Engl. J. Med., 260:*361 (1959).

13. Thompson, R. B., *et al.* Long-Term Trial of Oral Vitamin B_{12} in Pernicious Anemia. *Lancet, 2:*577 (1962).

14. Waife, S. O., *et al.* Oral Vitamin B_{12} Without Intrinsic Factor in the Treatment of Pernicious Anemia. *Ann. Intern. Med., 58:*810 (1963).

15. Kervans, J. R., *et al.* Influence of Certain Diseases on the Absorption of Vitamin B_{12} from the Gastrointestinal Tract. *J. Clin. Invest., 33:*949 (1954).

16. Hall, C. A. Long-Term Excretion of $Co^{57}B_{12}$ and Turnover within the Plasma. *Am. J. Clin. Nutr., 14:*156 (1964).

17. Heyssel, R. M., *et al.* Vitamin B_{12} Turnover in Man. The Assimilation of Vitamin B_{12} from Natural Foodstuff by Man and Estimates of Minimal Dietary Requirements. *Am. J. Clin. Nutr., 18:*176 (1966).

18. Helligers, A., *et al.* Vitamin B_{12} Absorption in Pregnancy and in the Newborn. *Am. J. Clin. Nutr., 5:*327 (1957).

19. Okuda, K., *et al.* Vitamin B_{12} Serum Level and Pregnancy. *Am. J. Clin. Nutr., 4:*440 (1956).

20. Baker, S. J., *et al.* Vitamin B_{12} Deficiency in Pregnancy and the Puerperium. *Brit. Med. J., i:*1658 (1962).

21. Ball, B. W., *et al.* Folic Acid and Vitamin B_{12} Levels in Pregnancy and Their Relation to Megaloblastic Anemia. *J. Clin. Pathol., 17:*165 (1964).

22. Glass, C. B. J., *et al.* Intestinal Absorption and Hepatic Uptake of Radioactive Vitamin B_{12} in Various Age Groups and the Effect of Intrinsic Factor Preparations. *Am. J. Clin. Nutr., 4:*124 (1956).

23. Mangay Chung, A. S., *et al.* Folic Acid, Vitamin B_6, Pantothenic Acid and Vitamin B_{12} in Human Dietaries. *Am. J. Clin. Nutr., 9:*573 (1961).

24. Yeh, S. D. J., *et al.* Vitamin B_{12} Absorption in Pyridoxine-Deficient Rats. *Am. J. Clin. Nutr., 7:*426 (1959).

25. Zalusky, R., *et al.* Cyanocobalamin Therapy Effect in Folic Acid Deficiency. *Arch. Intern. Med., 109:*545 (1962).

26. Smith, A. D. M. Veganism: A Clinical Survey with Observations on Vitamin B_{12} Metabolism. *Brit. Med. J., i:*1655 (1962).

27. Mehta, B. M., *et al.* Serum Vitamin B_{12} and Folic Acid Activity in Lactovegetarian and Nonvegetarian Healthy Adult Indians. *Am. J. Clin. Nutr., 15:*77 (1964).

Pantothenic Acid

1. Zook, E. G., *et al. Pantothenic Acid in Foods.* USDA Handbook No. 97 (1956).

2. Meyer, B. H., *et al.* Pantothenic Acid and Vitamin B_6 in Beef. *J. Am. Diet. Ass., 54:*122 (1960).

3. Calloway, D. H. Dehydrated Foods. *Nutr. Revs., 20:*257 (1962).

4. Schulman, M. P., *et al.* Heme Synthesis in Vitamin B_6 and Pantothenic Acid Deficiencies. *J. Biol. Chem., 226:*181 (1957).

5. Fidauza, A., *et al.* Influence of Deficiency of Pantothenic Acid, and of the Source of Dietary Fats, on the Fatty Acid Composition of Liver, Adrenals, and Plasma. Proceedings of the 6th International Congress of Nutrition. Edinburgh and London: E. & S. Livingstone, Ltd. (1964).

6. Review. Relation of Pantothenic Acid to Adrenal Cortical Function. *Nutr. Revs., 19:*79 (1961).

7. Hodges, R. E., *et al.* Factors Affecting Human Antibody Response. III. Immunologic Responses of Men Deficient in Pantothenic Acid. V. Combined Deficiencies of Pantothenic Acid and Pyridoxine. *Am. J. Clin. Nutr., 11:*85; 187 (1962).

8. Blunt, A. D., *et al.* Effect of Pantothenic Acid on Growth and Blood Picture in the Rat. *Brit. J. Nutr., 11:*62 (1957).

9. Pudelkewicz, C., *et al.* Interrelationships of Ascorbic Acid and Pantothenic Acid in the Young Guinea Pig. *J. Nutr., 81:*415 (1963).

10. Bean, W. B., *et al.* Human Pantothenic Acid Deficiency Produced by *Omega*-Methyl Pantothenic Acid. *J. Clin. Invest., 38:*1421 (1950).

11. Ralli, E. P. The Effect of Certain Vitamins on the Response of Normal Subjects to Cold Water Stress. *In* Nutrition Under Climatic Stress—A Symposium. Advisory Board on Quartermaster Research and Development, Committee on Foods. Washington, D.C.: NAS-NRC (1954).

12. Fox, H. M., *et al.* Pantothenic Acid Excretion on Three Levels of Intake. *J. Nutr., 75:*451 (1961).

13. Spies, T. D., *et al.* Pantothenic Acid in Human Nutrition. *J. Am. Med. Ass., 115:*523 (1940).

14. Williams, R. J. The Approximate Vitamin Requirements of Human Beings. *J. Am. Med. Ass., 119:*1 (1942).

15. Mangay Chung, A. S., *et al.* Folic Acid, Vitamin B$_6$, Pantothenic Acid, and Vitamin B$_{12}$ in Human Dietaries. *Am. J. Clin. Nutr., 9:*573 (1961).

16. Pace, J. K., *et al.* Metabolic Patterns in Preadolescent Children. V. Intake and Urinary Excretion of Pantothenic Acid and of Folic Acid. *J. Nutr., 74:*345 (1961).

Biotin

1. Sebrell, H. S., Jr., *et al.* Biotin. *The Vitamins,* II, 2nd ed. New York: Academic Press (1968).

2. Review. Mechanism of Action of Biotin-Enzymes. *Nutr. Revs., 21:*310 (1963).

3. Moat, A. G., *et al.* A Role for Biotin in Purine Biosynthesis. *J. Biol. Chem., 223:*985 (1956).

4. Landi, L., *et al.* Folic Acid and Biotin on the Metabolism of One Carbon Unit: Utilization of β-Carbon of Serine for the Synthesis of Methionine. *Experimenta., 22:*362 (1966).

5. Oxman, M. N., *et al.* Studies on the Metabolism of Adipose Tissue. VIII. Alterations Produced by Biotin Deficiency in the Rat. *Arch. Biochem. Biophys., 95:*99 (1961).

6. Oppel, T. W. Studies of Biotin Metabolism in Man. *Am. J. Med. Sci., 204:*856 (1942).

7. Baugh, C. M., *et al.* Human Biotin Deficiency, A Case History of Biotin Deficiency Induced by Raw Egg Consumption in a Cirrhotic Patient. *Am. J. Clin. Nutr., 21:*173 (1968).

8. Sydenstricker, V. P., *et al.* Observations on the Egg White Injury in Man and Its Cure With a Biotin Concentrate. *J. Am. Med. Ass., 118:*1199 (1942).

GENERAL REFERENCES

40. Agricultural Research Service. *Food Intake and Nutritive Value of Diets of Men, Women, and Children in the United States. Spring 1965.* USDA, ARS–62–18 (1969).

41. Beaton, G. H., and McHenry, E. W. (eds.), *Nutrition. A Comprehensive Treatise. Vol. II. Vitamins, Nutrient Requirements and Food Selections.* New York: Academic Press (1964).

42. Committee on Cereals, Food and Nutrition Board. *Cereal Enrichment in Perspective, 1958.* Washington, D.C.: NAS-NRC (1958).

43. National Food Situation. NFS–134, ERS, USDA (1970).

44. Food and Agricultural Organization of the United Nations. Report of a Joint FAO/WHO Expert Group. *Requirements of Vitamin A, Thiamine, Riboflavine, and Niacin.* FAO Nutrition Meetings Report Series No. 41, WHO Technical Report Series No. 362, Rome (1967).

45. Friend, B. Nutrients in United States Food Supply—A Review of Trends, 1909–1913 to 1965. *Am. J. Clin. Nutr., 20:*907 (1967).

46. Goldsmith, G. A. Human Requirements for Vitamin C and Its Use in Clinical Medicine. *Ann. N.Y. Acad. Sci., 92:*230 (1961).

47. Goldsmith, G. A. *Nutritional Diagnosis.* Springfield, Ill.: Thomas (1959).

48. Morgan, A. F. (ed.) *Nutritional Status U.S.A.* Berkeley: Calif. Agr. Experiment Station, Bulletin 769 (1959).

49. *Present Knowledge in Nutrition,* 3rd ed. New York: Nutrition Foundation (1967).

50. Sebrell, H. S., Jr., and Harris, R. S. (eds.), *The Vitamins, Vol. II,* 2nd ed. New York: Academic Press (1968).

51. United States National Agricultural Library. *Agricultural/Biological Vocabulary. Vol. 1. Categorized List; Vol. 2. Alphabetical List.* Washington, D.C. (1967).

52. Williams, R. R. *Toward the Conquest of Beriberi.* Cambridge: Harvard University Press (1961).

53. Wohl, M. G., and Goodhart, R. S. (eds.), *Modern Nutrition in Health and Disease,* 4th ed. Philadelphia: Lea & Febiger (1968), pp. 247–319.

Water
and
Electrolyte
Balance

The nutritional and physiological importance of water and the need to maintain the acid-base balance in tissues have been studied extensively. With imbalance between the fluids and the mineral elements within the cells, severe complications may arise. These may result from deficient or excessive intakes or from endogenous disturbances such as abnormal losses or retentions, defective absorption, or unusual distributions within body compartments.

The body's need for water is exceeded only by that for oxygen and its lack is felt more than that for food. The importance of this foodstuff was well established years ago by Rubner, when he showed that an animal in starvation can still live if he loses practically all glycogen and fat, and half the protein from his body, whereas a 10 per cent loss of water is very serious, and a 20 to 22 per cent decrease will result in death.

When water consumption is severely restricted, work output may suffer. Sir Edmund Hillary, whose ascent of Mount Everest was hailed as a remarkable accomplishment, credited the expedition's success largely to the normal hydration of the men's body tissues during the climb; this was the result of having a daily water supply of five to seven pints per person. Even mild dehydration during strenuous work may result in extreme fatigue.

Water intake is important not only in preventing dehydration but also in maintaining normal levels of electrolytes in the blood plasma. For example, when water intake is low in relation to that of sodium and chloride, the urine becomes highly concentrated and retentions of these two electrolytes may be sufficient to harm the body. During military maneuvers, especially in tropical countries, liberal water and salt intakes are essential and the transportation of enough water for the troops is a serious problem. This difficulty has resulted in the quantitative study of water requirement as related to salt consumption. Baker and associates (1) found that 4.69 liters of water are essential when the military ration contains 22 gm. of salt daily.

Early views of acid-base balance were based largely on the comparative amounts of the acid-forming elements (chlorine, phosphorus, and sulfur) and the base-forming elements (sodium, potassium, calcium, and magnesium) found in foods. With this in mind Sherman and his associates (2) calculated the comparative acid-base reactions of many common foods.

Later concepts advanced state that acids and bases are proton donors and acceptors, respectively, and that acidity is attributable not to single ions but to the collective proton activity of all the proton donors, both ions and molecules. Camien and co-workers (3), in an appraisal of acid-base balance, recommend that the terms "acid-base regulation" and "acid-base balance" be replaced with "acidity regulation" and "electrolyte balance."

Many substances, when ingested and excreted in urine and feces, are capable of influencing a person's acidity status. The potential acidity value of a substance can be determined by titration. The relation between intake and excretion indicates the regulation of acidity. This ash-total acidity value can be applied for foods, feces, and urine.

Water

THE WATER CONTENT OF THE BODY

Water is found in all parts of the body. The water within the cells (intercellular fluid) (4) comprises the largest part of the total amount and here, as in other parts, it furnishes an aqueous medium for the chemical reactions which constantly occur. Extracellular fluid is located largely in the interstitial spaces of tissues and organs (interstitial fluid), also in the blood plasma (intravascular fluid), and in lymph, cerebrospinal fluid, glandular and digestive secretions, and other body fluids (transcellular fluid).

When considered in relation to total body weight, water may vary from about 40 per cent in the very obese to 70 per cent in the very lean person. If lean body mass is the basis for study, the water content is comparatively constant and amounts to approximately 70 per cent.

To determine the transfer of water from one body compartment to another, a tracer substance (either deuterium or tritium) is employed, using a dilution technique. The isotope is given intravenously and the rate of its transfer from the serum is measured until water equilibrium is reached. This procedure may be used in studying the body composition of an obese subject.

Many variations in water content are to be expected. The percentage of water varies with age and sex. Between birth and one year, body water decreases from 80 to about 60 per cent of the body weight. In the male there appears to be a slight gain from then on until the early twenties;

in the female there is a steady decrease in water content, which is thought to be related to fat storage.

The different parts of the body vary markedly in their water content. Muscle has about 75 per cent water, and bone about 25 per cent. Blood plasma and red blood cells have about 92 and 60 per cent, respectively. Adipose tissue may vary from 10 to 30 per cent.

THE FUNCTIONS OF WATER

Water is a carrier of nutrients and waste. Water is the medium for transporting food materials to be used by the body. In a state of solution or suspension, simple sugars, amino acids, fats, minerals, and vitamins are passed through the intestinal walls and then carried to the cells by blood and lymph, the two most fluid tissues of the body. Waste products are carried and excreted in a similar manner. Oxygen and carbon dioxide also are transported by the bloodstream. After absorption, much fluid re-enters the alimentary tract, where it acts as a carrier of digestive enzymes. Large quantities of digestive juices are secreted daily by the body. It has been estimated that the 24-hour secretion of saliva, expressed in milliliters, is from 500 to 1500; of gastric juice, 1000 to 2500; of bile, 100 to 400; and of intestinal secretions, 700 to 3000. It also has been shown that in 24 hours as much as 170 liters of water may be filtered by the kidneys from the plasma; most of this is reabsorbed by the kidneys.

Water plays an important role as a regulator of body temperature. Water is an efficient heat conductor and serves to maintain the uniform body temperature essential for health. Evaporation of water from the skin provides one of the most important methods of removing surplus body heat. The perspiration which accompanies strenuous exercise and high environmental temperature is very noticeable. In the desert, losses through perspiration may amount to as much as 1200 ml. per hour. The resulting dehydration of tissues may have serious effects on the body.

Water has other functions. As a protector of internal organs, water is indispensable; it acts as a cushion and prevents transmission of shock from the outside. All the joints are kept lubricated and moist by the synovial fluid in them; the central nervous system is bathed by the cerebrospinal fluid.

Water occurs in a bound form in the tissues and its importance in maintaining equilibrium within the body is emphasized in certain diseases. In dehydration with its loss of water, the body attempts to counteract the decrease by excess combustion of food or body tissue; in edema due to excess sodium retention or to protein deficiency in the blood, the tissues retain extra water. Excess water is excreted to help eliminate acids and ketones in acidosis. These examples show that the body uses water in an effort to regulate its metabolism.

THE MAINTENANCE OF WATER BALANCE

The body secures water in many ways. It is more common practice to meet fluid needs through beverages such as coffee, tea, milk, juices, and soft drinks than by drinking water. Soup is another source of liquids, and a considerable percentage of the weight of fruits, vegetables, meat, and even the drier cereals and breads is water.

Food in oxidation furnishes water as well as carbon dioxide, ash, and nitrogenous compounds. An average of about 12 gm. of water per 100 calories may be expected, 10.3 gm. per 100 calories of protein, 13.9 gm. per 100 calories of carbohydrate, and 11.9 gm. per 100 calories of fat. During a 24-hour period this endogenous source of water, called "metabolic water," may amount to one pint, more or less.

Output regulates itself to intake. One means of excretion has already been mentioned—the perspiration which helps regulate body temperature. The amount of water lost in this way is determined by the body's need to lose heat, not by the water intake. The discomfort which can arise when water losses from this cause are excessive must be experienced to be appreciated. Besides evaporation from the skin, 400 to 500 ml. daily may be excreted in expired air; this loss varies with the atmospheric humidity.

Urinary loss of water in the healthy adult may amount to 1½ or 2 liters daily; 600 to 700 ml. are considered the minimal output if waste products are not to be retained. Variability in water intake is promptly reflected by urinary excretion. There will be a comparatively high concentration of solids and a small volume when little liquid is consumed, but a low specific gravity, light color, and large volume on a large intake.

In a diseased condition such as diabetes there may be a large urinary excretion; in chronic nephritis it may be low and retention of nitrogenous waste products may be excessive. Ordinarily there is little fluid in the feces but with diarrhea the loss may be great and result in dehydration of the tissues. Abnormal loss of water occurs also in cases of severe vomiting, hemorrhage, fever, and extensive burns. Edema is the result of retention of water by the body and may occur in some renal and heart disorders, in hypothyroidism, and malnutrition. The healthy individual of average weight, living under normal conditions of health and activity, maintains a fairly even balance between intake and output of water.

Water storage may obscure changes in weight. Sometimes on weight reduction regimes there may be alterations in the body's water content which obscure weight changes. A loss of as much as five to seven pounds in the first week or ten days may be due largely to water loss. In a study of water exchange in obese subjects Newburgh (5) found that on a subcalorie diet there may be a progressive retention of water for a time, which conceals the actual loss of fat tissue. After about two weeks, the water was eliminated and the body weight dropped. This accounts for certain puzzling cases of obese subjects who fail to lose weight for periods of as long as three weeks on a low-calorie diet. However, if underfeeding is continued, the water balance adjusts and the desired weight reduction is evident. Restriction of fluid in reducing diets is not necessary since this procedure does not prevent retention of water, nor does its use cause retention.

THE AMOUNT OF WATER NEEDED BY THE BODY

An ad libitum *supply of water is advised.* Because the sensation of thirst is, under most conditions, a safe guide to the requirement for water, it seems sensible to permit a person to drink water as he wishes. The FNB recommends 1 ml. water per calorie of food as a reasonable standard for calculating water allowances for all healthy individuals except infants. This includes fluids taken as water and in beverages and prepared foods, as well as the preformed water in foods and metabolic water. Infants require larger amounts of water than do either children or adults because infants have higher basal metabolic rates, proportionately greater surface area, and extra needs for tissue building. According to the FNB, infants' water requirements are met by mixtures which supply about 150 ml. water per 100 calories.

Recommendations for water intake also may be made in terms of the individual's weight. Table 13–1 shows appropriate allowances, as well as losses, based on body weight for infants, children, and adults. The figures

Table 13–1

Approximate Normal Losses and Allowances of Water Per Day*†

FOR PERSONS OF VARYING SIZE NOT SUBJECT TO EXERTION OR SWEATING

Size	Water loss ml.				Usual water allowance		
	Urine	Stool	Insensible**	Total	ml. per person	ml. per kg.	oz. per lb.
Infant, 2–10 kg.	200–500	25–40	75–300‡	300–840	330–1000	165–100	2.5–1.5
Child, 10–40 kg.	500–800	40–100	300–600	840–1500	1000–1800	100–45	1.5–0.7
Adolescent or adult, 60 kg.	800–1000	100	600–1000§	1500–2100	1800–2500	45–30	0.7–0.5

* Dauphinee, in *Clinical Nutrition,* 2nd ed., N. Jolliffe, editor. Courtesy Hoeber Medical Division, Harper & Row, Publishers, Inc., copyright © 1950, 1962, by Harper and Brothers.
† Including water content and water of oxidation of food which under normal circumstances, except for infants, approximates the insensible water loss.
** Insensible water loss includes that lost through perspiration and expired air.
‡ 1.3 ml. per kg. per hr.
§ 0.5 ml. per kg. per hr.

given for water allowances in ml. per person for the three age groups are in general agreement with those calculated on the basis of calorie intake.

Many factors affect the body's requirement for water. In addition to age, activity and environmental conditions are the most important variables in determining the body's need for water. Activity affects the water requirement to a great extent. Water loss is decreased during rest and sleep; light exercise in cool weather exerts only a slight effect. As activity becomes more intense, more water is needed to dissipate the heat produced.

The effect of environmental conditions on water requirement has been mentioned. High temperature and low relative humidity accelerate the demand for water, and these factors may be still more involved by presence or lack of air currents and amount and kind of clothing worn. The type of diet influences water intake. An excess of salt or other minerals or a high-protein diet will increase the need for liquid for elimination of waste. Consumption of concentrated sweets necessitates extra water for their dilution in the stomach. A sensation of thirst usually accompanies intake of such foods. Beverages such as tea, coffee, and cocoa, because of their xanthine derivatives, are diuretics and stimulate excretion of water through the kidneys, but the increase in excretion is temporary and is followed by a compensatory decrease in excretion.

Many people do not drink enough water. The daily water intake of many people probably is less than optimal (6). This is due both to a lack of realization of the importance of this foodstuff and to custom. Between-meal water drinking is not as common as it should be. Water consumption at meal time is now advised, provided the liquid is not used to wash down unchewed food. However, the mistaken belief still exists that water taken with the meal hinders digestion; its restriction at mealtime for children so they will drink milk is probably advisable, but drinking water between meals should be stressed. Limiting the water intake may be detrimental in that it affects the excreta, concentrating urine and making hard, dry feces.

Under certain conditions the amount of water consumed needs special consideration. Thirst or the desire for water may not take care of extra needs in fever, strenuous exercise, and at high environmental temperatures, or under such conditions as hyperthyroidism and low renal efficiency. The intake of water or fluid therefore may require special attention. Replacement of depleted liquid is especially important after a hemorrhage or a blood donation, and following extensive burns. Older persons often complain that they do not like water, in which case fruit juices and soft drinks may be prescribed. When the weather is very hot or when strenuous activity causes excess perspiration, salt as well as water is lost from the body; in certain heavy industries it has been found that there may be a loss of 1 liter of water per hour for an eight-hour day, and a daily total loss of 10 to 20 gm. of salt.

Electrolyte Balance

SOURCES OF ACID AND BASE

The products of metabolism are largely acidic. Most foods as they are eaten are neither acid nor basic. However, as the food materials are broken down by enzyme action in the digestive tract and by combustion in the cells, their comparative neutrality is changed and they exhibit reactions dependent on the products formed. Thus, carbohydrates in their catabolism form such acids as lactic and pyruvic, which ordinarily are broken down further to give carbon dioxide and water. Fats are split into fatty acids and glycerol and under normal conditions are oxidized to carbon dioxide and water. Under certain conditions, such as diabetes, fasting, or the consumption of a diet containing too low a ratio of carbohydrate to fat, the complete oxidation of the fatty acids is hindered and such products as acetone, acetoacetic acid, and β-hydroxybutyric acid accumulate. Proteins on hydrolysis yield amino acids which are deaminized to form ammonia and acid compounds, the latter of which are converted into carbon dioxide and water in the oxidation process. This brief review of the metabolism of the organic foodstuffs shows that large amounts of acid, mainly carbonic, and comparatively small quantities of base, such as ammonia, are formed.

The ash of foods which have been burned varies in reaction. After the combustion of foods within the body, an inorganic residue is left which may be more or less acidic. The reaction will be due to the relationship of proton donors to proton acceptors. Gonick and co-workers (7) used the direct titrametric method to analyze 18 foods commonly incorporated in hospital weighed diets (Table 13–2). It will be noted that most of the foods high in protein yield excess acid and that most fruits and vegetables are basic in reaction. Fruits and vegetables contain organic acids, most of which are oxidized in the body. A few organic acids do not undergo oxidation and therefore have an acid reaction; examples are tartaric acid, oxalic acid, and hippuric acid, found in prunes, plums, cranberries, and corn.

BODY ADJUSTMENTS TO VARIATIONS IN ACID AND BASE

There is a constancy in reaction of the blood. Despite the large amounts of acids formed in the body, the reaction of the tissues is very slightly alkaline and remains markedly constant. In normal subjects the hydrogen

Table 13–2

Excess Acid or Base in Individual Foods*

Food	Weight gm.	Phosphorus mg.	Sulfate meq.	Excess Acid meq.	Excess Base meq.
Eggs	100	216	8.3	11.9	
Steak	100	215	7.1	10.9	
Ground beef	100	235	7.1	11.4	
American cheese	100	429	7.1		7.1
Cottage cheese	100	159	2.3	5.5	
Milk	100 (ml)	103	1.8		2.7
White bread	100	177	6.8	5.0	
Whole wheat bread	100	217	7.9	6.7	
Salt-free bread	100	105	6.3	7.6	
Potato, raw	100	73	4.6		5.6
Lettuce	100	18	1.2		1.8
String beans	100	22	1.2		4.9
Peas	100	71	1.6		1.2
Peaches	100	10	1.5		4.8
Pears	100	8	0.8		1.0
Orange juice	100 (ml)	6	0.6		3.4
Tomatoes	100	20	0.7		6.5
Apple juice	100 (ml)	10	0.3		0.2

* From Gonick, H. C., *et al.* Re-examination of the Acid-Ash Content of Several Diets. *Am. J. Clin. Nutr.*, 21:898 (1968).

ion concentration of the blood and other body tissues lies within a range of pH 7.35 to 7.43*; this is found to vary a little during the day. The limits of normality are pH 7.32 to 7.47. Ordinarily a pH of 7.55 in the blood is thought to indicate the condition known as alkalosis, one below 7.3, acidosis; but both these states are quite rare.

The body has several ways of maintaining its constant reaction. One is the buffer action of proteins in the blood; the most important proteins in this respect are the two hemoglobins. As stated earlier, oxy-hemoglobin is a stronger acid than reduced hemoglobin; it therefore has a greater tendency to form salts. When it is present in the blood in larger amounts than reduced hemoglobin, the proportion of salt to acid is greater. In the change of oxy-hemoglobin to the reduced form, enough alkali is freed to neutralize much of the carbon dioxide present, and when the reduced hemoglobin is oxidized in the lungs, it reacts with the bicarbonate and liberates carbon dioxide which is then exhaled. Thus, protein serves in two ways—as a buffer to increase the carbon dioxide capacity of the

* Hydrogen ion concentration refers to the concentration of active ions per liter of a material. The term "pH" is the negative logarithm corresponding to the given concentration. For instance, a solution with a pH of 4 is 1/10,000 normal, one with a pH of 5 is 1/100,000 normal. A neutral substance has a pH of 7. All pH values above 7 represent alkalinity and all those below represent acidity.

blood and as a means of freeing base when carbon dioxide is liberated in the lungs.

The phosphates and carbonates in the system also act as buffers and neutralize the acid formed in metabolism. These salts are less efficient buffers than are the proteins—the phosphates because of their small concentration, the carbonates because they do not tend to dissociate at the hydrogen ion concentration found in the blood. The bicarbonate-carbonic acid system functions in maintaining acid-base balance in the body in a more efficient way than as buffer. Because the acid formed from bicarbonate is volatile, and the carbon dioxide from it is constantly being excreted through the lungs, bicarbonate plays a most important role by supplying a base which may combine with all other acids. For this reason bicarbonates are called the alkaline reserve and represent to a large extent the base available for body use. Since the carbon dioxide-combining power of the blood depends on the amount of alkali present, analysis of the carbon dioxide in the blood is considered a means of determining normality of reaction. In acidosis the alkali reserve is depleted, in alkalosis there is an excess.

The chloride shift is another way of maintaining a pH of about 7.35 in the tissues. Chloride as well as bicarbonate is found in smaller amounts in the corpuscles than in the blood plasma. When the carbon dioxide tension of the blood increases, the concentration of chloride in the cells increases, since it diffuses from the plasma; the bicarbonate increases proportionately more in the plasma, thus increasing the potential alkalinity of the blood. Sulfate and phosphate ions diffuse as well as chloride, but since there is more chloride in the blood, its action in this regard is considered more important.

It must be understood that the carbon dioxide tension of the blood tends to be kept nearly constant in an effort to eliminate excesses of the waste product. Thus, if an acid condition prevails in the tissues, there is a tendency to lower the carbon dioxide tension in the lungs, and this in turn lowers the concentration in the blood, which brings about decreased acidity in the tissues. The stimulation of the respiratory center which occurs at such times favors breathing and elimination of the extra carbon dioxide.

The body normally maintains an alkali reserve. The body's alkali reserve can be greatly depleted, since, when the base is drawn from the volatile bicarbonate to combine with a fixed acid, it forms a salt which may be excreted through the kidneys. The body can control this loss of base in several ways. First, the urine is much more acid than is the blood, thus sparing the base to some extent. Second, there is a tendency for ammonia, formed in catabolism of protein, to replace the basic part of the salt, which is then excreted as an ammonium compound, the freed base remaining in the blood stream as a bicarbonate. A third way of conserving the bicarbonate base involves the phosphates which are found in larger amounts in urine than in blood and which represent by far the greatest proportion of acid elements in the urine. When the urine acidity is low, a pH of 7.4, it has been estimated that about 80 per cent of the phosphate in the blood is present as dibasic salts, and in a urine of pH 4.8, about 99 per cent of the total phosphate is found as mono-basic salts. Thus the body tends to conserve the alkali reserve by excreting the more acid salt in the urine and retaining the more or less basic salts. Organic acids may be excreted in varying amounts in the urine but usually are oxidized in the body or, if excreted unchanged, are present in too small quantity to influence markedly the acid-base balance. Citric, malic, and tartaric acids ingested in foods are among those utilized by the body; those which are not used include benzoic and oxalic. The body's great tolerance for citric and tartaric acids has been shown by Blatherwick and Long (8). They found that normal human subjects could consume as much as 2400 ml. of orange juice or 1 liter of grape juice without increasing the urine's acidity. In fact, use of these fruits tends to decrease the hydrogen ion concentration of the urine, since their sourness is due to acid salts, such as potassium acid tartrate and calcium acid citrate, which on oxidation contribute to the total base in the body.

When the body cannot adjust, certain conditions arise. There are several evidences of strain on the body mechanism when the system is greatly taxed. These may be caused largely by interference with excretion and also, possibly, by an unusual intake of fixed acids and by abnormal metabolism. Under such circumstances there may be very rapid respiration, a rise in urinary ammonium salts, increased acidity of the urine, and a fall in the alkaline reserve. Clinical acidosis does not occur until the mechanisms prove unequal to meeting the strains put on them. A secondary result, associated with the more acid urine, is decreased solubility of uric acid, in which state it is held within the body and deposited largely in the joints.

The body can adjust to ordinary variations in diet. It has been a common practice in the past to attribute various bodily ills to poor adjustment of the diet with reference to the acid-base balance. Bischoff and co-workers (9) studied the effect of acid ash and alkaline ash foodstuffs on man's acid-base equilibrium. In a series of short-time experiments, six subjects were fed diets made excessively acid by the addition of 1 pound of beefsteak, or excessively alkaline by including 1 pound of bananas, 1 quart of orange juice, or 1 quart of milk. Determinations of the plasma bicarbonate and pH made at intervals during an eight-hour period following ingestion of each diet showed no significant alteration from the values for fasting blood. Reaction of the urine was influenced, but it was emphasized that this does not necessarily imply changes in the blood. The results of these experiments verify Bischoff's earlier statement that the alkali reserve of healthy human beings is not shifted outside the so-called normal limits by ingestion of foodstuffs, either acid or alkaline. The diet adequate in other respects need not be balanced as to acid and base reaction. However, to treat renal acidosis it has been recommended that the amount of protein in the diet be limited to 40 gm. per day. Gonick and co-workers analyzed several hospital diets containing variable levels of protein. Those with 60 to 100 gm. protein were found to be neutral in reaction, whereas those with 40 gm. protein were basic.

REFERENCES

1. Baker, E. M., *et al.* Water Requirements of Men as Related to Salt Intake. *Am. J. Clin. Nutr., 12:*394 (1963).
2. Sherman, H. C. Nutritional Aspects of Acid-Base Balance. *Chemistry of Food and Nutrition,* 8th ed. New York: Macmillan (1952).
3. Camien, M. N., *et al.* A Critical Reappraisal of "Acid-Base" Balance. *Am. J. Clin. Nutr., 22:*786 (1969).
4. Siri, W. E. Gross Composition of the Body. *Advan. Biol. Med. Phys., IV:*239. New York: Academic Press (1956).
5. Newburgh, L. H. The Cause of Obesity. *J. Am. Med. Ass., 97:*1659 (1931).
6. Ashe, B. I., *et al.* Protein, Salt, and Fluid Consumption of One Thousand Residents of New York. *J. Am. Med. Ass., 108:*1160 (1937).
7. Gonick, H. C., *et al.* Re-examination of the Acid-Ash Content of Several Diets. *Am. J. Clin. Nutr., 21:*898 (1968).
8. Blatherwick, N. R., *et al.* Studies of Urinary Acidity. I. Some Effects of Drinking Large Amounts of Orange Juice and Sour Milk. *J. Biol. Chem., 53:*103 (1922).
9. Bischoff, F., *et al.* The Effect of Acid Ash and Alkaline Ash Foodstuffs on the Acid-Base Equilibrium of Man. *J. Nutr., 7:*51 (1934).

GENERAL REFERENCES

10. Alper, C. Fluid and Electrolyte Balance. *In* M. G. Wohl and R. S. Goodhart (eds.), *Modern Nutrition in Health and Disease,* 4th ed. Philadelphia: Lea and Febiger, 1968.
11. Hardy, J. D., *et al.* Measurement of Body Water: Techniques and Practical Implications. *J. Am. Med. Ass., 149:*1113 (1952).

Nutrition During the Reproductive Period

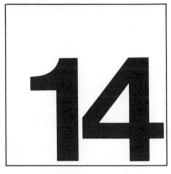

A woman's nutriture during the pre-pregnancy period affects her success in child bearing. Studies indicate that the adolescent girl frequently fails to meet the recommended allowances for various nutrients and that she has the poorest food habits in her family. Today many girls still in their teens marry and bear children. Their own physical growth is not yet complete, and this fact, along with an inadequate diet and the extra demands of pregnancy and lactation, adds to the metabolic burdens on the body.

Throughout the reproduction period many changes occur within the woman's body, conditions involving growth and development of the tissues concerned with maternal and infant well-being. Following the first two weeks after conception, the pre-implantation period, comes a critical interval, lasting to the eighth week, during which major organogenesis occurs. The metabolic changes which result from the implantation of the fertilized ovum are marked and apt to result in poor appetite, disturbances of digestion, nausea, and vomiting. The hormones specifically related to reproduction become very active; others, such as the thyroid gland hormones, are formed at an increased rate. The placenta, which nourishes the fetus until delivery, develops rapidly and reaches its maximal size early in gestation. This tissue also plays protective and excretory roles and controls the passage of nutrients and waste materials according to the needs of mother and child.

Many investigations have been conducted to relate general and specific dietary lacks during pregnancy to such faulty performances as nausea and pernicious vomiting, pre-eclampsia, prematurity, and stillbirths, as well as to weight and length of the infant at birth and success in lactation. Although the findings have not always demonstrated consistent significant correlation between the occurrence of such conditions and the maternal diet, there is no doubt concerning the importance of nutrition in pregnancy. Both the course of pregnancy and the health of the offspring can be affected by maternal nutritional deficiencies. In extreme malnutrition congenital malformations may be evident in the skeleton, soft tissues, brain, and other parts of the body, but this degree of poor nutrition is thought to be very uncommon. The extent of deficiency which may be reached without immediate evidence of harm to mother or infant is not known.

It has been customary to think that the pregnant woman must eat a total equivalent to her nonpregnant needs and to those of her accessory tissues and the developing fetus. The idea has been advanced that, because a pregnant woman is physiologically quite different from her nonpregnant self, her dietary needs may also be altered through a process of nutritional adaptation. This concept has been demonstrated in women in the case of several nutrients. Examples of such adaptations will be given in the following discussion.

Pregnancy

THE REQUIREMENTS FOR ENERGY AND THE LIPIDS DURING PREGNANCY

The basal metabolic rate changes during pregnancy. During the third to fourth month of gestation the basal fuel need falls to a subnormal level and from then on advances steadily. By the end of gestation the rate may have increased by 20 per cent. Growth of the fetus and of the placenta and other maternal tissues which have high metabolic activity is largely responsible for this increase; it is greater than would be expected from the increase in body weight. Experiments by Carpenter and Murlin (1), who studied three women by means of a bed calorimeter at the Carnegie Nutrition Laboratory, showed that the increase in metabolic activity is due largely to the active protoplasmic tissue of the fetus. They found that the basal rate of the pregnant subject just before parturition was equal to that of the mother and child taken separately three to ten days after delivery. The basal rate of the newborn infant, per kg. of body weight, was two and one-half times that of the mother after delivery. The increased activity of the glands of internal secretion is another cause of the higher basal rate. More thyroid activity is indicated by the rise in blood iodine which is observed beginning with the second month of pregnancy; iodine in the blood decreases in the first two weeks after delivery.

Total energy needs vary. Although the basal metabolic rate increases markedly and there is a gain in body weight, the total energy requirement is not expected to show a comparable rise. This is true because the woman's physical activity is reduced and she leads a more leisurely life.

The FNB recommends 200 calories per day extra during pregnancy. This increase is thought to be especially important for the active, immature young woman undergoing her first pregnancy.

Weight control is advised. The expected weight gain includes, for the first four months, a total of about 3 pounds and from then on about 0.8 pound per week. If the woman is underweight a greater gain may be advised and if she is obese, less. In investigations of mothers and their infants, Macy (2) found negligible correlations between median birth weights and lengths of infants and diet ratings and prenatal care of the women.

In a study of 1570 prenatal patients at Philadelphia Lying-In Hospital Tompkins and co-workers (3) secured data on the relation between gain in weight of the women and prematurity (weight of 5.5 pounds or less at birth) of their infants. They plotted a curve of expected weight gain at monthly intervals and found that during the first trimester a maternal gain of approximately 3 pounds was to be expected, by the end of the second trimester, about 14 pounds, and at term, 24 pounds. When a patient gained less than was predicted, there was a tendency for premature birth. Tompkins and associates also found that toxemia incidence was greater among women 20 per cent or more overweight or 15 per cent or more underweight at the beginning of pregnancy; excess weight gain during the first and second trimesters was associated with a higher rate of toxemia. These trends show the importance of weight control both before and during pregnancy.

Fats and fatty acids are important considerations. Both the quantity and quality of the fat intake should be considered. Under usual conditions of health, fat should contribute about 30 per cent of the total calories. A satisfactory P/S ratio should be maintained now as at other times of life. A study made by Hansen and co-workers (4) of 30 pregnant women compared constituents in the diet during the third trimester with serum lipids. Calories, protein, total fat, unsaturated fat, and linoleic acid were determined and compared with serum cholesterol, total fatty acids, linoleic acid, and arachidonic acid. No significant correlations were found between the pregnant woman's diet and the lipids in her serum nor between her diet and the lipids in the serum of the infant at birth. However, the prospective mother's serum was significantly higher than the newborn's in cholesterol, total fatty acids, and linoleic acid and lower in arachidonic acid.

PROTEIN ADAPTATIONS DURING PREGNANCY

Protein is stored during this period. Many studies made on pregnant human beings and animals indicate an increase in body nitrogen during pregnancy and an amount retained which tends to be above that needed for fetal growth and the accessory tissues. This net gain is more likely to occur when the protein intake is high. However, work on animals shows that the condition occurs also on restricted protein intake, possibly because of decreased nitrogen excretion and more economical utilization of protein. It is suggested that growth hormones may be involved in these alterations.

Plasma proteins are lowered during pregnancy. The investigations by Macy and her associates (2) on large groups of women during the prenatal period were referred to in Chapter 1. The large number of carefully selected cases, the seriatim data secured throughout the successful period of pregnancy, and the objective and careful control of data accumulated make this study of great value both to research workers and to women who may profit from the findings. A group of 425 women was chosen on the basis that they were healthy and without defects which might impair their general well-being. They completed gestation successfully and delivered healthy full-term infants weighing at least 5.5 pounds. These women were compared with 48 equally carefully chosen nonpregnant women. To avoid inclusion of extreme values which are not typical, the investigators eliminated extremes and included ranges from the 10th to the 90th percentiles. They stated medians and ranges for six components of the blood. Data from the Macy studies on plasma proteins and the changes which may be expected during reproduction will be discussed in this section.

The levels of total plasma protein were lower in pregnant than in nonpregnant women and the amounts decreased throughout pregnancy. The protein levels of the babies were even lower than were those of their respective mothers.

Electrophoretic methods made it possible to secure accurate estimations of the various components of the blood proteins. In an uncomplicated pregnancy Macy and co-workers (5) found that the levels of total serum protein, albumin, and five globulin fractions were distributed in a characteristic and predictable pattern and that the different protein fractions varied in amounts during the three trimesters. When the blood proteins of the pregnant women were compared with those of the nonpregnant female, it was found that the albumin and the γ-globulin concentrations tended to be lower, whereas the other globulin fractions were higher.

Reboud and co-workers (6) studied the plasma proteins, including the lipoprotein fractions, of pregnant women. The total levels of protein fell throughout the period, but as was found in the Macy investigation, the individual fractions varied, some increasing, some decreasing, some not changing significantly. Reboud suggests that there are three protein phases in a normal pregnancy. The first is a period of adaptation during which decreases in the albumins, lipoproteins, and lipids occur. The second, one of balance which continues to about the 32nd week, is marked by a continued low for the albumins, but there is a rise to above normal for the lipoproteins. The third period, designated as preparation for delivery, tends to be a reversal to a state more similar to that of the nonpregnant woman. Knowledge of these alterations in plasma proteins should be useful in studying the pathological conditions which may occur during reproduction.

An increase in dietary protein is recommended. The greater requirement at this time is related largely to the demands of the fetal and accessory tissues. This is estimated to be about 950 gm. during the last six weeks of gestation. The FNB recommends that an extra 10 gm. of protein per day be included in the diet during pregnancy. This extra allows for fetal needs; expected variations in ultilization and in protein quality have already been included in the recommendations for the nonpregnant woman.

A low-protein maternal diet at this time may not only affect milk secretion after delivery but also may cause anemia, nutritional edema, poor muscular tone of the uterus, and lowered resistance. In order to obtain the desired amount of protein the daily diet should include 1 quart of milk, 6 to 8 ounces of lean meat, or its equivalent in protein, and 1 egg, as well as the usual amounts of whole grain or enriched cereal products, fruits, and vegetables.

Few studies have been made of amino acid needs during pregnancy. Sheft and Oldham (7) investigated the intakes and excretions of ten amino acids in 13 pregnant women. Intakes of methionine, phenylalanine, and tryptophan ranked low when compared with the amounts ordinarily recommended. Excretions of threonine, methionine, and histidine were markedly higher in these pregnant women than in nonpregnant subjects. Comparatively large amounts of these amino acids are found in meat, milk, and egg proteins, which are important in the diet during the reproductive period.

The value of liberal protein during pregnancy is widely accepted but sometimes the importance of calories in the utilization of protein is ignored. These relationships were discussed in Chapter 6. In the investigation by Oldham and Sheft (8) negative nitrogen balances were common even though the protein intakes seemed adequate. This condition was associated with low calorie consumption which averaged about 1850 calories per day, and, in the case of four of the women, was 1000 calories or less.

THE SPECIAL IMPORTANCE OF THE MINERALS DURING PREGNANCY

Calcium and phosphorus are necessary for bone and tooth growth. Early in pregnancy ossification of fetal bone centers takes place and by the fourth month, most of the bones are undergoing calcium and phosphorus deposition and the teeth are forming. In actual amount, comparatively little calcium is deposited in the fetus during the first trimester but as more rapid growth occurs the rate of uptake is greater. According to Needham (9) at three months in a fetus weighing 36 gm. there is only

0.25 mg. of calcium; at five, six, seven, and eight months, as the body increased from 330 gm. to 600, to 1000, to 1500 gm., the calcium content increases from 3.3 gm. to 7.5, to 11.6, to 20.4 gm., and to 25 gm. at term. By the end of the prenatal period the temporary teeth are well formed in the jaw and calcification of the first permanent molars has begun. Since skeletal growth is of vital concern even at this early stage, the bone-building foods should be supplied liberally throughout the entire child bearing period.

In pregnancy there is evidence of increased efficiency of calcium absorption. Calcium metabolism during pregnancy has been studied by means of radioactive calcium. The placenta rapidly transfers this mineral from maternal to fetal circulation and at a high rate when compared with the calcium in the mother's blood stream. It is estimated that every hour the rapidly growing fetus takes about 7 per cent of the calcium from the maternal blood; regular replenishment through diet is important to avoid draining calcium from the maternal skeleton. Several extensive investigations have been made to determine mineral behavior during pregnancy. Toverud and Toverud (10) studied calcium and phosphorus metabolism during four-day periods, in one woman from the third month of pregnancy to its completion, in several other women during the last two or three months of pregnancy. In 21 out of 27 experiments they found negative calcium and phosphorus balances but succeeded in getting a positive balance by increasing calcium to 1.7 gm., and phosphorus to 1.6 gm. daily. Milk and calcium lactate were fed as supplements. Macy and co-workers (11) in their studies on three women determined calcium and phosphorus balances at four-week intervals throughout the last half of pregnancy. Their diets, considered to be abundant in food essentials, contained daily 2400 to 3600 kcal, 72.5 to 147.5 gm. of protein, 1.5 to 2.7 gm. of calcium, and 1.5 to 3.0 gm. of phosphorus. Even on these intakes excessive excretion of calcium occurred during varying periods of the pregnancies, but phosphorus showed comparatively better retention.

Kerr and co-workers (12) studied serum calcium and phosphate in 24 pregnant and 32 nonpregnant women. A drop in blood calcium levels during the reproductive period was associated with a decrease in the protein-bound fraction but not in free calcium; this decrease may be related to the low serum albumin level. Kerr's investigation also considered means of raising the serum calcium. After fasting blood samples were taken, each pregnant woman was given orally one of four supplements each containing 2 gm. calcium; blood and urine samples were taken at intervals. Calcium lactate raised both calcium and phosphate levels in the serum and increased the urinary excretion of calcium. Calcium sulfate and di-calcium phosphate caused no change in either blood or urine. The fourth supplement, nonfat milk powder, had no effect on serum concentration but increased urinary calcium excretion.

Therefore, calcium lactate was considered the best supplement if one is needed during the reproductive period.

During pregnancy, the FNB recommends that an additional 0.4 gm. of calcium be included in the daily diet. The Board also recommends that the phosphorus intake be equivalent to that of calcium at this time. One quart of milk, supplying almost nine-tenths of the needed calcium, as well as considerable phosphorus and protein, should be incorporated into the day's dietary. Calcium pills should not be substituted for the milk, unless an allergy prevents its use, since milk is so valuable in other nutrients. Cheese, eggs, meat, and vegetables may complete the day's need.

The pregnant body conserves iron. There are several ways in which the woman adapts in this respect. The first relates to the saving of iron through cessation of menstruation. A second means of conservation results from improved absorption of iron during pregnancy; studies using radioactive iron have demonstrated that there is a three- to fourfold increase in absorption of this mineral in the last trimester. Beaton (13) suggests that this efficiency is related to the increase in the amount of plasma transferrin, the iron-transport protein.

Table 14–1 gives data on iron requirements during pregnancy, presented by The Committee on Iron Deficiency of the American Medical Association (14). The Committee states that a daily replacement of from 2 to 5 mg. iron (mean, 3.5 mg.) is needed to fulfill these requirements during gestation. Greater need occurs during the last six months of pregnancy since red cell volume increases begin at about the fourth month. The Committee estimates a requirement of 20 to 48 mg. per day, amounts which would be very difficult to obtain through diet. Since iron is seldom stored in the body, the Committee recommends supple-

Table 14–1

Iron Requirements for Pregnancy *

	Average mg.	*Range* mg.
External iron loss	170	150–200
Expansion of red cell mass	450	200–600
Fetal iron	270	200–370
Iron in placenta and cord	90	30–170
Blood loss at delivery	150	90–310
Total requirement[1]	980	580–1340
Cost of pregnancy[2]	680	440–1050

* Committee on Iron Deficiency, American Medical Association. *J. Am. Med. Ass. 203:*407 (1968)
1 Blood loss at delivery not included.
2 Expansion of red cell mass not included.

mentary iron therapy during the last half of pregnancy if stores are depleted.

Macy and her associates (2) in their investigation of the metabolic state during reproduction found that the hemoglobin level of the blood fell during the first five months of gestation and remained low. This may be explained by the increase in blood volume at this time. Actually, the hemoglobin content of the red cells shows little or no change and, since the number of red blood cells actually increases during pregnancy, the total hemoglobin may be greater. The seeming drop by Macy's subjects was not considered to be related to a corresponding lack of dietary iron but rather to hemodilution. The placenta tends to conserve iron for the infant's needs. The Macy study showed that hemoglobin is much more concentrated in the blood of the infant at birth than in that of the woman at any time during gestation; the median levels were approximately 50 per cent higher than were those of their respective mothers.

The FNB estimates increased needs of 2 to 4 mg. iron per day during the latter part of pregnancy. However, since it recommends an allowance of 18 mg. per day for all women of child-bearing age, it believes that this amount should allow enough accumulation of iron stores so that more during pregnancy will not be necessary. As sources of dietary iron, nutritionists advise liberal amounts of lean meat (including liver), eggs, leafy green vegetables, legumes, dried fruits, whole grain and enriched cereal products, and molasses.

The supply of other minerals is important. During pregnancy the concentration of iodine in the blood gradually increases; by the third trimester this exceeds the normal range found in the nonpregnant woman. In the chapter on iodine it was stated that the need for this mineral depends largely on the locality in which the individual lives and that pregnancy is one period of susceptibility to goiter. It has been found that myxedema to a large extent prevents conception, and that when pregnancy does occur, the glandular disorder frequently is inherited by the offspring.

The type of thyroid disorder most common during pregnancy is simple goiter. In regions where it is endemic, from 40 to 60 per cent of the pregnant women have this deficiency disease and some enlargements of the thyroid glands are observed even in nongoitrous localities. Therefore frequent examinations by a physician are advised. The FNB sets the daily allowance for iodine during pregnancy at 125 mg. This is 25 mg. more than that of the nonpregnant woman of 22 years.

Little is known about the amount of magnesium needed during pregnancy. The RDA is 450 mg., as compared with 300 mg. for the nonpregnant woman of 22 years.

Among other trace minerals which may need special consideration is zinc. Geographic and socioeconomic factors were considered by Sarram and co-workers (15) in a study of zinc nutrition in Iran. They found a decreased concentration of zinc in the blood plasma and hair of pregnant women living in rural areas. The diet of these women contained few foods of animal origin; it was mostly bread.

Sodium intake should be considered. The amount of sodium in the diet of the pregnant woman sometimes is limited as a means of preventing edema and hypertension, conditions associated with the toxemia of this period. Pike and co-workers (16) found in experiments with pregnant rats that a low sodium diet resulted in decrease in plasma sodium and increase in potassium; the animals showed signs of sodium deficiency and their young were small and immature compared with those of normal animals. In pregnant rats on a higher sodium level and in nonpregnant animals there were no such effects; the rats were able to regulate sodium retention and maintain desired concentrations in the body's tissues and fluids. The adrenal cortex hormone, aldosterone, is thought to be involved through its effect on the reabsorption of sodium by the kidney. When there is a need to conserve this element, more of the hormone is secreted. Watambe and associates (17), working with pregnant women, found changes in rate of secretion of aldosterone during pregnancy that were related to the amount of sodium ingested; on a low sodium intake more of the hormone was secreted. This results in more reabsorption by the kidney and less sodium in the urine.

THE VITAMIN NEEDS DURING PREGNANCY

The fat-soluble vitamins are especially important. In the Macy studies (2), serum vitamin A, carotenoids, and alkaline phosphatase were determined. The serum levels of vitamin A and its precursors tend to be somewhat higher in the woman than in the infant. These relationships are associated with their special functions in respect to epithelial cells during organogenesis, to bone and tooth formation, and to vision. The role of vitamin A in synthesis of mucopolysaccharides found in connective tissues and cartilage is important during this period of building fetal tissues.

The FNB advises 6000 IU of vitamin A value daily. Whole milk, butter or fortified margarine, eggs, liver, and leafy green and yellow vegetables taken in recommended amounts will care for the body's extra needs at this time. In setting the allowance, it is assumed that about two-thirds of the vitamin A requirement comes from carotene.

In the Macy studies the serum alkaline phosphatase showed a different trend from that of vitamin A. Concentration of this aid to calcium and phosphorus utilization more nearly paralleled growth of the fetal skeleton and storage of the minerals in the woman.

Although clinical symptoms of vitamin D deficiency during pregnancy are rare in the United States and Europe, the effects of lack are evident in the infant, largely as poor calcification of the bones. Since pregnancy is a time of great calcium and phosphorus demand, vitamin D is included as a dietary requirement, and 400 IU is the quantity advocated by the FNB. Vitamin D milk, when taken in the amount considered essential to meet the calcium needs, will supply the vitamin D requirement; fish liver oils or their concentrates often are prescribed by the physician and will add to the day's supply of vitamin A. The amount needed will vary considerably depending on the product's potency. The rays of the sun, by activating the precursor in the skin, may furnish enough vitamin D; however, this means of securing the requirement is apt to be less reliable and should not ordinarily be counted on during pregnancy.

Pregnancy's effects on the requirement for vitamin E have not been established. However, the recommended allowance for this vitamin is increased to 30 IU per day. No RDA for vitamin K has been set. Neonatal hemorrhage which may occur in some infants is treated directly, not by giving vitamin K to the mother shortly before labor.

The water-soluble vitamins are also important at this time. The sixth component of the blood studied by Macy and her associates was vitamin C. During pregnancy the concentrations were lower than those in the non-pregnant woman. The levels decreased throughout the gestation period and into postpartum. In the infants the average serum concentrations were two to four times those of the mothers. The placenta favors passage of ascorbic acid into fetal blood but may act as a barrier and prevent reentrance to the mother's blood stream.

In a cooperative study made by Martin and co-workers (18) at Vanderbilt University School of Medicine, 2129 pregnant women were included. Intakes of ascorbic acid were recorded and medians for the second and third trimesters estimated. It was found that 14 per cent of the women had daily intakes of less than 40 mg. and only 15 per cent consumed 80 mg. or more daily during both these periods. A correlation was found between intake of the vitamin and its level in the serum.

The FNB recommends an allowance of 60 mg. ascorbic acid daily. Eight ounces of orange juice, or the vitamin C equivalent, are advised to meet this requirement.

The allowances for thiamin and niacin equivalent are increased by 0.1 and 2.0 mg., respectively. These figures are based on the greater calorie intake. The daily riboflavin intake should be increased by 0.3 mg. The larger increase for riboflavin is due to greater metabolic size resulting from growth of the fetus and related tissues. Meat, milk, eggs, and whole grain and enriched breads and cereals are valuable sources of these three vitamins.

Investigations on riboflavin indicate a tendency toward decreased excretion during the latter part of pregnancy; this is to be expected during this time of greater nitrogen storage and utilization. In a study of tryptophan-niacin relationships in pregnancy, Wertz and co-workers (19) determined the excretion of these two nutrients and niacin metabolites in 12 women. Urinary losses were found to be higher during pregnancy. When a tryptophan supplement was given, urinary excretion of this amino acid decreased significantly, indicating a more efficient conversion of tryptophan into niacin in the pregnant than in the nonpregnant woman.

The FNB recommends a daily allowance of 0.8 mg. folacin. Deficiency of this vitamin is fairly common during the last trimester of pregnancy, as evidenced by the prevalence of megaloblastic anemia (20). Folacin is necessary for synthesis of nucleic acids, and lack of it is serious for the rapidly growing fetus. There also is some evidence that a folate deficiency may result in fetal malformation, abortion, hemorrhage, and prematurity. Since placentation and formation of the fetus occur early in pregnancy, supplementation with folacin early in pregnancy or before conception is frequently recommended. A daily supplement of 1 mg. folacin has been suggested. Since undiagnosed pernicious anemia is very rare among pregnant women, use of this level of folic acid is not considered a hazard (21).

The FNB recommends 8 μg vitamin B_{12} daily during pregnancy. There is often a gradual fall of this vitamin in the woman's serum, due possibly to hemodilution, possibly to an excessive demand by the fetus.

Little is known about specific needs for vitamin B_6 during pregnancy. However, in pregnant women there is considerable evidence of biochemical abnormalities which may be corrected when the vitamin is administered. Vitamin B_6 is transported actively by the placenta so that fetal blood contains about five times as much of the vitamin as maternal blood (22). To meet fetal needs the FNB suggest addition of 0.5 mg. vitamin B_6 daily, making a total of 2.5 mg. Sometimes, a multivitamin supplement is prescribed to furnish an extra margin of safety for all the B-complex vitamins. This supplement should be one to two times the RDA.

SPECIAL DIETARY PROBLEMS

Elimination must be considered. Pregnant women tend to suffer from constipation, since the enlarged uterus may press against the intestines and hinder normal motility. Too, there may be an inclination to decrease activity. This is not advisable, since the usual amount of exercise not only favors elimination but also keeps the body fit generally. Treatment of constipation by diet is better than by medicine. The pregnant woman will doubtless find that the means which were efficacious at other times in her life will be helpful now. For most women inclusion of ample fluids, plenty of fruits and vegetables, and some whole grain cereal products in the diet will suffice. If more is needed, the physician should be consulted.

The teeth require special attention. The teeth have greater tendency to decay during pregnancy than at other times. The Council on Dental Therapeutics, while recognizing the importance of a good diet to the mother's well-being, maintains that integrity of the teeth is primarily a matter of prompt attention by the dentist.

The roles of protein, minerals, and vitamins in building teeth and fetal bones were discussed earlier. If the water is not fluoridated, sodium fluoride tablets may be prescribed; the fluoride is absorbed through the placenta and is useful to the fetus. The supplement is considered beneficial to the growing body from the standpoint of both sodium and fluoride.

It is thought that vitamin B_6 may have a caries-inhibiting effect. In one investigation, Hillman, Caboud, and Schenone (23) studied 540 pregnant women. The group which received supplementary vitamin B_6 had a smaller increase in DMF (decayed, missing, filled) rating than did the group which received a placebo.

Nausea and pre-eclampsia may occur. Nausea or morning sickness is common during the first three or four months of pregnancy. Pernicious vomiting also may occur. Possible causes of this condition include nervous disturbances, placental protein intoxication, and a derangement in carbohydrate metabolism. Frequent small high-carbohydrate feedings may be advised as a means of control.

An overweight condition sometimes is associated with pre-eclampsia. This disorder is indicated by edema, headache, proteinuria, and increased blood pressure. These are considered warning signs of toxemia, in which convulsions and coma occur. As a way to control toxemia, Little (24) suggested a diet containing 0.75 gm. sodium and 2000 calories. Laboratory evidence indicates that vitamin B_6 requirement may be increased in toxemic subjects, but in practice supplementary vitamin B_6 has not been found to influence the frequency or course of the disorder.

Anemia may be the result of any of several lacks. Anemia is commonly observed during pregnancy and may be associated with both fetal and maternal complications. Kelsay (25), who made a compendium of nutritional status studies conducted in the United States, 1957–67, stated that approximately 20 per cent of more than 5000 pregnant women had less than 10 gm. hemoglobin per 100 ml. blood and that serum folate levels were also low in anemic pregnant women. Some of the cases so diagnosed may not actually be anemia but are due to hemodilution. However, in many cases a fall in hemoglobin can be controlled by adequate and timely use of iron. If absorption of the mineral is faulty, parenteral therapy may be effective. In some cases of anemia, extra protein, ascorbic acid, folic acid, and vitamin B_{12} may be indicated.

Certain foods are advised daily. The diet recommended is based on the special nutrient needs of this period. The foods listed in Table 14–2 may be used as a guide but should be adapted for individual cases.

Studies made on pregnant women have indicated a tendency to inadequacy of food intake. Stevens and Ohlson (26) in 1967 reported an investigation on the estimated diets of 129 medically indigent women in Iowa. With the exception of calcium and iron, the mean intakes of nutrients exceeded the recommended allowances of 1968. The mean calcium intake (1.21 ± 0.518 gm.) barely met the standard. The mean iron intake was low, 14.3 ± 3.67 mg. More subjects under 20 and over 30

Table 14–2

A Daily Food Guide in Pregnancy

Foods	Amounts	Comments
Milk	1 quart	Use as a beverage, in hot drinks, or in cooking. Nonfat (skim) milk may be used for weight control. Dry milk solids may be substituted for fresh milk or used as a supplement. 1 ounce cheddar cheese may be substituted for 1 cup milk.
Meat, fish, poultry	1–2 servings, 6 to 8 ounces	Use lean meats. Organ meats, such as liver, should be eaten at least once a week.
Eggs	1–2 eggs	
Fruit	2 or more servings	One serving should be citrus, such as 1 orange, ½ grapefruit, or 4 ounces citrus fruit juice. 8 ounces tomato juice may be substituted for 4 ounces citrus fruit juice.
Potato	1 medium	
Other vegetables	2 or more servings	Use raw, cooked, or in salads. At least one serving (1 cup) should be dark-green or deep-yellow.
Bread and cereal	3 servings	Use whole grain or enriched products. One serving is equal to 1 slice bread or ½ cup cereal, macaroni, spaghetti, or rice.
Margarine (fortified), butter, oil	3 to 6 teaspoons	Use plain or in cooking.
Desserts	1 serving, if desired	Use simple desserts, which include milk, eggs, fruit.
Vitamin D	400 IU	This may be secured in milk, either whole or skim.

years of age had lower intakes of some of the nutrients than did those aged 20 to 30. Mean weight gains of the women and mean birth weights of the babies were within normal range.

Lactation

THE ENERGY REQUIREMENT DURING LACTATION

Secretion of milk requires fuel. The body has a threefold demand for calories during lactation. First, enough fuel is needed to permit the woman to carry on her ordinary daily activity. In addition are two requirements peculiar to the period. The smaller one is associated with the activity of the mammary glands themselves, the larger is related to the energy value of the milk secreted. The FAO Committee on Calorie Requirements (1) tentatively estimates that the calorie efficiency of human milk production is about 60 per cent; in other words, if the nursing mother's body stores are not to be drawn from, she will require 1000 extra calories in her diet to supply 600 calories of milk. The FNB likewise recommends an additional 1000 calories during lactation. This figure is based on the assumption that the woman will produce 850 ml. of milk daily, and that it equals approximately 120 calories per 100 ml. of milk supplied. A study made in Macy's laboratory (2) showed the efficiency of some women in converting food into milk; the three women in the study were high milk-producers and were able not only to nurse their own babies but also to sell the excess to the Mother's Milk Bureau. It has been found that the specific functions of lactation will proceed for a time, despite a shortage of calories, at the expense of the mother's reserves. Loss of weight during lactation is fairly common.

The quantity of milk produced may be related to the energy intake. It is sometimes said that there is a relationship between the intake of food and the quantity of milk secreted. This matter has been investigated in dairy cattle; calories in excess of the requirements failed to change the composition of milk or to stimulate its secretion. Underfeeding retarded the flow, especially after a period of time; the lack of sufficient food first caused a depletion of maternal tissue in an effort to maintain the milk supply. The remarkable power to secrete milk for some time on inadequate rations is a valuable means of protecting the young. It is well known that many women cannot produce a large supply of milk, regardless of what they eat, since there are inherited tendencies in this respect as in others. However, an optimal diet will favor secretion to the individual's greatest capacity.

DIETARY FAT IN RELATION TO HUMAN MILK

The fat content of human milk is reflected by the mother's diet. Variations may be expected in the composition of human milk as well as in the quantity produced. Differences are due to the stage of lactation; colostrum contains much less fat than does the mature milk. Even during a single nursing period, as well as at different times of day, and between the two breasts, variations are noticeable. Also, to some extent, the maternal diet is reflected in the milk; this is true for both fats and fatty acids.

The mean linoleic acid content of human milk amounts to over 10 per cent of the total fatty acids present. In cow's milk this essential fatty acid is only about 2 per cent of the total.

The enzymes in human milk have been studied. Human milk is known to contain lipases, esterases, and acid and alkaline phosphatases; these enzymes are thought to be important for newborn babies. In a study made in India on 60 healthy lactating women, Karmarkar and Rama-khrishnan (3) analyzed diets for fat. They found that as the dietary fat increased up to about 70 gm. daily, there was a slight but significant increase in the amount of milk fat and a larger increase in the activity of the milk for total lipase, esterase, and alkaline phosphatase. This stimulus to enzyme activity is thought to be closely related to the amount of fat in the diet.

PROTEIN NEEDS DURING LACTATION

A liberal protein intake is advised. Even more of this nutrient is recommended during lactation than during pregnancy. The amount, related to the protein content of the milk, is approximately 12 gm. per liter; the mother's milk daily output averages 850 ml., with an upper limit of 1200 ml. Human milk on the average contains 1.2 gm. protein per 100 ml. At the upper level of output the additional amount of ideal protein needed by the nursing mother would be approximately 15 gm. An extra 5 gm. protein is advised to allow for the fact that the quality of protein in her diet may not be ideal, making the RDA during lactation 20 gm. above that of the nonpregnant woman. A dietary study by Macy, Shukers, and associates (2) indicated that the comparatively large amount of protein is favored. They found the protein as well as the calorie intake of their subjects to be high. The voluntary intakes for the three subjects contained an average of 160, 165, and 150 gm. of protein daily. Their respective milk outputs represented 33, 25, and 18 gm. of protein, or 21, 15, and 12 per cent, respectively, of the intake.

Certain proteins favor elaboration of milk. The amino acids of the blood are used by the mammary gland in milk formation and the quality as well as the quantity of these compounds in the blood is influenced by diet. Therefore, it is logical to assume that those proteins containing large amounts of the essential amino acids should be superior during lactation. That this is true has been demonstrated often in animal experiments.

Animal protein has been shown to be more efficient for human milk production than plant protein. It is of interest that Macy's superior milk-producers derived 55 to 75 per cent of their protein from animal sources, chiefly milk. From these investigations it seems advisable for the nursing mother to consume a diet rich in the more adequate forms of protein.

MINERAL REQUIREMENTS OF THIS PERIOD

Positive balances of calcium and phosphorus are difficult to attain. The women in Macy's study (4) tended to be in negative calcium and phosphorus balance throughout lactation, despite liberal intakes of these minerals. Macy and associates also found that daily supplements of cod liver oil (15 gm.) and yeast (10 gm.) improved calcium and phosphorus retentions. In several cases the balances were brought from negative to positive.

To care for the increase in calcium and phosphorus requirements during lactation, the FNB recommends that the daily calcium and phosphorus intakes be increased by 0.5 gm. over those of the nonpregnant woman.

The need for iron is continued. Nature has provided iron for the infant through storage in the fetus rather than through milk. The statement is made that, at birth, the human child has three times as much iron, in proportion to weight, as at maturity. This store is sufficient to last for several months. The FNB advises continuance of the 18 mg. allowance approved during pregnancy. This should care amply for the iron in human milk, which may amount to 1 mg. daily.

Anemia may occur during lactation. Mackay (5) tested the blood of 50 outpatient mothers, selected at random, all of whose babies were under ten months. She found a range of hemoglobin from 62 to 96 per cent, and an average of 75 per cent; in 29 cases, the test showed a level below 80 per cent. She later treated 44 anemic cases with ferric ammonium citrate and compared their blood and that of their infants with 37 untreated anemic cases. Although the iron salt had a gradual regenerative effect on the women's blood, the results on the infants were negative. She thought this due partly to the short period of treatment, but more, probably, to the mother's inability to transmit iron through her milk. For the mother's own well-being, her food should be rich in iron.

Iodine deficiency in the young may be treated through the mother. The FNB recommends 150 µg. iodine daily during lactation. Although the percentages of iron and copper in milk cannot be affected by dietary means, this is not true for iodine. During lactation iodine passes into the milk; it has been estimated that at the period of maximal milk flow the minimal iodine requirement would be doubled. The popular treatment, both prophylactic and curative, for the breast-fed infant is administration of some form of this mineral to the mother. Protection is afforded by its passage through her blood stream into the milk. Iodine plays a role in lactation and, when given as a supplement to nursing mothers, has been shown to cause increased milk output. There is no convincing proof that hyperthyroidism may be induced by increasing iodine intake, and use of iodized salt is approved at this time.

VITAMIN NEEDS DURING LACTATION

Vitamin A needs during lactation are even higher than those of pregnancy. The FNB recommends 8000 IU of vitamin A value daily for nursing mothers. This is 2000 IU more than is advised during pregnancy. The increased amount is suggested because of the comparatively small storage of the factor in the infant at birth and the high vitamin A content of breast milk. Human colostrum contains two to three times as much vitamin A as does the later secretion; mature human milk contains, on an average, half again as much of vitamin A as cow's milk.

Vitamin D is important during lactation. The nursing period is a great strain on the woman's metabolic processes. Since vitamin D aids in calcium utilization, the FNB recommends 400 IU of the vitamin daily; 1 quart of milk fortified with the antirachitic factor is advised.

Human milk may be deficient in vitamin D. The assertion is frequently made that human milk is a perfect food, and many mothers have relied upon the veracity of this statement. Consequently, it has been a surprise to many to find that breast-fed infants may have rickets. Macy and co-workers (6) found that 100 ml. of human milk contain from 0.4 to 10 USP units of vitamin D and 100 ml. of cow's milk, from 0.5 to 4.0 units. Both contain amounts too small to prevent rickets. It is believed that neither administration of vitamin D to the mother nor exposure of her body to ultraviolet rays will protect the baby from this disease since the factor is not secreted into the milk in sufficient amounts. Administration of some form of vitamin D directly to the young is the generally accepted precaution.

The requirement for vitamin E during lactation has not been determined. The same amount is recommended during lactation as during pregnancy. No recommendation is made for vitamin K.

The body continues to require extra vitamin C during lactation. During pregnancy the mother's system is partially depleted of this vitamin to supply fetal blood, in which the level of vitamin C is higher than in maternal blood. Human milk contains, on an average, more than twice as much ascorbic acid as cow's milk and there is less chance of loss of the vitamin in human milk because of environmental factors such as oxidation and heat treatment. The FNB recommends 60 mg. ascorbic acid daily while the mother is nursing her baby.

Requirements for the B-complex vitamins are great during lactation. The increased allowance for thiamin is based on the amount of the calorie increase; this is 0.5 mg. thiamin per 1000 kcal. Actually, the amount of thiamin in human milk varies, depending on intake of the nutrient. Mature human milk contains an average of 0.015 mg. thiamin per 100 ml. milk, so if 850 ml. of milk is secreted daily the thiamin output would be approximately 0.13 mg.

The FNB recommends an additional daily intake of approximately 0.5 mg. riboflavin during lactation. This figure is based on the riboflavin content of human milk (approximately 40 μg. per 100 ml.), the amount of milk secreted (approximately 850 ml.), and the per cent utilization of the additional riboflavin for milk production (approximately 70 per cent). This makes a total allowance of 2.0 mg. riboflavin.

The FNB recommends 20 mg. equivalents of niacin during lactation, an increase consistent with that for calories. Human milk has an average of 0.17 mg. niacin and 22 mg. tryptophan per 1000 ml.: this amounts to about 0.5 mg. of niacin equivalent per 100 ml., or 8 equivalents per 1000 kcal.

Increased intakes of biotin, vitamin B_6, folacin, and vitamin B_{12} also are recommended by the FNB. For biotin and vitamin B_6 the amounts are associated with those in human milk, approximately 4 μg. and 0.1 mg. per liter, respectively. The FNB has not recommended allowances for biotin. For vitamin B_6 it approves 2.5 mg. daily, the same as in pregnancy. For folacin and vitamin B_{12} the recommendations are 0.5 mg. and 6 μg., respectively. The increase in folacin is associated with increased demands on body stores.

Macy and co-workers have conducted many studies on the relationships of lactation to metabolism of the B-complex vitamins (7, 8, 9). Thiamin, riboflavin, niacin, pantothenic acid, and biotin intakes have been compared with secretion in milk during different stages of milk production, e.g., early (one to five days postpartum), transitional (six to ten days postpartum), and mature. It has been found that secretion of the B vitamins in milk tends to be low at first and to rise fairly rapidly; however, the percentage of the intake secreted in mature milk is comparatively small.

When vitamin B-complex supplements were given to ten healthy lactating women no stimulation to milk production resulted. However, more thiamin, riboflavin, and niacin were secreted in the milk. The amounts of pantothenic acid and biotin in milk were not affected.

FACTORS INVOLVED IN MILK SECRETION

Marked variations in milk secretion occur. There may be many variations in milk flow in the same individual. Production of milk tends to increase as lactation progresses; in late lactation the amount decreases. Not only are there differences in secretion from day to day, but from hour to hour. These are both quantitative and qualitative in nature and may influence the baby's rate of development. Emptying the breasts completely is important in stimulating secretion. This may be definitely increased by removal of milk, whereas accumulation in the breasts discourages secretion. Expression by hand or by a breast pump of any milk remaining after nursing stimulates a greater flow.

Nervous strain and overactivity are detrimental to optimal milk production. A calm, quiet life favors maximal secretion of milk. On the other hand, fear, grief, worry, anxiety, excitement, and anger retard its flow. Although a moderate amount of exercise favors milk production, excessive or heavy work has a depressing effect.

An optimal diet favors milk secretion and maternal well-being. The relationship of diet to successful lactation and to the woman's health has been discussed. The diet during lactation is quite similar to that of the pregnant woman. One difference is the quantity; since during lactation the demands are great and there is less probability of harm from excess, a more liberal calorie consumption may be advised. The extra nutrients needed may be obtained from vegetables, fruits, whole grain or enriched cereal products, and milk. Selection may be from a great variety of foods, but a few may have to be eliminated because they cause discomfort. Wholesome and simply-cooked meals will help maintain physical health for the mother and also build a strong body for the child.

PROBLEMS

1. Plan a day's diet for a pregnant woman which will meet the recommended dietary allowances in all respects and which will be appetizing.
2. Outline a lesson to be given at a prenatal clinic on the general subject of food in relation to weight control. Suggest some menus.
3. Prepare a leaflet on diet during lactation with special consideration for the woman whose milk secretion is limited.
4. Make a trip to a prenatal clinic.

REFERENCES

Pregnancy

1. Carpenter, T. M., *et al.* Energy Metabolism of Mother and Child Just Before and After Birth. *Arch. Intern. Med., 7:*184 (1911).
2. Macy, I. G., *et al.* Physiological Adaptation and Nutritional Status During and After Pregnancy. *J. Nutr., 52:* Supp. 1:1 (1954).
3. Tompkins, W. T., *et al.* Maternal and Newborn Nutrition Studies at Philadelphia Lying-In Hospital. Maternal Studies. II. Prematurity and Maternal Nutrition. *Milbank Memorial Fund Proceedings of 1954 Conference.*

4. Hansen, A. E., *et al.* Influence of Diet on Blood Serum Lipids in Pregnant Women and Newborn infants. *Am. J. Clin. Nutr., 15:*11 (1964).

5. Macy, I. G., *et al. Physiological Changes in Plasma Proteins. Characteristics of Human Reproduction.* Detroit: Children's Fund of Michigan (1952).

6. Reboud, P., *et al.* The Influence of Normal Pregnancy and the Postpartum State of Plasma Proteins and Lipids. *Am. J. Obstet. Gynecol., 86:*820 (1963).

7. Sheft, B. B., *et al.* Amino Acid Intakes and Excretions During Pregnancy. *J. Am. Diet. Ass., 28:*313 (1952).

8. Oldham, H., *et al.* Effect of Caloric Intake on Nitrogen Utilization During Pregnancy. *J. Am. Diet. Ass., 27:*847 (1951).

9. Needham, J. *Chemical Embryology.* Cambridge, Eng.: Cambridge University Press (1931).

10. Toverud, K. U., *et al.* Mineral Metabolism During Pregnancy and Lactation with Special Regard to Prevention of Rickets and Dental Caries. *Norsk Mag Laegevidenskap, 90:*1245 (1929).

11. Macy, I. G., *et al.* Metabolism of Women During the Reproductive Cycle. I. Calcium and Phosphorus Utilization in Pregnancy. *J. Biol. Chem., 86:*17 (1930).

12. Kerr, C., *et al.* Calcium and Phosphorus Dynamics in Pregnancy. *Am. J. Obstet. Gynecol., 83:*2 (1962).

13. Beaton, G. H. Nutritional and Physiological Adaptations in Pregnancy. *Fed. Proc., 20:*196 (1961).

14. A Report of The Committee on Iron Deficiency, Council on Foods and Nutrition, American Medical Association. *Iron Deficiency in the United States. J. Am. Med. Ass., 203:*407 (1968).

15. Sarram, M., *et al.* Zinc Nutrition in Pregnancy in Iran. *Am. J. Clin. Nutr., 22:*726 (1969).

16. Pike, R. L. Sodium Intake During Pregnancy. *J. Am. Diet. Ass., 44:*176 (1964).

17. Watambe, M., *et al.* Secretion Rate of Aldosterone in Normal Pregnancy. *J. Clin. Invest., 42:*1619 (1963).

18. Martin, M. P., *et al.* The Vanderbilt Cooperative Study of Maternal and Infant Nutrition. X. Ascorbic Acid. *J. Nutr., 62:*201 (1957).

19. Wertz, A. A., *et al.* Tryptophan-Niacin Relationships in Pregnancy. *J. Nutr., 64:*339 (1958).

20. Reviews. Folic Acid and Pregnancy I, II. *Nutr. Revs., 25:*325 (1967) and *26:*5 (1968).

21. Pritchard, J. A. Folic Acid Requirements in Pregnancy-Induced Megaloblastic Anemia. *J. Am. Med. Ass., 203:*1163 (1969).

22. Karlin, R., *et al.* Contribution to the Study of Vitamin B_6 Levels During Childbirth in the Total Blood of the Mother and in Total Cord Blood. *Gynecol. Obstet., 62:*281 (1963).

23. Hillman, R. W., *et al.* The Effects of Pyridoxine Supplements on the Dental Caries Experience of Pregnant Women. *Am. J. Clin. Nutr., 10:*512 (1962).

24. Little, B. Treatment of Pre-eclampsia. *New Engl. J. Med., 270:*94 (1964).

25. Kelsay, J. H. A Compendium of Nutritional Status Studies and Dietary Evaluation Studies Conducted in the United States, 1957–1967. *J. Nutr., 99:*Supp. 1, Part II:123 (1969).

26. Stevens, H. A., *et al.* Nutritive Value of the Diets of Medically Indigent Pregnant Women. *J. Am. Diet. Ass., 50:*290 (1967).

Lactation

1. Food and Agricultural Organization of the United Nations. Report of the Second Committee on Calorie Requirements. *Calorie Requirements.* FAO Nutritional Studies No. 15, Rome (1957).

2. Shukers, C. F., *et al.* A Quantitative Study of the Dietary of the Human Mother with Respect to the Nutrients Secreted into Breast Milk. *J. Nutr., 5:*127 (1932).

3. Karmarkar, M. G., *et al.* Relation Between Dietary Fat, Fat Content of Milk and Concentration of Certain Enzymes in Human Milk. *J. Nutr., 69:*274 (1959).

4. Macy, I. G., *et al.* Metabolism of Women During the Reproductive Cycle. III. Calcium, Phosphorus, and Nitrogen Utilization in Lactation Before and After Supplementing the Usual Home Diets with Cod Liver Oil and Yeast. *J. Biol. Chem., 86:*59 (1930).

5. Mackay, H. M. M. *Nutritional Anemia in Infancy.* London: Medical Research Council, Special Series, Rept. No. 157 (1931).

6. Macy, I. G., *et al. The Composition of Milks.* Bull. No. 119. Washington, D.C.: NAS-NRC (1950).

7. Roderuck, C. E., *et al.* Human Milk Studies. XXIII. Free and Total Thiamine Contents of Colostrum and Mature Human Milk. *Am. J. Dis. Childr., 70:*162 (1945).

8. Roderuck, C. E., *et al.* Human Milk Studies. XXIV. Free and Total Riboflavin Contents of Colostrum and Mature Human Milk. *Am. J. Dis. Childr., 70:*171 (1945).

9. Coryell, M. N., *et al.* Human Milk Studies. XXII. Nicotinic Acid, Pantothenic Acid and Biotin Contents of Colostrum and Mature Human Milk. *Am. J. Dis. Childr., 70:*150 (1945).

GENERAL REFERENCES

27. Macy, I. G., *et al.* Physiological Adaptation & Nutritional Status During and After Pregnancy. *J. Nutr., 52,* Supp. 1:1 (1954).

28. Moyer, E. Z., *et al.* Nutritional Status of Mothers and Their Infants. Detroit: Children's Fund of Michigan (1954).

29. Toverud, K. U., *et al. Maternal Nutrition and Child Health, An Interpretive Review,* Bull. No. 1230. Washington, D.C.: NAS-NRC (1950).

30. WHO Expert Committee. *Nutrition in Pregnancy and Lactation.* Tech. Report Series No. 302, Geneva (1965).

31. Food and Nutrition Board, NAS-NRC, Committee on Maternal Nutrition. *Maternal Nutrition and the Course of Pregnancy.* Washington, D.C. (1970).

Nutrition During Infancy

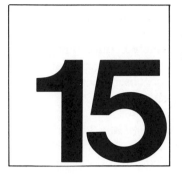

The early years of a child's life are closely associated in nutritional importance with the months of pregnancy. Growth is very rapid, particularly during the first year, and dietary adaptations are needed frequently. In the first few months of life, adjustments in homeostasis also are made; these relate especially to digestion and excretion, and to hormone secretion. Breast feeding is considered especially important at this time. Since infants vary considerably in rate of growth and development, it is unwise to make comparisons and to expect that every child will reach a particular stage in development at a specific age. Instead, the child should be examined frequently by a physician, and it is important that his advice on foods and changes in daily routines be followed.

THE NUTRIENT REQUIREMENTS OF THE INFANT

Energy needs are great. Studies on basal and total energy requirements have shown that, in terms of body weight, the calorie requirements of infants are considerably higher than those of the adult.

Basal metabolism is high at birth and increases rapidly during the first nine months. Thereafter, except for a rise for a few years at puberty, it gradually diminishes throughout life. The infant's growth rate also affects his calorie needs which increase as the weight curve goes up and diminish when he grows less rapidly. Activity is the factor which makes for the greatest individual variation in fuel needs, and expenditures for this purpose may vary widely. In detailed studies on the energy needs of infants, Benedict and Talbot (1) found that the quiet baby required 15 per cent of the total calories for activity, the usually active infant, 25 per cent, and the extremely active infant, 40 per cent. These researchers showed that there is an average increase in energy metabolism of 65 per cent as a result of strenuous crying and kicking in a newborn baby: in some cases, the increase amounted to over 200 per cent. As the infant becomes older and more active, total fuel requirements increase, and frequently the child who is learning to crawl or walk will not make normal weight gain because of lack of additional calories.

Rose and Mayer (2) made a detailed study of 29 infants during the ages of four to six months, determining dietary intake, weight and height gain, triceps skinfold thickness, and activity; the latter was measured by a device called an actometer. They found that calorie intake was related more to degree of activity than to size or rate of growth. About one-fourth of the total energy output was due to physical activity.

The FNB recommends that calorie allowances for infants be reduced in suitable steps from a level of 120 calories per kg. per day at birth to 100 calories per kg. per day by the end of the first year. If the baby is breast fed, it is assumed that 850 ml. of human milk daily will furnish the energy requirements of the first few months. However, the calorie needs of each individual child must be considered, since many factors may alter the total energy requirement. The FNB suggests that infants' calorie adjustments be made on the basis of observations of growth, appetite, activity, and extent of body fat deposits.

The essential fatty acid content of the diet is important. Linoleic acid is important in the infant's nutriture. Hansen, Wiese, and co-workers (3) found that infants maintained on diets adequate in all nutrients except fat developed skin lesions, diarrhea, and perianal irritation. Also, growth was retarded. When given fat containing linoleic acid, the symptoms disappeared. When the amount of linoleic acid was varied to determine how much was needed, no signs of deficiency occurred in infants receiving from 1.3 to 7.3 per cent of the total calories as linoleic acid. In another study, Wiese, Hanson, and Adam (4) maintained 21 healthy infants under one year of age on milk mixtures which varied in linoleic acid content. Linoleic acid supplied less than 0.1 per cent of the total calories in the skim milk, 0.9 per cent in the evaporated milk, and 4.0 per cent in the breast milk. The levels of the di- and tetraenoic acids were higher and those of the trienoic acids lower in the infants fed breast milk than in those receiving either skim or evaporated milk.

The FNB states that the minimum requirement for linoleic acid appears to be near 2 per cent of the calorie intake. In infants this is considered the lowest level of linoleate at which the serum triene:tetraene ratio remains constant. To provide for this and a reserve against stress the Board recommends that 3 per cent of the calories in the infant's formula should be in the form of linoleate.

Protein and amino acid needs are associated with the growth rate. The protein and calorie requirements of infants are relatively higher than those of adults; this is because of the increased demands for growth. During infancy the quality of the protein intake is as important as the quantity. Holt, Snyderman, and associates (5) conducted many studies on infants' protein and essential amino acid requirements. The synthetic diets used were based on the amino acid pattern of human milk, the only variable being the amino acid under investigation. They found that histidine, a nonessential amino acid for the human adult, is necessary for growth and maintenance of health in infants. Table 15–1 shows the requirements for essential amino acids for adults, schoolboys aged ten to 12 years, and infants, and lists the amino acids supplied by breast milk and cow's milk fed at levels compatible with health. The results of these studies indicate that the requirements for essential amino acids are affected by the amounts of protein-sparing nutrients, the ratio of essential to nonessential amino acids, and the pattern of essential amino acids in the diet. These workers state that the benefits of supplementation are attributable more to a correction of amino acid imbalance than to meeting a lack in absolute requirement.

The protein RDA for infants are based on the composition of human milk and are set at 1.8 gm. per 100 kcal. If computed according to body weight the allowance is 2.2 gm. per kg. during the first two months, 2.0 gm. per kg. from then to six months, and 1.8 gm. per kg. for the rest of the first year. It is assumed that mother's milk is 100 per cent utilized. Formulas prescribed in place of breast milk are planned to

Table 15–1

Requirements of Essential Amino Acids, and Intakes of Infants*

	Essential Amino Acid Requirements, Mg. Per Kg. Body Weight Daily			Intakes, Mg. Daily, of Infants Receiving	
Amino acid	Adults	School-boys 10 to 12 years	Infants	Human milk, 155 ml. per kg. daily	Cow's milk, amounts providing 2 gm. protein per kg. daily
Histidine	—	—	34	32	45
Isoleucine	7.8	28	119	123	128
Leucine	8.5	49	150	230	216
Lysine	6.1	59	103	112	156
Methionine	3.9§	27‡	45†	73	52
Phenylalanine	3.7§	27#	90§	92	104
Threonine	5.0	34	87§	80	92
Tryptophan	2.5	37	22	31	30
Valine	9.0	33	105	128	138

* Adapted from Holt and Snyderman, in *Nutrition Abstracts and Reviews,* 35: 1–13, 1965. Courtesy of the authors and *Nutrition Abstracts and Reviews.*
† In presence of cystine.
‡ In absence of cystine.
§ In presence of tyrosine.
# In absence of tyrosine.

simulate human milk. From one year on, as the diet contains protein of less optimal quality, the amount of the nutrient consumed should be proportionately higher. If infants under one year are fed regular mixed diets the quality conversion factor of 100/70, based on human milk should be applied.

The supply of minerals is important during infancy. The baby's rapid growth requires comparatively large amounts of calcium and phosphorus. Adequate prenatal nutrition will supply a store of bone minerals to prevent rickets, provided postnatal care furnishes a liberal supply of calcium and phosphorus. At first a very large percentage of the calcium a breast-fed baby receives is retained.

The thriving breast-fed infant receives daily approximately 0.06 gm. of calcium per kg. of body weight; the infant who is fed 100 ml. of cow's milk per kg. gets 0.12 gm. of calcium per kg. The latter retains more calcium, but despite this seeming advantage of cow's milk, the breast-fed baby's rate of growth is excellent. It has been demonstrated that the calcium of human milk is used more efficiently than is that of cow's milk. Beal (6) reported on calcium and phosphorus intakes of 94 children whom she followed serially from birth to two years. She calculated intakes from nutritional histories. Data were presented in terms of percentiles. Calcium and phosphorus intakes both increased in the first six to nine months; from then on into the preschool years calcium consumption decreased due to less use of milk. In Beal's study more girls than boys tended to be in the lower percentiles of intake of both calcium and phosphorus, but wide variations were noted. Dietary calcium:phosphorus ratios decreased steadily from one month to two years.

Kahn and co-workers (7) made carefully controlled balance studies on 30 healthy infants of one to 11 months, each balance period lasting for 28 days, and run consecutively in most subjects for eight to ten months. These studies were conducted in the home under careful supervision. Formula milk consumption averaged 654 ml. per day during the second month and fell gradually to 590 ml. per day by the tenth month as solid food intake increased. Calcium intake averaged 500 mg. per day throughout the study period. The lower-than-expected calcium intakes were associated with the use of pre-modified milk formulas which contained less calcium than cow's milk. Phosphorus intake rose from an average of 391 mg. per day in the second month to 519 mg. by the tenth month. Calcium and phosphorus retentions both increased with greater intake but at a less rapid rate as intake increased.

Hanna (8), who studied calcium absorption in term infants fed either human milk or prepared formulas, found that the fatty acid composition of the formula affected absorption of this mineral, and that a high content of palmitic and stearic acids had an adverse effect.

Dietary iron is the mineral most likely to be lacking, especially after the first few months. At birth the body of a healthy infant contains approximately 75 mg. iron per kg., about three times that of an adult, based on body weight. Approximately 55 mg. per kg. are found in the infant's red cells. During the first three to four months the baby's blood volume doubles and the concentration of iron in hemoglobin falls to about half that present at birth. This explains why the infant may get along without depending on dietary iron while he is doubling his birth weight. A low-birth-weight infant or one whose total hemoglobin mass is low at birth needs food iron earlier in life. The FNB advises 2 mg. per kg. per day soon after birth for this infant whereas the normal-term infant maintains optimal hemoglobin levels if he receives 1 mg. per kg. per day starting at about three months. The RDA is based on an average need, during the first year, of 1.5 mg. per kg. per day.

The high incidence of hypochromic anemia in infants, found after the fetal store of iron is depleted, is related to the proportionately greater need for iron during growth and probably to an inadequate dietary supply. The Committee on Nutrition of the American Academy of Pediatrics (9) states that a good mixed diet for an infant contains a maximum of 6 mg. iron per 1000 kcal unless foods are artificially fortified. Since eggs, meat, and green vegetables, the best sources of iron, are not consumed in sufficient amounts, enriched cereals should be used. These contain 8.6 to 22 mg. iron per ounce of dry cereal. The Committee recommends large-scale fortification of milk and grain products for infants who have outgrown baby foods but still do not consume large quantities of other foods.

Little research has been done on other minerals in the infant's diet. Of the trace elements, only sodium has been considered a matter of concern, and this in regard to an over- rather than an under-supply. Guthrie (10) considered this problem in relation to the use of processed baby foods which currently are salted. This practice caters more to the parent's taste than to the infant's nutritive needs. The intake of sodium by a breast-fed infant is less than one-third that of one fed cow's milk; this smaller amount is considered adequate. Young animals fed proportionately high salt diets have been found to have permanent, often fatal, hypertension.

A liberal supply of vitamins is necessary. Vitamin D is essential for utilization and retention of calcium and phosphorus. Since neither human nor cow's milk contains enough of the vitamin to assure prevention of rickets, a supplemental source is recommended for both breast-fed and formula-fed infants. In the past it was common to prescribe fish liver oils. Now the use of preparations in aqueous solution is preferred in order to avoid the possibility of lipoid pneumonia which may result from aspiration of oil by the very young infant. The water-miscible form combines very easily with milk formulas and the infant appears to use the vitamin more efficiently when it is dissolved in water rather than in oil. The FNB recommends a daily intake of 400 IU of vitamin D for both breast-fed and formula-fed infants. This amount is thought to permit excellent retention of calcium during infancy, provided the calcium intake is sufficient.

The use of vitamin D requires two precautions. The first relates to the time for beginning administration. During the first week of life feeding vitamin D tends to cause hypocalcemia, possibly because it aggravates the hypoparathyroid state which is evident at this time; this effect was demonstrated by Pincus and co-workers (11) in studies on newborn infants. The second precaution relates to dosage. Hypercalcemia occurs when excess of vitamin D is given. In severe cases renal function may be impaired and there may be an aortic systolic murmur. Because of these and other effects which may be related to excessive intake or defective metabolism the Committee on Nutrition of the American Academy of Pediatrics (12) recommends restricted use of vitamin D supplements in foods.

Most vitamin D preparations also contain vitamin A, which is essential as a growth promoter. The 1500 IU recommended by the FNB for the child under one year ordinarily are secured from either breast or cow's milk; breast milk contains more of the vitamin, especially in the early stages of lactation. Since cow's milk may at times furnish insufficient amounts of vitamin A, many pediatricians advise supplementing the baby's formula at an early age with egg yolk, green and yellow vegetables, and a concentrate containing vitamin A. Vitamin A, like vitamin D, is absorbed better from aqueous solution than from a fat medium. Excessive intake of vitamin A is not safe; it is thought that symptoms of excess appear more rapidly in the young infant than at a later age. Anorexia, hyperirritability and desquamation of the skin, bone decalcification, and increased intracranial pressure may be noted.

Since cow's milk is a poor and variable source of vitamin E satisfying the requirement for this vitamin presents problems. Variable intakes during pregnancy and inefficient placental transfer complicate the matter, especially in the newborn and premature baby (13). The FNB recommends 5 IU vitamin E daily during the first year. Since modified formulas and cereals are the main source of vitamin E for the young infant, Dicks-Bushnell and co-workers (14) analyzed six of the former and ten of the latter for both total- and α-tocopherol. Wide ranges were found. The amount of total tocopherol in the formulas was 0.08 to 3.86 mg. per 100 gm.; of α-tocopherol, 0.08 to 1.06 mg. In the ten cereals, total tocopherol was 0.03 to 1.80 mg.; α-tocopherol was 0.03 to 0.49 mg. Since considerable destruction may occur during processing these workers suggest supplementation with α-tocopherol.

Some infant formulas contain vegetable oils as a fat source. The relationship between PUFA and vitamin E requirement was discussed in Chapter 11. Hassan and co-workers (15) found a syndrome consisting of edema, skin lesions, an elevated platelet count, and morphologic changes in erythrocytes in premature infants fed formula mixtures containing relatively high PUFA. These abnormalities disappeared rapidly when vitamin E was given.

As explained in Chapter 11, the newborn is susceptible to hemorrhage caused by lack of vitamin K. The breast-fed baby is more susceptible than the artificially-fed. Deficiency of this vitamin is more likely to occur in premature or anoxic infants and those born to mothers who have received anticoagulants (16, 17). A single dose of 1 mg. of a water-miscible form of vitamin K_1 immediately after birth is considered adequate to prevent hemorrhage; excessive doses may be harmful.

Human milk contains, on an average, more than twice as much ascorbic acid as does cow's milk but some supplementary form of the vitamin is given customarily to all infants, since even the mother's milk may be lacking in the factor if her diet is poor. Vitamin C should be included early, always before the second month, and in sufficient amounts. Many physicians prescribe a concentrate of ascorbic acid or a bland fruit juice such as apple juice fortified with ascorbic acid instead of orange juice. The FNB recommends 35 mg. of ascorbic acid daily during the first year. In cases of nutritional anemia larger amounts may be prescribed because this vitamin, together with vitamin E, improves the response to iron therapy.

With the exception of niacin and inositol there are, on an average, larger quantities of the B-complex vitamins in cow's milk than in human milk. Even when heated, cow's milk is a better source of thiamin than human milk. For both bottle- and breast-fed infants an early supplement of thiamin is approved; enriched cereals and citrus fruit help to furnish the 0.4 mg. per 1000 calories recommended by the FNB for the child under one year. Milk is an excellent source of riboflavin and both breast-fed and formula-fed babies probably get enough of this factor if the milk intake is sufficient. In calculating the recommended allowance of riboflavin for infants the FNB assumes that 0.1 mg./kg.$^{0.75}$ is required to maintain tissue saturation. This amounts to 0.4 mg. per day at two months, 0.5 mg. at two to six months, and 0.6 mg. at six months to one year.

The niacin requirement is conditional on the intake of tryptophan. Provided no niacin is fed, the infant's need can be met by tryptophan from which niacin can be synthesized. Human milk is an excellent source of tryptophan and contains some niacin. One liter of human milk contains an average of 22 mg. tryptophan and 0.17 mg. niacin, making a total of niacin equivalent of 8 mg. per 1000 kcal. The daily requirement set by the FNB increases from 5 to 8 mg. equivalents during the first year of life.

The amount of vitamin B_6 in human milk is very low—only 0.01 to 0.03 mg. per liter during the first month. It gradually increases to 0.1 mg. per liter. At birth the infant has a store of vitamin B_6, due to a concentrating mechanism of the placenta. Since the baby's intake of milk increases and the concentration of protein in breast milk is low, the vitamin B_6 coenzymatic activity is not great enough to produce clinical signs of lack. However, the relationship of protein to vitamin B_6 is critical, and in cases where breast milk remains low in the vitamin, the protein may overtax the coenzymatic capacity. Convulsions result (18). In cow's milk with a protein content of 3.3 gm. per 100 gm. the vitamin B_6 level is also increased to 0.35–0.6 mg. per liter and no deficiency syndrome is manifest. In proprietary formulas the ratio of this vitamin to protein should be at least 0.015 mg. to 1 gm.

The infant's RDA for vitamin B_{12} is 1.0 to 2.0 μg. per day. Little is known about specific needs during infancy for the other water-soluble vitamins. According to Holt and Snyderman (5) a requirement for folic acid need not be considered if the diet contains enough ascorbic acid and if no antibiotics are taken. These workers also state that if the methionine intake is sufficient choline intake is not important. Pantothenic acid, biotin, and inositol are important as catalysts but are not known to be essential for the infant.

Table 15–2 lists the RDA of 16 nutrients for infants, expressed in amounts approved for 100 kcal of formula.

The requirements of the premature infant need special consideration. The premature infant has greater nutritional requirements because it is

Table 15–2

Recommended Dietary Allowances for Infants Expressed in Relation to Energy Needs (amounts per 100 kcal) *

	unit	*0–1/6 yr*	*1/6–1/2 yr*	*1/2–1 yr*
Protein	gm	1.8	1.8	1.8
Vitamin A	IU	300	200	170
Vitamin D	IU	80	50	45
Vitamin E	IU	1	1	1
Ascorbic Acid	mg	7	5	4
Folacin	mg	0.01	0.01	0.01
Niacin	mg-equiv.	1.0	0.9	0.9
Riboflavin	mg	0.08	0.07	0.07
Thiamin	mg	0.05	0.05	0.05
Vitamin B_6	mg	0.04	0.04	0.04
Vitamin B_{12}	μg	0.2	0.2	0.2
Calcium	mg	80	70	70
Phosphorus	mg	40	50	60
Iodine	μg	5	5	5
Iron	mg	1.2	1.3	1.7
Magnesium	mg	8	8	8

* Recommended Dietary Allowances, Seventh Revised Edition. Washington, D.C.: FNB, NAS-NRC Publ. 1694 (1968).

born with an inadequate store of nutrients and grows at a relatively rapid rate. During the first two weeks of life when the basal metabolic rate is low and there is little body activity, the calorie intake is not a primary concern; overfeeding is to be avoided. After two weeks, from 55 to 60 calories per pound of body weight are recommended to promote the growth rate expected in this baby. Since the ability to digest and absorb fat is thought to be below average, the formula prescribed is low in fat and proportionately high in carbohydrate. This reduction in fat intake may necessitate tocopherol supplementation; also, the increase in calories from carbohydrate may result in need for additional thiamin.

Studies on blood serum levels of calcium in premature and full-term infants have shown that the calcium content of blood is considerably lower and fluctuates more in premature than in full-term infants (19). Breast-milk feeding of premature babies appears to result in consistent increases in serum calcium levels. There is more lactose in human milk than in cow's milk, and this carbohydrate enhances calcium utilization.

To increase the protein and calcium intakes of the premature baby dry nonfat milk may be added to the human milk, expressed by hand because the infant is too weak to nurse. Casein hydrolysates and strained meats also have been used to supplement the milk supply and both result in favorable nitrogen retention. However, since the casein product is a better source of calcium, meat is advocated only for infants unable to take milk.

The premature infant is anemic. A low level of red blood cells and hemoglobin may be expected for about 12 weeks, when a slow but spontaneous rise will occur. Various preparations have been used to stimulate blood formation. Gorten and Cross (20) found that addition of 12 mg. of ferrous iron per quart of formula is effective prophylaxis against iron-deficiency anemia in premature infants.

Some authorities believe that premature infants require more vitamins A and D than do full-term infants because their absorption of fats is poor and growth needs are greater. As much as 2500 IU of vitamin A and 1000 IU of vitamin D daily in a water-miscible preparation have been recommended. However, since 1500 IU of vitamin A and 400 IU of vitamin D are considered very liberal for the full-term infant, other authorities do not think it necessary to give more than these amounts to the premature.

Vitamins E and K both need special consideration at this period. It is important not to use formulas high in PUFA or, if such formulas are prescribed, to give extra vitamin E (21). Although vitamin K may be needed to prevent hemorrhage, the fact that an excess may result in kernicterus must be remembered.

More ascorbic acid is needed because the premature infant does not metabolize the aromatic amino acids as completely as does the infant born at term, and because a high-protein diet is administered at this time. It has been shown that both tyrosine and phenylalanine are incompletely broken down by the premature infant when the ascorbic acid in the diet is not increased. From 50 to 100 mg. daily of the factor are advocated by Crosse (22), the larger amount for the infant on the higher protein diet. It is believed that both breast and cow's milk provide enough of the B-complex vitamins to promote growth in the premature baby.

It has been a common practice to delay the first feeding of the premature baby, who may exhibit a gag reflex and is susceptible to aspiration. Beard and co-workers (23) contrasted the effect of withholding food and liquid with that of early feeding of glucose solution and milk formula. One group of 69 infants was fasted for 72 hours. Another group of 60 was fed at six hours of age; on the first day, a glucose solution; on the second, half-strength milk formula; on the third, full-strength formula. In the first group hypoglycemia, ketonuria, and diminished liver glycogen stores were evident, in contrast to a normal state in the second group.

BREAST FEEDING VERSUS BOTTLE FEEDING

Many nutrition authorities advocate breast feeding. Certain advantages of human milk over cow's milk are well known. Colostrum, the first secretion of the mammary glands, is of great value to the baby. Table 15–3 shows its superior nutritive value in protein and in some of the minerals and vitamins. Colostrum also is rich in enzymes and immune bodies, all of which may be significant in the growth and health of newborns.

Some of the advantages attributed to breast feeding are no longer pertinent. One is rate of growth. Beal (24), who took nutritional histories serially on 95 infants over a two-year period, found that 68 per cent of the group were breast-fed at the beginning and, in 25 per cent of these, breast feeding was continued past two months. The other infants received either whole milk or evaporated milk formulas. There was no consistent relationship of physical growth to the type of feeding. Supplementing all three types of feeding with semisolid or solid foods and cow's milk at an early age tended to diminish differences which might otherwise have been significant.

The fact that human milk is more easily digested has been used as an argument for breast feeding. However, the curd of cow's milk, coarser and less flocculent than that of human milk, can be processed (by boiling or autoclaving) so that it is easily broken down and efficiently utilized. The fat of human milk is in a finer emulsion and contains more short-chain and unsaturated fatty acids than does cow's milk. This may account for easier digestion and assimilation, especially in premature and newborn infants. Tomarelli and co-workers (25) found that the most important factors adversely affecting total fat absorption were the content of palmitic acid in the 1,3 positions and the total stearic acid content.

Other considerations affect the type of feeding used. Breast feeding has been advocated because it has been found to reduce both morbidity and

Table 15–3

Composition of Milks Used in Infant Feeding*

PER 100 ML. OF WHOLE MILK

Nutrient	Human			Cow	Goat
	Colostrum (1–5 Days)	Transitional (6–10 Days)	Mature	Mature	Mature
Energy, cal.	58.0	74.0	71.0	69.0	76.0
Fat, gm.	2.9	3.6	3.8	3.7	4.1
Lactose, gm.	5.3	6.6	7.0	4.8	4.7
Protein, gm.	2.7	1.6	1.2	3.3	3.3
Casein, gm.	1.2	0.7	0.4	2.8	2.5
Lactalbumin, gm.		0.8	0.3	0.4	0.4
Minerals, gm.	0.33	0.24	0.21	0.72	0.77
Calcium, mg.	31.0	34.0	33.0	125.0	130.0
Phosphorus, mg.	14.0	17.0	15.0	96.0	106.0
Iron, mg.	0.09	0.04	0.15	0.10	0.05
Vitamins					
A, μg.	89.0	88.0	53.0	34.0	
Carotenoids, μg.	112.0	38.0	27.0	38.0	
D, U.S.P. units			0.42	2.36†	
E, mg.	1.28	1.32	0.56	0.06	
K, Dam-Glavind units‡			26.0	100.0	
Ascorbic acid, mg.	4.4	5.4	4.3	1.6	1.4
Biotin, μg.	0.1	0.4	0.4	3.5	6.3
Choline, mg.			9.0	13.0	
Folic acid, μg.	0.05	0.02	0.18	0.23	0.03
Inositol, mg.			39.0	13.0	21.0
Nicotinic acid, μg.	75.0	175.0	172.0	85.0	273.0
Pantothenic acid, μg.	183.0	288.0	196.0	350.0	289.0
Pyridoxine, μg.			11.0	48.0	7.0
Riboflavin, μg.	29.6	33.2	42.6	157.0	114.0
Thiamin, μg.	15.0	6.0	16.0	42.0	48.0
B_{12}, μg.	0.045	0.036	Trace	0.56	0.024

* Data from *The Composition of Milks*. FNB, NAS–NRC Publ. 254. Washington, D.C.: (Revised 1953).

† Based on mid-point of range.

‡ One Dam-Glavind unit equals the activity of 0.083 μg. of vitamin K_1.

mortality in infants. This is especially true when the bacteriologic safety of the substitute is questionable. Clinical observations have demonstrated that infants fed human milk have increased resistance to intestinal disorders and to respiratory diseases, including otitis media. György (26) suggests that the prevalence of *Lactobacillus bifidus* in the intestinal flora of infants fed human milk may play a role in promoting a healthier nutritional status. Human milk contains much more of a factor which promotes the growth of *Lactobacillus bifidus*. However, György believes that all the requirements of the young infant, at least until four to six months of life, can be met by either breast milk or a cow's milk formula when daily supplements of vitamin D, ascorbic acid, and iron are included. He also recommends addition of the B-complex vitamins to a cow's-milk formula.

Many psychological factors may be involved in the type of feeding chosen. A desirable relationship between mother and child may be favored through the act of nursing. There is little scientific support to the theory that the breast-fed baby is better adjusted to life than the bottle-fed child. Other reasons for breast feeding include a saving in time and labor, and elimination of sanitation problems and formula errors.

Breast feeding is not common today. This may be because of the mother's disinterest, or possibly, also, of the physician's lack of concern. Often the mother who attempts to nurse her baby will find she has an adequate supply of milk by the fifth day. If at first the output of milk is not sufficient, the flow often may be increased by complete drainage of the milk from the breast by manual expression after each nursing. Including more liquid and more protein in the diet may stimulate the flow. Avoiding undue fatigue, nervous strain, and overwork are important considerations. However, if nursing the baby is too great a strain on the mother's health, she is reassured by knowing that a formula on which the baby will thrive is obtainable.

The longitudinal study by Beal (27) between 1946 and 1966 gives data on the actual practices used by families of middle- and upper-middle socioeconomic levels who attended the Child Research Council of the School of Medicine, University of Colorado. Ninety-five infants were followed, most for their first two years. Serial nutritional histories were taken by a carefully developed technique. Average daily nutrient intakes were calculated; physical examination, anthropometric measurements, x-rays of long bones, and other physical and physiologic tests were administered. The children were under the care of 49 physicians in private practice. The results of this investigation are indicative of current practices. Of the 64 infants started on breast feeding, 34 were still breast fed at one month, 17 at three months; beyond six months, only nine were still breast fed. Solid foods and cow's milk were used to supplement the diet of both breast- and formula-fed infants. In the first month of life only nine infants received no food except breast milk; in the second month, only three. By the third month nursing infants received from other foods a median of 20 per cent of the total calories or protein intake of the formula-fed child.

PRACTICAL PROBLEMS OF FEEDING

The self-demand plan is favored by many pediatricians. In the past a feeding schedule was arbitrarily imposed upon an infant. Four-hour feeding intervals were usually considered most desirable. This practice is still followed in some hospitals until mother and baby are discharged. Once at home, the current trend is to let the infant determine how often and when he wants to be fed. For the self-demand method to be successful, the mother must be able to recognize hunger symptoms and she must be sure that the baby is really satisfied at the end of nursing. The majority of infants quickly adjust to receiving no food at night and make normal weight gains. Observations made by the Department of Pediatrics of the University of Chicago (28) indicate that most infants want to be fed five or six times in 24 hours and that, on the self-demand schedule, a reasonable interval is usually held, except during the late afternoon and evening when the demand is apt to be greater. On such a schedule most babies double their birth weight in less than five months and are not excessively fat and flabby. There is a marked reduction in amount of fussing and crying, and the immediate effect on the baby is favorable.

The self-demand plan may not work for premature and sickly infants. Too, a baby may suddenly increase his feedings to more than the usual number. If continued, this may be associated with disease or abnormality in the infant. In such cases, the physician should always be consulted.

The length of the nursing time varies. The baby usually takes 15 to 20 minutes to nurse. A study made on infants to determine the optimal feeding time showed that the average baby received three-fourths of his total intake during the first five minutes of nursing. This would indicate that the time suggested as the maximum is long enough for the average infant. To determine whether the period should be lengthened, the doctor may want data on the amount of milk the baby gets in the allotted time. This is accomplished by weighing the baby before and after nursing. When the self-demand method of feeding is used, a period of nursing of more than 30 to 40 minutes, or a demand to be fed more than seven or eight times a day, indicates that the milk supply is not sufficient. Ordinarily the child is nursed on one breast only, the other being used for the next period. If the child does not thrive on one breast, both should be offered. If this does not bring the desired results, a supplementary feeding is indicated.

The baby should be held while being fed. One argument advanced for breast feeding is the favorable emotional effect on child and mother. The mother-child relationship is improved by the close contact of the nursing period. If the infant is bottle-fed, he should be held in his mother's arms, not left in the crib.

Certain conditions contraindicate breast feeding. It sometimes happens that, even though she desires to nurse her infant, a mother is advised not to do so. Among the contraindications to breast feeding is a severe maternal illness, especially if fever or infection is present. If another pregnancy intervenes during lactation, nursing should be stopped to relieve the strain on the mother and to give both the new fetus and the young infant a better opportunity to develop. If the child is too weak to nurse or cannot because of harelip or cleft palate, the breast milk may be extracted, then administered to the baby with a medicine dropper. The premature infant often is fed this way.

Supplementing the mother's diet and the breast feedings may be preferred to complete weaning. Many women feel that an inadequate flow of milk is sufficient reason for putting the baby on a formula. This is not necessarily true since scientific investigations have shown that milk secretion often may be augmented. The sensible mother, under her physician's direction, will attempt to increase her supply; a few means of stimulation have been mentioned.

If the baby does not thrive on breast milk, the mother may continue to nurse it and, with the pediatrician's advice, replace one or more breast feedings with a formula and supplements such as orange and vegetable juices and vitamin B-complex preparations.

Weaning the breast-fed baby is best done gradually. The best time to wean an infant should be determined in consultation with the physician. If possible, weaning should be a gradual process. Some doctors suggest substitution of one breast feeding with a formula feeding, either in a bottle or by cup. This helps train the baby and also relieves the mother. In a day or two, an additional bottle or cup feeding is introduced. Sufficient intervals should be allowed for adjustment. With this procedure weaning is usually accomplished within a two- or three-week period.

PREPARATION OF THE FORMULA IN THE HOME

Many forms of milk are available. Fresh pasteurized and evaporated milks are most often used in preparing the formula at home. If the former is used, homogenized is preferred because its fat globules are fine and well dispersed throughout the liquid, and the curd is soft. Skim or partially-skimmed milk are prescribed on occasion. Many pediatricians advise evaporated milk because of its uniform composition, ease of digestion, and sterility. Vitamin D is already added to it. Condensed milk should not be confused with evaporated. The high sugar content of condensed milk makes its use inadvisable except in certain feeding problems and it is then used under the pediatrician's supervision. Dry milk, whole or skim, is used more often in making proprietary foods than in formulas prepared at home.

Occasionally, an infant does not thrive on cow's milk, and another milk source must be used. Difficult feeding cases, especially those involving milk idiosyncrasy, have been brought to a normal condition by use of goat's milk. The quantitative composition of goat's and cow's milk is quite similar (Table 15–3). The fat in goat's milk is more highly emulsified than the fat in cow's milk, and the curd formed from goat's milk tends to be granular rather than elastic. These characteristics make it an easily digested product. Another advantage is that it does not carry the tubercle bacillus. However, goat's milk must be pasteurized lest it transmit undulant fever. In some countries the milk of other mammals such as the ass, camel, llama, reindeer, sheep, or water buffalo is available.

Cow's milk must be modified because of its composition. Comparison of the constituents of cow's and human milk shows numerous differences (Table 15–3). Since cow's milk has about three times as much protein and ash, it might seem logical to dilute in a ratio of 1:3 to make it equivalent to the human product. However, this amount of dilution does not promote normal development in the infant. The trend now is to modify cow's milk so that the formula approaches human milk in protein and mineral content; calories are restored by adding carbohydrate and fat rich in the essential fatty acids. An allowance of from 1½ to 2 ounces of cow's milk per pound of body weight has been found to supply sufficient protein.

Dilution of the milk according to protein needs involves lowering the other constituents as well. The fat is considerably reduced, which may be an advantage, since fat is difficult for the baby to digest. The fat in cow's milk contains a higher percentage of volatile fatty acids than the fat in human milk (10 per cent compared to 1.5 per cent). These fatty acids have been shown to be irritating to the alimentary tract and to hinder the digestive processes. Thus dilution of cow's milk is necessary to produce a formula that will be well tolerated and digested with comparative ease.

The carbohydrate in both types of milk is lactose. Cow's milk contains about two-thirds as much lactose as human milk, and this is further reduced on dilution. In order to increase the energy value of the formula, some form of carbohydrate is added. Sucrose and corn syrup are most often used. They are usually well tolerated and less expensive than other sugars. In case of unusual gas production, lactose or dextrimaltose may be substituted. Several dextrimaltose compounds are on the market. Some contain no ash, some have sodium chloride, and some have a potassium salt. The latter type is used in certain proprietary foods because cow's milk is deficient in potassium and because the salt acts as a laxative.

The total amount of carbohydrate recommended for the infant is 4 to 6 gm. per pound per day. When the quantity contained in milk is calculated, it will be found that an additional 0.1 ounce of sugar per pound of body weight will be sufficient. Pediatricians usually set 1.5 ounces per day as the upper limit of sugar addition, since an excess may cause diarrhea and will result in a craving for sweets.

The mineral content of cow's and human milk varies in both quantity and quality. Table 15–4 gives the comparative amounts of minerals in the two milks. With the exception of iron, zinc, and copper, cow's milk con-

Table 15–4

The Mineral Content of Mature Human and Cow's Milk*

EXPRESSED IN MG. PER 100 ML. OF WHOLE MILK

Mineral	Human Milk	Cow's Milk
Calcium	33	125
Magnesium	4	12
Potassium	55	138
Sodium	15	58
Phosphorus	15	96
Sulfur	14	30
Chlorine	43	103
Zinc	0.53	0.38
Iron	0.15	0.10
Copper	0.04	0.03
Iodine	0.007†	0.021

* Data from *The Composition of Milks.* FNB, NAS–NRC Publ. 254. Washington, D.C. (Revised 1953).
† From analysis of skimmed human milk.

tains more of all the minerals, and a dilution of 1 to 1 still leaves as much ash as is found in human milk. The proportion of phosphorus is high in cow's milk due to its greater casein content. Comparisons made of the absorption and retention of ash by breast-fed infants and those receiving whole cow's milk showed that the bottle-fed baby absorbed 60 per cent of the total ash and retained only about 15 per cent, whereas the breast-fed baby absorbed 80 per cent of the ash and retained 40 to 50 per cent. It appears that the ash of human milk is superior to that of cow's for infant feeding.

Whole milk modification is frequently used. Whole cow's milk, diluted with water and reinforced with carbohydrate, may be recommended for the normal bottle-fed infant. The following guides are suggested for formula preparations:

1. *For protein:* Allow 1½ to 2 ounces of milk per pound of body weight. If sudden weaning is necessary, only 1 ounce of milk per pound is advocated, with a gradual increase to 1½ ounces. In some cases, an infant may need 2½ ounces per pound for normal growth.
2. *For carbohydrate:* Add 0.1 ounce of sugar per pound of body weight.
3. *For total liquid:* Allow 2 ounces more of fluid per feeding than the baby is months old until the age of six months. By this time, the infant will be receiving other foods so that feedings larger than 8 ounces are not needed. The total fluid requirement may be met by giving water and fruit or vegetable juices between feedings.

4. *For calories:* Allow 45 to 55 per pound daily during the first year. The total should be sufficient to permit normal growth. The milk formula will supply most of the calories during the first three or four months. From then on the gradual supplementation with solid foods will provide additional calories.

An acid milk formula is prescribed for some infants. Acid is usually combined with evaporated milk and corn syrup in amounts determined by the physician. Lactic acid is used more often than are other acids, such as hydrochloric, acetic in vinegar, or citric in fruit juices. Probably the most important advantage of this type of formula is its aid in digesting protein. Cow's milk is digested more slowly and less completely than human milk due largely to its high buffer content, that is, its capacity to bind a large amount of the hydrochloric acid normally secreted in the infant's stomach. Acid may need to be added to counteract the neutralizing effect of cow's milk. Another important function of the acid is to precipitate the casein in very fine soft curds which are more quickly digested than are the typical casein curds.

Because of its greater ease of digestion, it is common to feed acid milk in undiluted form, thus increasing the formula's calorie value. For this reason the acid milk formula is frequently given to premature and to malnourished babies, and to those who have limited gastric capacity and who regurgitate when a large quantity of food is fed.

Many proprietary foods are available. These are planned in relation to human milk which, with the exception of iron and vitamin D, is thought to meet the needs of a normal infant. Manufacturers approach the problem through addition, elimination, and alteration. Some physicians prefer these proprietary products to those made at home. According to Owen (29), about half the babies who are not breast fed at four months receive these products.

Owen describes three general types of proprietary foods based on cow's milk. The first, which is currently fed to less than 1 per cent of infants, consists of the protein, fat, minerals, and carbohydrate of cow's milk but the fat content is reduced and some carbohydrate is added: vitamins also are added to meet the requirements. In another type, the butterfat is replaced by vegetable oil, usually corn or coconut. The concentrations of protein, carbohydrate, and vitamins are also adjusted. About 30 per cent of the four-month-old infants in the United States receive this type of feeding. The third type of proprietary food differs from the others in two main ways. Butterfat is replaced by a vegetable oil, and the mineral and protein concentrations are changed to make them similar to human milk. This is done by using a mixture of partially demineralized whey proteins and skim milk, with appropriate amounts of mineral salts. More detailed information on these products may be obtained in Owen's article or from specific product labels.

ADDITION OF FOODS DURING THE FIRST YEAR

Water is the earliest addition. Even more essential to the body than food is water, a constituent of its structure and a regulator of its activities. The water requirements of infants are relatively higher than those of adults and special attention must be given to guard against dehydration. The total amount of liquid required daily by the very young infant is equal to approximately 3 ounces per pound of body weight. By the last months of the first year, 2 ounces per pound is sufficient. Part of this fluid is included in the regular feedings. In addition, sterile lukewarm water should be given at intervals daily from birth on and may be fed from a teaspoon or bottle.

Vitamin supplements are the next additions. Some source of vitamin D and of ascorbic acid should be included early in the diet of both breast- and bottle-fed infants. Administration of vitamin D usually begins within two weeks to a month after birth, reaches the maximal dosage within the third month, and is continued for two or more years. It is not thought wise to give vitamin D during the first week of life because of its hypocalcemic effect. The amount of vitamin D is prescribed by the physician. When the baby adjusts to this supplement, ascorbic acid is given; if the pure vitamin is prescribed, it is usually added to the formula. If orange juice is the choice, 1 teaspoon diluted in an equal amount of sterile water is thought to be sufficient at first and may be gradually increased until the infant receives 2 ounces or more of juice a day. It may be fed from spoon or bottle and later from a cup, either just before a feeding period or between periods. Tomato juice, if used for economy, should not be spiced and more should be given, since it has approximately only half the ascorbic acid content of orange juice. Apple juice fortified with ascorbic acid is tolerated well by many infants.

Some pediatricians prescribe a multivitamin preparation containing ascorbic acid, vitamins A and D, and members of the B complex. This practice may simplify the mother's work and may tend to insure the daily intake of these nutrients. Other specialists favor use of the natural sources, believing that the infant should learn early to take a variety of flavors, textures, and consistencies, which the multivitamin product does not provide.

The timing of additions of solid foods to the diet of the infant varies. Today there is a trend toward offering the infant solid foods at an early age, sometimes within a few weeks of birth. Guthrie (30) reported on the use of solid foods, both as to timing and nutrient contribution. Of 129 infants, about half were breast fed. Of the remaining 56, 32 per cent had been offered solid food by three weeks of age. By nine weeks all infants received solid foods. However, these food supplements added little to the calorie intake. At three weeks they supplied an average of

5 per cent of the calories, at seven weeks, 12 per cent, at 13 weeks, 21 per cent. Iron and thiamin were the important contributions from the solid foods.

The times of introducing new foods suggested in this chapter are conservative; they may be changed on the advice of the pediatrician. During the second, third, or fourth month both bottle- and breast-fed babies usually are given cereal daily. Specially formulated infant cereals or strained well-cooked regular cereals diluted with formula or milk should be served at first. Later, perhaps by the fifth month, unstrained cereals may be fed. The variety of cooked cereals may be increased as the baby grows older, so that the child will become accustomed to different textures and learn to like a number of foods. Cereals are given for their fuel value, for their aid in elimination, and if whole grain or enriched products, for their contribution of iron and vitamins.

Some authorities advocate giving vegetables and fruits before cereals. However, a more common practice is to include these foods after cereals, at about four or five months. Vegetables usually are introduced before fruits. Spinach, carrots, green beans, and peas are among the first vegetables given, but others may be used for variety. Ripe mashed bananas, cooked strained apricots, applesauce, peaches, pears, and prunes are the first fruits added. Strained fruits and vegetables specially prepared for infant feeding may be purchased or the foods may be prepared at home by cooking until very soft, straining, and for vegetables, seasoning lightly with salt. If the new flavor or texture proves objectionable, the food may be mixed with cereal or diluted with milk or formula.

The amounts of cereal, vegetables, and fruit to be fed cannot be stated in specific figures. Probably a teaspoonful a day of each is enough at first. As the child becomes accustomed to the foods, the quantity may be increased until good-sized servings are fed. They may be given before the breast or bottle feeding and at a time when the appetite tends to be keen. Cereal might be given before the 10 A.M. feeding, and fruit or vegetable before the 2 P.M. feeding. Special care must be taken so that the amount is not enough to cause a sensitization of food or diarrhea. If diarrhea does occur, the food responsible should be omitted from the diet until the child is again normal and administered in a smaller quantity the next time it is offered. Because of the laxative quality of fruits and vegetables the change from sieved to unsieved form must be gradual and should be determined by the roughage content of each food.

Foods should be given to aid in the eruption of teeth. Teething begins at about the fifth or sixth month and the infant may want to put things in his mouth. At this time strips of hard dry toast or zwieback may be given; later, graham crackers may be offered. Very little toast will be consumed at first, but the sucking and chewing processes will help develop the gums and assist in eruption of teeth. When the child learns to swallow the food, the calorie intake will be increased.

Egg yolk may be added between the third and fifth months. Egg yolk is given to the young child because it is a source of iron, vitamin A, and the B-complex vitamins. Ordinarily, the physician will prescribe only ¼ teaspoon daily for the first few days. This small quantity may be increased gradually until the baby gets the whole yolk; then small portions of the white may be included. Because egg white may lead to protein sensitization, the daily intake should be small at first, then increased cautiously. Egg yolk may be served in a variety of ways: soft cooked, hard cooked and grated, or in combination with such other foods as milk, cereal, fruit, or vegetable. Some pediatricians advise the inclusion of egg yolk before addition of cereals and vegetables or fruits.

Meat is advocated in the infant's diet. Meat may be included as early as the second month. Some pediatricians recommend canned pureed meats, meat soups, or scraped lean meat mixed with cereal as soon as the infant can eat from a spoon. Later, ground broiled meat, including liver, beef, lamb, veal, pork, and poultry, may be fed. The intakes of protein, iron, and some vitamins are increased by addition of meats.

Variety in foods is important. When variety in the diet is stressed, a child tends to have fewer dislikes and develops a natural interest in the new and unknown. On the other hand, when the same foods are served every day a feeding problem may result. However, it is important to introduce new foods gradually and to allow the infant to become familiar with one food before introducing another. The wise mother will begin early to alternate foods and to encourage the child to eat at least a little of several foods.

Some early additions to the baby's diet are baked potato, cream soups, thoroughly boned flaked fish and canned salmon and tuna, scraped apple, junket, custard, and cornstarch pudding. Butter or margarine may be used in moderation. Bacon, cooked crisp, may be given. Sugar should be used sparingly, not because it is a harmful food, but because it detracts from the original flavor and creates a "sweet tooth" in the baby. Whole grain cereals and breads may be given as soon as the child's digestive tract will accept the roughage, but the transition should be gradual.

The infant may take whole undiluted milk at six months or even earlier. This practice is often followed at a very early age when reconstituted evaporated milk is given. In such a case, the infant's fluid needs must still be met. A change also must be made from the self-demand schedule to three meals a day with a lunch in midmorning and afternoon. This will simplify the mother's problem in feeding her family. The baby may eat breakfast and the noon meal with the family if the atmosphere is calm, but, because his food is simple and his bedtime is early, he should have his night meal separately.

The feeding of every infant should be watched by a competent pediatrician. Infant welfare clinics, supported by municipal health departments and private organizations, aim to provide this supervision for infants whose families cannot afford private care. Excellent bulletins on infant feeding are available from federal and state sources.

INDICATIONS OF HEALTH IN AN INFANT

The most common criterion is regular gain in weight. The infant's weight is a useful indication of progress. At birth the average baby weighs 7 to 7.5 pounds, about one-tenth of which is lost during the first few days but usually regained in about two weeks. From this time on, the infant should gain consistently. At first the breast-fed infant gains more rapidly and uniformly, but by the end of the year the bottle-fed baby will have made an equivalent growth. In the past it was expected that a healthy baby should double his weight in six months and treble it in a year; today, many infants double their birth weight in three to four months. A stationary weight or a gain of only 2 or 3 ounces a week implies that something is wrong; on the other hand, an increment in excess of 8 ounces a week may not be considered wise, since retarded bone growth and slow physical development may be associated with it. Gastrointestinal disturbances in the second year may result from previous overfeeding.

The increase in height, while proportionately much less than that in weight, is also a sign of health and should be fairly regular. From about 20 inches at birth, the baby will increase to 30 or more by the end of the first year. Modern babies grow taller than their parents. Height is less affected by nutrition disorders than is weight; however, stunted growth may result from lack of minerals and vitamins.

Adequate nutrition is indicated by other physical signs. Rosy cheeks, bright eyes, good muscle tonus, and a firm layer of subcutaneous fat are signs of health in an infant. Eruption of teeth begins at about the fifth month. The girl's teeth usually appear earlier than those of the boy, those of the breast-fed infant before those of the bottle-fed. By the end of the first year from six to 12 teeth may be expected.

During the first few months the infant will sleep much of the 24 hours, awakening only to be fed. Exercising arms and legs is a part of normal development, as is a lusty cry when the child is hungry. With physical wants satisfied, the child will sleep through the night without demanding attention. A well baby is a happy one.

Elimination is an indication of health. The stools of a breast-fed infant are normally soft in consistency, yellow in color, and slightly aromatic in odor. Sometimes they contain small soft fat curds and an excess of mucus and are greenish in color. However, if the infant is healthy in other respects, these slight abnormalities should be ignored. On a diet of cow's milk the bowel movements will be fewer in number than the two or three eliminated daily by the breast-fed infant. They are firmer in consistency, a lighter yellow in color, and more offensive in odor, due to the larger amount of protein in the milk. Again mucus and curds may be present and, if accompanied by poor gain in weight, may indicate a need for a dietary change. Constipation is more likely in the bottle-fed baby because of such contributing factors as the lower amount of lactose and the alkalinity of the fecal mass. Treatment under the direction of a doctor should be largely dietary and may involve a change in the type of carbohydrate used, addition of cereal or vegetable, or increase in orange and other fruit pulps. Correcting constipation before the habit becomes fixed is important and essential for the baby's optimal health.

PROBLEMS

1. Calculate milk modification formulas for normal infants of different ages according to rules given in the text. Compare with the suggestions for the bottle feeding of normal infants in the Children's Bureau bulletin, *Infant Care,* and similar bulletins from state departments.
2. Plan formulas for babies of different ages with the following variables:
   a. Whole milk with different carbohydrate supplements.
   b. Dried milk.
   c. Evaporated milk.
   d. Proprietary foods.
   Calculate the amount of calories, protein, carbohydrate, fat, calcium, phosphorus, iron, and vitamins for each of the day's formulas.
3. Visit a well-baby clinic, observe the babies as they are weighed, and if permitted, listen to the conference between the mother and doctor, nurse, or nutritionist.

REFERENCES

1. Benedict, F. G., *et al. The Gaseous Metabolism of Infants.* Washington, D.C.: Carnegie Institution of Washington, Publ. 201 (1914).
2. Rose, H. E., *et al.* Activity, Calorie Intake, Fat Storage, and the Energy Balance of Infants. *Pediat., 41:*18 (1968).
3. Hansen, A. E., *et al.* Role of Linoleic Acid in Infant Nutrition. *Pediat., 31:*171 (1963).
4. Wiese, H. F., *et al.* Essential Fatty Acids in Infant Nutrition. *J. Nutr., 66:*345 (1958).
5. Holt, L. E., *et al.* Nutrition in Infancy and Adolescence. *In* M. G. Wohl and R. S. Goodhart (eds.), *Modern Nutrition in Health and Disease,* 4th ed. Philadelphia: Lea & Febiger (1968).
6. Beal, V. A. Calcium and Phosphorus in Infancy. *J. Am. Diet. Ass., 53:*450 (1968).
7. Kahn, B., *et al.* Intake and Excretion of Calcium and Phosphorus by Infants: Calcium Retention and Model. *Pediat., 43:*668 (1969).
8. Hanna, F. M., *et al.* Calcium—Fatty Acid Absorption in Term Infants Fed Human Milk and Prepared Formulas Simulating Human Milk. *Pediat., 45:*216 (1970).

9. Committee on Nutrition of the American Academy of Pediatrics. Iron Balance and Requirements in Infancy. *Pediat., 43:*134 (1969).

10. Guthrie, H. A. Infant Feeding Practices—A Predisposing Factor in Hypertension? *Am. J. Clin. Nutr., 21:*863 (1968).

11. Pincus, J. B., *et al.* Effects of Vitamin D on the Serum Calcium and Phosphorus Levels in Infants During the First Week of Life. *Pediat., 13:*178 (1954).

12. Committee on Nutrition of the American Academy of Pediatrics. The Relation Between Infantile Hypercalcemia and Vitamin D—Public Health Implications in North America. *Pediat., 40:*1050 (1967).

13. Herting, D. C. Perspective in Vitamin E. *Am. J. Clin. Nutr., 19:*210 (1966).

14. Dicks-Bushnell, M. W., *et al.* Vitamin E Content of Infant Formulas and Cereals. *Am. J. Clin. Nutr., 20:*262 (1967).

15. Hassam, H., *et al.* Syndrome in Premature Infants Associated with Low Plasma Vitamin E Levels and High Polyunsaturated Fatty Acid Diet. *Am. J. Clin. Nutr., 19:*147 (1966).

16. Sutherland, J. M., *et al.* Hemorrhagic Disease of the Newborn. Breast Feeding as a Necessary Factory in Pathogenesis. *Am. J. Dis. Childr., 113:*524 (1967).

17. Committee on Nutrition of the American Academy of Pediatrics. Vitamin K Compounds and the Water-Soluble Analogues. *Pediat., 28:*501 (1961).

18. Bessey, O. A., *et al.* Intake of Vitamin B_6 and Infantile Convulsions: A First Approximation of Requirements of Pyridoxine in Infants. *Pediat., 20:*33 (1957).

19. Bruck, E., *et al.* Serum Calcium and Phosphorus in Premature and Full-Term Infants. *Am. J. Dis. Childr., 90:*653 (1955).

20. Gorten, M. K., *et al.* Iron Metabolism in Premature Infants. II. Prevention of Iron Deficiency. *J. Pediat., 64:*509 (1964).

21. Hanna, F. M., *et al.* Vitamin E in the Nutrition of the Premature Newborn Infant. *Am. J. Clin. Nutr., 16:*384 (1965).

22. Crosse, V. M. The Feeding of Premature Infants. *Brit. J. Nutr., 6:*230 (1952).

23. Beard, A. G., *et al.* Prenatal Stress and the Premature Neonate. *J. Pediat., 68:*329 (1966).

24. Beal, V. A. Breast- and Formula-Feeding of Infants. *J. Am. Diet. Ass., 55:*31 (1969).

25. Tomarelli, R. M., *et al.* Effect of Positional Distribution on the Absorption of the Fatty Acids of Human Milk and Infant Formulas. *J. Nutr., 95:*583 (1968).

26. György, P. Orientation in Infant Feeding. *Fed. Proc., 20:* No. 1, Part III, Supp. No. 7:169 (1961).

27. Beal, V. A. The Nutritional History in Longitudinal Research, *J. Am. Diet. Ass., 51:*426 (1967).

28. Aldrich, C. A., *et al.* A Self-Regulating Feeding Program for Infants. *J. Am. Med. Ass., 135:*340 (1947).

29. Owen, G. M. Modification of Cow's Milk for Infant Formulas: Current Practices. *Am. J. Clin. Nutr., 22:*1150 (1969).

30. Guthrie, H. A. Effect of Early Feeding of Solid Foods on Nutritive Intake of Infants. *Pediat., 38:*879 (1966).

Nutrition During Childhood, Adolescence, and the Later Years

16

Throughout childhood and adolescence, intricate adjustments occur, involving changes in body size, shape, and proportion, all easily observable. Later, the more active processes of growth characteristic of youth are replaced by those that involve preservation of the integrity of the body tissue and maintenance of metabolic activities. Since 1900 the average life expectancy has risen in the United States from 49 to over 70 years. As a result, the nutritional needs and practices of the elderly are receiving increased attention.

Development of good food habits and nutrition practices in early childhood establish the foundation for adult health. The nutrients discussed earlier are necessary for maintenance of health and well-being, but requirements for specific nutritional factors vary as the metabolic demands change during successive periods of life. In recent years several groups of investigators have initiated longitudinal studies, in which the variables studied have included body build, physiological vs. chronological age, socioeconomic status, and ethnic background. Dietary, clinical, and biochemical findings have been used in assessing nutritional status. Some of these studies will be mentioned in this chapter.

Childhood and Adolescence

GROWTH AND DEVELOPMENT OF CHILDREN AND ADOLESCENTS

Rates of growth and development are less rapid after the first year but are equally important. Never again during life does growth continue so rapidly as during the first year. From about one year until adolescence, the rate of growth in both weight and height declines. Then comes a period of acceleration, between age 11 and 13 in girls and age 13 to 15 in boys. Following this is another decline in rate until, at about 17 for girls and 19 for boys, skeletal growth is completed.

Certain variations in growth must be considered. Throughout childhood boys are taller and heavier than girls, the one exception being at age 11 to 12 when girls mature more rapidly and exceed boys. A table in the Appendix gives average weight and height for boys and girls ages four to 17. It has been shown that the child who is superior physically is likely to mature at an earlier age and will achieve full growth and stature sooner than the child whose physical status is sub-optimum.

Studies have been made on body composition. During growth and maturation the relative amounts of water, sodium, and chlorine decrease whereas nitrogen, calcium, phosphorus, potassium, and magnesium increase (1). During adolescence the fat-free content of the boy's body increases to a greater extent than the girl's (2). By age 20 the girl's body fat content is one and one-half to two times that of the boy's. Young and co-workers (3) determined body density, skinfold thickness, and anthropometric measurements of 102 normal girls aged nine through 16. These workers developed regression equations to predict specific gravity which may be used to indicate total body fatness. They found that fatness is more closely related to physiological than chronological age and that there is a marked difference between children depending on sexual development.

Studies of rate of growth show that weight increment is not uniform throughout the year but proceeds irregularly, being greater during the fall and early winter months and less in the late winter and spring. Possible causes of this variability are diet, sunshine, exercise, nervous tension, and susceptibility to infectious disease. Nationality and type of build are influential factors in growth, in both height and weight, and an evaluation of nutrition by means of weight that does not consider these facts is unreliable. Normal children grow at different rates and the most rapid rate may not always be best in the long run. Weight gain may result merely from increased calorie intake and may not be an indication of healthy growth. Studies by Mitchell (4) have shown that improved nutrition can affect stature in a national group. She found that improved nutrition practices in Japan since 1948 have resulted in increased stature of school children. In 1962 boys of age 14 were 3 inches taller and girls of age 11 were 2½ inches taller than were children of those ages in 1948.

Investigators of children's physical growth have set up a variety of standards for assessing individual progress. The standards may be expressed in graphs, tables, or in the case of bone growth, in x-rays, and may be based on various body parts such as weight of the body, standing height, stem length, girth of chest, pelvis, arm or calf, breadth of pelvis or chest, and development of the carpal bones and epiphyses of the hand.

Macy and Kelly (5), who have appraised skeletal growth and development with x-rays, stress the fact that assessments of both growth and development should be included since each contributes to the general picture. They also advise that these and other measurements be made throughout the entire period of childhood and, if possible, each time by the same assessors. Other means of investigating the ways in which a child grows and develops include psychometric observations, anthropometric measurements, chemical and metabolic assessments, urinary excretion, hematological changes, gastrointestinal activity, and tooth development.

Appearance and attitudes indicate the child's state of nutrition. Certain outward signs of well-being are associated with a healthy child. These include:

Hair—smooth and lustrous.
Eyes—bright and clear with no dark circles under them.
Skin—clear, smooth and slightly moist; mucous membranes pink.
Subcutaneous fat—abundant and firm.
Muscles—well-developed throughout the body; with good tonus.
Skeletal structure—bones of legs and arms straight with no enlargement of joints; chest broad and deep with room for lung expansion; pelvic arch of optimal measurement; skull and jaw well-shaped and developed; teeth well-formed, well-placed, and without cavities.
Posture—head erect, chest out, abdomen in, feet parallel.

There also must be evidences of normal functioning such as are shown by good mastication, digestion, absorption, and elimination. Sleep and rest, exercise, relaxation, sunshine, and good sanitation are essential parts of a regime which will be reflected in the child's appearance as well as in his reactions toward life.

THE ENERGY REQUIREMENT

The basal needs have been determined. Since there is an intensive stimulus to cellular activity in the child, the basal metabolism is higher than that of the adult. It is also known that the relatively greater surface area contributes to the increased rate. Studies on the basal metabolism of children and adolescents have been conducted in a number of laboratories in various parts of the world and basal metabolism standards have been formulated from the resulting data. Table 3–1 (p. 37) shows that the metabolism of girls is lower than that of boys at all age levels.

The total calorie needs vary at different ages and with different activities. Many dietary studies have been made in which calorie intakes were estimated for children of different ages, and as would be expected, wide individual variations are noted depending on age, weight, and activity. In recent years when the dangers of obesity in adult life have been emphasized, it is natural that this condition in children should be investigated. Some of the obesity in children is associated more with inactivity than with overeating (6). In estimating any individual's calorie need, activity as well as weight and age should be considered.

The FNB recommends about 80 kcal per kg. for the child up to ten years and then gradual decrease to 50 kcal per kg. for adolescent boys and 35 kcal per kg. for adolescent girls. These average figures may not apply to an individual child who varies depending on the amount and intensity of physical activity. Variations are also marked due to the onset of adolescence. During both childhood and adolescence the test of a sufficiency in calorie intake depends on the extent to which growth needs and other signs of physical health are met.

Taylor and co-workers (7) investigated the total energy requirements of children from the activity standpoint. Studies were performed on boys and girls of seven to 14 years, and from seven to 20 children were used for each activity. The basal metabolic rates of the nine- to 11-year-old children ranged from 1.42 to 1.60 calories per kg. per hour for the boys, and 1.41 to 1.49 for the girls. In general, it was found that the more strenuous activities demanded more fuel and that the younger children required more kcal per kg. of weight for an activity.

The importance of sufficient calorie intake for growth, both visible and invisible, was demonstrated by Macy and Hunscher (8) in a study on ten healthy children, four to nine years old, over 45 consecutive five-day balance periods. The diet was adequate and contained 1 quart of milk per child daily; protein furnished 14 to 16 per cent of the calories. Despite inclusion of this amount of protein, nitrogen retention was depressed when the calorie consumption was not sufficient to promote a satisfactory gain in body weight. A difference as little as 10 kcal per kg. was sufficient to cause failure in growth.

THE PROTEIN AND MINERAL REQUIREMENTS

The protein demand per unit of body weight decreases. This is more marked than that of calories since the need for protein is not affected by activity. The total protein allowance set by the FNB increases from 25 gm. for the two-year-old to 40 gm. for the eight- to ten-year-old. Thereafter, allowances for the two sexes differ. By 18 the boy's allowance is set at 60 gm. per kilo, that of the girl, at 55 gm. Increments for growth were added to the maintenance protein requirement based on the fact that gain in body weight is 18 per cent protein.

One of the most extensive investigations of protein intake of children was conducted by Stearns and associates (9)—458 studies on 51 children, one to four years old, and 481 studies on 67 children, four to ten years old. Creatinine excretion was studied as a measure of skeletal muscle growth, as well as of nitrogen retention in relation to intake. Growth of skeletal muscle exceeds that of the body as a whole in children of these ages and will be sacrificed to avoid loss of nitrogen from other more vital tissues if protein intake is insufficient. As a result of these investigations Stearns and co-workers recommend 3 to 3.5 gm. of protein per kg. per day during the preschool years and from then on a gradual decline not to reach 2.5 gm. per kg. per day until after the tenth year. By this time the adult proportion of skeletal muscle to total body weight should be attained. Another argument for liberal protein is its beneficial effect on bone development; in extreme protein malnutrition the bones tend to be smaller, less well-calcified, and with fewer trabeculae.

Biochemical tests have been used to ascertain the protein nutriture of adolescent and preadolescent children. Hodges and Krehl (10) found that about 8 per cent of a large group of teenagers in Iowa had total protein below 6 gm./100 ml. blood; this marks a deficient level. Christakis and co-workers (11) studied 642 children, ten to 13 years old, in New York City. In 7 per cent the ratio of serum amino acids was 2.0 or more, indicating probable protein malnutrition. This ratio, determined by chromatographic technique, involves the essential amino acids leucine, isoleucine, valine, and methionine in the denominator and the nonessential amino acids glycine, serine, glutamine, and taurine in the numerator. In protein malnutrition the essential amino acids in the serum are lowered, while the nonessential amino acids are almost unchanged (12).

Quality of protein in the diet influences growth. The choice of protein sources is especially important for children of all ages and must be considered in deciding on the kind and amount of protein to be included in the diet. When a larger proportion of the less adequate sources is used, a greater total amount is required. However, since protein is so vital a building food, it seems especially wise to include in children's diets a liberal supply of those kinds which have high biological value. The amino acid requirements during growth and the comparative values of different proteins in this respect were discussed in Chapter 6. The importance of good quality protein was demonstrated in a nitrogen balance study by Abernathy and co-workers (13) on 15 healthy children, seven to nine years old. Diets were developed to simulate those of many low-income Southern families: one diet contained 25 gm. protein, a second, 46 gm. On the lower protein diet there was poor retention of nitrogen, on the other, adequate retention. The low sulfur amino acid content was considered the main reason for failure of the first diet.

Calcium and phosphorus requirements of children and adolescents are high. As skeletal growth continues comparatively rapidly, the needs for liberal amounts of calcium and phosphorus may be expected. Leitch and Aitken (14) estimated that approximately 1200 gm. of calcium are accumulated in the human body from birth to age 20. The daily retention for skeletal growth is thought to be between 75 and 150 mg. per day from the first to the eighth years of life, and it may be as great as 400 mg. per day during the prepubertal and pubertal periods. The FNB believes that these requirements will be more than adequately met by daily calcium allowances of 800 mg. for the two- to six-year-old child, gradually increasing to 1200 mg. by the tenth to 12th year, and 1300 and 1400 mg. for 12- to 18-year-old girls and boys, respectively. An equal amount of phosphorus should be included in the diet.

Among the first studies on calcium were those by Sherman and Hawley (15); in 1922 they performed metabolism studies on 12 children from three to 13 years old. They found that retention of the mineral increased with age and with size of child as well as with milk intake. Positive calcium balances were secured on intakes of 450 mg. of calcium per day in all children but retentions were low; intakes of 750 mg. of calcium daily improved retentions in all cases and a further increase to 1000 mg. of calcium was considered beneficial although not essential for all.

Considerable research has been conducted on children of different ages. The time and rate of ossification of various bone centers have been used to predict skeletal age, one of the bases used to ascertain a child's nutritional status. Under normal conditions the metacarpal and metatarsal centers ossify at certain chronological ages; boys have been shown to be slower than girls in this respect. X-rays of these centers are taken by some investigators; others study the bone contours of the hand, elbow, knee, foot, hip, and shoulder as indications of skeletal maturation. Dreizen and co-workers (16) studied 160 children with chronic nutritive failure and found that the bone centers of the hands and wrists were retarded in maturation; when some of these children were given milk supplements their response in ossification was greater than it was in those who were not given the milk.

More recent work has related calcium retention to the state of depletion or saturation of skeletal tissues and the individual's capacity to assimilate. Ohlson and Stearns (17) reported studies of calcium, phosphorus, and nitrogen retentions on children and adolescents on adequate and borderline diets over a long period of time. They found that it took six months on a good diet for the subjects who had been on borderline diets to equal the retentions of the previously well-fed subjects. These investigators emphasize that an habitually poor diet prior to conception increases the rates of stillbirths and neonatal mortality. They also found that emotional disturbances may decrease calcium retention, even when the diet is adequate in calcium. In the past, 3 to 4 cups of milk daily were advocated for children and 1 quart for teenagers. Since the allowances for calcium were reduced by the FNB in the 1963 and 1968 revisions of the recommendations, the USDA suggests daily consumption of 2 to 3 cups of milk by children under nine years of age, 3 or more cups by those nine to 12 years, and 4 or more cups by teenagers. Some nutrition authorities do not agree with these suggestions. They believe that the diets of children under nine years should include the equivalent of 3 or more cups of milk and those of older children and adolescents, 4 or more cups.

The child's iron needs are very high. In the latest revision of RDA the amounts of iron advised have been increased, especially during the preschool years and adolescence. From one to three years, 15 mg. daily are recommended, from three to ten years, 10 mg. daily. Boys from 12 to 18 and girls from ten to 18 are advised to have as much iron as do their mothers—18 mg. daily.

Owen and co-workers (18), who are studying the nutritional status of preschool children, have reported on 725 children, aged one to six years, in a national cross-sectional sample. They found that iron deficiency was a common occurrence in this age group regardless of socioeconomic level but that the incidence was greatest among the poor. Approximately 7 per cent of these children had hemoglobin levels below 11 gm. per 100 ml., and 45 per cent were considered iron-deficient on the basis of insufficient saturation of transferrin.

THE VITAMIN NEEDS OF CHILDREN AND ADOLESCENTS

Nutritional status has been related to vitamin intake. Several studies show the importance of past and present diet in determining nutritional status. Both clinical and biochemical signs of a below-par condition have been investigated. Myers and associates (19) studied 322 Boston children living in a depressed urban district. They found the following conditions: 93 per cent showed dental pathology; 62 per cent had acute gingivitis, 52 per cent, dry scaling skin; 25 per cent, follicular keratosis; 25 per cent, tongue involvement; 13 per cent, eye signs; and 15 per cent, bow legs. Hemoglobin and hematocrit values were low in 22 and 13 per cent of the children respectively. Group averages for both serum vitamin A and carotene were in a lower range of the "acceptable" ICNND standards. Urinary determinations expressed in relation to creatinine excretion indicated that 20 per cent of the children were in the "low" thiamin excretion range; riboflavin and N^1-methylnicotinamide levels were within normal limits. Other biochemical data were not given. The dietary records revealed inadequate intakes of protein, iron, and vitamins A and C.

Kerry and Crispin (20) reported dietary and biochemical findings in a group of 40 Nebraska preschool children, 20 of higher and 20 of lower socioeconomic status. Calculations of three-day diet records indicated that the RDA standards (1964) were met, with the exception of low iron and slightly low calories in both groups. Urinary excretions of thiamin, riboflavin, niacin, and pantothenic acid indicated that levels of these four vitamins were better in the higher socioeconomic group even though dietary intakes were somewhat better in the lower group.

The more favorable nutritional status of the higher group was associated with better dietary intakes over the entire lifetime rather than with intakes found at the time the biochemical tests were made.

Another study by Owen and co-workers (21) was made on 585 preschool children in rural Mississippi; this was a pilot study in preparation for one of national scope. This investigation included assessment of nutrient intakes and laboratory tests on blood and urine. The children were divided into four groups according to family income: those from families with (1) less than $500; (2) from $500 to $1000; (3) from $1000 to $1500; and (4) more than $1500 per person per year. In general, it was found that calorie, calcium, and ascorbic acid intakes were inadequate for the lowest income children. A majority of all the children were ingesting less than the RDA for iron. Anemia was common, particularly among the poor. Low hemoglobin, serum iron and ascorbic acid, and urinary riboflavin excretion levels were found in from one-fourth to one-third of the children from the families with the lowest incomes. None of the children had signs of malnutrition, but there was a relation between poverty and biochemical evidence of suboptimal nutrition.

The FNB has listed allowances for ten vitamins. For vitamin A, interpolated estimated allowances are based on average body weights plus additional arbitrary amounts to satisfy growth needs. It is considered that about one-half of the vitamin A intake is in the form of the provitamin.

The Board recommends 400 IU vitamin D for children through adolescence, a requirement which is influenced by degree of access to sunlight. This amount is considered ample to sustain normal skeletal growth, provided the diet includes enough calcium and phosphorus. The allowance may be met easily by using fortified milk which contains 400 IU of vitamin D per quart because milk is an excellent carrier of the vitamin and of calcium and phosphorus. Often the vitamin D concentrate prescribed for an infant is continued during early childhood. In such cases, inclusion of vitamin D-fortified foods must be carefully considered, to avoid possible vitamin D toxicity.

For children from one to 12 years, 40 mg. ascorbic acid daily are approved. From then on through adolescence 45 to 55 mg. are recommended. The figures for children beyond 12 years were calculated as 2.5 mg. per kg. body weight$^{0.75}$. For thiamin, allowances are calculated as 0.5 mg. per 1000 kcal. This amount maintains whole-blood thiamin levels and permits relatively high thiamin excretions. Riboflavin allowance is related to metabolic body size; to age ten, requirements to maintain tissue saturation are 0.1 mg. per kg.$^{0.75}$, from ten to 12 and 12 to 14 the allowances are set at 0.09 and 0.08 mg. riboflavin per kg.$^{0.75}$, respectively. The recommended allowances of niacin equivalent for children of all ages are 6.6 mg. per 1000 kcal. Vitamin B_6 allowances were set for the first time in the seventh edition of RDA, since data had become available in sufficient quality and quantity. Allowances gradually increase from 0.5 mg. daily for the one- to two-year-old child to 1.2 mg. daily for the eight- to ten-year-old and to 1.8 and 2.0 mg. for the 18-year-old male and female, respectively. Recommendations are also made for the first time in the 1968 RDA for vitamin E, folacin, and vitamin B_{12}. Vitamin E requirements, like ascorbic acid and riboflavin, are related to metabolic size. Allowances are set at 10 IU daily for the one- to two-year-old and increase to 25 IU for the adolescent. Folacin and vitamin B_{12} allowances are 0.1 mg. and 2.0 μg., respectively, for the one- to two-year-old and gradually increase to adult levels of 0.4 mg. and 5 μg., respectively.

OTHER ASPECTS OF CHILD AND ADOLESCENT NUTRITION

During the growth period control of dental caries is very important. The relationships of calcium and phosphorus, fluoride, vitamin A, vitamin D, and ascorbic acid to the development of the teeth and gums have been discussed. Dental caries which occur largely as a result of nutritional lacks is a common occurrence. Caries may occur in both enamel and dentine. The result is disintegration of dental tissue, which may have very serious and far-reaching effects. Much research is being conducted on this complicated and subtle problem as it relates to diet and tooth decay. Many factors are involved. It is known that microorganisms are required to cause caries. Too, the amount and consistency of the saliva are significant; a watery saliva of low viscosity favors a low incidence of caries. In experimental animals fed purified diets, mono- and disaccharides were found to cause a higher caries incidence than did the polysaccharide dextrin (22). The form in which sugar is fed was studied in an experiment conducted on mentally retarded patients in a Swedish hospital (23). The control group on the basal diet of typical Swedish foods had an average per person per year of 0.3 tooth surface which had become carious. The other two groups received sugar, 300 gm. daily (equal to a year's supply of approximately 200 pounds), either in solution with meals or in a sticky form between meals; the carious surfaces averaged 0.67 for the first group, 4.0 for the second. Pectin, which adheres to the enamel of the tooth surfaces and adsorbs fermentative sugars, also gives a medium favorable for bacterial action. Rate of clearance and consumption with or between meals were factors in determining extent of decay.

Some research indicates that the factors involved are systemic rather than acting directly through the mouth. Differences have been found in cariogenicity of diets in which the sucrose content is the same. Two diets have been used in rat experiments; both contained the same high per cent of sucrose and the same amount of salt mixture composed of adequate amounts of the minerals recognized as essential. The diet used in the Emory University laboratories resulted in a lower incidence of carious lesions than did that used in research at the Harvard School of Dental Medicine, and workers in these two laboratories have conducted detailed investigations to determine the cause or causes of this difference (24). They have eliminated magnesium, manganese, iron, sodium, potassium, yeast and liver extract, and vitamin mixtures as possible causes of the differences and suggest that trace minerals as yet unidentified may be implicated.

McClure (25) has associated a lack of lysine with rat caries; when the cariogenic diet containing mixtures of wheat and sugar was autoclaved there was an increased incidence of severe, smooth-surface caries. Addition of lysine reduced this condition.

Constant and associates (26) studied the effect of various mineral supplements fed to cotton rats. Supplements of citrate, lactate, or acetate did not alter the occurrence of tooth decay, but those of calcium carbonate, disodium phosphates, and various mixtures, with and without calcium, retarded the development rate of decay in erupted teeth. Studies on human beings have been less conclusive. In one study on children (7) 1 per cent sodium dihydrogen phosphate was added to breakfast cereal and fed to a large number of subjects. A control group received the unsupplemented cereal. Examination of the teeth over a two-year period indicated consistently lower increments of dental caries in the supplemented group. Most striking results were noted in proximal surfaces of the teeth.

Because of the difficulties in studying children directly, long-time studies have been made on rats which are susceptible to caries. Shaw and co-workers (28) used 699 rats in a study of the post-eruptive and developmental influence of some dairy products, using them as supplements to a cariogenic diet. Either milk, chocolate drink, chocolate milk, a mixture of milk, vanilla ice cream, and cheddar cheese, or a mixture of chocolate milk, vanilla ice cream, and cheddar cheese was used in amounts which approximated levels of human consumption. When fed on a post-eruptive basis, all supplements resulted in major reductions in incidence of caries, but none had a detectable effect on development of teeth which would be less susceptible to caries.

It is difficult to conduct an investigation on the relationship of the human diet to the teeth because human teeth develop over long periods of time and rigid control of food intake is required. However, a long series of studies, conducted by Boyd and co-workers (29), showed striking results in caries prevention in children who were fed diets high in minerals and vitamins and low in carbohydrate. These investigators worked with diabetic children, with children suffering from celiac disease, and with those in an orthopedic ward of a hospital, as well as with normal children living in their own homes. The caries-preventive diet they suggested includes daily: 1 quart of milk, 1 egg, 1 teaspoonful of cod liver oil, 1 ounce of butter, 1 orange, 2 or more servings each of succulent vegetables and fruits, and other foods desired by the child. Candy, if allowed at all, is given only after meals.

Today dentists and health authorities advocate brushing the teeth immediately after eating as a means of dissolving and washing away the food particles; rinsing the mouth with water is recommended when brushing is not possible.

During adolescence special problems arise. The growth rate during adolescence is higher than at any other time except infancy, and requirements for most nutrients are greater than during adulthood. However, as the young person's desire to assert authority and gain independence increases, food habits often are changed and unbalanced diet may result. The food and eating habits of older children are common discussion topics. Nutrient intakes and eating practices of teenagers were investigated by Huenemann, Hampton, and co-workers (30, 31) as part of a four-year longitudinal study. They found that calcium and iron were the most neglected nutrients; to a lesser degree, ascorbic acid and vitamin A were lacking. The 122 boys and girls who completed the four-week diet study were grouped as lean, average, and obese. Average-weight boys and lean girls tended to have higher intakes of calories and nutrients than did the others; in general, a higher calorie intake was associated with a higher intake of protein, minerals, and vitamins. Obese boys and girls tended to eat less frequently and to skip meals more frequently than did the others. The most frequently skipped meal was lunch. Snacking was a common practice and tended to improve nutrient intakes. Great variations were noted in calorie intakes from individual to individual and from day to day for each individual.

One problem resulting from poor food habits among adolescents is the increased incidence of tuberculosis in this age group. The relationship between susceptibility to tuberculosis and nutritional status in youth has been explored in considerable detail. Tuberculosis has been found to occur more frequently in the underweight and in those whose diets are inadequate in protein and calcium.

The trend toward early marriage and early parenthood is a matter of concern. Today half of the first-time marriages involve girls under 20 years and an estimated one-third to one-half of them are pregnant. This adds physiological stress for the teenage girl whose body still requires a generous supply of nutrients to complete its own growth. Studies on obstetrical performance have shown that the incidence of eclampsia, toxemia, miscarriage, and prematurity is higher among teenagers than among older women. Girls with poor nutritional histories are even poorer obstetrical risks. It has been found, also, that the babies of teenagers frequently have inadequate nutritional stores to protect them during the first days of neonatal life. The high nutrient needs of the adolescent girls themselves, coupled with the increase in teenage pregnancies, emphasize the importance of sound teenage nutrition training.

Obesity in childhood poses problems. Juvenile onset of obesity tends to result in an adult obesity which is more severe and more resistant to treatment (32). Also, in childhood obesity there may be a tendency to hyperglycemia. Teenage overweight is an increasing problem. It has been estimated that between 20 and 30 per cent of adolescents are significantly overweight; many, to the extent that they can be classed as medical problems. Studies have shown that this occurs more frequently in girls than in boys. In addition to the health hazards of obesity, tensions and stresses are built up among teenagers which often make the problem worse.

The relation of calorie consumption to the occurrence of obesity in young people has been studied extensively. The data have shown that the average calorie intake is often below that recommended by the FNB. Evidence from studies by Bullen and Mayer (33) on obese teenagers matched for age with controls of normal weight indicates that the obese subjects actually eat less than the nonobese and that they also exercise less. Obese teenage girls have been found to be inactive 60 to 70 per cent of the time during a tennis game or while engaged in other sports. In comparison, their nonobese counterparts were inactive only 10 to 20 per cent of the time.

Supplementation of home meals is a way to improve the child's nutritional status. In more and more schools the noon lunch is becoming an integral part of the educational program. In the United States each year millions of children and adolescents receive well-balanced lunches at school.

In 1943 as part of the wartime food program the federal government began to provide money and foods for distribution to schools which met certain school lunch standards. The National School Lunch Act became law in 1946, and two types of lunches were recommended—a "Type A" lunch planned to furnish at least one-third of the day's nutrient requirements for the ten- to 12-year-old child, and a "Type B" lunch intended to supplement food brought from home. The Type B lunch program was discontinued in 1958. The following foods are required in the Type A lunch:

½ pt. fluid whole milk, served as a beverage
2 oz. (edible portion as served) of lean meat, poultry, or fish; or
    2 oz. cheese; or 1 egg; or ½ c. cooked dry beans or peas; or 4
    tablespoons peanut butter; or an equivalent of any combination
    of the above foods. To be counted in meeting this requirement,

these foods must be served in a main dish or in a main dish and one other menu item.

¾ c. serving of two or more vegetables or fruits or both. A serving (¼ c. or more) of full-strength vegetable or fruit juice may be used to meet not more than ¼ c. of this requirement.

1 slice whole grain or enriched bread: or a serving of other bread, such as cornbread, biscuits, rolls, or muffins made with whole grain or enriched meal or flour.

2 teaspoons butter or fortified margarine. In January, 1970, this was changed to one teaspoon.

It is also recommended that lunches include a food for ascorbic acid each day, a food for vitamin A twice a week, and several foods for iron each day. Smaller portions may be served to children under ten years of age and larger portions to those over 12 and to adolescents. However, every lunch must include one half-pint of milk.

Both money and surplus commodities are available from the federal government for school systems which serve lunches that meet the Type A lunch minimum requirements. Except in needy or depressed areas, the state must match the federal financial support.

The study by Murphy and associates (34, 35, 36, 37) of the nutritive content of Type A lunches as served to sixth-graders in 300 schools from 19 states was mentioned in Chapters 7 and 10. Energy value, protein, lipids, five major minerals, ten trace minerals, and seven vitamins were determined in aliquots of the meals as served. One-third of the RDA was set as the goal to be attained. It was found that, on the average, the goals were met or exceeded in protein, calcium, phosphorus, iron for the boys, and the seven vitamins analyzed. The average lunch failed to meet the goals for kcal magnesium, and iron for the girls. No RDA have been set for several of the minerals but, except for zinc, they were considered marginal or low. The total fat in the average lunch represented 39 per cent of the meal's calories. There were averages of 14.6 gm. saturated fatty acids, 10.2 gm. mono-unsaturated fatty acids (of which 9.5 gm. were oleic acid), and 3.8 gm. PUFA (of which 2.99 gm. were linoleic acid). The P/S ratio averaged 0.27. The linoleic acid accounted for about 10 per cent of the total fatty acids, or about 4 per cent of the calories in the lunch. In about one-third of the schools linoleic acid accounted for less than 3 per cent of the calories.

A midmorning school lunch is sometimes advocated as a way to promote growth in children. This often is recommended and in some cases is beneficial, especially if the supplement increases the intake of an essential food lacking in the home diet without disturbing the appetite for meals. Milk is the most commonly served lunch. However, Chaney (38) found that orange juice as the supplement promoted growth better than did milk in a group of over 200 California children belonging mostly to families of higher economic levels. In another study made on children from homes of low-level incomes, milk was superior to oranges in promoting weight gain. Although some children gain well, have better appetites for meals, and eat balanced diets without a midmorning lunch, others, particularly the active, need something to eat in the middle of the morning. Many schools, both public and private, participate in the Special Milk Program of the USDA. This program is designed to increase milk consumption by students in elementary and secondary schools. Part of the cost of the milk is paid by the federal government so that milk may be sold to the children at a reduced price.

Today, more and more young children eat at least one meal outside the home—in what are variously called day nurseries, child-care centers, day-care centers, or nursery schools. Usually, the noon meal is provided in these centers, and in many instances the menu is reported to the home. Recommendations for morning and evening meals sometimes are made by the nutritionist at the center so that the child will receive the needed nutrients each day.

Particular study is made of the child's psychological reaction to the important process of eating. Many influences, good and bad, are continually at work. The aim is to make these constructive in every way possible. Attention which is evident to the child is avoided. Foods are prepared and served attractively. Helping to prepare the meal often proves an incentive for consuming the product. The wise practices of the center should be adopted in the home if the child is to have a wholesome attitude toward his food, since they will contribute much to his future well-being and happiness.

GENERAL RULES FOR FEEDING CHILDREN

The diet should be adequate in quantity and quality. The intelligent mother first will consider selection of food so as to supply the materials essential for growth and health. Protein adequate in quantity and quality may be supplied by milk, meat, fish, poultry, eggs, and cheese. In addition to the amount of milk recommended, the preschool child should have two small servings of protein-rich foods, the size of the servings being increased as the child becomes older. For calcium, the suggested amount of milk supplies a sufficiency; for phosphorus, meat, eggs, whole grains, and vegetables will supplement the milk which furnished the basic portion of the total needed. Special consideration must be given to iron which is likely to be lacking in the child's diet; meat, sometimes liver, should be given as soon as the child can chew it. Eggs, green leafy vegetables, whole and enriched grains, and certain fruits are other iron-rich foods which may be included frequently in the diet. Most of the foods mentioned above will furnish one or more of the vitamins; since cooking is likely to destroy ascorbic acid, oranges or tomatoes should be supplied in liberal amounts. Ripe banana is another valuable source of ascorbic acid. When the child is about 18 months old, finger foods such as carrot and celery sticks, and sandwiches of chopped cabbage and chopped lettuce may be given. Proper elimination is usually maintained by a daily diet of two fruits, two vegetables, and whole grain products; the liquid requirement is furnished by milk and water. Sufficient calories for optimal growth are the last dietary essential to be mentioned, but not the least in importance for the growing child.

The diet should include a variety of foods. Instead of serving oatmeal week in, week out, just because it is the favorite, wheat cereals or rice should be substituted occasionally so the child will not suddenly tire of the one variety and consequently refuse to eat any cereal. Frequent change is likely to furnish a well-balanced diet. For the same reasons a variety of vegetables is advised; if the young child is encouraged to try each new food as it is introduced, the dislike which so frequently accompanies the unknown will be prevented. The child who is taught to eat everything on his plate is much more likely to enjoy optimal health than is the one who picks and chooses. Different cooking methods and new attractive combinations make an appeal and encourage enjoyment of all wholesome foods.

Use of some foods is restricted. Certain foods are in themselves or because of their method of preparation not suitable for a child. Among these are stimulating foods, such as those seasoned with pepper and other spices. Although the child may seem to tolerate them, they are usually less popular and after a period of time are likely to result in digestive upsets. Tea and coffee are not allowed, as much because they usurp the place of milk as because they overstimulate the system. Even when taken in small amounts in milk, they create a desire for artificial flavors and destroy the liking for natural food. Fried foods, especially when allowed to soak in the fat, unripe bananas and apples, and corn with its cellulose coating should be avoided. For the younger child foods such as nuts and navy beans which are difficult to chew are omitted; however, peanut butter and a soup made of the bean pulp may be given early. Several fruits are restricted until the digestive tract can care for them: berries, watermelon and cantaloup are likely to cause digestive upsets. Rich dishes which contain cream, much butter, or concentrated sugar are limited for the preschool child. Simple desserts such as angel food or sponge cake, milk puddings, custard, ice cream without nuts, and plain cookies are allowed. Candy should be permitted sparingly and given at the end of the meal.

The psychological approach is important. Provision of the correct foods for the child, regularity of meal times, correct cooking methods, and attractive service are all important in securing proper food intake and developing good food habits. Parents should avoid showing worry about a child's food consumption as youngsters quickly sense the feeling and take advantage of the situation. A discussion of disliked foods is always out of place, especially in front of finicky eaters. Encouragement and praise go much further than nagging. A good example set by the rest of the family is important; it cannot be expected that a vegetable refused by the father will be eaten by his admiring son. A small serving of the disfavored food appetizingly prepared and accompanied by a favorite dessert will encourage the child to eat it. Distraction by interesting conversation is much to be preferred to coaxing or games which center around the child. These general principles for securing his cooperation will do more than any amount of scolding, punishing, or forcing.

The Later Years

THE AGING PROCESS

Aging is continuous. This process is in operation from the beginning of life to the end, and it varies in acceleration, particularly in the later years. Shock and associates (39) at the Gerontology Research Center of the National Institutes of Child Health and Human Development are conducting a longitudinal study to investigate in quantitative terms the changes in various organ systems which occur in normal individuals and the conditions which may affect these changes. Some 700 men, aged 20 to 96 years, are being subjected at regular intervals to physiologic, biochemical, clinical, and psychologic tests.

Biological age differs from chronological age. Shock has found gradual decrements in many physiologic functions and marked differences in individuals in the effects of age. Physiologic stresses may reduce the reserve capacity of many organ systems. Decreases are due partly to the loss of functioning cells in organs and tissues, partly to reductions in cellular metabolism and enzymatic activity. The reasons for these differences, when known, will advance the fields of gerontology (the study of aging) and of geriatrics (the study of the prevention and treatment of the diseases of the elderly).

The influence of heredity and environment, including nutrition and the relative roles of exogenous and endogenous factors, are of practical concern. Early investigations by Sherman (40) on rats demonstrated that diet throughout the early years is important in retaining the vital characteristics of youth into the later years and in lengthening the life span. McCay (41) showed that rats on diets restricted in quantity lived almost 50 per cent longer than did those on *ad libitum* diets.

More recently Ross (42) studied the activity of hepatic enzymes in the aging rat; he used approximately 1000 male animals, aged 21 to

1000 days. When the age-associated activity of the enzymes was modified by dietary changes there were corresponding modifications in the length of life. Rapid growth rates, associated with increased enzyme activity, were not commensurate with a long life span. Long-term calorie restriction promoted the longest life span and the lowest incidence of disease.

NUTRITIONAL REQUIREMENTS

Calorie needs decrease with age. The metabolically active tissue mass decreases. Basal metabolism, affected by a lower surface area, diminishes progressively. The resting rate falls by about 2 per cent per decade in adults (43). Bodily activity usually declines with advancing years. The FNB proposes that calorie allowances be reduced by 3 per cent for each decade between ages 35 and 55, by 5 per cent per decade from ages 55 to 75, and by 7 per cent for ages 75 and over. The 1968 adjustments for age are less than those recommended in the 1963 RDA, based on the assumption that many individuals who are already sedentary do not decrease their activity further as they grow still older.

Adjustments in calorie intake must be made on an individual basis in order to maintain normal body weight. Obesity, frequently a problem in late middle age, increases susceptibility to the so-called degenerative diseases, including hypertension, coronary artery disease, atherosclerosis, and diabetes. Extreme underweight, on the other hand, is more prevalent than obesity in those over age 70. Since a continuous supply of energy is required for the biochemical reactions involved in the life processes, insufficient intake of calories will cause a breakdown in cell metabolism. The lessened vigor and sense of well-being, and the lack of interest in life exhibited by many elderly people is often due to calorie deprivation.

The effects aging has on protein requirement are being investigated. Many studies have been made to determine whether the protein needs during the later years are greater, less, or the same as in a younger adult. Tuttle and co-workers (44) demonstrated that total essential amino acid needs were greater in four out of five older subjects and that both methionine and lysine were required in greater amounts to maintain nitrogen balance. Wannemacher and associates (45), working on young and old dogs, found that the amount of nitrogen required for maintenance in a young adult may not adequately fill the protein reserves to provide for old age, at which time there is a decreased rate of protein anabolism.

However, daCosta and Moorhouse (46) found that a habitually low protein intake did not significantly affect such indices of human well-being as serum albumin, total plasma amino acids, lean body mass, metacarpal bone cortical thickness, or dorsal hand skinfold thickness. In their study on 28 males and 15 females, 73 to 87 years of age, the protein intake ranged from 41 to 80 gm. in men and 33 to 60 gm. in women. This represented from 8 to 14 per cent of the day's calories.

The FNB, assuming that older people utilize protein as efficiently as younger adults, recommends no change in the amount of protein for various ages of adults. The figure is set as approximately 0.9 gm. protein per kg. body weight. Since the calorie allowance is lessened after 55 years and the total amount of food consumed is apt to be less, the proportion of protein in the diet may need to be increased.

Fat and carbohydrate intakes may need to be adjusted. Because the incidence of degenerative diseases of the cardiovascular system is common among older people, it has been recommended that their total intake of fat be limited. Some authorities suggest that the amounts of animal fats in the diet should be reduced and emphasis placed on the inclusion of fats from plant sources. Thus, the ratio of polyunsaturated to saturated fatty acids would be increased. On the other hand, the Council on Foods and Nutrition of the American Medical Association (47) states that, since no direct causal relationship between dietary fat, serum lipid concentration, and atherosclerosis has been proved, any recommendations for alterations in fat intake in the prevention and treatment of atherosclerosis should be considered as experimental. However, it is recognized that the ability to digest and absorb fats diminishes with advancing age. Therefore, most authorities recommend that for the average older person not more than 30 per cent of the total calories should be supplied by fat and that part of the fat calories should come from plant sources rich in PUFA.

Impaired glucose tolerance is fairly common in older people (48). In a five-hour oral glucose tolerance test conducted on 20 men and 20 women, nondiabetic patients, 68 to 91 years old, a 72.5 per cent incidence of impaired tolerance was found; this was associated with a delayed insulin response. The abnormal glucose tolerance was much more common in women than in men. This condition, if present, often is controlled by restricting carbohydrate intake.

Special emphasis should be placed on the intake of some minerals, particularly calcium and iron. The prevalence of osteoporosis among the older population is related to many factors; among them are hormonal changes, inactivity, and low protein and calcium intakes. Data from studies by Roberts and co-workers (49) and by Swanson and associates (50) indicate that the calcium requirement of older women may be greater than that of older men. Whether this is a sex difference associated with hormonal secretions or is due to long-term inadequate intakes of calcium among women has not been established definitely. Whedon and associates (51) found that individual requirements for calcium vary widely and that increasing the intake results in improved calcium storage among patients with osteoporosis. The FNB does not recommend any increase in the daily calcium intake for older persons. However, they suggest that the 800 mg. daily allowance may afford little margin of safety for the female who is at greater risk of developing osteoporosis than the male.

The use of fluoride may be advocated. Bernstein and co-workers (52), who studied 1015 North Dakota subjects over 45 years old, compared the bone densities of the 715 who lived where the fluoride content of the water was low (0.15 to 0.3 ppm.) with those residing where the water contained 4 to 5.8 ppm. fluoride. In the former group they found a higher incidence of osteoporosis, reduced bone density, and more collapsed vertebrae. This was true especially of the women.

Absorption of iron is often impaired in the elderly, due partly to diminished gastric secretion of hydrochloric acid. Iron deficiency anemias frequently result. A daily intake of 10 mg. of iron is recommended by the FNB. This amount is thought to meet the needs of the average adult male and of the post-menopausal female. The needs for other minerals during the later years for the normal healthy individual are essentially similar to those of the younger adult.

Knowledge of the vitamin requirements of older persons is inconclusive. The vitamin needs with advancing years have been the subject of many studies but specific changes in requirements for older persons have been limited because of conflicting evidence. In 1968 the FNB changed some of its recommendations for adults of 55 years and over, and it has included figures for some of the vitamins not previously listed; these include vitamin E, folic acid, vitamin B_6, and vitamin B_{12}. In this latest revision ascorbic acid allowances for older people have been reduced, with women getting less than men. Thiamin and riboflavin allowances have been increased over amounts previously advised. Horwitt (53) favors setting the riboflavin allowance in relation to protein rather than calories since fuel needs are decreased in older adults. On the basis of studies on the absorption, metabolism, and excretion of vitamin B_{12} by old and young subjects, Watkin and associates (54) suggest the possibility of an age-dependent decrement in the vitamin B_{12} binding capacity of tissues. Since there is evidence that the ability to absorb vitamin B_{12} decreases with age, it may be advisable for older persons to increase their intake of the vitamin. The FNB recommends 6 μg. daily for adults over age 55.

No change was made in the allowance for vitamin A. No recommendation is made for including vitamin D in the diet of the elderly. However, Exton-Smith and associates (55), who studied British women over 70 years old, found that low skeletal density was associated with serum calcium and serum phosphorus under 30 and with high serum alkaline phosphatase values. These women had very low vitamin D intakes, and it was concluded that this was an important factor in producing skeletal rarefaction.

Dietary and biochemical studies are used in determining the adequacy of the diets and nutritional status of older people. Interest in these problems has increased in recent years. In 1948 Gillum and Morgan (56) began a detailed study of the blood and diet of older persons living in San Mateo County, California; resurveys of the diet, morbidity, and mortality of this population were made in 1952 and 1962 (57). When the dietary intakes are compared with the 1968 RDA, about one-half of the women and one-fourth of the men had less than two-thirds of the calcium allowance, about one-fourth of both men and women had low intakes of vitamin A, and some had insufficient intakes of ascorbic acid.

Swanson and associates (50) surveyed the food intakes of a group of women representing an area probability sample of all women 30 years old and over in Iowa at the time of the survey. They found that the calories, protein, and calcium in the daily diets, self-chosen by these women, decreased as age progressed. The low consumption of milk and of meat, fish, poultry, and protein extenders in the self-chosen diets indicated that intakes of protein and calcium were low.

Dibble, Brin, and associates (58) investigated the nutritional status of 214 senior citizens residing in public housing units. Iron, thiamin, and riboflavin intakes were found to be suboptimal in 43, 41, and 17 per cent, respectively. The women were more overweight than the men and had lower hematocrit values and higher levels of plasma ascorbic acid, urinary thiamin, and urinary riboflavin. After 70 years there were less overweight conditions and a decrease in plasma ascorbic acid.

McGandy and co-workers (59) secured dietary records from 252 healthy men, 20 to 99 years old. They also determined basal oxygen consumption and estimated their physical activity. These subjects participated in the Baltimore longitudinal study mentioned at the beginning of this chapter and came from a comparatively high socioeconomic level. The decrement in total caloric intake was accounted for by decrease in basal metabolic rate and by energy spent for physical activity. Calcium, vitamin A, and ascorbic acid intakes did not follow the caloric pattern of a progressive fall with age. Intakes of iron, thiamin, riboflavin, and niacin showed progressive decreases with age but the amounts were not statistically significant. With the possible exception of calcium, the RDA (1964) were met by the large majority of these subjects. The percentage of calories derived from protein was remarkably constant throughout this age span—approximately 16 per cent—but fat calories dropped from 42 per cent in the 45- to 54-year-old group to 36 per cent in the 80-year-old group and calories from carbohydrates increased from 42 to 48 per cent in these two age groups. Cholesterol intakes during the same period fell from a mean of 620 mg. to 480 mg. This decrease was related to the reduced use of meat (excluding poultry and fish) in the older group.

In the 1965 nationwide survey of diet in the United States (60) it was found that persons of 55 years and older tended to decrease the adequacy of their diets as expressed in percentage of the RDA. However, the decreases were not great except for calcium, which barely met the standard for two-thirds of the RDA.

PLANNING MEALS FOR THE AGING POPULATION

The living situation of the older age group must be considered. As the number of persons over 65 years of age increases, consideration of their living situation in relation to their nutritional needs becomes increasingly important. Many live alone, sometimes with limited facilities; others live in nursing homes or homes for the aged. Home-care programs and services such as "meals-on-wheels" provide needed nutritional assistance to the elderly who are either disabled or shut-in. Although more emphasis should be placed on the nutritional care of patients in nursing homes and in other such institutions, the custom of making mealtime a social hour also has considerable beneficial effects on the total nutrient intake and the nutritional status of the patients.

When the elderly person lives with the family, attention should be given to his changing physiologic state. Meals planned to meet the specific needs of the older person, served in a pleasant, attractive atmosphere, do much to aid in proper digestion and adequate nutrient intake.

Older people tend to be susceptible to food fads. Because older persons are concerned about their health, interested in retaining youthful characteristics, or anxious about a chronic ailment, they are easy prey for the promoter of the so-called "health foods." There is no evidence that any particular food will restore lost youth or relieve such diseases as arthritis, diabetes, or heart ailments. Special products advertised as "health foods" and multivitamin and mineral mixtures may do no harm in themselves, but they are expensive. Well-balanced, varied meals composed of the foods available in the ordinary market will supply all the essential nutrients for the healthy elderly person. Those who have special dietary problems should follow their physician's advice.

The emotional as well as the physiological and nutritional needs of the individual must be met by the food served. In planning meals for the older person, consideration should be given to the foods to which he has been accustomed throughout his life. Introduction of new and unfamiliar foods in the diet of a person over 70 may be traumatic. If problems involving dentition or digestive disabilities occur, it may be advisable to provide soft, simple foods and to include milk beverages between meals.

The influence of psychological factors such as fear, worry, anxiety, or loneliness have been shown to affect not only actual dietary intake but also utilization of nutrients. In studies with older women, Swanson reported negative nitrogen and calcium balances during anxiety episodes over the terminal illness of a relative and during periods of living alone. Imposition of drastic changes in types of food and in meal patterns also often results in reduced food intake due to appetite failure or rejection of food.

Economic factors influence the diets and nutritional status of the elderly.
Many people when they reach retirement age must adjust to living on
incomes lower than those to which they were accustomed and some
become overly concerned about finances. These factors influence the
amounts and kinds of food purchased and may lead to dietary practices
which result in nutritional deficiencies.

Dietary surveys indicate that nutritional lacks are more closely related to income level and educational background than to age. In the
1965 nationwide dietary survey, the percentage of households with good
diets increased with income. Poor diets were four times as frequent
among households whose incomes were under $3000 per year as those
whose incomes were $10,000 and over. In the NNS now being conducted,
over 39 per cent of the 8000 persons over 60 with annual incomes under
$5000 consumed less than half the approved allowance for vitamin A,
and 30 per cent had less than half that for ascorbic acid, according to
preliminary data.

Many bulletins and pamphlets which give helpful information for
planning simple, attractive, nutritious meals are available. Table 16–1
gives sample low-cost menus for a week. These menus are easy to prepare
and include planning left-overs, as for example, preparation of enough
stew for the Monday evening meal and for Tuesday noon meal as well.

PROBLEMS

1. Plan a menu for a three-year-old child. Calculate the amount of animal
   and vegetable protein in it. Determine the intake of protein per kg. of
   body weight.
2. Plan two days' menus for a child who dislikes milk. Include in each menu
   at least 3 cups of milk concealed in some way.
3. Give directions in leaflet form for sensible food for a child on a picnic.
4. Write a week's menus for a summer camp of 9- to 12-year-old boys. Limit
   the cost of food according to the range of local prices. Plan the market
   order for the week.
5. Plan a day's menus for each of 2 teenagers, a boy and a girl, which include
   between meal snacks. Calculate the amounts of calcium and protein.
6. Plan menus for 2 days for a 75-year-old woman who has difficulty chewing and dislikes fluid milk.

REFERENCES

1. Speckman, E. W., *et al.* The Effect of Nutrition on Body Composition.
   *Nutr. Revs., 25:*1 (1967).
2. Forbes, G. W. Growth of the Lean Body Mass During Childhood and
   Adolescence. *J. Pediat., 64:*822 (1964).

Table 16–1

*Sample Low-Cost Menus for a Week**

BUTTER OR MARGARINE WOULD BE SERVED WITH THESE MEALS, A GLASS OF MILK AT LEAST ONCE A DAY, TEA OR COFFEE AS DESIRED

Sunday	Monday	Tuesday	Wednesday	Thursday	Friday	Saturday
Orange juice Scrambled egg Toast	Orange juice Oatmeal Milk Toast	Prunes French toast Sirup	Orange slices Soft-cooked egg Toasted rolls	Prunes Ready-to-eat cereal Milk Peanut butter biscuits	Tomato juice Milk toast Jelly	Orange juice Oatmeal Milk Toasted corn muffins
Swiss steak Mashed potatoes Broccoli Bread Chocolate pudding	Frankfurters stuffed with mashed potatoes and cheese Scalloped tomatoes Hot rolls Apple brown betty	Lamb stew Beets Tossed green salad Bread Rice and raisin pudding	Meat loaf Scalloped potatoes Steamed cabbage Peanut butter biscuits Fruit in season	Cream of tomato soup Egg salad–shredded lettuce sandwich Gingerbread	Creamed egg and mushrooms on noodles Cabbage, carrot, raisin salad	Braised liver Potatoes boiled in jackets Green peas Grated carrot salad Bread Orange-milk sherbet
Welsh rarebit Crisp bacon strip Apple-raisin salad Ice cream Cookies	Lamb stew with potatoes Snap beans Bread Chocolate pudding	Spaghetti, tomato, chopped meat casserole Broccoli Bread Grapefruit segments	Cheese fondue Snap beans Bread Peaches Gingerbread	Meat loaf— tomato sauce Creamed potatoes Spinach Bread Tapioca pudding	Baked fish Baked potato slices Green peas Corn muffins Tapioca pudding	Vegetable-bean soup Toasted cheese sandwich Fruit in season

* From *Food Guide for Older Folks*, Home and Garden Bulletin No. 17, Agricultural Research Service, United States Department of Agriculture, Revised 1963.

3. Young, C. M., *et al.* Body Composition Studies of Preadolescent and Adolescent Girls. III. Predicting Specific Gravity. *J. Am. Diet. Ass., 53:*469 (1968).

4. Mitchell, H. S. Protein Limitation and Human Growth. *J. Am. Diet. Ass., 44:*165 (1964).

5. Macy, I. G., *et al.* Body Composition in Childhood. *Human Biol., 28:*291 (1956).

6. Mayer, J. Some Aspects of Obesity in Children. *Postgrad. Med., 34:*83 (1963).

7. Taylor, C. M., *et al.* The Energy Expenditure of Boys and Girls. *J. Nutr., 35:*511 (1948); *36:*123 (1948); *38:*1 (1949); *44:*275, 295 (1951).

8. Macy, I. G., *et al.* Calories—A Limiting Factor in the Growth of Children. *J. Nutr., 45:*189 (1951).

9. Stearns, G., *et al.* The Protein Requirements of Children from One to Ten Years of Age. *Ann. N.Y. Acad. Sci., 69:*857 (1958).

10. Hodges, R. E., *et al.* Nutritional Status of Teenagers in Iowa. *Am. J. Clin. Nutr., 17:*20 (1965).

11. Christakis, G. A., *et al.* A Nutritional Epidemiologic Investigation of 642 New York City Children. *Am. J. Clin. Nutr., 21:*107 (1968).

12. Whitehead, R. G., *et al.* Serum Amino Acids in Kwashiorkor. I. Relationship to Clinical Condition. *Am. J. Clin. Nutr., 14:*313 (1964).

13. Abernathy, R. P., *et al.* Nitrogen Balance Studies with Children Fed Foods Representing Diets of Low Income Southern Families. *Am. J. Clin. Nutr., 23:*408 (1970).

14. Leitch, I., *et al.* The Estimation of Calcium Requirement: A Re-examination. *Nutr. Abstr. Revs., 29:*393 (1959).

15. Sherman, H. C., *et al.* Calcium and Phosphorus Metabolism in Children. *J. Biol. Chem., 53:*375 (1922).

16. Dreizen, S., *et al.* Maturation of Bone Centers in Hand and Wrist of Children with Chronic Nutritive Failure. *Am. J. Dis. Childr., 87:*429 (1954).

17. Ohlson, M. A., *et al.* Calcium Intake of Children and Adults. *Fed. Proc., 18:*1076 (1959).

18. Owen, G. M., *et al.* Nutritional Status of Preschool Children: Hemoglobin, Hematocrit, and Plasma Iron Values. *J. Pediat., 76:*761 (1970).

19. Myers, M. L., *et al.* A Nutritional Study of School Children in a Depressed Urban District. II. Physical and Biochemical Findings. *J. Am. Diet. Ass., 53:*226; 234 (1968).

20. Kerry, E., *et al.* Nutritional Status of Preschool Children. I. Dietary and Biochemical Findings. *Am. J. Clin. Nutr., 21:*1274 (1968).

21. Owen, G. M., *et al.* Nutritional Status of Mississippi Preschool Children —A Pilot Study. *Am. J. Clin. Nutr., 22:*1444 (1969).

22. Schweigert, B. S., *et al.* Dental Caries in the Cotton Rat. III. Effect of Different Dietary Carbohydrates on the Incidence and Extent of Dental Caries. *J. Nutr., 29:*405 (1945).

23. Gustafsson, B. E., *et al.* The Vipeholm Dental Caries Study: The Effect of Different Levels of Carbohydrate Intake on Caries Activity in 436 Individuals Observed for Five Years. *Acta. Odont. Scand., 11:*232 (1954).

24. Wynn, W., *et al.* Further Studies on the Difference in Cariogenicity of Two Diets Comparable in Sucrose Content. *J. Nutr., 67:*569 (1959).

25. McClure, F. J. Wheat Cereal Diets, Rats Caries, Lysine, and Minerals. *J. Nutr., 65:*619 (1958).

26. Constant, M. A. Dental Caries in the Cotton Rat. XIV. Further Studies of Caries Production by Natural Diets with Especial Reference to the Role of Minerals, Fat, and the Stage of Refinement of Cereals. *J. Nutr., 53:*17 (1954).

27. Stookey, G. K., *et al.* The Clinical Effectiveness of Phosphate-Enriched Breakfast Cereal on the Incidence of Dental Caries in Children. *J. Am. Dent. Ass., 74:*752 (1967).

28. Shaw, J. H., *et al.* Studies on the Relation of Dairy Products to Dental Caries in Caries-Susceptible Rats. *J. Nutr., 67:*253 (1959).

29. Boyd, J. D., *et al.* Dietary Control of Dental Caries. *Am. J. Dis. Childr., 38:*721 (1920).

30. Hamptom, M. C., *et al.* Caloric and Nutrient Intakes of Teenagers. *J. Am. Diet. Ass., 50:*385 (1967).

31. Huenemann, R. L., *et al.* Food and Eating Practices of Teen-Agers. *Am. J. Am. Diet. Ass., 53:*17 (1968).

32. Heald, F. P. Natural History and Physiological Basis of Adolescent Obesity. *Fed. Proc., 25:*4 (1966).

33. Bullen, B. A., *et al.* Physical Activity of Obese and Non-Obese Adolescent Girls Appraised by Motion Picture Sampling. *Am. J. Clin. Nutr., 14:*211 (1964).

34. Murphy, E. W., *et al.* Nutritive Content of Type A School Lunches. *School Lunch J., 22:*11 (1968).

35. Murphy, E. W., *et al.* Vitamin Content of Type A School Lunches. *J. Am. Diet. Ass., 55:*372 (1969).

36. Murphy, E. W., *et al.* Lipid Components of Type A School Lunches. *J. Am. Diet. Ass., 56:*504 (1970).

37. Murphy, E. W., *et al.* Trace Minerals in Type A School Lunches. *J. A. Diet. Ass., 58:*115 (1971).

38. Chaney, M. S. Comparison of the Value of Milk and Oranges as Supplementary Lunch for Underweight Children. *Am. J. Dis. Childr., 26:*337 (1923).

39. Shock, N. W. Physiological Aspects of Aging. *J. Am. Diet. Ass., 56:*491 (1970).

40. Sherman, H. C., *et al.* Effects of Increasing the Calcium Content of a Diet in which Calcium is One of the Limiting Factors. *J. Nutr., 10:*363 (1935).

41. McCay, C. M., *et al.* Growth, Aging, Chronic Disease, and Life Span in Rats. *Arch. Biochem., 2:*469 (1943).

42. Ross, M. H. Aging, Nutrition, and Hepatic Enzyme Activity Patterns in the Rat. *J. Nutr., 97:*565 (1969).

43. Durnin, J. V. G. A. *Energy, Work, and Leisure.* London: Heineman Educational Books (1967).

44. Tuttle, S. G., *et al.* Further Observations on the Amino Acid Requirements of Older Men. I. Effects of Non-Essential Nitrogen Supplements Fed with Different Amounts of Essential Amino Acids. II. Methionine and Lysine. *Am. J. Clin. Nutr., 16:*225, 229 (1965).

45. Wannamacher, R. W., Jr., *et al.* Determination of Optimal Dietary Protein Requirements of Young and Old Dogs. *J. Nutr., 88:*66 (1966).

46. daCosta, F., *et al.* Protein Nutrition in Aged Individuals on Self-Elected Diets. *Am. J. Clin. Nutr., 22:*1618 (1969).

47. Council on Foods and Nutrition, American Medical Association. The Regulation of Dietary Fat. *J. Am. Med. Ass., 181:*411 (1962).

48. Zeytinoglu, I. Y., *et al.* The Process of Aging: Serum Glucose and Immunoreactive Insulin Levels During the Oral Glucose Tolerance Test. *J. Am. Geriat. Soc., 17:*1 (1969).

49. Roberts, P. H., *et al.* Nutritional Status of Older Women—Nitrogen, Calcium, Phosphorus Retentions of 9 Women. *J. Am. Diet. Ass., 24:*292 (1948).

50. Swanson, P. Adequacy in Old Age. Part I. Role of Nutrition. Part II. Nutrition Education Programs for the Aging. *J. Home Econ., 56:*651, 728 (1964).

51. Whedon, G. D. Effects of High Calcium Intakes on Bones, Blood, and Soft Tissues: Relationship of Calcium Intake to Balance in Osteoporosis. *Fed. Proc., 18:*1112 (1959).

52. Bernstein, D. G., *et al.* Prevalence of Osteoporosis in High- and Low-Fluoride Areas in North Dakota. *J. Am. Med. Ass., 198:*499 (1966).

53. Horwitt, M. K. Nutritional Requirements of Man, with Special Reference to Riboflavin. *Am. J. Clin. Nutr., 18:*458 (1966).

54. Watkin, D. M. New Findings in the Nutrition of Older People. *Am. J. Pub. Health, 55:*548 (1965).

55. Exton-Smith, A. N., *et al.* Nutrition and Metabolic Bone Disease in Old Age. *Lancet, 2:*999 (1966).

56. Gillum, H. L., *et al.* Nutritional Status of the Aging. *J. Nutr., 55:*265, 289, 431, 449, 655, 671 (1955).

57. Steinkamp, R. C., *et al.* Resurvey of an Aging Population—Fourteen-Year Follow-Up. *J. Am. Diet. Ass., 46:*103 (1965).

58. Dibble, M. V., *et al.* Evaluation of the Nutritional Status of Elderly Subjects, with a Comparison Between Fall and Spring. *J. Am. Geriat. Soc., 15:*1031 (1967).

59. McGandy, R. B., *et al.* Nutrient Intakes and Energy Expenditure in Men of Different Ages. *J. Gerontol., 21:*581 (1966).

60. Consumer and Food Economics Research Division, Agricultural Research Service, USDA. *Food Intake and Nutritive Value of Diets of Men, Women, and Children in the United States, Spring, 1965. A Preliminary Report, 1969.* No. 62–18. Washington, D.C.: ARS, USDA.

GENERAL REFERENCES

61. Moyer, E. Z., *et al. Basic Data on Metabolic Patterns in 7- to 10-Year-Old Girls in Selected Southern States.* Washington, D.C.: Home Economics Research Rept. No. 33 A.R.S. (1967).

62. Shaw, J. K. Nutrition in Relation to Dental Medicine. In M. G. Wohl and R. S. Goodhart (eds.), *Modern Nutrition in Health and Disease,* 4th ed. Philadelphia: Lea & Febiger (1968).

Nutrition
Today

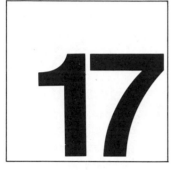

The science of nutrition is a complex subject which cuts across many disciplines. In the twentieth century the increase in information on human nutritional needs has been outstanding. Almost the entire knowledge of essential nutrients has been obtained in this century. The combined efforts of research workers in the biological, physical, and social sciences have greatly improved the nutritional status of human beings. Now, through research in molecular biology and molecular genetics, the mechanisms of protein synthesis and transfer of genetic information are being elucidated.

Throughout the preceding chapters the relation of nutrition to health and well-being has been discussed. The known functions of the nutrients, the interrelationships among them, and their food sources have been considered. However, much still needs to be learned about them. Although the amounts of the various nutrients required to prevent the classical deficiency diseases are known, knowledge is still limited as to what constitutes optimum levels of intake. More information is needed on the effects of new processing procedures on the nutritional value of foods, on the availability of some nutrients that occur in "bound" forms in foods, and on the composition and nutritive value of foods available in parts of the world where food supplies are limited and malnutrition is prevalent.

Advances in agriculture and food technology involving the production, processing, marketing, and preparation of foods, exploration into space, nuclear testing with attendant hazards of fall-out radiation, population growth, and economic status all have broad implications for those concerned with the health and welfare of people of all nations. Some current nutrition problems will be mentioned in this chapter. This may serve to unify specific discussions of past chapters and to stress the importance of nutrition in the world situation.

WORLD PROBLEMS RELATED TO NUTRITION

One of the major concerns in the world today is the adequacy of the food supply in relation to population growth. The world population now numbers about 3.5 billion people, and it is said that between two-thirds and four-fifths of them are either undernourished, malnourished, or both. By 1985, it is estimated that there will be five billion people on this planet, and that by the year 2000 there may be over seven billion (1). Progress is being made in agriculture and in food technology, and the world's food supply is being increased in both quality and quantity. However, a wide gap between agricultural and population expansion still remains in the less well-developed regions of the world, and, thus, a nutritional crisis exists. The benefits of agricultural and industrial improvements often are offset by rapid population growth. Whereas in the more advanced countries average annual rates of population increase are 0.5 to 1.5 per cent, the rates in many developing countries are 2.6 to 3.8 per cent (2).

Technical assistance and food aid are provided to developing regions by a variety of programs and agencies. Among them are the Food for Peace Program of the United States, the World Food Program and the Freedom from Hunger Campaign of FAO, the programs of other United Nations agencies such as UNICEF and UNESCO. In addition, there are the people-to-people projects of civic, private, professional, and religious groups, and of foundations such as the Ford, Macy, and Rockefeller Foundations. Food production is increasing as a result of the technical assistance programs. However, the Panel on World Food Supply (1) has estimated that, unless the rate of population increase is reduced considerably, all efforts to augment agricultural and economic development will be ineffective and population increase will continue to outpace food supply.

Protein and calorie deficiencies are common. One of the most serious problems in the technically underdeveloped countries is that of protein and calorie malnutrition (3, 4). Kwashiorkor and marasmus, previously described in Chapter 6, are diseases caused by inadequate intake of good quality protein and of inadequate calories and protein, respectively. These nutritional deficiency diseases are common in Latin America, Africa, the Near and Far East, and within recent years even have been found in the United States.

Kwashiorkor occurs among infants and children, usually between the ages of one and four, and most frequently in infants following weaning when they are put on diets of cereal products that are low in quality and quantity of protein. Marasmus, a form of semistarvation, results from the mother's failure to nurse her baby and the substitution of feedings that are inadequate in both calories and protein.

In regions where kwashiorkor occurs it has been estimated that, for every case of the disease, there are 100 cases of protein malnutrition that result in retarded physical growth and psychomotor development. Schrimshaw and co-workers (5) in studies in Guatemala found that young children suffering from protein malnutrition are more susceptible to infections and diarrheal disease than are well-nourished children.

WHO, FAO, and INCAP (Institute of Nutrition of Central America and Panama) are working together, and with nutrition teams from many universities, on extensive programs to improve the nutritional quality as well as the quantitative adequacy of diets in the underdeveloped countries (Figure 17–1). Some of the practical applications of these efforts were discussed in Chapter 6 as they relate to development of low-cost protein-rich foods for supplementary feeding of infants and young children.

Figure 17–1
In Mexico to increase the consumption of food rich in protein content, particularly dried fish, FAO nutritionists, working with the Department of Education and the Institute of Nutrition, organized a yearly "fish week" in the secondary schools. Here these young students are learning to prepare tamales *containing fish.* (*From* World Food Problems, No. 2: Man and Hunger, *Revised 1961. Courtesy of the Food and Agriculture Organization of the United Nations.*)

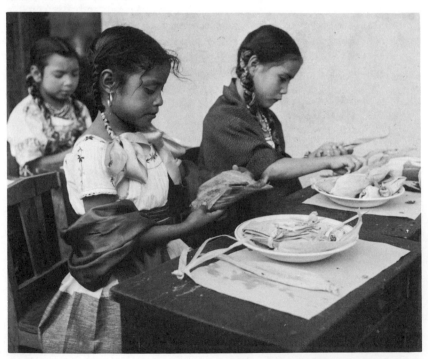

Another promising means of combating protein malnutrition is supplementation of the natural food supply with one or more of the amino acids known to be lacking. Since populations groups in many parts of the world subsist almost exclusively on grains with lesser amounts of pulses, it has been suggested that the available plant sources be fortified with amino acids to improve their quality. The addition in correct proportions of lysine to wheat, millet, teff, barley, or sorghum, of lysine and tryptophan to corn, and of lysine and threonine to rice would do much to alleviate protein malnutrition (6). These amino acids can be produced at low cost and in large amounts. Improvement in the protein quality of cereals and of cereal-vegetable mixtures when the principal limiting amino acids are added has been demonstrated (7).

Development of high-lysine corn by genetic improvement has spurred the search for a similar gene in other grains. If grains, dietary staples for a large segment of the world's population, can be produced with well-balanced protein in sufficient amounts, much progress will be made toward solution of the global nutrition problem (8).

Improved agricultural practices are increasing the indigenous production of food crops in some developing countries. High-yielding varieties of wheat and rice have been developed in Mexico and the Philippines, respectively. These varieties permit harvesting of two or sometimes even three crops per year. High-yielding types of corn, sorghum, and millet are being studied in India under the leadership of the Rockefeller Foundation.

Deficiency diseases due to inadequate intakes of vitamins occur in many areas. In many countries, and often in specific areas within a country, severe manifestations of vitamin malnutrition are found. In the Third World Food Survey conducted by FAO (9), vitamin A deficiency was reported to be a public health problem in Indonesia, mainland China, Burma and other parts of the Far East, in parts of Latin America, and in the semiarid zones of Africa. Vitamin A lack was evidenced by night blindness, skin disorders, and xerophthalmia often resulting in permanent blindness, especially among children. These conditions were found to be due mainly to insufficient intakes of such foods as green and yellow vegetables, milk, eggs, butter, fish-liver oils, and carotene-containing vegetable oils. However, symptoms of vitamin A deficiency were not found in the humid coastal zones of West Africa, where the supplies of red palm oil, which is rich in carotene, are ample and its use widespread.

The findings from the ICNND surveys mentioned in Chapter 1 have shown that avitaminosis A is prevalent in many countries (10); in some it is a general problem, while in others, it is a problem in special areas of the country or within special groups.

Both FAO and ICNND surveys have shown that nutritional diseases due to lack of the B vitamins and of vitamin C also occur in most of the less-developed areas of the world. Beriberi is found in population groups that subsist on diets of highly polished rice. The disease is common and is a major cause of death among infants two to five months old in Burma, Thailand, Vietnam, the south mainland of China, East Pakistan, and in some parts of India. In recent years the incidence of beriberi has been reduced in areas where government regulations require only partial milling or enrichment of rice or where the practice of not washing parboiled rice before cooking is common. On the other hand, the occurrence of thiamin deficiency disease has increased in some parts of the world because of the introduction of machine milling which has led to availability and consumption of highly polished rice.

The nutritional disease most frequently discovered in the countries studied has been ariboflavinosis. This deficiency syndrome has been reported to occur in individuals who consume diets limited in leafy vegetables and pulses or legumes and devoid of animal proteins. Among the most frequently observed signs of lack of riboflavin are sore lips and sore tongues. These conditions result from the use of starchy staple foods and the concomitant low consumption of dairy products and fresh leafy vegetables.

Pellagra occurs in corn-eating areas of the world, particularly in regions where sources of protein which include the essential amino acid tryptophan are limited. Nutritional status surveys have shown that the basic causes of this disease are inadequate supplies and intakes of good quality protein and of niacin-containing foods. The relationship of protein intake to niacin nutriture was discussed in Chapter 12.

Scurvy occurs in many parts of the world where adults consume diets limited in fruits and vegetables and where infants are weaned from breast feeding to high carbohydrate diets.

Endemic goiter and nutritional anemia are problems in some areas. According to the reports of studies by FAO, WHO, and INCAP, endemic goiter is a significant problem in many parts of the world. As was pointed out in Chapter 9, it is a nutritional deficiency disease found in areas where soil and drinking water are low in iodine content. The disease is more common in females ages 12 to 18 years and in males ages nine to 13 years than in adults. Field studies conducted in Latin America by INCAP under the directorship of Scrimshaw (11) showed that addition of potassium iodate to table salt is effective in treatment and prevention of goiter. Legislation requiring iodization of all salt has been passed in many Central and South American countries but as yet has not been enforced in all of them.

Nutritional anemia is widespread in those parts of the world where diets are marginal in protein, iron, folic acid, and less frequently, in vitamin B_{12}. Darby and associates (12) in investigations carried out in the Jordanian sector of Jerusalem and in Egypt, reported an association between vitamin E nutriture and the occurrence of macrocytic anemia in malnourished infants. They found the anemia was not readily correctable by usual dietary treatment or by administration of common hemopoietic agents but that it did respond to tocopherol therapy.

Nutritional anemia is of special concern during periods of growth and reproduction and may result either in high maternal and infant mortality or in a chronic condition with many insidious side-effects. Anemia, commonly found in tropical areas, is often associated with malaria and with parasitic infections, and with zinc deficiency (13).

NUTRITION PROBLEMS IN THE UNITED STATES

Nutritional deficiencies are known to exist. In the past few years much concern has been expressed about the nutritional status of segments of the population in the United States. As a result, in late 1967, Congress directed the Department of Health, Education, and Welfare to conduct a National Nutrition Survey (NNS). This survey, which was begun in 1968, was mentioned in Chapter 1. Low-income areas of ten states were selected for the initial phase of the survey. So that all results will be comparable, each survey is being conducted according to the procedures outlined in the ICNND Manual for Nutrition Surveys (14).

Preliminary findings include enlargement of the thyroid in 5 per cent of the sample, anemia in between 5 and 10 per cent, low serum vitamin A and ascorbic acid levels in from 5 to 20 per cent, and low urinary riboflavin and thiamin excretions in from 9 to 15 per cent. Clinical manifestations of vitamin D and protein-calorie deficiencies also were found. A high prevalence of decayed and missing teeth and abnormal changes in gum tissue were found. The reports to date stress the fact that the findings are preliminary and that they should not be construed to represent the national picture or even the situation in one state (15, 16, 17).

Dietary studies over the past two decades have shown repeatedly that inadequate intakes of ascorbic acid, calcium, iron, and vitamin A occur among all age groups. These deficiencies are associated most frequently with low consumption of milk and cheese, and of fruits and vegetables, particularly those rich in ascorbic acid and vitamin A value. As was discussed in Chapter 16, teenage girls tend to have the poorest diets.

Biochemical and clinical evidence of iodine, iron, ascorbic acid, riboflavin, and thiamin deficiencies has been reported from a survey of 1000 school children, ages ten to 16 years, in five rural areas of southern Louisiana (18). Extensive studies in various parts of the country have shown that hypochromic microcytic anemia due to iron deficiency is common among infants and preschool children.

Osteoporosis, which occurs frequently in the elderly, was mentioned in earlier chapters. It appears to be associated with low calcium intake over many years as well as with hormonal changes that affect calcium metabolism.

Overnutrition is a cause for concern. Reference was made to the country-wide survey reported in *Nutritional Status U.S.A.* (19). One earlier significant finding in this investigation was the high incidence of caloric overnutrition. Overweight was found to a considerable extent in all age groups; however, the degree and occurrence varied in different regions of the country.

The preliminary findings from the NNS (17) indicate that a relatively large number of persons, particularly women, are in the overweight category. Of the women studied, over 50 per cent of those over age 30 weighed 20 per cent or more above that considered desirable for their age and height. Obesity is one of the major nutritional diseases in the United States and actually is a form of malnutrition. The hazards of obesity were discussed in Chapter 3.

The dangers from large intakes of fat, the toxic effects of excessive amounts of vitamins A and D, and the possibility of masking some symptoms of pernicious anemia with folic acid supplements also were mentioned in preceding chapters.

It is not known to what extent an individual adapts to increased intakes of specific nutrients or how long a time is required for such an adjustment to be made. A guide for use in interpreting intake data for eight nutrients has been prepared by ICNND (Table 17–1). The figures, intended primarily for use in population groups of physically active young adult males, may also be used as a basis for judging the adequacy of diets of other subjects. Instead of set figures, ranges are proposed which have the advantage of allowing for individual variation. Some of the "accept-

Table 17–1

Suggested Guide to Interpretation of Nutrient Intake Data for "Reference" Man[*][†]

Nutrient	Deficient	Low	Acceptable	High
Protein				
(gm. per kg. body weight)	<.5[a]	0.5–0.9	1.0–1.4	≧1.5[b]
Calcium (gm. per day)	<.3	0.30–0.39	0.4–0.7	≧.8
Iron (mg. per day)	<6.0	6–8	9–11	≧12
Vitamin A (I.U. per day)	<2,000	2,000–3,499	3,500–4,999	≧5,000
Ascorbic acid (mg. per day)	<10	10–29	30–49	≧50
Thiamine				
(mg. per 1,000 calories)	<.2	0.2–0.29	0.3–0.4	≧.5
Riboflavin (mg. per day)	<.7	0.7–1.1	1.2–1.4	≧1.5
Niacin (mg. per day)	<5	5–9	10–14	≧15

[*] From the *Manual for Nutrition Surveys.* Interdepartmental Committee on Nutrition for National Defense (now Nutrition Section, Office of International Research, National Institutes of Health, United States Department of Health, Education, and Welfare). 2nd edition, 1963.
[†] The "reference" man is a physically active young adult, 25 years old, and weighing 65 kg. See the discussion in Chapter 3 of standards used for the daily energy requirement in group studies.
[a] < — less than; [b] ≧ — equal to or more than.

able" intake figures are below the RDA for these nutrients. However, it must be remembered that the recommended allowances are levels of nutrient intake judged to be adequate for maintenance of good nutrition of people in the United States, whereas the guidelines proposed by ICNND are for evaluating and interpreting dietaries in relation to nutritional status throughout the world.

Some authorities believe that a maximal or top limit of safety should be set, as well as a minimal. But there still is no scientific evidence to show what are optimum levels of intake and what figures should be listed as maximal. Nutrition research is increasingly concerned with the problems of obesity, atherosclerosis, and other degenerative diseases, and the role of overnutrition in their incidence. When it is possible to obtain large amounts of food, accepted policy seems to be to continue the present plan of liberal consumption of most nutrients, to reduce the percentage of calories from fat, and to rely upon clinical observations and biochemical tests to furnish warnings of excess intakes. Habits of eating a wide variety of foods and avoiding extremes should be developed early and continued throughout life.

Nutrition education must consider many factors. The relatively poor nutritional status of some groups and in some areas of the United States has been found to be related to levels of income and education, housing, and cultural background. Too, psychological factors are often involved. Nutrition education programs that take these influences into consideration and translate the current knowledge of nutrition into practical terms of foods and meals should do much to improve nutritional well-being.

The Interagency Committee on Nutrition education (ICNE) coordinated by the USDA (20) formulated some basic concepts in nutrition for use in education programs. These concepts are fundamental ideas about food and nutrition, not facts to be presented and taught as such (Table 17–2). In addition (21), concepts and generalizations about foods and nutrition have been developed as part of the national study on the home economics curriculum in secondary schools under the sponsorship of the Office of Education of the United States Department of Health, Education, and Welfare. Use of these basic ideas in the planning and conduct of all types of nutrition education programs is being encouraged. It is thought that teaching by the concept approach will be effective in conveying sound nutrition information to people, both young and old. More importantly it should stimulate them to want to put the knowledge gained into practice in their daily lives.

Food faddism is a serious problem. Mention was made in Chapter 1 of the impact of food fads on the present nutritional scene. Since earliest recorded history, magical qualities have been attributed to certain foods and an aura of mystery has surrounded many of them. As knowledge of nutritional requirements has increased, people generally have become

Table 17–2

Basic Nutrition Concepts*

> 1. *Nutrition is the food you eat and how the body uses it.*
>   - We eat food to live, to grow, to keep healthy and well, and to get energy for work and play.
> 2. *Food is made up of different nutrients needed for growth and health.*
>   - All nutrients needed by the body are available through food.
>   - Many kinds and combinations of food can lead to a well-balanced diet.
>   - No food, by itself, has all the nutrients needed for full growth and health.
>   - Each nutrient has specific uses in the body.
>   - Most nutrients do their best work in the body when teamed with other nutrients.
> 3. *All persons, throughout life, have need for the same nutrients, but in varying amounts.*
>   - The amounts of nutrients needed are influenced by age, sex, size, activity, and state of health.
>   - Suggestions for the kinds and amounts of food needed are made by trained scientists.
> 4. *The way food is handled influences the amount of nutrients in food, its safety, appearance, and taste.*
>   - Handling means everything that happens to food while it is being grown, processed, stored, and prepared for eating.

* Formulated by the Interagency Committee on Nutrition Education. Reported by Hill, M. M., in *Nutrition Program News,* United States Department of Agriculture, November–December, 1964.

more aware of the importance of food, but they are still susceptible to false claims about the food supply. According to the FDA, the four myths which nutrition education must combat are claims that all disease is due to faulty diet, that malnutrition is caused by soil depletion, that the use of chemical fertilizers is detrimental to health, and that foods are overprocessed.

The FDA estimates that over half a million dollars is spent annually in the United States on nonprescribed special food supplements, vitamin and mineral products, and the so-called "natural" foods. Faddism abounds particularly in the area of weight control and among the elderly. In some instances, use of these special products involves only a waste of money; in other cases, their cost is so high that insufficient money is left for purchasing foods necessary for an adequate diet (22). Some fads actually are harmful. Exploitation of the public by the purveyors of "miracle" foods credited with therapeutic values for the cure of organic diseases is a serious matter. Use of these special food supplements often is substituted for medical advice and serious illness results.

OTHER NUTRITIONAL CONCERNS OF TODAY

Interrelationhips between nutrients are important. Throughout the discussions in the text, reference was made to the effects of certain nutrients in helping or hindering the use of others in metabolic processes. For example, the interactions between protein, carbohydrate, and fat which may result in formation of muscle and other important tissues or in fat storage were considered. Synthesis of essential from nonessential substances and formation of vitamins from precursors were discussed. Other interrelationships between nutrients were explained, including those of calcium, phosphorus and vitamin D; iron and copper, the B vitamins and ascorbic acid; vitamin E and selenium; vitamin B_6 and protein and fat; and folic acid and vitamin B_{12}, to mention a few. Functional relationships, such as the use of ascorbic acid and vitamin E as antioxidants, vitamin D and fluorides as an aid in calcification and in prevention of dental caries, and the trace minerals and the B-complex vitamins as parts of various enzyme systems were explained. Interplay between nutrients, including the amino acids, fatty acids, the less well-known minerals and the vitamins, is being investigated in many laboratories. Findings from these studies undoubtedly will introduce new problems and should serve to stimulate students to read professional journals regularly in order to keep abreast of the latest reliable information. A list of periodicals in which reports of such investigations appear is included in the Appendix.

The quality of the food supply is also important. Agriculture and the food industry are making many contributions. The first link in the chain of availability of superior foods today is controlled by the farmer. Guided by the results of agricultural research, the farmer plants improved seeds in proper soil, uses fertilizers balanced according to specific needs, harvests crops at their prime, and feeds balanced rations to animals and poultry.

Transportation is another important link. Current practices are based on the realization that quality affects nutritive value and that packaging and shipping methods have significant effects on nutrient retention. Precooling of fruits and vegetables, vacuum packaging, and storing in refrigerated compartments favor successful shipping over long distances. Transportation of perishable produce by air freight is another important factor in preserving the quality and in varying the food supply.

The distribution link is the final one in the chain. Foods to be sold fresh may have to be held for periods of time prior to sale. As a result, refrigerated display cases and iced fruit and vegetable counters are used in food markets. Storage of fresh produce in an atmosphere controlled as to temperature and humidity, often with increased carbon dioxide content, has resulted in greatly extended storage life, and it is a means of retaining some types of produce in their original states.

Today most foods are packaged. The procedures used before packaging to maintain freshness may affect nutritive value. Sorbic acid sprayed on cheese or its wrapper in controlled amounts retards mold growth. Antioxidants prevent rancidity in fats and foods high in fat content. A solution of aureomycin in which poultry is dipped after it is dressed retards growth of microorganisms. Radiation pasteurization keeps potatoes and onions from sprouting, kills trichinae in pork, destroys insects in grain products, and extends the shelf-life of prepackaged fresh meats. The low level of radiation used in this process does not actually destroy all microorganisms, but it is considered a safe procedure from the standpoint of the consumer's health. The use of any of these treatments or addition of any additive or chemical in any packaged food must be printed on the label. The habit of reading labels should be acquired by all food purchasers.

Much of the food available to the consumer has been preserved in order to destroy or inhibit the growth of microorganisms. Three preservation methods are commonly used: canning, freezing, and dehydration. Modern canning methods include use of pressure chambers and agitator cookers which are types of presterilization or aseptic canning. These are high-temperature techniques which markedly increase the rate of destruction of bacterial spores. The comparatively short time required for these procedures results in retention of color, flavor, and nutritive value which approximate those of freshly cooked foods.

One new development in freezing is dehydrofreezing. About half the water in fresh food is evaporated before freezing. The quality of the finished product is not affected, and packaging and storage costs are reduced. Frozen and freeze-dehydrated foods have excellent nutritive values which compare well with those of fresh foods even after cooking.

In recent years many improvements have been made in dehydration methods. These include procedures which speed the drying and cooling processes and result in retention of the volatile flavoring constituents in the dried foods.

Drying in a vacuum, which prevents oxidative changes and puts food products into a form which reconstitutes quickly, is one advance of food science and technology. Dried milk which may be reconstituted "instantly" is an example of the effectiveness of the dehydration process and of the contribution of food technology to improved nutritional status of people.

Radiation preservation of food is still in its experimental stages. Problems have arisen in relation to retention of color, flavor, odor, and texture of irradiated foods (23). Also, the health safety of foods processed by ionizing energy is being questioned. The potential health problems include production of toxic agents and of induced radioactivity, carcinogenicity, chromosome aberrations in plant materials resulting from the irradiation and autoclaving of sucrose, mutagenic changes in pathogenic bacteria, and shifts in microbial flora not recognized through odor before toxins are produced.

The nutritive quality of foods exposed to ionizing energy is reduced. The extent of the destruction of nutrients depends on the dosage applied and the relative sensitivity of a given nutrient to radiation. Radiation sterilization of a food results in greater destruction of vitamins, especially of thiamin, than radiation pasteurization. Sterilization and pasteurization are differentiated by the level of radiation dose and the resulting shelf-life of the product. The Joint Expert Committee of FAO/IAEA/WHO (24) has concluded that, although irradiation is a promising method for protecting and preserving food, it must be carefully controlled and more fully studied.

In the United States the food irradiation research program is broad in scope and is being conducted principally by the Atomic Energy Commission (AEC) and the Army (25, 26). The AEC has been concerned with radiation pasteurization of eggs, fish, fruits, vegetables, and poultry in order to extend their shelflife in conjunction with refrigeration. In contrast, the Army has concentrated on radiation sterilization of meats, poultry, and shrimp in order to produce packaged foods with a storage life of two years without refrigeration.

Chemical compounds are added to foods. Some chemicals are added intentionally, to control plant diseases and infestations by insects and rodents which can be detrimental to foods during growing periods or distribution. Since these substances may be toxic if ingested in large amounts, their concentration in food is carefully controlled.

There are about 700 functional and intentional additives. These have been studied and classified by the Food Protection Committee of the FNB of the National Research Council (27). The main reason for their use is to provide more food at lower unit cost to producer and to consumer. Some additives are used when the nutritive value of foods has been decreased during processing or refining. Important nutrient additions are thiamin, riboflavin, niacin, and iron which are required to enrich white flour and white bread. Now 28 states have mandatory bread-enrichment legislation and in the others enrichment is practiced widely. In some states corn, rice, and macaroni products must be enriched also. Voluntary enrichment is carried on by many cereal product manufacturers. Approximately all the margarine sold is fortified with vitamin A. Milk is the approved carrier of vitamin D; if skim, it usually also has vitamin A added to it. Additions of iodides to salt and fluorides to the public water supplies are other examples which, when properly controlled, are valuable additives. However, it is becoming increasingly evident that consumption of cereals and milk is declining and, therefore, questions are being raised as to the efficacy of the enrichment or fortification of these foods. It has been suggested that consideration be given to increasing the nutrients added to some foods and to encouraging use of fortified foods such as vitamin-D milk and iodized salt, and of enriched cereals and breads (15). The value of amino acids as supplements to cereals and to cereal-vegetable mixtures has been mentioned. However, when animal protein is available and is consumed in sufficient amounts, addition of amino acids to foods seems unnecessary.

A few chemical additives indirectly may have a beneficial effect on nutritional status. Meat tenderizers by softening connective tissue have been shown to make animal protein more available for use. The antioxidants used to prevent deterioration of fats have resulted in retention of vitamin A value.

False or biased opinions expressed by individuals in the press or other communication media may frighten or prejudice the public so that they will not use what they think of as food adulterants. Actually, lives have been saved by the use of chemical additives, and the nutritional status of many persons has been raised (28). It seems wise to follow the lead of federal, state, and local public health authorities who may be expected to make cautious and wise decisions in regard to the use of these additives.

The nutritional problems associated with care of the handicapped and of the mentally ill need consideration. In general, the nutritional needs of the handicapped are similar to needs of those who have no infirmities, but special adjustments may have to be made depending on the nature of the handicap. Work simplification and calorie intake may be problems for the crippled person. The individual who has rheumatic fever, arthritis, epilepsy, cleft palate, impaired vision, or a heart condition also may have nutrition problems.

The relationship of nutrition to mental health is an almost untouched field of research. Some work is being done on the status of B-vitamin nutriture and the psychological factors involved in the relation of food habits to mental illness. Although it is not assumed that diet plays a direct role in mental health, indirectly it may be significant. It has been suggested that some of the malnutrition being revealed in the preliminary findings of the NNS is caused by psychiatric disease (29).

The causes of disease as they relate to nutrient intake are being investigated. One of the more recent approaches to the study of the causes of disease in man is that not only pathogenic agents but also the environmental situation—including biological, physical, and social factors— are involved. Studies on the syndrome of weaning diarrhea which is endemic in most of the technically underdeveloped areas of the world have shown that there is a synergism between malnutrition and infection. The diarrhea occurs when the supply of breast milk is no longer adequate for the child, when the supplementary or substitute feeding is grossly deficient in protein and other nutrients, or when this feeding is contaminated because of poor sanitation.

Resistance to such infectious diseases as measles has been found to be related to nutritive state. The mortality rate among children from this communicable disease has been reported to be 90 times higher in Mexico and 189 times higher in Guatemala than in the United States (5). Economic and social factors which result in extensive malnutrition are considered responsible in these Latin-American countries.

Inborn errors of metabolism frequently lead to severe nutritional disease (30). These errors are inherited and originate in one or more mutations of a gene. The mutations may alter the metabolism of specific amino acids, carbohydrates, lipids, or minerals. Some of them, if not treated early, may result in mental retardation. In recent years many new inborn errors of metabolism have been identified, some of which can be treated successfully by dietary measures.

The stress of flight into space poses nutritional problems. The space ventures of astronauts in recent years have raised many questions about the nutritional needs of space explorers (31, 32). A new interdisciplinary technology which has been called "gastronautics" has developed. Johnson has suggested that the regulation of diet consistent with normal metabolic function and with food habits should be termed "astrophysiological dietetics." However, little is understood about the physiological response to nutrient intake during periods of weightlessness. It is thought that reduction of gravitational force may result in metabolic responses similar to those observed in patients at bed rest. These include excessive losses of calcium, phosphorus, sodium, and postassium, and possibly of other electrolytes. Evidence is accumulating that astronauts also may need additional magnesium in their food. Although precise data are lacking to support the need for increases in nutrient intake, studies on animals exposed to high altitudes indicate that increased intakes of some minerals and of ascorbic acid, vitamin E, and possibly of thiamin are beneficial. The combined efforts of research in engineering, food science, sociology, and nutrition are being directed to development of food systems that will be nutritionally adequate and acceptable to astronauts in space (33).

Nutritional knowledge needs to be brought to the lay person in a meaningful way. Solution of the many problems related to food and nutrition rests ultimately with those involved in the *science* of nutrition and those involved in the *practice* of nutrition (34). The *science* of nutrition is concerned with nutritional requirements and the factors that influence these needs. The *practice* of nutrition is involved with application of the fundamental knowledge gained through research in the science of nutrition. Students of nutrition have the responsibility to continue to expand and quantify more accurately the knowledge we have on human nutritional needs and the factors that influence these needs. Also, they have the responsibility of applying this knowledge toward solution of the international problem of malnutrition and undernutrition. An interdisciplinary approach is required if the world's food and nutrition needs are to be met. Chemists, biochemists, biologists, economists, food technologists, anthropologists, physicians, dentists, home economists, dietitians, nutritionists, and social workers all must be involved and work together. All have many contributions to make. Much has been accomplished in this century to improve the health and well-being of people throughout the world by the efforts and work of those trained in the science and practice of nutrition. The need for more persons trained in nutrition knowledge and interested in its application is much greater than the supply. The satisfaction of a life and work that is devoted to helping people solve problems related to emotional, economic, physiological, psychological, and social needs is a goal worth striving for and attaining.

REFERENCES

1. Panel on the World Food Supply, President's Science Advisory Committee. *The World Food Problem,* Vol. I and II. Washington, D.C.: Govt. Printing Office (1967).

2. Goldsmith, G. A. *World Food Supply and Population Increase.* Proc. Western Hemisphere Nutrition Congress II. Chicago: Am. Med. Ass., pg. 4 (1969).

3. Jansen, G. R., *et al.* World Problems in Protein Nutrition. *Am. J. Clin. Nutr., 15:*262 (1964).

4. Jelliffe, D. B. *Child Nutrition in developing Countries.* U.S. Public Health Service Pub. No. 1822. Washington, D.C.: Govt. Printing Office, 1968.

5. Scrimshaw, N. S. Ecological Factors in Nutritional Disease. *Am. J. Clin. Nutr., 14:*112 (1964).

6. Stare, F. J. Nutritional Improvement and World Health Potential. *J. Am. Diet. Ass., 57:*107 (1970).

7. Scrimshaw, N. S. Nature of Protein Requirements. Ways They Can Be Met in Tomorrow's World. *J. Am. Diet. Ass., 54:*94 (1969).

8. Butz, E. L. Our Daily Bread. *J. Am. Diet. Ass., 56:*107 (1970).

9. Food and Agriculture Organization of the United Nations. *Third World Food Survey.* Freedom from Hunger Campaign Basic Study No. 11. Rome (1963).

10. Schaefer, A. E. Nutritional Deficiencies in Developing Countries. *J. Am. Diet. Ass., 42:*295 (1963).

11. Scrimshaw, N. S. Endemic Goiter in Latin America. *Pub. Health Reports, 75:*731 (1960).

12. Darby, W. J. Research Developments in International Nutrition. *Am. J. Pub. Health, 53:*1789 (1963).

13. Prasad, A. S. A Century of Research on the Metabolic Role of Zinc. *Am. J. Clin. Nutr., 22:*1215 (1969).

14. International Committee on Nutrition for National Defense. *Manual for Nutrition Surveys,* 2nd. ed. Bethesda, Md.: Nat'l. Inst. of Health (1963).

15. Schaefer, A. E., *et al.* Are We Well Fed? The Search for the Answer. *Nutr. Today, 4, No. 1:*2 (1969).

16. McGanity, W. J. Preliminary Findings: Nutrition Survey in Texas. *Texas Med., 65:*40 (1969).

17. Schaefer, A. E. The National Nutrition Survey. *J. Am. Diet. Ass., 54:*371 (1969).

18. Goldsmith, G. A. Clinical Nutrition Problems in the United States Today. *Nutr. Revs., 23:*1 (1965).

19. Morgan, A. F., (ed.), *Nutritional Status U.S.A.* Berkeley: Calif. Agr. Sta. Bull. 769 (1959).

20. Hill, M. M. *Basic Nutrition Concepts—Their Use in Program Planning and Evaluation.* Nutr. Program News, USDA, Nov-Dec., 1964.

21. Hill, M. M. *Nutrition Education—An Integral Part of Consumer Education.* Nutr. Program News, USDA, May-June, 1970.

22. Wagner, M. G. The Irony of Affluence. *J. Am. Diet. Ass., 57:*311 (1970).

23. Goldblith, S. A. SANE Perspectives Regarding Radiation Effects. *Food Tech., 24:*44 (1970).

24. Food and Agriculture Organization and World Health Organization of the United Nations. *The Technical Basis for Legislation on Irradiated Food.* WHO Technical Report Series No. 316 and FAO Atomic Energy Series No. 6. Rome (1965).

25. Josephson, E. S., *et al.* Engineering and Economics of Food Irradiation. *Trans. N.Y. Acad. Sci.,* Series II, *30:*600 (1968).

26. Goldblith, S. A. Possible Applications to Food of Ionizing and Non-Ionizing Radiation. *J. Am. Diet. Ass., 51:*233 (1967).

27. National Academy of Sciences-National Research Council, Food Protection Committee, FNB. *Chemicals Used in Food Processing.* NRC Publ. 1274. Washington, D.C. (1965).

28. Coon, J. M. Protecting Our Internal Environment. *Nutr. Today,* 5, No. *2:*14 (1970).

29. Kampmeier, R. H. Mental Disease: A Cause of Malnutrition. *Nutr. Today,* 4, No. *1:*12 (1969).

30. Craig, J. W. Present Knowledge of Nutrition in Inborn Errors of Metabolism. *Nutr. Rev., 26:*161 (1968).

31. Calloway, D. H. Nutritional Aspects of Gastronautics. *J. Am. Diet. Ass., 40:*528 (1962).

32. Johnson, R. E. Calorie Requirements Under Adverse Conditions. *Fed. Proc., 22:*262 (1963).

33. Nanz, R. A., *et al.* Acceptability of Food Items Developed for Space Flight Feeding. *Food Tech., 21:*71 (1967).

34. Harper, A. E. Nutrition: Where Are We? Where Are We Going? *Am. J. Clin. Nutr., 22:*87 (1969).

GENERAL REFERENCES

35. Agricultural Research Service, USDA, *Toward the New: A Report on Better Foods and Nutrition from Agricultural Research.* Agriculture Information Bulletin No. 341. Washington, D.C. (1970).

36. Aykroyd, W. R. *Wheat in Human Nutrition.* FAO Nutritional Studies No. 23. FAO, Rome (1970).

37. Bing, F. C. Chemicals and Other Additives to Foods. *In* M. G. Wohl and R. S. Goodhart (eds.), *Modern Nutrition in Health and Disease,* 4th ed. Philadelphia: Lea & Febiger (1968).

38. Davis, R. A., *et al.* Review Studies of Vitamin and Mineral Nutrition in the United States (1950–1969). *J. Nutr. Ed., 1, No. 2, Supp. 1* (1969).

39. Food and Agricultural Organization of the United Nations. *Manual on Food and Nutrition Policy.* FAO Nutritional Studies No. 22. FAO, Rome (1969).

40. Food and Agriculture Organization of the United Nations. *Specifications for the Identity and Purity of Food Additives and Their Toxicological Evaluation: Some Emulsifiers and Stabilizers and Certain Other Substances; Some Flavouring Substances and Non-Nutritive Sweetening Agents; Some Antibiotics; Some Food Colours, Emulsifiers, Stabilizers, Anticaking Agents, and Certain Other Substances.* FAO Nutrition Meetings Reports Nos. 43, 44, 46, and WHO Technical Report Series Nos. 373, 383, 430, 445. Rome (1967, 1968, 1969, 1970).

41. Holmes, A. C. *Visual Aids in Nutrition Education. A Guide to Their Preparation and Use.* FAO, Rome (1968).

42. Kelsay, J. H. A Compendium of Nutritive Status Studies and Dietary Evaluation Studies Conducted in the United States, 1957–1967. *J. Nutr., 99:Supp. 1, Part II:* 123 (1969).

43. National Academy of Sciences-National Research Council. *Pre-School Child Malnutrition. Primary Deterrent to Human Progress.* NRC Pub. 1282. Washington, D.C. (1966).

44. National Academy of Sciences-National Research Council. *Some Considerations in the Use of Human Subjects in Safety Evaluation of Pesticides and Food Chemicals.* NRC Pub. 1270. Washington, D.C. (1965).

45. Nutrition Programs Service Unit, Consumer and Food Economics Research Division, ARS, USDA. *Proceedings of Nutrition Education Conference, Theme. Effective Communication.* Misc. Pub. No. 1075. Washington, D.C. (1968).

46. Ritchie, J. A. S. Learning Better Nutrition: *A Second Study of Approaches and Techniques.* FAO Nutritional Studies No. 21. FAO, Rome (1968).

Appendix

General References

BOOKS

Ackroyd, W. R. *Food for Man.* Long Island City, N.Y. Pergamon Press (1964).

Beaton, G. H. *Nutrition, A Comprehensive Treatise in Three Volumes:* I. *Macronutrients and Nutrient Elements,* 1964. II. *Vitamins, Nutrient Requirements, and Food Selection,* 1964. III. *Nutritional Status: Assessment and Applications,* 1966. New York: Academic Press.

Bogert, L. J., Briggs, G. M., and Calloway, D. H. *Nutrition and Physical Fitness,* 8th ed. Philadelphia: Saunders (1966).

Bourne, G. H. (ed.), *World Review of Nutrition and Dietetics,* Annual. White Plains, N.Y. Albert J. Phiebig (U.S. distributor).

Davidson, S., and Passmore, R. *Human Nutrition and Dietetics,* 4th ed. Baltimore: Williams & Wilkins (1969).

Guthrie, H. A. *Introductory Nutrition,* 2nd ed. St. Louis: Mosby (In preparation, 1970).

Hayes, J. (ed.), *Protecting Our Food: The Yearbook of Agriculture, 1966.* Washington, D.C.: USDA (1966).

Heald, F. P. (ed.), *Adolescent Nutrition and Growth.* New York: Appleton-Century-Crofts (Meredith) (1969).

Jolliffe, N. (ed.), *Clinical Nutrition,* 2nd ed. New York: Harper & Row (1962).

Lowenberg, M. E., Todhunter, E. N., Wilson, E. D., Feeney, M. C., and Savage, J. R. *Food & Man.* New York: Wiley (1968).

McCollum, E. V. *A History of Nutrition.* Boston: Houghton Mifflin (1957).

McHenry, E. W. *Basic Nutrition,* rev. ed. Philadelphia: Lippincott (1963).

Pike, R. L., and Brown, M. L. *Nutrition: An Integrated Approach.* New York: Wiley (1967).

Robinson, C. H. *Fundamentals of Nutrition.* New York: Macmillan (1968).

Robinson, C. H. *Proudfit-Robinson's Normal and Therapeutic Nutrition,* 13th ed. New York: Macmillan (1967).

Sebrell, W. H., Haggerty, J. J., and Editors of *Life. Food and Nutrition.* New York: Life Science Library Time Inc. (1967).

Stefferud, A. (ed.), *Food: The Yearbook of Agriculture, 1959.* Washington, D.C.: USDA (1959).

Taylor, C. M., and Pye, O. F. *Foundations of Nutrition,* 6th ed. New York: Macmillan (1966).

Williams, S. *Nutrition and Diet Therapy.* St. Louis: Mosby (1969).

Wilson, E. D., Fisher, K. H., and Fuqua, M. E. *Principles of Nutrition,* 2nd ed. (3rd ed. in preparation), New York: Wiley (1965).

Wohl, M. G., and Goodhart, R. S. (eds.), *Modern Nutrition in Health and Disease,* 4th ed. Philadelphia: Lea & Febiger (1968).

The abbreviations in parentheses have been used in the end-of-chapter reference lists of this text.

REVIEW PUBLICATIONS

Annual Review of Biochemistry	(Ann. Rev. Biochem.)
Annual Review of Physiology	(Ann. Rev. Physiol.)
Nutrition Abstracts and Reviews	(Nutr. Abstr. Revs.)
Nutrition Reviews	(Nutr. Revs.)
Physiological Reviews	(Physiol. Revs.)
Vitamins and Hormones	(Vitamins Hormones)

RESEARCH AND PROFESSIONAL JOURNALS

Acta Medica Scandinavia	(Acta Med. Scand.)
Acta Obstetrics and Gynecology Scandinavia	(Acta Obstet. Gynecol. Scand.)
Acta Odontologica Scandinavica	(Acta. Odont. Scand.)
Advances in Biological and Medical Physics	(Adv. Biol. Med. Phys.)
Advances in Metabolic Disorders	(Adv. Metab. Disord.)
American Journal of Clinical Nutrition	(Am. J. Clin. Nutr.)
American Journal of Digestive Diseases	(Am. J. Dig. Dis.)
American Journal of Diseases of Children	(Am. J. Dis. Childr.)
American Journal of Epidemiology	(Am. J. Epidemiol.)
American Journal of Medical Science	(Am. J. Med. Sci.)
American Journal of Medicine	(Am. J. Med.)
American Journal of Nursing	(Am. J. Nursing)
American Journal of Obstetrics and Gynecology	(Am. J. Obstet. Gynecol.)
American Journal of Physiology	(Am. J. Physiol.)
American Journal of Public Health	(Am. J. Pub. Health)
Annals of Internal Medicine	(Ann. Intern. Med.)
Annals of the New York Academy of Sciences	(Ann. N.Y. Acad. Sci.)
Archives of Biochemistry and Biophysics *until 1951, Archives of Biochemistry*	(Arch. Biochem. Biophy.) (Arch. Biochem.)
Archives of Diseases of Children	(Arch. Dis. Childr.)
Archives of Internal Medicine	(Arch. Intern. Med.)
Archives of International Medicine	(Arch. International Med.)
Biochemica et Biophysica Acta	(Biochem. Biophys. Acta)
Biochemical Journal	(Biochem. J.)
Blood	(Blood)
British Journal of Hematology	(Brit. J. Hematol.)

British Journal of Nutrition	(Brit. J. Nutr.)
British Medical Journal	(Brit. Med. J.)
Canadian Medical Association Journal	(Can. Med. Ass. J.)
Bulletin New York Academy of Medicine	(Bull. N.Y. Acad. Med.)
Cereal Chemistry	(Cereal Chem.)
Circulation	(Circula.)
Dental Progress	(Dent. Progress)
Diabetes	(Diabetes)
Endocrinology	(Endocrin.)
Experimenta	(Experimenta)
Federation Proceedings	(Fed. Proc.)
Food Research	(Food Research)
Food Technology	(Food Tech.)
Geriatrics	(Geriat.)
Gynecology and Obstetrics	(Gynecol. Obstet.)
Human Biology	(Human Biol.)
Journal of the American Chemical Society	(J. Am. Chem. Soc.)
Journal of the American Dental Association	(J. Am. Dent. Ass.)
Journal of the American Dietetic Association	(J. Am. Diet. Ass.)
Journal of the American Geriatrics Society	(J. Am. Geriat. Soc.)
Journal of the American Medical Association	(J. Am. Med. Ass.)
Journal of Applied Physiology	(J. Appl. Physiol.)
Journal of Atherosclerosis Research	(J. Ather. Res.)
Journal of Bacteriology	(J. Bact.)
Journal of Bone and Joint Surgery	(J. Bone Joint Surg.)
Journal of Biological Chemistry	(J. Biol. Chem.)
Journal of Clinical Investigation	(J. Clin. Invest.)
Journal of Clinical Pathology	(J. Clin. Pathol.)
Journal of Experimental Biology	(J. Expl. Biol.)
Journal of Experimental Medicine	(J. Expl. Med.)
Journal of Gerontology	(J. Gerontol.)
Journal of Home Economics	(J. Home Econ.)
Journal of Hygiene	(J. Hyg.)
Journal of Laboratory and Clinical Medicine	(J. Lab. Clin. Med.)
Journal of Lipid Research	(J. Lipid Res.)
Journal of Nutrition	(J. Nutr.)
Journal of Nutrition Education	(J. Nutr. Ed.)
Journal of Pediatrics	(J. Pediat.)

Journal of Physiology	(J. Physiol.)
Journal of the American Office of Agricultural Chemists	(J. Am. Off. Agr. Chem.)
Lancet	(Lancet)
Medicine	(Med.)
Milbank Memorial Fund Quarterly	(Milbank Mem. Fund Quart.)
New England Journal of Medicine	(New Eng. J. Med.)
New Zealand Medical Journal	(New Zealand Med. J.)
Nutrition Today	(Nutr. Today)
Pediatric Research	(Pediat. Res.)
Pediatrics	(Pediat.)
Postgraduate Medicine	(Postgrad. Med.)
Proceedings of the Society for Experimental Biology and Medicine	(Proc. Soc. Expl. Biol. Med.)
Public Health Reports	(Pub. Health Repts.)
Scandinavian Journal of Haematology, Series Haematologica	(Ser. Haematol.)
School Lunch Journal	(School Lunch J.)
Science	(Sci.)
Texas Medicine	(Texas Med.)
Transactions of the New York Academy of Science	(Trans. N.Y. Acad. Sci.)

Supplementary List of Food Composition Tables

GENERAL USE IN THE UNITED STATES

Agricultural Research Service. *Nutritive Value of Foods.* USDA, Home and Garden Bull. No. 72 Revised 1970; Slightly Revised, Jan., 1971.

Bunnell, R. H., *et al.* Alpha-Tocopherol Content of Foods. *Am. J. Clin. Nutr., 17:*1 (1965).

Chilean Iodine Educational Bureau. *Iodine Content of Foods: Annotated Bibliography 1825.* London (1952).

Church, C. F. *Food Values of Portions Commonly Used. Bowes and Church,* 11th ed. Philadelphia: Lippincott (1970).

Dicks, M. W. *Vitamin E Content of Foods and Feeds for Human and Animal Consumption.* Laramie: Wyoming Agr. Exp. Sta. Bull. 435 (1966).

Feeley, R. M., *et al.* Nutritive Values of Foods Distributed under USDA Food Assistance Programs. *J. Am. Diet. Ass., 57:*528 (1970).

Franz, M., *et al.* Calcium, Phosphorus, Magnesium, Sodium, and Potassium Composition of 95 Foods. *J. Am. Diet. Ass., 35:*1170 (1959).

Hardinge, M. G., *et al.* Lesser Known Vitamins in Foods. *J. Am. Diet. Ass., 38:*240 (1961).

Hardinge, M. G., *et al.* Carbohydrates in Foods. *J. Am. Diet. Ass., 46:*197 (1965).

McCance, R. A., *et al. The Composition of Foods,* 3rd rev. ed. Medical Research Council Spec. Rept. Series No. 297 (1960).

McCarthy, M. A., *et al.* Phenylalanine and Tyrosine in Fruits and Vegetables. *J. Am. Diet. Ass., 52:*130 (1968).

Merrill, A. L., *et al. Procedures for Calculating Nutritive Values of Home-Prepared Foods: as Used in Agriculture Handbook No. 8, Composition of Foods—raw, processed, prepared* (revised 1963). USDA, ARS 62–13 (1966).

Meyer, B. H., *et al.* Pantothenic Acid and Vitamin B_6 in Beef. *J. Am. Diet. Ass., 54:*122 (1969).

Milhanich, P., *et al.* Fatty Acids in Newer Brands of Margarine. *J. Am. Diet. Ass., 56:*29 (1970).

Orr, M. L. *Pantothenic Acid, Vitamin B_6, and Vitamin B_{12} in Foods.* USDA, Home Econ. Research Rept. No. 36 (1969).

Orr, M. L., *et al. Amino Acid Content of Foods.* USDA, Home Econ. Research Rept. No. 4 (1957).

Toepfer, E. W., *et al. Folic Acid Content of Foods—Microbiological Assay by Standardization Methods and Compilation of Data from the Literature.* USDA, Agr. Handbook No. 29 (1951).

Watt, B. K., *et al. Composition of Foods—raw, processed, prepared.* USDA, Agr. Handbook No. 8 (Revised 1963). (*Note:* In addition to the general tables on composition of foods, this handbook contains specific tables on selected fatty acids in foods, cholesterol in foods, and magnesium in foods.)

Zook, E. G., *et al.* Mineral Composition of Fruits. *J. Am. Diet. Ass., 52:*225 (1968).

Zook, E. G., *et al.* Total Diet Study: Content of Ten Minerals—Alumimum, Calcium, Phosphorus, Sodium, Potassium, Boron, Copper, Iron, Manganese, and Magnesium. *J. Ass. Off. Agric. Chem., 48:*850 (1965).

RELATED TO OTHER COUNTRIES

Aykroyd, W. R., *et al. The Nutritive Value of Indian Foods and the Planning of Satisfactory Diets.* Indian Council Med. Res. Bull. 23 (1956).

Bocobo, D. L., *et al. Food Composition Tables Recommended for Use in the Philippines.* Inst. of Nutrition, Dept. of Health, Handbook No. 1, Manila (1951).

Chatfield, C. *Food Composition Tables for International Use.* FAO, UN Nutritional Studies No. 3, Rome (1949).

Chatfield, C. *Food Composition Tables—Minerals and Vitamins—for International Use.* FAO, UN Nutritional Studies No. 11, Rome (1954).

Food and Agriculture Organization of the United Nations. *The Amino Acid Content of Foods and Biological Data on Proteins.* Food Policy and Food Science Service, Nutrition Division, No. 24, Rome (1970).

Food and Agriculture Organization of the United Nations. *Food Composition Tables—Annotated Bibliography.* Nutrition Information Documents Series. No. 1. Rome (1970). (Obtainable from UNIPUB, Inc., P.O. Box 443, New York.)

Leung, W. W. Food Composition Table for Use in Africa. Nutrition Program, National Center for Chronic Disease Control. Bethesda, Md. (1968). (Copies are obtainable from the Nutrition Program, National Center for Chronic Disease Control, Health Services and Mental Health Admin., Public Health Service, US Dept. of Health, Education & Welfare, Bethesda, Md.)

Leung, W. W., *et al.* INCAP-ICNND. *Food Composition Table for Use in Latin America.* Interdepartmental Comm. on Nutrition for Natl. Defense, Natl. Inst. of Health, Bethesda, Md. (1961).

Leung, W. W., *et al. Composition of Foods Used in Far Eastern Countries.* USDA, Agr. Handbook No. 34 (1952).

Miller, C. D., *et al. Nutritive Values of Some Hawaii Foods in Household Units and Common Measures.* Hawaii Agric. Expt. Sta. Circ. 52 (1957).

Platt, B. S. *Tables of Representative Values of Foods Commonly Used in Tropical Countries.* Med. Research Council Spec. Rept. Series No. 302. London: H. M. Stationery Off. (1962).

Schlosser, G. C., *et al.* Cottonseed Flour, Peanut Flour, and Soy Flour: Formulas and Procedures for Family and Institutional Use in Developing Countries. USDA, ARS No. 61–7 (1969).

Table A–1

*Minimum Daily Requirements of Specific Nutrients Established
by the United States Food and Drug Administration**†

Subjects	Cal-cium	Phos-phorus	Iron	Iodine	Vita-min A	Thia-min	Ribo-flavin	Niacin	Vita-min C	Vita-min D
					U.S.P.					U.S.P.
	mg.	mg.	mg.	mg.	units	mg.	mg.	mg.	mg.	units
Infants										
Not more than 12 months	—	—	—	—	1500	0.25	0.6	—	10	400
Children										
Less than 6 years	750	750	7.5	0.1	3000	0.50	0.9	5.0	20	400
6 years or more	750	750	10.0	0.1	3000	0.75	0.9	7.5	20	400
Adults										
12 years or more	750	750	10.0	0.1	4000	1.0	1.2	10.0	30	400
Pregnant women	1500	1500	15.0	0.1	4000	1.0	1.2	10.0	30	400

* Adapted from Code of Federal Regulations, Title 21, Sections 125.1, 125.3, 125.4. Washington, D.C., 1964. U.S. Government Printing Office.
† Table prepared by Patterson, M. L., and Marble, B. B., in *American Journal of Clinical Nutrition, 16:* 440–444, 1965. Courtesy of the authors and *American Journal of Clinical Nutrition.*

Table A–2

Body Weights in Kilograms (kg) and kg$^{3/4}$

	kg	kg$^{3/4}$		kg	kg$^{3/4}$
Infants	4	2.8	Males	35	14.4
	7	4.3		43	16.8
	9	5.2		59	21.3
Children	12	6.4		67	23.4
	14	7.2		70	24.2
	16	8.0	Females	44	17.1
	19	9.1		52	19.4
	23	10.5		54	19.9
	28	12.2		58	21.0

Recommended Dietary Allowances, Seventh Revised Edition. Washington, D.C.: FNB, NAS-NRC Publ. 1694 (1968).

Table A–3 / Recommended Daily Dietary Allowances,* Revised 1968

Food and Nutrition Board, National Academy of Sciences-National Research Council

DESIGNED FOR THE MAINTENANCE OF GOOD
NUTRITION OF PRACTICALLY ALL HEALTHY PEOPLE IN THE U.S.A.

	Age† (years) From Up to	Weight (kg)	(lbs)	Height cm	(in.)	kcal	Protein (gm)	Vita-min A Activity (IU)	Vita-min D (IU)	Vita-min E Activity (IU)
Infants	0–1/6	4	9	55	22	kg × 120	kg × 2.2||	1,500	400	5
	1/6–1/2	7	15	63	25	kg × 110	kg × 2.0||	1,500	400	5
	1/2–1	9	20	72	28	kg × 100	kg × 1.8||	1,500	400	5
Children	1–2	12	26	81	32	1,100	25	2,000	400	10
	2–3	14	31	91	36	1,250	25	2,000	400	10
	3–4	16	35	100	39	1,400	30	2,500	400	10
	4–6	19	42	110	43	1,600	30	2,500	400	10
	6–8	23	51	121	48	2,000	35	3,500	400	15
	8–10	28	62	131	52	2,200	40	3,500	400	15
Males	10–12	35	77	140	55	2,500	45	4,500	400	20
	12–14	43	95	151	59	2,700	50	5,000	400	20
	14–18	59	130	170	67	3,000	60	5,000	400	25
	18–22	67	147	175	69	2,800	60	5,000	400	30
	22–35	70	154	175	69	2,800	65	5,000	—	30
	35–55	70	154	173	68	2,600	65	5,000	—	30
	55–75+	70	154	171	67	2,400	65	5,000	—	30
Females	10–12	35	77	142	56	2,250	50	4,500	400	20
	12–14	44	97	154	61	2,300	50	5,000	400	20
	14–16	52	114	157	62	2,400	55	5,000	400	25
	16–18	54	119	160	63	2,300	55	5,000	400	25
	18–22	58	128	163	64	2,000	55	5,000	400	25
	22–35	58	128	163	64	2,000	55	5,000	—	25
	35–55	58	128	160	63	1,850	55	5,000	—	25
	55–75+	58	128	157	62	1,700	55	5,000	—	25
Pregnancy						+200	65	6,000	400	30
Lactation						+1,000	75	8,000	400	30

* The allowance levels are intended to cover individual variations among most normal persons as they live in the United States under usual environmental stresses. The recommended allowances can be attained with a variety of common foods, providing other nutrients for which human requirements have been less well defined.
† Entries on lines for age range 22–35 years represent the reference man and woman at age 22. All other entries represent allowances for the midpoint of the specified age range.

Table A–3 (continued)

Ascorbic Acid (mg)	Folacin‡ (mg)	Niacin (mg equiv)§	Riboflavin (mg)	Thiamin (mg)	Vitamin B_6 (mg)	Vitamin B_{12} (μg)	Calcium (g)	Phosphorus (g)	Iodine (μg)	Iron (mg)	Magnesium (mg)
35	0.05	5	0.4	0.2	0.2	1.0	0.4	0.2	25	6	40
35	0.05	7	0.5	0.4	0.3	1.5	0.5	0.4	40	10	60
35	0.1	8	0.6	0.5	0.4	2.0	0.6	0.5	45	15	70
40	0.1	8	0.6	0.6	0.5	2.0	0.7	0.7	55	15	100
40	0.2	8	0.7	0.6	0.6	2.5	0.8	0.8	60	15	150
40	0.2	9	0.8	0.7	0.7	3	0.8	0.8	70	10	200
40	0.2	11	0.9	0.8	0.9	4	0.8	0.8	80	10	200
40	0.2	13	1.1	1.0	1.0	4	0.9	0.9	100	10	250
40	0.3	15	1.2	1.1	1.2	5	1.0	1.0	110	10	250
40	0.4	17	1.3	1.3	1.4	5	1.2	1.2	125	10	300
45	0.4	18	1.4	1.4	1.6	5	1.4	1.4	135	18	350
55	0.4	20	1.5	1.5	1.8	5	1.4	1.4	150	18	400
60	0.4	18	1.6	1.4	2.0	5	0.8	0.8	140	10	400
60	0.4	18	1.7	1.4	2.0	5	0.8	0.8	140	10	350
60	0.4	17	1.7	1.3	2.0	5	0.8	0.8	125	10	350
60	0.4	14	1.7	1.2	2.0	6	0.8	0.8	110	10	350
40	0.4	15	1.3	1.1	1.4	5	1.2	1.2	110	18	300
45	0.4	15	1.4	1.2	1.6	5	1.3	1.3	115	18	350
50	0.4	16	1.4	1.2	1.8	5	1.3	1.3	120	18	350
50	0.4	15	1.5	1.2	2.0	5	1.3	1.3	115	18	350
55	0.4	13	1.5	1.0	2.0	5	0.8	0.8	100	18	350
55	0.4	13	1.5	1.0	2.0	5	0.8	0.8	100	18	300
55	0.4	13	1.5	1.0	2.0	5	0.8	0.8	90	18	300
55	0.4	13	1.5	1.0	2.0	6	0.8	0.8	80	10	300
60	0.8	15	1.8	+0.1	2.5	8	+0.4	+0.4	125	18	450
60	0.5	20	2.0	+0.5	2.5	6	+0.5	+0.5	150	18	450

‡ The folacin allowances refer to dietary sources as determined by *Lactobacillus casei* assay. Pure forms of folacin may be effective in doses less than ¼ of the RDA.

§ Niacin equivalents include dietary sources of the vitamin itself plus 1 mg equivalent for each 60 mg of dietary tryptophan.

‖ Assumes protein equivalent to human milk. For proteins not 100 percent utilized factors should be increased proportionately.

The Nutritive Value of Foods

EXPLANATION OF TABLE A–4

This table of nutritive values for common household measures of foods was prepared by the home economists of the USDA and published in Home and Garden Bulletin, No. 72, Nutritive Value of Foods. Reproduced here is the third edition of the table, revised in August, 1970, and slightly revised in January, 1971.

Foods listed: The table lists the food values of over 600 items commonly used in the United States. Some of the food items listed in previous editions were dropped because they are no longer in general use. More than 150 other items have been added and values for all foods reviewed and updated as necessary. Weight in grams is shown for an approximate measure of each food as it is described; if inedible parts are included in the description, both measure and weight include these parts.

The approximate measure shown for each food is in cups, ounces, pounds, a piece of a certain size, or some other well-known unit. The measure shown can be calculated readily to larger or smaller amounts by multiplying or dividing. However, because the measures are approximate (some are rounded for convenient use), calculated nutritive values for very large quantities of some food items may be less representative than those for smaller quantities.

The cup measure refers to the standard measuring cup of 8 fluid ounces or ½ liquid pint. The ounce refers to 1/16 of a pound avoirdupois, unless fluid ounce is indicated. The weight of a fluid ounce varies according to the food measured.

Food values: Values are shown for food energy, protein, fat, fatty acids, carbohydrate, calcium, iron, vitamin A value, thiamin, riboflavin, preformed niacin, and ascorbic acid. Water content is given also because the percentage of moisture present is needed for identification and comparison of many food items.

For many of the prepared items, values have been calculated from the ingredients in typical recipes. (See Merrill, A. L., *et al.* Procedures for Calculating Nutritive Values of Home-Prepared Foods. ARS, USDA, 62–13 (1966).

Values for vegetables and toast are without fat added, either during preparation or at the table. Some destruction of vitamins, especially of ascorbic acid, may occur when foods are cut or shredded. Such losses are variable, and no deduction for these losses has been made. Values for meat are as cooked and drained without drippings. For many cuts, values are for the meat both with and without the fat that can be trimmed either in preparation or after service.

Table A–4
Nutritive Values of the Edible Part of Foods

[Dashes in the columns for nutrients show that no suitable value could be found although there is reason to believe that a measurable amount of the nutrient may be present]

Food, approximate measure, and weight (in grams)		Water	Food energy	Protein	Fat	Fatty acids			Carbohydrate	Calcium	Iron	Vitamin A value	Thiamin	Riboflavin	Niacin	Ascorbic acid
						Saturated (total)	Unsaturated									
							Oleic	Linoleic								
	Grams	Percent	Calories	Grams	Grams	Grams	Grams	Grams	Grams	Milligrams	Milligrams	International units	Milligrams	Milligrams	Milligrams	Milligrams
MILK, CHEESE, CREAM, IMITATION CREAM; RELATED PRODUCTS																
Milk:																
Fluid:																
1 Whole, 3.5% fat----- 1 cup-----	244	87	160	9	9	5	3	Trace	12	288	0.1	350	0.07	0.41	0.2	2
2 Nonfat (skim)------ 1 cup-----	245	90	90	9	Trace				12	296	.1	10	.09	.44	.2	2
3 Partly skimmed, 2% nonfat milk solids added. 1 cup-----	246	87	145	10	5	3	2	Trace	15	352	.1	200	.10	.52	.2	2
Canned, concentrated, undiluted:																
4 Evaporated, unsweetened 1 cup-----	252	74	345	18	20	11	7	1	24	635	.3	810	.10	.86	.5	3
5 Condensed, sweetened 1 cup-----	306	27	980	25	27	15	9	1	166	802	.3	1,100	.24	1.16	.6	3
Dry, nonfat instant:																
6 Low-density (1⅓ cups needed for reconstitution to 1 qt.) 1 cup-----	68	4	245	24	Trace				35	879	.4	¹20	.24	1.21	.6	5
7 High-density (⅞ cup needed for reconstitution to 1 qt.). 1 cup-----	104	4	375	37	1				54	1,345	.6	¹30	.36	1.85	.9	7
Buttermilk:																
8 Fluid, cultured, made from skim milk. 1 cup-----	245	90	90	9	Trace				12	296	.1	10	.10	.44	.2	2
9 Dried, packaged------- 1 cup-----	120	3	465	41	6	3	2	Trace	60	1,498	.7	260	.31	2.06	1.1	------
Cheese:																
Natural:																
Blue or Roquefort type:																
10 Ounce---------- 1 oz.-----	28	40	105	6	9	5	3	Trace	1	89	.1	350	.01	.17	.3	0
11 Cubic inch------- 1 cu. in.	17	40	65	4	5	3	2	Trace	Trace	54	.1	210	.01	.11	.2	0

¹ Value applies to unfortified product; value for fortified low-density product would be 1500 I.U. and the fortified high-density product would be 2290 I.U.

Table A–4 (continued)

Nutritive Values of the Edible Part of Foods

[Dashes in the columns for nutrients show that no suitable value could be found although there is reason to believe that a measurable amount of the nutrient may be present]

	Food, approximate measure, and weight (in grams)		Water	Food energy	Pro-tein	Fat	Fatty acids Satu-rated (total)	Fatty acids Unsaturated Oleic	Fatty acids Unsaturated Lin-oleic	Carbo-hy-drate	Cal-cium	Iron	Vita-min A value	Thia-min	Ribo-flavin	Niacin	Ascor-bic acid
		Grams	Per cent	Calo-ries	Grams	Grams	Grams	Grams	Grams	Grams	Milli-grams	Milli-grams	Inter-national units	Milli-grams	Milli-grams	Milli-grams	Milli-grams
	MILK, CHEESE, CREAM, IMITATION CREAM; RELATED PRODUCTS—Con. Cheese—Continued Natural—Continued																
12	Camembert, pack-aged in 4-oz. pkg. with 3 wedges per pkg. 1 wedge	38	52	115	7	9	5	3	Trace	1	40	0.2	380	0.02	0.29	0.3	0
	Cheddar:																
13	Ounce 1 oz.	28	37	115	7	9	5	3	Trace	1	213	.3	370	.01	.13	Trace	0
14	Cubic inch 1 cu. in.	17	37	70	4	6	3	2	Trace	Trace	129	.2	230	.01	.08	Trace	0
	Cottage, large or small curd: Creamed:																
15	Package of 12-oz., net wt. 1 pkg.	340	78	360	46	14	8	5	Trace	10	320	1.0	580	.10	.85	.3	0
16	Cup, curd pressed down. 1 cup	245	78	260	33	10	6	3	Trace	7	230	.7	420	.07	.61	.2	0
	Uncreamed:																
17	Package of 12-oz., net wt. 1 pkg.	340	79	290	58	1	1	Trace	Trace	9	306	1.4	30	.10	.95	.3	0
18	Cup, curd pressed down. 1 cup	200	79	170	34	1	Trace	Trace	Trace	5	180	.8	20	.06	.56	.2	0
	Cream:																
19	Package of 8-oz., net wt. 1 pkg.	227	51	850	18	86	48	28	3	5	141	.5	3,500	.05	.54	.2	0
20	Package of 3-oz., net wt. 1 pkg.	85	51	320	7	32	18	11	1	2	53	.2	1,310	.02	.20	.1	0
21	Cubic inch 1 cu. in.	16	51	60	1	6	3	2	Trace	Trace	10	Trace	250	Trace	.04	Trace	0
	Parmesan, grated:																
22	Cup, pressed down. 1 cup	140	17	655	60	43	24	14	1	5	1,893	.7	1,760	.03	1.22	.3	0
23	Tablespoon 1 tbsp.	5	17	25	2	2	1	Trace	Trace	Trace	68	Trace	60	Trace	.04	Trace	0
24	Ounce 1 oz.	28	17	130	12	9	5	3	Trace	1	383	.1	360	.01	.25	.1	0
	Swiss:																
25	Ounce 1 oz.	28	39	105	8	8	4	3	Trace	1	262	.3	320	Trace	.11	Trace	0
26	Cubic inch 1 cu. in.	15	39	55	4	4	2	1	Trace	Trace	139	.1	170	Trace	.06	Trace	0

No.	Food, approximate measure, and weight	Measure	Grams	Water (pct.)	Food energy (cal.)	Protein (g)	Fat (g)	Saturated (total) (g)	Unsat. Oleic (g)	Unsat. Linoleic (g)	Carbohydrate (g)	Calcium (mg)	Iron (mg)	Vitamin A (I.U.)	Thiamine (mg)	Riboflavin (mg)	Niacin (mg)	Ascorbic acid (mg)
	Pasteurized processed cheese:																	
	American:																	
27	Ounce	1 oz.	28	40	105	7	9	5	3	Trace	1	198	.3	350	.01	.12	Trace	0
28	Cubic inch	1 cu. in.	18	40	65	4	5	3	2	Trace	Trace	122	.2	210	Trace	.07	Trace	0
	Swiss:																	
29	Ounce	1 oz.	28	40	100	8	8	4	3	Trace	1	251	.3	310	Trace	.11	Trace	0
30	Cubic inch	1 cu. in.	18	40	65	5	5	3	2	Trace	Trace	159	.2	200	Trace	.07	Trace	0
	Pasteurized process cheese food, American:																	
31	Tablespoon	1 tbsp.	14	43	45	3	3	2	1	Trace	1	80	.1	140	Trace	.08	Trace	0
32	Cubic inch	1 cu. in.	18	43	60	4	4	2	1	Trace	1	100	.1	170	Trace	.10	Trace	0
33	Pasteurized process cheese spread, American.	1 oz.	28	49	80	5	6	3	2	Trace	2	160	.2	250	Trace	.15	Trace	0
	Cream:																	
34	Half-and-half (cream and milk).	1 cup	242	80	325	8	28	15	9	1	11	261	.1	1,160	.07	.39	.1	2
35	Light, coffee or table	1 tbsp.	15	80	20	1	2	1	1	Trace	1	16	Trace	70	Trace	.02	Trace	Trace
36	Light, coffee or table	1 cup	240	72	505	7	49	27	16	1	10	245	.1	2,020	.07	.36	.1	2
37		1 tbsp.	15	72	30	1	3	2	1	Trace	1	15	Trace	130	Trace	.02	Trace	Trace
38	Sour	1 cup	230	72	485	7	47	26	16	1	10	235	.1	1,930	.07	.35	.1	2
39		1 tbsp.	12	72	25	Trace	2	1	1	Trace	1	12	Trace	100	Trace	.02	Trace	Trace
40	Whipped topping (pressurized).	1 cup	60	62	155	2	14	8	5	Trace	6	67	---	570	Trace	.04	---	---
41		1 tbsp.	3	62	10	Trace	Trace	Trace	Trace	Trace	Trace	3	---	30	Trace	Trace	Trace	---
	Whipping, unwhipped (volume about double when whipped):																	
42	Light	1 cup	239	62	715	6	75	41	25	2	9	203	.1	3,060	.05	.29	.1	2
43		1 tbsp.	15	62	45	Trace	5	3	2	Trace	1	13	Trace	190	Trace	.02	Trace	Trace
44	Heavy	1 cup	238	57	840	5	90	50	30	3	7	179	.1	3,670	.05	.26	.1	2
45		1 tbsp.	15	57	55	Trace	6	3	2	Trace	1	11	Trace	230	Trace	.02	Trace	Trace
	Imitation cream products (made with vegetable fat):																	
	Creamers:																	
46	Powdered	1 cup	94	2	505	4	33	31	1	0	52	21	.6	²200	---	Trace	Trace	---
47		1 tsp.	2	2	10	Trace	1	Trace	Trace	0	1	1	Trace	²Trace	---	---	---	---
48	Liquid (frozen)	1 cup	245	77	345	3	27	25	1	0	25	29	---	²100	0	0	0	---
49		1 tbsp.	15	77	20	Trace	2	1	Trace	0	2	2	.1	²10	0	0	0	---
50	Sour dressing (imitation sour cream) made with nonfat dry milk.	1 cup	235	72	440	9	38	35	1	Trace	17	277	Trace	10	.07	.38	.2	1
51		1 tbsp.	12	72	20	Trace	2	2	Trace	Trace	1	14	Trace	Trace	Trace	Trace	---	Trace
	Whipped topping:																	
52	Pressurized	1 cup	70	61	190	1	17	15	1	0	9	5	---	²340	---	0	0	---
53		1 tbsp.	4	61	10	Trace	1	1	Trace	0	Trace	Trace	Trace	²20	---	0	0	---

² Contributed largely from beta-carotene used for coloring.

Table A–4 *(continued)*

Nutritive Values of the Edible Part of Foods

[Dashes in the columns for nutrients show that no suitable value could be found although there is reason to believe that a measurable amount of the nutrient may be present]

#	Food, approximate measure, and weight (in grams)	Water (Percent)	Food energy (Calories)	Protein (Grams)	Fat (Grams)	Fatty acids Saturated (total) (Grams)	Fatty acids Unsaturated Oleic (Grams)	Fatty acids Unsaturated Linoleic (Grams)	Carbohydrate (Grams)	Calcium (Milligrams)	Iron (Milligrams)	Vitamin A value (International units)	Thiamin (Milligrams)	Riboflavin (Milligrams)	Niacin (Milligrams)	Ascorbic acid (Milligrams)
	MILK, CHEESE, CREAM, IMITATION CREAM; RELATED PRODUCTS—Con.															
	Whipped topping—Continued															
54	Frozen ---- 1 cup ---- 75	52	230	1	20	18	Trace	0	15	5	---	[2]560	---	0	---	0
55	1 tbsp ---- 4	52	10	Trace	1	1	Trace	0	1	Trace	---	[2]30	---	0	---	0
56	Powdered, made with whole milk. 1 cup ---- 75	58	175	3	12	10	1	Trace	15	62	Trace	[2]330	.02	.08	.1	Trace
57	1 tbsp ---- 4	58	10	Trace	1	1	Trace	Trace	1	3	Trace	[2]20	Trace	Trace	Trace	Trace
	Milk beverages:															
58	Cocoa, homemade ---- 1 cup ---- 250	79	245	10	12	7	4	Trace	27	295	1.0	400	.10	.45	.5	3
59	Chocolate-flavored drink made with skim milk and 2% added butterfat. 1 cup ---- 250	83	190	8	6	3	2	Trace	27	270	.5	210	.10	.40	.3	3
	Malted milk:															
60	Dry powder, approx. 1 oz ---- 28. 3 heaping teaspoons per ounce.	3	115	4	2	---	---	---	20	82	.6	290	.09	.15	.1	0
61	Beverage ---- 1 cup ---- 235	78	245	11	10	---	---	---	28	317	.7	590	.14	.49	.2	2
	Milk desserts:															
62	Custard, baked ---- 1 cup ---- 265	77	305	14	15	7	5	1	29	297	1.1	930	.11	.50	.3	1
	Ice cream:															
63	Regular (approx. 10% fat). ½ gal ---- 1,064	63	2,055	48	113	62	37	3	221	1,553	.5	4,680	.43	2.23	1.1	11
64	1 cup ---- 133	63	255	6	14	8	5	Trace	28	194	.1	590	.05	.28	.1	1
65	3 fl. oz. cup ---- 50	63	95	2	5	3	2	Trace	10	73	Trace	220	.02	.11	.1	1
66	Rich (approx. 16% fat). ½ gal ---- 1,188	63	2,635	31	191	105	63	6	214	927	.2	7,840	.24	1.31	1.2	12
67	1 cup ---- 148	63	330	4	24	13	8	1	27	115	Trace	980	.03	.16	.1	1
	Ice milk:															
68	Hardened ---- ½ gal ---- 1,048	67	1,595	50	53	29	17	2	235	1,635	1.0	2,200	.52	2.31	1.0	10
69	1 cup ---- 131	67	200	6	7	4	2	Trace	29	204	.1	280	.07	.29	.1	1
70	Soft-serve ---- 1 cup ---- 175	67	265	8	9	5	3	Trace	39	273	.2	370	.09	.39	.2	2

No.	Food, approximate measure		Grams	Water (pct)	Food energy	Protein	Fat	Saturated	Oleic	Linoleic	Carbohydrate	Calcium	Iron	Vit. A	Thiamine	Riboflavin	Niacin	Ascorbic acid
	Yoghurt:																	
71	Made from partially skimmed milk.	1 cup	245	89	125	8	4	2	1	Trace	13	294	.1	170	.10	.44	.2	2
72	Made from whole milk.	1 cup	245	88	150	7	8	5	3	Trace	12	272	.1	340	.07	.39	.2	2
	EGGS																	
	Eggs, large, 24 ounces per dozen:																	
	Raw or cooked in shell or with nothing added:																	
73	Whole, without shell	1 egg	50	74	80	6	6	2	3	Trace	Trace	27	1.1	590	.05	.15	Trace	0
74	White of egg	1 white	33	88	15	4	Trace	---	---	---	Trace	3	Trace	0	Trace	.09	Trace	0
75	Yolk of egg	1 yolk	17	51	60	3	5	2	2	Trace	Trace	24	.9	580	.04	.07	Trace	0
76	Scrambled with milk and fat.	1 egg	64	72	110	7	8	3	3	Trace	1	51	1.1	690	.05	.18	Trace	0
	MEAT, POULTRY, FISH, SHELLFISH; RELATED PRODUCTS																	
77	Bacon, (20 slices per lb. raw), broiled or fried, crisp.	2 slices	15	8	90	5	8	3	4	1	1	2	.5	0	.08	.05	.8	---
	Beef,[3] cooked:																	
	Cuts braised, simmered, or pot-roasted:																	
78	Lean and fat	3 ounces	85	53	245	23	16	8	7	Trace	0	10	2.9	30	.04	.18	3.5	---
79	Lean only	2.5 ounces	72	62	140	22	5	2	2	Trace	0	10	2.7	10	.04	.16	3.3	---
	Hamburger (ground beef), broiled:																	
80	Lean	3 ounces	85	60	185	23	10	5	4	Trace	0	10	3.0	20	.08	.20	5.1	---
81	Regular	3 ounces	85	54	245	21	17	8	8	Trace	0	9	2.7	30	.07	.18	4.6	---
	Roast, oven-cooked, no liquid added:																	
	Relatively fat, such as rib:																	
82	Lean and fat	3 ounces	85	40	375	17	34	16	15	1	0	8	2.2	70	.05	.13	3.1	---
83	Lean only	1.8 ounces	51	57	125	14	7	3	3	Trace	0	6	1.8	10	.04	.11	2.6	---
	Relatively lean, such as heel of round:																	
84	Lean and fat	3 ounces	85	62	165	25	7	3	3	Trace	0	11	3.2	10	.06	.19	4.5	---
85	Lean only	2.7 ounces	78	65	125	24	3	1	1	Trace	0	10	3.0	Trace	.06	.18	4.3	---
	Steak, broiled:																	
	Relatively fat, such as sirloin:																	
86	Lean and fat	3 ounces	85	44	330	20	27	13	12	1	0	9	2.5	50	.05	.16	4.0	---
87	Lean only	2.0 ounces	56	59	115	18	4	2	2	Trace	0	7	2.2	10	.05	.14	3.6	---
	Relatively lean, such as round:																	
88	Lean and fat	3 ounces	85	55	220	24	13	6	6	Trace	0	10	3.0	20	.07	.19	4.8	---
89	Lean only	2.4 ounces	68	61	130	21	4	2	2	Trace	0	9	2.5	10	.06	.16	4.1	---
	Beef, canned:																	
90	Corned beef	3 ounces	85	59	185	22	10	5	4	Trace	0	17	3.7	20	.01	.20	2.9	---
91	Corned beef hash	3 ounces	85	67	155	7	10	5	4	Trace	9	11	1.7	---	.01	.08	1.8	---
92	Beef, dried or chipped	2 ounces	57	48	115	19	4	2	2	Trace	0	11	2.9	---	.04	.18	2.2	---
93	Beef and vegetable stew	1 cup	235	82	210	15	10	5	4	Trace	15	28	2.8	2,310	.13	.17	4.4	15

[2] Contributed largely from beta-carotene used for coloring.

[3] Outer layer of fat on the cut was removed to within approximately ½-inch of the lean. Deposits of fat within the cut were not removed.

Table A–4 (continued)
Nutritive Values of the Edible Part of Foods

[Dashes in the columns for nutrients show that no suitable value could be found although there is reason to believe that a measurable amount of the nutrient may be present]

	Food, approximate measure, and weight (in grams)		Water	Food energy	Protein	Fat	Fatty acids			Carbohydrate	Calcium	Iron	Vitamin A value	Thiamin	Riboflavin	Niacin	Ascorbic acid
							Saturated (total)	Unsaturated									
								Oleic	Linoleic								
		Grams	Percent	Calories	Grams	Grams	Grams	Grams	Grams	Grams	Milligrams	Milligrams	International units	Milligrams	Milligrams	Milligrams	Milligrams
	MEAT, POULTRY, FISH, SHELLFISH; RELATED PRODUCTS—Continued																
94	Beef potpie, baked, 4¼-inch diam., weight before baking about 8 ounces. 1 pie ---	227	55	560	23	33	9	20	2	43	32	4.1	1,860	0.25	0.27	4.5	7
	Chicken, cooked:																
95	Flesh only, broiled --- 3 ounces ---	85	71	115	20	3	1	1	1	0	8	1.4	80	.05	.16	7.4	---
	Breast, fried, ½ breast:																
96	With bone --- 3.3 ounces ---	94	58	155	25	5	1	2	1	1	9	1.3	70	.04	.17	11.2	---
97	Flesh and skin only --- 2.7 ounces ---	76	58	155	25	5	1	2	1	1	9	1.3	70	.04	.17	11.2	---
	Drumstick, fried:																
98	With bone --- 2.1 ounces ---	59	55	90	12	4	1	2	1	Trace	6	.9	50	.03	.15	2.7	---
99	Flesh and skin only --- 1.3 ounces ---	38	55	90	12	4	1	2	1	Trace	6	.9	50	.03	.15	2.7	---
100	Chicken, canned, boneless 3 ounces ---	85	65	170	18	10	3	4	2	0	18	1.3	200	.03	.11	3.7	3
101	Chicken potpie, baked 4¼-inch diam, weight before baking about 8 ounces. 1 pie ---	227	57	535	23	31	10	15	3	42	68	3.0	3,020	.25	.26	4.1	5
	Chili con carne, canned:																
102	With beans --- 1 cup ---	250	72	335	19	15	7	7	Trace	30	80	4.2	150	.08	.18	3.2	---
103	Without beans --- 1 cup ---	255	67	510	26	38	18	17	1	15	97	3.6	380	.05	.31	5.6	---
104	Heart, beef, lean, braised --- 3 ounces ---	85	61	160	27	5			1	1	5	5.0	20	.21	1.04	6.5	1
	Lamb,[3] cooked:																
105	Chop, thick, with bone, broiled. 1 chop, 4.8 ounces.	137	47	400	25	33	18	12	1	0	10	1.5	---	.14	.25	5.6	---
106	Lean and fat --- 4.0 ounces ---	112	47	400	25	33	18	12	1	0	10	1.5	---	.14	.25	5.6	---
107	Lean only --- 2.6 ounces ---	74	62	140	21	6	3	2	Trace	0	9	1.5	---	.11	.20	4.5	---
	Leg, roasted:																
108	Lean and fat --- 3 ounces ---	85	54	235	22	16	9	6	Trace	0	9	1.4	---	.13	.23	4.7	---
109	Lean only --- 2.5 ounces ---	71	62	130	20	5	3	2	Trace	0	9	1.4	---	.12	.21	4.4	---
	Shoulder, roasted:																
110	Lean and fat --- 3 ounces ---	85	50	285	18	23	13	8	1	0	9	1.0	---	.11	.20	4.0	---
111	Lean only --- 2.3 ounces ---	64	61	130	17	6	3	2	Trace	0	8	1.0	---	.10	.18	3.7	---

Item No.	Food, approximate measure	Grams	Water (%)	Food energy (cal.)	Protein (g)	Fat (g)	Fatty acids — Saturated (total) (g)	Unsaturated — Oleic (g)	Unsaturated — Linoleic (g)	Carbohydrate (g)	Calcium (mg)	Iron (mg)	Vitamin A (I.U.)	Thiamine (mg)	Riboflavin (mg)	Niacin (mg)	Ascorbic acid (mg)
112	Liver, beef, fried — 2 ounces	57	57	130	15	6	—	—	—	3	6	5.0	30,280	.15	2.37	9.4	15
113	Pork, cured, cooked: Ham, light cure, lean and fat, roasted. — 3 ounces	85	54	245	18	19	7	8	2	0	8	2.2	0	.40	.16	3.1	—
114	Luncheon meat: Boiled ham, sliced — 2 ounces	57	59	135	11	10	4	4	1	0	6	1.6	0	.25	.09	1.5	—
115	Canned, spiced or unspiced. — 2 ounces	57	55	165	8	14	5	6	1	1	5	1.2	0	.18	.12	1.6	—
116	Pork, fresh,[3] cooked: Chop, thick, with bone. — 1 chop, 3.5 ounces.	98	42	260	16	21	8	9	2	0	8	2.2	0	.63	.18	3.8	—
117	Lean and fat — 2.3 ounces	66	42	260	16	21	8	9	2	0	8	2.2	0	.63	.18	3.8	—
118	Lean only — 1.7 ounces	48	53	130	15	7	2	3	1	0	7	1.9	0	.54	.16	3.3	—
119	Roast, oven-cooked, no liquid added: Lean and fat — 3 ounces	85	46	310	21	24	9	10	2	0	9	2.7	0	.78	.22	4.7	—
120	Lean only — 2.4 ounces	68	55	175	20	10	3	4	1	0	9	2.6	0	.73	.21	4.4	—
121	Cuts, simmered: Lean and fat — 3 ounces	85	46	320	20	26	9	11	2	0	8	2.5	0	.46	.21	4.1	—
122	Lean only — 2.2 ounces	63	60	135	18	6	2	3	1	0	8	2.3	0	.42	.19	3.7	—
123	Sausage: Bologna, slice, 3-in. diam. by ⅛ inch. — 2 slices	26	56	80	3	7	—	—	—	Trace	2	.5	—	.04	.06	.7	—
124	Braunschweiger, slice 2-in. diam. by ¼ inch. — 2 slices	20	53	65	3	5	2	2	Trace	Trace	2	1.2	1,310	.03	.29	1.6	—
125	Deviled ham, canned — 1 tbsp.	13	51	45	2	4	—	2	—	0	1	.3	—	.02	.01	.2	—
126	Frankfurter, heated (8 per lb. purchased pkg.). — 1 frank.	56	57	170	7	15	—	—	—	1	3	.8	—	.08	.11	1.4	—
127	Pork links, cooked (16 links per lb. raw). — 2 links	26	35	125	5	11	4	5	1	Trace	2	.6	0	.21	.09	1.0	—
128	Salami, dry type — 1 oz.	28	30	130	7	11	—	—	—	Trace	4	1.0	—	.10	.07	1.5	—
129	Salami, cooked — 1 oz.	28	51	90	5	7	—	—	—	Trace	3	.7	—	.07	.07	1.2	—
130	Vienna, canned (7 sausages per 5-oz. can). — 1 sausage	16	63	40	2	3	—	—	—	Trace	1	.3	—	.01	.02	.4	—
131	Veal, medium fat, cooked, bone removed: Cutlet. — 3 oz.	85	60	185	23	9	5	4	Trace	0	9	2.7	—	.06	.21	4.6	—
132	Roast. — 3 oz.	85	55	230	23	14	7	6	Trace	0	10	2.9	—	.11	.26	6.6	—
133	Fish and shellfish: Bluefish, baked with table fat. — 3 oz.	85	68	135	22	4	—	—	—	0	25	.6	40	.09	.08	1.6	—
134	Clams: Raw, meat only — 3 oz.	85	82	65	11	1	—	—	—	2	59	5.2	90	.08	.15	1.1	8
135	Canned, solids and liquid. — 3 oz.	85	86	45	7	1	—	—	—	2	47	3.5	—	.01	.09	.9	—
136	Crabmeat, canned — 3 oz.	85	77	85	15	2	—	—	—	1	38	.7	—	.07	.07	1.6	—

[3] Outer layer of fat on the cut was removed to within approximately ½-inch of the lean. Deposits of fat within the cut were not removed.

Table A–4 (continued)

Nutritive Values of the Edible Part of Foods

[Dashes in the columns for nutrients show that no suitable value could be found although there is reason to believe that a measurable amount of the nutrient may be present]

	Food, approximate measure, and weight (in grams)	Water	Food energy	Protein	Fat	Fatty acids			Carbohydrate	Calcium	Iron	Vitamin A value	Thiamin	Riboflavin	Niacin	Ascorbic acid
						Saturated (total)	Unsaturated									
							Oleic	Linoleic								
		Per cent	Calories	Grams	Grams	Grams	Grams	Grams	Grams	Milligrams	Milligrams	International units	Milligrams	Milligrams	Milligrams	Milligrams
	MEAT, POULTRY, FISH, SHELLFISH; RELATED PRODUCTS—Continued															
	Fish and shellfish—Continued															
137	Fish sticks, breaded, cooked, frozen; stick 3¾ by 1 by ½ inch. 10 sticks or 8 oz. pkg. 227	66	400	38	20	5	4	10	15	25	0.9	-----	0.09	0.16	3.6	-----
188	Haddock, breaded, fried 3 oz. 85	66	140	17	5	1	3	Trace	5	34	1.0	-----	.03	.06	2.7	-----
189	Ocean perch, breaded, fried 3 oz. 85	59	195	16	11	-----	-----	-----	6	28	1.1	-----	.08	.09	1.5	-----
140	Oysters, raw, meat only (13–19 med. selects). 1 cup 240	85	160	20	4	-----	-----	-----	8	226	13.2	740	.33	.43	6.0	-----
141	Salmon, pink, canned 3 oz. 85	71	120	17	5	1	1	Trace	0	4167	.7	60	.03	.16	6.8	-----
142	Sardines, Atlantic, canned in oil, drained solids. 3 oz. 85	62	175	20	9	-----	-----	-----	0	372	2.5	190	.02	.17	4.6	-----
143	Shad, baked with table fat and bacon. 3 oz. 85	64	170	20	10	-----	-----	-----	0	20	.5	20	.11	.22	7.3	-----
144	Shrimp, canned, meat 3 oz. 85	70	100	21	1	-----	-----	-----	1	98	2.6	50	.01	.03	1.5	-----
145	Swordfish, broiled with butter or margarine. 3 oz. 85	65	150	24	5	-----	-----	-----	0	23	1.1	1,750	.03	.04	9.3	-----
146	Tuna, canned in oil, drained solids. 3 oz. 85	61	170	24	7	2	1	1	0	7	1.6	70	.04	.10	10.1	-----
	MATURE DRY BEANS AND PEAS, NUTS, PEANUTS; RELATED PRODUCTS															
147	Almonds, shelled, whole 1 cup 142	5	850	26	77	6	52	15	28	332	6.7	0	.34	1.31	5.0	Trace
	Beans, dry: Common varieties as Great Northern, navy, and others: Cooked, drained:															
148	Great Northern 1 cup 180	69	210	14	1	-----	-----	-----	38	90	4.9	0	.25	.13	1.3	0

No.	Food, approximate measure	Measure	Grams	Water (%)	Food energy (cal.)	Protein (g)	Fat (g)	Saturated (g)	Oleic (g)	Linoleic (g)	Carbohydrate (g)	Calcium (mg)	Iron (mg)	Vitamin A (I.U.)	Thiamine (mg)	Riboflavin (mg)	Niacin (mg)	Ascorbic acid (mg)
149	Navy (pea)	1 cup	190	69	225	15	1	---	---	---	40	95	5.1	0	.27	.13	1.3	0
	Canned, solids and liquid: White with—																	
150	Frankfurters (sliced)	1 cup	255	71	365	19	18	---	---	---	32	94	4.8	330	.18	.15	3.3	Trace
151	Pork and tomato sauce	1 cup	255	71	310	16	7	2	3	1	49	138	4.6	330	.20	.08	1.5	5
152	Pork and sweet sauce	1 cup	255	66	385	16	12	4	5	1	54	161	5.9	---	.15	.10	1.3	---
153	Red kidney	1 cup	255	76	230	15	1	---	---	---	42	74	4.6	10	.13	.10	1.5	---
154	Lima, cooked, drained	1 cup	190	64	260	16	1	---	---	---	49	55	5.9	---	.25	.11	1.3	---
155	Cashew nuts, roasted	1 cup	140	5	785	24	64	11	45	4	41	53	5.3	140	.60	.35	2.5	---
	Coconut, fresh, meat only:																	
156	Pieces, approx. 2 by 2 by ½ inch	1 piece	45	51	155	2	16	14	1	Trace	4	6	.8	0	.02	.01	.2	1
157	Shredded or grated, firmly packed	1 cup	130	51	450	5	46	39	3	Trace	12	17	2.2	0	.07	.03	.7	4
158	Cowpeas or blackeye peas, dry, cooked	1 cup	248	80	190	13	1	---	---	---	34	42	3.2	20	.41	.11	1.1	Trace
159	Peanuts, roasted, salted, halves	1 cup	144	2	840	37	72	16	31	21	27	107	3.0	---	.46	.19	24.7	0
160	Peanut butter	1 tbsp.	16	2	95	4	8	2	4	2	3	9	.3	---	.02	.02	2.4	0
161	Peas, split, dry, cooked	1 cup	250	70	290	20	1	---	---	---	52	28	4.2	100	.37	.22	2.2	---
162	Pecans, halves	1 cup	108	3	740	10	77	5	48	15	16	79	2.6	140	.93	.14	1.0	2
163	Walnuts, black or native, chopped	1 cup	126	3	790	26	75	4	26	36	19	Trace	7.6	380	.28	.14	.9	---
	VEGETABLES AND VEGETABLE PRODUCTS																	
	Asparagus, green: Cooked, drained:																	
164	Spears, ½-in. diam. at base	4 spears	60	94	10	1	Trace	---	---	---	2	13	.4	540	.10	.11	.8	16
165	Pieces, 1½ to 2-in. lengths	1 cup	145	94	30	3	Trace	---	---	---	5	30	.9	1,310	.23	.26	2.0	38
166	Canned, solids and liquid	1 cup	244	94	45	5	1	---	---	---	7	44	4.1	1,240	.15	.22	2.0	37
	Beans:																	
167	Lima, immature seeds, cooked, drained	1 cup	170	71	190	13	1	---	---	---	34	80	4.3	480	.31	.17	2.2	29
	Snap: Green:																	
168	Cooked, drained	1 cup	125	92	30	2	Trace	---	---	---	7	63	.8	680	.09	.11	.6	15
169	Canned, solids and liquid	1 cup	239	94	45	2	Trace	---	---	---	10	81	2.9	690	.07	.10	.7	10

[4] If bones are discarded, value will be greatly reduced.

Nutritive Values of the Edible Part of Foods

[Dashes in the columns for nutrients show that no suitable value could be found although there is reason to believe that a measurable amount of the nutrient may be present]

Food, approximate measure, and weight (in grams)		Water	Food energy	Protein	Fat	Fatty acids			Carbohydrate	Calcium	Iron	Vitamin A value	Thiamin	Riboflavin	Niacin	Ascorbic acid
						Saturated (total)	Unsaturated Oleic	Linoleic								
	Grams	Per cent	Calories	Grams	Grams	Grams	Grams	Grams	Grams	Milligrams	Milligrams	International units	Milligrams	Milligrams	Milligrams	Milligrams
VEGETABLES AND VEGETABLE PRODUCTS—Continued																
Beans—Continued																
Snap—Continued																
Yellow or wax:																
170 Cooked, drained... 1 cup	125	93	30	2	Trace	-----	-----	-----	6	63	0.8	290	0.09	0.11	0.6	16
171 Canned, solids and liquid. 1 cup	239	94	45	2	1	-----	-----	-----	10	81	2.9	140	.07	.10	.7	12
172 Sprouted mung beans, cooked, drained. 1 cup	125	91	35	4	Trace	-----	-----	-----	7	21	1.1	30	.11	.13	.9	8
Beets:																
173 Cooked, drained, peeled: Whole beets, 2-in. diam. 2 beets	100	91	30	1	Trace	-----	-----	-----	7	14	.5	20	.03	.04	.3	6
174 Diced or sliced 1 cup	170	91	55	2	Trace	-----	-----	-----	12	24	.9	30	.05	.07	.5	10
175 Canned, solids and liquid. 1 cup	246	90	85	2	Trace	-----	-----	-----	19	34	1.5	20	.02	.05	.2	7
176 Beet greens, leaves and stems, cooked, drained. 1 cup	145	94	25	3	Trace	-----	-----	-----	5	144	2.8	7,400	.10	.22	.4	22
Blackeye peas. See Cowpeas.																
Broccoli, cooked, drained:																
177 Whole stalks, medium size. 1 stalk	180	91	45	6	1	-----	-----	-----	8	158	1.4	4,500	.16	.36	1.4	162
178 Stalks cut into ½-in. pieces. 1 cup	155	91	40	5	1	-----	-----	-----	7	136	1.2	3,880	.14	.31	1.2	140
179 Chopped, yield from 10-oz. frozen pkg. 1⅜ cups	250	92	65	7	1	-----	-----	-----	12	135	1.8	6,500	.15	.30	1.3	143
180 Brussels sprouts, 7-8 sprouts (1¼ to 1½ in. diam.) per cup, cooked. 1 cup	155	88	55	7	1	-----	-----	-----	10	50	1.7	810	.12	.22	1.2	135
Cabbage:																
Common varieties:																

No.	Food	Measure	Weight (g)	Water (%)	Food energy	Protein (g)	Fat (g)				Carbohydrate (g)	Calcium (mg)	Iron (mg)	Vitamin A (I.U.)	Thiamine (mg)	Riboflavin (mg)	Niacin (mg)	Ascorbic acid (mg)
	Raw:																	
181	Coarsely shredded or sliced.	1 cup	70	92	15	1	Trace	---	---	---	4	34	.3	90	.04	.04	.2	33
182	Finely shredded or chopped.	1 cup	90	92	20	1	Trace	---	---	---	5	44	.4	120	.05	.05	.3	42
183	Cooked.	1 cup	145	94	30	2	Trace	---	---	---	6	64	.4	190	.06	.06	.4	48
184	Red, raw, coarsely shredded.	1 cup	70	90	20	1	Trace	---	---	---	5	29	.6	30	.06	.04	.3	43
185	Savoy, raw, coarsely shredded.	1 cup	70	92	15	2	Trace	---	---	---	3	47	.6	140	.04	.06	.2	39
186	Cabbage, celery or Chinese, raw, cut in 1-in. pieces.	1 cup	75	95	10	1	Trace	---	---	---	2	32	.5	110	.04	.03	.5	19
187	Cabbage, spoon (or pakchoy), cooked.	1 cup	170	95	25	2	Trace	---	---	---	4	252	1.0	5,270	.07	.14	1.2	26
	Carrots:																	
	Raw:																	
188	Whole, 5½ by 1 inch, (25 thin strips).	1 carrot	50	88	20	1	Trace	---	---	---	5	18	.4	5,500	.03	.03	.3	4
189	Grated.	1 cup	110	88	45	1	Trace	---	---	---	11	41	.8	12,100	.06	.06	.7	9
190	Cooked, diced.	1 cup	145	91	45	1	Trace	---	---	---	10	48	.9	15,220	.08	.07	.7	9
191	Canned, strained or chopped (baby food).	1 ounce	28	92	10	Trace	Trace	---	---	---	2	7	.1	3,690	.01	.01	.1	1
192	Cauliflower, cooked, flowerbuds.	1 cup	120	93	25	3	Trace	---	---	---	5	25	.8	70	.11	.10	.7	66
	Celery, raw:																	
193	Stalk, large outer, 8 by about 1½ inches, at root end.	1 stalk	40	94	5	Trace	Trace	---	---	---	2	16	.1	100	.01	.01	.1	4
194	Pieces, diced.	1 cup	100	94	15	1	Trace	---	---	---	4	39	.3	240	.03	.03	.3	9
195	Collards, cooked.	1 cup	190	91	55	5	1	---	---	---	9	289	1.1	10,260	.27	.37	2.4	87
	Corn, sweet:																	
196	Cooked, ear 5 by 1¾ inches.[5]	1 ear	140	74	70	3	1	---	---	---	16	2	.5	[6]310	.09	.08	1.0	7
197	Canned, solids and liquid.	1 cup	256	81	170	5	2	---	---	---	40	10	1.0	[6]690	.07	.12	2.3	13
198	Cowpeas, cooked, immature seeds.	1 cup	160	72	175	13	1	---	---	---	29	38	3.4	560	.49	.18	2.3	28
	Cucumbers, 10-ounce; 7½ by about 2 inches:																	
199	Raw, pared.	1 cucumber	207	96	30	1	Trace	---	---	---	7	35	.6	Trace	.07	.09	.4	23
200	Raw, pared, center slice ⅛-inch thick.	6 slices	50	96	5	Trace	Trace	---	---	---	2	8	.2	Trace	.02	.02	.1	6
201	Dandelion greens, cooked.	1 cup	180	90	60	4	1	---	---	---	12	252	3.2	21,060	.24	.29	---	32

[5] Measure and weight apply to entire vegetable or fruit including parts not usually eaten.

[6] Based on yellow varieties; white varieties contain only a trace of cryptoxanthin and carotenes, the pigments in corn that have biological activity.

Table A-4 (continued)

Nutritive Values of the Edible Part of Foods

[Dashes in the columns for nutrients show that no suitable value could be found although there is reason to believe that a measurable amount of the nutrient may be present]

	Food, approximate measure, and weight (in grams)	Water	Food energy	Protein	Fat	Fatty acids Saturated (total)	Unsaturated Oleic	Unsaturated Linoleic	Carbohydrate	Calcium	Iron	Vitamin A value	Thiamin	Riboflavin	Niacin	Ascorbic acid
		Per cent	Calories	Grams	Grams	Grams	Grams	Grams	Grams	Milligrams	Milligrams	International units	Milligrams	Milligrams	Milligrams	Milligrams
	VEGETABLES AND VEGETABLE PRODUCTS—Continued															
202	Endive, curly (including escarole). 2 ounces 57	93	10	1	Trace				2	46	1.0	1,870	0.04	0.08	0.3	6
203	Kale, leaves including stems, cooked. 1 cup 110	91	30	4	1				4	147	1.3	8,140				68
	Lettuce, raw:															
204	Butterhead, as Boston types; head, 4-inch diameter. 1 head 220	95	30	3	Trace				6	77	4.4	2,130	.14	.13	.6	18
205	Crisphead, as Iceberg; head, 4¾-inch diameter. 1 head 454	96	60	4	Trace				13	91	2.3	1,500	.29	.27	1.3	29
206	Looseleaf, or bunching varieties, leaves. 2 large 50	94	10	1	Trace				2	34	.7	950	.03	.04	.2	9
207	Mushrooms, canned, solids and liquid. 1 cup 244	93	40	5	Trace				6	15	1.2	Trace	.04	.60	4.8	4
208	Mustard greens, cooked. 1 cup 140	93	35	3	1				6	193	2.5	8,120	.11	.19	.9	68
209	Okra, cooked, pod 3 by ⅝ inch. 8 pods 85	91	25	2	Trace				5	78	.4	420	.11	.15	.8	17
	Onions:															
	Mature:															
210	Raw, onion 2½-inch diameter. 1 onion 110	89	40	2	Trace				10	30	.6	40	.04	.04	.2	11
211	Cooked. 1 cup 210	92	60	3	Trace				14	50	.8	80	.06	.06	.4	14
212	Young green, small, without tops. 6 onions 50	88	20	1	Trace				5	20	.3	Trace	.02	.02	.2	12
213	Parsley, raw, chopped. 1 tablespoon 4	85	Trace	Trace	Trace				Trace	8	.2	340	Trace	.01	Trace	7
214	Parsnips, cooked. 1 cup 155	82	100	2	1				23	70	.9	50	.11	.12	.2	16
	Peas, green:															
215	Cooked. 1 cup 160	82	115	9	1				19	37	2.9	860	.44	.17	3.7	33
216	Canned, solids and liquid. 1 cup 249	83	165	9	1				31	50	4.2	1,120	.23	.13	2.2	22

No.	Food	Measure																
217	Canned, strained (baby food).	1 ounce	28	86	15	1	Trace	---	---	---	3	3	.4	140	.02	.02	.4	3
218	Peppers, hot, red, without seeds, dried (ground chili powder, added seasonings).	1 tablespoon	15	8	50	2	2	---	---	---	8	40	2.3	9,750	.03	.17	1.3	2
	Peppers, sweet:																	
	Raw, about 5 per pound:																	
219	Green pod without stem and seeds.	1 pod	74	93	15	1	Trace	---	---	---	4	7	.5	310	.06	.06	.4	94
220	Cooked, boiled, drained	1 pod	73	95	15	1	Trace	---	---	---	3	7	.4	310	.05	.05	.4	70
	Potatoes, medium (about 3 per pound raw):																	
221	Baked, peeled after baking.	1 potato	99	75	90	3	Trace	---	---	---	21	9	.7	Trace	.10	.04	1.7	20
	Boiled:																	
222	Peeled after boiling	1 potato	136	80	105	3	Trace	---	---	---	23	10	.8	Trace	.13	.05	2.0	22
223	Peeled before boiling	1 potato	122	83	80	2	Trace	---	---	---	18	7	.6	Trace	.11	.04	1.4	20
	French-fried, piece 2 by ½ by ½ inch:																	
224	Cooked in deep fat	10 pieces	57	45	155	2	7	2	2	4	20	9	.7	Trace	.07	.04	1.8	12
225	Frozen, heated	10 pieces	57	53	125	2	5	1	1	2	19	5	1.0	Trace	.08	.01	1.5	12
	Mashed:																	
226	Milk added	1 cup	195	83	125	4	1	1	---	---	25	47	.8	50	.16	.10	2.0	19
227	Milk and butter added	1 cup	195	80	185	4	8	4	3	Trace	24	47	.8	330	.16	.10	1.9	18
228	Potato chips, medium, 2-inch diameter.	10 chips	20	2	115	1	8	2	2	4	10	8	.4	Trace	.04	.01	1.0	3
229	Pumpkin, canned	1 cup	228	90	75	2	1	---	---	---	18	57	.9	14,590	.07	.12	1.3	12
230	Radishes, raw, small, without tops.	4 radishes	40	94	5	Trace	Trace	---	---	---	1	12	.4	Trace	.01	.01	.1	10
231	Sauerkraut, canned, solids and liquid.	1 cup	235	93	45	2	Trace	---	---	---	9	85	1.2	120	.07	.09	.4	33
	Spinach:																	
232	Cooked	1 cup	180	92	40	5	1	---	---	---	6	167	4.0	14,580	.13	.25	1.0	50
233	Canned, drained solids	1 cup	180	91	45	5	1	---	---	---	6	212	4.7	14,400	.03	.21	.6	24
	Squash:																	
	Cooked:																	
234	Summer, diced	1 cup	210	96	30	2	Trace	---	---	---	7	52	.8	820	.10	.16	1.6	21
235	Winter, baked, mashed.	1 cup	205	81	130	4	1	---	---	---	32	57	1.6	8,610	.10	.27	1.4	27
	Sweetpotatoes:																	
	Cooked, medium, 5 by 2 inches, weight raw about 6 ounces:																	
236	Baked, peeled after baking.	1 sweet-potato.	110	64	155	2	1	---	---	---	36	44	1.0	8,910	.10	.07	.7	24
237	Boiled, peeled after boiling.	1 sweet-potato.	147	71	170	2	1	---	---	---	39	47	1.0	11,610	.13	.09	.9	25

Table A–4 (continued)

Nutritive Values of the Edible Part of Foods

[Dashes in the columns for nutrients show that no suitable value could be found although there is reason to believe that a measurable amount of the nutrient may be present]

	Food, approximate measure, and weight (in grams)	Water	Food energy	Pro-tein	Fat	Fatty acids Satu-rated (total)	Unsaturated Oleic	Unsaturated Lin-oleic	Carbo-hy-drate	Cal-cium	Iron	Vita-min A value	Thia-min	Ribo-flavin	Niacin	Ascor-bic acid
		Per-cent	*Calo-ries*	*Grams*	*Grams*	*Grams*	*Grams*	*Grams*	*Grams*	*Milli-grams*	*Milli-grams*	*Inter-national units*	*Milli-grams*	*Milli-grams*	*Milli-grams*	*Milli-grams*
	VEGETABLES AND VEGETABLE PRODUCTS—Continued															
	Sweetpotatoes—Continued															
238	Candied, 3½ by 2¼ inches. 1 sweet-potato. *Grams* 175	60	295	2	6	2	3	1	60	65	1.6	11,030	0.10	0.08	0.8	17
239	Canned, vacuum or solid pack. 1 cup 218	72	235	4	Trace	----	----	----	54	54	1.7	17,000	.10	.10	1.4	30
	Tomatoes:															
240	Raw, approx. 3-in. diam. 2⅛ in. high; wt, 7 oz. 1 tomato 200	94	40	2	Trace				9	24	.9	1,640	.11	.07	1.3	7 42
241	Canned, solids and liquid. 1 cup 241	94	50	2	1				10	14	1.2	2,170	.12	.07	1.7	41
	Tomato catsup:															
242	Cup 1 cup 273	69	290	6	1				69	60	2.2	3,820	.25	.19	4.4	41
243	Tablespoon 1 tbsp 15	69	15	Trace	Trace				4	3	.1	210	.01	.01	.2	2
	Tomato juice, canned:															
244	Cup 1 cup 243	94	45	2	Trace	----	----	----	10	17	2.2	1,940	.12	.07	1.9	39
245	Glass (6 fl. oz.) 1 glass 182	94	35	2	Trace	----	----	----	8	13	1.6	1,460	.09	.05	1.5	29
246	Turnips, cooked, diced 1 cup 155	94	35	1	Trace	----	----	----	8	54	.6	Trace	.06	.08	.5	34
247	Turnip greens, cooked 1 cup 145	94	30	3	Trace	----	----	----	5	252	1.5	8,270	.15	.33	.7	68
	FRUITS AND FRUIT PRODUCTS															
248	Apples, raw (about 3 per lb.).[5] 1 apple 150	85	70	Trace	Trace	----	----	----	18	8	.4	50	.04	.02	.1	3
249	Apple juice, bottled or canned. 1 cup 248	88	120	Trace	Trace	----	----	----	30	15	1.5	-------	.02	.05	.2	2
	Applesauce, canned:															
250	Sweetened 1 cup 255	76	230	1	Trace	----	----	----	61	10	1.3	100	.05	.03	.1	8 3
251	Unsweetened or artifi-cially sweetened. 1 cup 244	88	100	1	Trace	----	----	----	26	10	1.2	100	.05	.02	.1	8 2

No.	Food, approximate measure, and weight (in grams)	Grams	Water (%)	Food energy	Protein	Fat (total)	Saturated	Oleic	Linoleic	Carbohydrate	Calcium	Iron	Vitamin A	Thiamine	Riboflavin	Niacin	Ascorbic acid
	Apricots:																
252	Raw (about 12 per lb.)[6] 3 apricots ---	114	85	55	1	Trace				14	18	.5	2,890	.03	.04	.7	10
253	Canned in heavy sirup-- 1 cup ---	259	77	220	2	Trace				57	28	.8	4,510	.05	.06	.9	10
254	Dried, uncooked (40 halves per cup). 1 cup ---	150	25	390	8	1				100	100	8.2	16,350	.02	.23	4.9	19
255	Cooked, unsweetened, fruit and liquid. 1 cup ---	285	76	240	5	1				62	63	5.1	8,550	.01	.13	2.8	8
256	Apricot nectar, canned--- 1 cup ---	251	85	140	1	Trace				37	23	.5	2,380	.03	.03	.5	[8] 8
	Avocados, whole fruit, raw:[6]																
257	California (mid- and late-winter; diam. 3⅛ in.). 1 avocado ---	284	74	370	5	37	7	17	5	13	22	1.3	630	.24	.43	3.5	30
258	Florida (late summer, fall; diam. 3⅝ in.). 1 avocado ---	454	78	390	4	33	7	15	4	27	30	1.8	880	.33	.61	4.9	43
259	Bananas, raw, medium size.[5] 1 banana ---	175	76	100	1	Trace				26	10	.8	230	.06	.07	.8	12
260	Banana flakes--- 1 cup ---	100	3	340	4	1				89	32	2.8	760	.18	.24	2.8	7
261	Blackberries, raw--- 1 cup ---	144	84	85	2	1				19	46	1.3	290	.05	.06	.5	30
262	Blueberries, raw--- 1 cup ---	140	83	85	1	1				21	21	1.4	140	.04	.08	.6	20
263	Cantaloups, raw; medium, ½ melon; 5-inch diameter about 1⅔ pounds.[5] ½ melon ---	385	91	60	1	Trace				14	27	.8	[9] 6,540	.08	.06	1.2	63
264	Cherries, canned, red, sour, pitted, water pack. 1 cup ---	244	88	105	2	Trace				26	37	.7	1,660	.07	.05	.5	12
265	Cranberry juice cocktail, canned. 1 cup ---	250	83	165	Trace	Trace				42	13	.8	Trace	.03	.03	.1	[10] 40
266	Cranberry sauce, sweetened, canned, strained. 1 cup ---	277	62	405	Trace	1				104	17	.6	60	.03	.03	.1	6
267	Dates, pitted, cut--- 1 cup ---	178	22	490	4	1				130	105	5.3	90	.16	.17	3.9	0
268	Figs, dried, large, 2 by 1 in. 1 fig ---	21	23	60	1	Trace				15	26	.6	20	.02	.02	.1	0
269	Fruit cocktail, canned, in heavy sirup. 1 cup ---	256	80	195	1	Trace				50	23	1.0	360	.05	.03	1.3	5

[5] Measure and weight apply to entire vegetable or fruit including parts not usually eaten.

[7] Year-round average. Samples marketed from November through May, average 20 milligrams per 200-gram tomato; from June through October, around 52 milligrams.

[8] This is the amount from the fruit. Additional ascorbic acid may be added by the manufacturer. Refer to the label for this information.

[9] Value for varieties with orange-colored flesh; value for varieties with green flesh would be about 540 I.U.

[10] Value listed is based on products with label stating 30 milligrams per 6 fl. oz. serving.

Nutritive Values of the Edible Part of Foods

[Dashes in the columns for nutrients show that no suitable value could be found although there is reason to believe that a measurable amount of the nutrient may be present]

	Food, approximate measure, and weight (in grams)		Water	Food energy	Protein	Fat	Fatty acids			Carbohydrate	Calcium	Iron	Vitamin A value	Thiamin	Riboflavin	Niacin	Ascorbic acid
							Saturated (total)	Unsaturated Oleic	Linoleic								
		Grams	Percent	Calories	Grams	Grams	Grams	Grams	Grams	Grams	Milligrams	Milligrams	International units	Milligrams	Milligrams	Milligrams	Milligrams
	FRUITS AND FRUIT PRODUCTS—Con.																
	Grapefruit:																
	Raw, medium, 3¾-in. diam.[5]																
270	White___ ½ grapefruit.	241	89	45	1	Trace	---	---	---	12	19	0.5	10	0.05	0.02	0.2	44
271	Pink or red___ ½ grapefruit.	241	89	50	1	Trace	---	---	---	13	20	0.5	540	0.05	0.02	0.2	44
272	Canned, sirup pack___ 1 cup	254	81	180	2	Trace	---	---	---	45	33	.8	30	.08	.05	.5	76
	Grapefruit juice:																
273	Fresh___ 1 cup	246	90	95	1	Trace	---	---	---	23	22	.5	(11)	.09	.04	.4	92
	Canned, white:																
274	Unsweetened___ 1 cup	247	89	100	1	Trace	---	---	---	24	20	1.0	20	.07	.04	.4	84
275	Sweetened___ 1 cup	250	86	130	1	Trace	---	---	---	32	20	1.0	20	.07	.04	.4	78
	Frozen concentrate, unsweetened:																
276	Undiluted, can, 6 fluid ounces. 1 can	207	62	300	4	1	---	---	---	72	70	.8	60	.29	.12	1.4	286
277	Diluted with 3 parts water, by volume. 1 cup	247	89	100	1	Trace	---	---	---	24	25	.2	20	.10	.04	.5	96
278	Dehydrated crystals___ 4 oz	113	1	410	6	1	---	---	---	102	100	1.2	80	.40	.20	2.0	396
279	Prepared with water 1 cup (1 pound yields about 1 gallon).	247	90	100	1	Trace	---	---	---	24	22	.2	20	.10	.05	.5	91
	Grapes, raw:[5]																
280	American type (slip skin). 1 cup	153	82	65	1	1	---	---	---	15	15	.4	100	.05	.03	.2	3
281	European type (adherent skin). 1 cup	160	81	95	1	Trace	---	---	---	25	17	.6	140	.07	.04	.4	6
	Grapejuice:																
282	Canned or bottled___ 1 cup	253	83	165	1	Trace	---	---	---	42	28	.8	----	.10	.05	.5	Trace
	Frozen concentrate, sweetened:																
283	Undiluted, can, 6 fluid ounces. 1 can	216	53	395	1	Trace	---	---	---	100	22	.9	40	.13	.22	1.5	(12)

No.	Food	Measure														
284	Diluted with 3 parts water, by volume.	1 cup	250	86	135	1	Trace	---	33	8	.3	10	.05	.08	.5	(¹²)
285	Grapejuice drink, canned.	1 cup	250	86	135	Trace	Trace	---	35	8	.3	---	.03	.03	.3	(¹²)
286	Lemons, raw, 2⅛-in. diam, size 165.⁵ Used for juice.	1 lemon	110	90	20	1	Trace	---	6	19	.4	10	.03	.01	.1	39
287	Lemon juice, raw	1 cup	244	91	60	1	Trace	---	20	17	.5	50	.07	.02	.2	112
	Lemonade concentrate:															
288	Frozen, 6 fl. oz. per can.	1 can	219	48	430	Trace	Trace	---	112	9	.4	40	.04	.07	.7	66
289	Diluted with 4⅓ parts water, by volume.	1 cup	248	88	110	Trace	Trace	---	28	2	Trace	Trace	Trace	.02	.2	17
	Lime juice:															
290	Fresh	1 cup	246	90	65	1	Trace	---	22	22	.5	20	.05	.02	.2	79
291	Canned, unsweetened	1 cup	246	90	65	1	Trace	---	22	22	.5	20	.05	.02	.2	52
	Limeade concentrate, frozen:															
292	Undiluted, can, 6 fluid ounces.	1 can	218	50	410	Trace	Trace	---	108	11	.2	Trace	.02	.02	.2	26
293	Diluted with 4⅓ parts water, by volume.	1 cup	247	90	100	Trace	Trace	---	27	2	Trace	Trace	.02	Trace	Trace	5
294	Oranges, raw, 2⅝-in. diam., all commercial, varieties.⁵	1 orange	180	86	65	1	Trace	---	16	54	.5	260	.13	.05	.5	66
295	Orange juice, fresh, all varieties.	1 cup	248	88	110	2	1	---	26	27	.5	500	.22	.07	1.0	124
296	Canned, unsweetened	1 cup	249	87	120	2	Trace	---	28	25	1.0	500	.17	.05	.7	100
	Frozen concentrate:															
297	Undiluted, can, 6 fluid ounces.	1 can	213	55	360	5	Trace	---	87	75	.9	1,620	.68	.11	2.8	360
298	Diluted with 3 parts water, by volume.	1 cup	249	87	120	2	Trace	---	29	25	.2	550	.22	.02	1.0	120
299	Dehydrated crystals	4 oz.	113	1	430	6	2	---	100	95	1.9	1,900	.76	.24	3.3	408
300	Prepared with water (1 pound yields about 1 gallon).	1 cup	248	88	115	2	1	---	27	25	.5	500	.20	.07	1.0	109
301	Orange-apricot juice drink	1 cup	249	87	125	1	Trace	---	32	12	.2	1,440	.05	.02	.5	¹⁰40

⁵ Measure and weight apply to entire vegetable or fruit including parts not usually eaten.

¹⁰ Value listed is based on product with label stating 30 milligrams per 6 fl. oz. serving.

¹¹ For white-fleshed varieties value is about 20 I.U. per cup; for red-fleshed varieties, 1,080 I.U. per cup.

¹² Present only if added by the manufacturer. Refer to the label for this information.

Table A-4 (continued)

Nutritive Values of the Edible Part of Foods

[Dashes in the columns for nutrients show that no suitable value could be found although there is reason to believe that a measurable amount of the nutrient may be present]

	Food, approximate measure, and weight (in grams)		Water	Food energy	Protein	Fat	Fatty acids Saturated (total)	Fatty acids Unsaturated Oleic	Fatty acids Unsaturated Linoleic	Carbohydrate	Calcium	Iron	Vitamin A value	Thiamin	Riboflavin	Niacin	Ascorbic acid
		Grams	Per cent	Calories	Grams	Grams	Grams	Grams	Grams	Grams	Milligrams	Milligrams	International units	Milligrams	Milligrams	Milligrams	Milligrams
	FRUITS AND FRUIT PRODUCTS—Con.																
	Orange and grapefruit juice: Frozen concentrate:																
302	Undiluted, can, 6 fluid ounces. 1 can	210	59	330	4	1	---	---	---	78	61	0.8	800	0.48	0.06	2.3	302
303	Diluted with 3 parts water, by volume. 1 cup	248	88	110	1	Trace	---	---	---	26	20	.2	270	.16	.02	.8	102
304	Papayas, raw, ½-inch cubes. 1 cup	182	89	70	1	Trace				18	36	.5	3,190	.07	.08	.5	102
	Peaches: Raw:																
305	Whole, medium, 2-inch diameter, about 4 per pound.[5] 1 peach	114	89	35	1	Trace				10	9	.5	[13]1,320	.02	.05	1.0	7
306	Sliced. 1 cup	168	89	65	1	Trace				16	15	.8	[13]2,230	.03	.08	1.6	12
	Canned, yellow-fleshed, solids and liquid: Sirup pack, heavy:																
307	Halves or slices. 1 cup	257	79	200	1	Trace	---	---	---	52	10	.8	1,100	.02	.06	1.4	7
308	Water pack. 1 cup	245	91	75	1	Trace	---	---	---	20	10	.7	1,100	.02	.06	1.4	7
309	Dried, uncooked. 1 cup	160	25	420	5	1				109	77	9.6	6,240	.02	.31	8.5	28
310	Cooked, unsweetened, 10–12 halves and juice. 1 cup	270	77	220	3	1				58	41	5.1	3,290	.01	.15	4.2	6
	Frozen:																
311	Carton, 12 ounces, not thawed. 1 carton	340	76	300	1	Trace	---	---	---	77	14	1.7	2,210	.03	.14	2.4	[14]135
	Pears:																
312	Raw, 3 by 2½-inch diameter.[5] 1 pear	182	83	100	1	1				25	13	.5	30	.04	.07	.2	7
	Canned, solids and liquid: Sirup pack, heavy:																
313	Halves or slices. 1 cup	255	80	195	1	1				50	13	.5	Trace	.03	.05	.3	4

No.	Food, approximate measure		Grams	Water (%)	Food energy (cal.)	Protein (g)	Fat (g)	Carbohydrate (g)	Calcium (mg)	Iron (mg)	Vit. A (I.U.)	Thiamine (mg)	Riboflavin (mg)	Niacin (mg)	Ascorbic acid (mg)
	Pineapple:														
314	Raw, diced	1 cup	140	85	75	1	Trace	19	24	.7	100	.12	.04	.3	24
	Canned, heavy sirup pack, solids and liquid:														
315	Crushed	1 cup	260	80	195	1	Trace	50	29	.8	120	.20	.06	.5	17
316	Sliced, slices and juice	2 small or 1 large	122	80	90	Trace	Trace	24	13	.4	50	.09	.03	.2	8
317	Pineapple juice, canned	1 cup	249	86	135	1	Trace	34	37	.7	120	.12	.04	.5	[8]22
	Plums, all except prunes:														
318	Raw, 2-inch diameter, 1 plum about 2 ounces.[5]	1 plum	60	87	25	Trace	Trace	7	7	.3	140	.02	.02	.3	3
319	Canned, sirup pack (Italian prunes): Plums (with pits) and juice.[5]	1 cup	256	77	205	1	Trace	53	22	2.2	2,970	.05	.05	.9	4
	Prunes, dried, "softenized", medium:														
320	Uncooked[5]	4 prunes	32	28	70	1	Trace	18	14	1.1	440	.02	.04	.4	1
321	Cooked, unsweetened, 17–18 prunes and ⅓ cup liquid.[5]	1 cup	270	66	295	2	1	78	60	4.5	1,860	.08	.18	1.7	2
322	Prune juice, canned or bottled.	1 cup	256	80	200	1	Trace	49	36	10.5	------	.03	.03	1.0	[8]5
	Raisins, seedless:														
323	Packaged, ½ oz. or 1½ tbsp. per pkg.	1 pkg	14	18	40	Trace	Trace	11	9	.5	Trace	.02	.01	.1	Trace
324	Cup, pressed down	1 cup	165	18	480	4	Trace	128	102	5.8	30	.18	.13	.8	2
	Raspberries, red:														
325	Raw	1 cup	123	84	70	1	1	17	27	1.1	160	.04	.11	1.1	31
326	Frozen, 10-ounce carton, not thawed.	1 carton	284	74	275	2	1	70	37	1.7	200	.06	.17	1.7	59
327	Rhubarb, cooked, sugar added.	1 cup	272	63	385	1	Trace	98	212	1.6	220	.06	.15	.7	17
	Strawberries:														
328	Raw, capped	1 cup	149	90	55	1	1	13	31	1.5	90	.04	.10	1.0	88
329	Frozen, 10-ounce carton, not thawed.	1 carton	284	71	310	1	1	79	40	2.0	90	.06	.17	1.5	150
330	Tangerines, raw, medium, 2⅜-in. diam., size 176.[5]	1 tangerine	116	87	40	1	Trace	10	34	.3	360	.05	.02	.1	27
331	Tangerine juice, canned, sweetened.	1 cup	249	87	125	1	1	30	45	.5	1,050	.15	.05	.2	55
332	Watermelon, raw, wedge, 4 by 8 inches (⅟₁₆ of 10 by 16-inch melon, about 2 pounds with rind).[5]	1 wedge	925	93	115	2	1	27	30	2.1	2,510	.13	.13	.7	30

[5] Measure and weight apply to entire vegetable or fruit including parts not usually eaten.

[8] This is the amount from the fruit. Additional ascorbic acid may be added by the manufacturer. Refer to the label for this information.

[13] Based on yellow-fleshed varieties; for white-fleshed varieties value is about 50 I.U. per 114-gram peach and 80 I.U. per cup of sliced peaches.

[14] This value includes ascorbic acid added by manufacturer.

Nutritive Values of the Edible Part of Foods

[Dashes in the columns for nutrients show that no suitable value could be found although there is reason to believe that a measurable amount of the nutrient may be present]

	Food, approximate measure, and weight (in grams)	Water	Food energy	Protein	Fat	Fatty acids			Carbohydrate	Calcium	Iron	Vitamin A value	Thiamin	Riboflavin	Niacin	Ascorbic acid
						Saturated (total)	Unsaturated									
							Oleic	Linoleic								
		Percent	Calories	Grams	Grams	Grams	Grams	Grams	Grams	Milligrams	Milligrams	International units	Milligrams	Milligrams	Milligrams	Milligrams
	GRAIN PRODUCTS															
	Bagel, 3-in. diam.:															
333	Egg _____ 1 bagel _____ 55	32	165	6	2	--	--	--	28	9	1.2	30	0.14	0.10	1.2	0
334	Water _____ 1 bagel _____ 55	29	165	6	2	--	--	--	30	8	1.2	0	.15	.11	1.4	0
335	Barley, pearled, light, uncooked. 1 cup _____ 200	11	700	16	2	Trace	1	1	158	32	4.0	0	.24	.10	6.2	0
336	Biscuits, baking powder from home recipe with enriched flour, 2-in. diam. 1 biscuit _____ 28	27	105	2	5	1	2	1	13	34	.4	Trace	.06	.06	.1	Trace
337	Biscuits, baking powder from mix, 2-in. diam. 1 biscuit _____ 28	28	90	2	3	1	1	1	15	19	.6	Trace	.08	.07	.6	Trace
338	Bran flakes (40% bran), added thiamin and iron. 1 cup _____ 35	3	105	4	1	--	--	--	28	25	12.3	0	.14	.06	2.2	0
339	Bran flakes with raisins, added thiamin and iron. 1 cup _____ 50	7	145	4	1	--	--	--	40	28	13.5	Trace	.16	.07	2.7	0
	Breads:															
340	Boston brown bread, slice 3 by ¾ in. 1 slice _____ 48	45	100	3	1	--	--	--	22	43	.9	0	.05	.03	.6	0
	Cracked-wheat bread:															
341	Loaf, 1 lb. _____ 1 loaf _____ 454	35	1,190	40	10	2	5	2	236	399	5.0	Trace	.53	.41	5.9	Trace
342	Slice, 18 slices per loaf. 1 slice _____ 25	35	65	2	1	--	--	--	13	22	.3	Trace	.03	.02	.3	Trace
	French or vienna bread:															
343	Enriched, 1 lb. loaf. 1 loaf _____ 454	31	1,315	41	14	3	8	2	251	195	10.0	Trace	1.27	1.00	11.3	Trace
344	Unenriched, 1 lb. loaf. 1 loaf _____ 454	31	1,315	41	14	3	8	2	251	195	3.2	Trace	.36	.36	3.6	Trace
	Italian bread:															
345	Enriched, 1 lb. loaf. 1 loaf _____ 454	32	1,250	41	4	Trace	1	2	256	77	10.0	0	1.32	.91	11.8	0
346	Unenriched, 1 lb. loaf. 1 loaf _____ 454	32	1,250	41	4	Trace	1	2	256	77	3.2	0	.41	.27	3.6	0
	Raisin bread:															
347	Loaf, 1 lb. _____ 1 loaf _____ 454	35	1,190	30	13	3	8	2	243	322	5.9	Trace	.23	.41	3.2	Trace

No.	Food	Measure																
348	Slice, 18 slices per loaf	1 slice	25	35	65	2	1	--	--	--	13	18	.3	Trace	.01	.02	.2	Trace
	Rye bread:																	
	American, light (⅓ rye, ⅔ wheat):																	
349	Loaf, 1 lb	1 loaf	454	36	1,100	41	5	--	--	--	236	340	7.3	0	.82	.32	6.4	0
350	Slice, 18 slices per loaf	1 slice	25	36	60	2	Trace	--	--	--	13	19	.4	0	.05	.02	.4	0
351	Pumpernickel, loaf, 1 lb	1 loaf	454	34	1,115	41	5	--	--	--	241	381	10.9	0	1.04	.64	5.4	0
	White bread, enriched: [15]																	
	Soft-crumb type:																	
352	Loaf, 1 lb	1 loaf	454	36	1,225	39	15	3	8	2	229	381	11.3	Trace	1.13	.95	10.9	Trace
353	Slice, 18 slices per loaf	1 slice	25	36	70	2	1	--	--	--	13	21	.6	Trace	.06	.05	.6	Trace
354	Slice, toasted	1 slice	22	25	70	2	1	--	--	--	13	21	.6	Trace	.06	.05	.6	Trace
355	Slice, 22 slices per loaf	1 slice	20	36	55	2	1	--	--	--	10	17	.5	Trace	.05	.04	.5	Trace
356	Slice, toasted	1 slice	17	25	55	2	1	--	--	--	10	17	.5	Trace	.05	.04	.5	Trace
357	Loaf, 1½ lbs	1 loaf	680	36	1,835	59	22	5	12	3	343	571	17.0	Trace	1.70	1.43	16.3	Trace
358	Slice, 24 slices per loaf	1 slice	28	36	75	2	1	--	--	--	14	24	.7	Trace	.07	.06	.7	Trace
359	Slice, toasted	1 slice	24	25	75	2	1	--	--	--	14	24	.7	Trace	.07	.05	.6	Trace
360	Slice, 28 slices per loaf	1 slice	24	36	65	2	1	--	--	--	12	20	.7	Trace	.06	.05	.7	Trace
361	Slice, toasted	1 slice	21	25	65	2	1	--	--	--	12	20	.6	Trace	.06	.05	.6	Trace
	Firm-crumb type:																	
362	Loaf, 1 lb	1 loaf	454	35	1,245	41	17	4	10	2	228	435	11.3	Trace	1.22	.91	10.9	Trace
363	Slice, 20 slices per loaf	1 slice	23	35	65	2	1	--	--	--	12	22	.6	Trace	.06	.05	.6	Trace
364	Slice, toasted	1 slice	20	24	65	2	1	--	--	--	12	22	.6	Trace	.06	.05	.6	Trace
365	Loaf, 2 lbs	1 loaf	907	35	2,495	82	34	8	20	4	455	871	22.7	Trace	2.45	1.81	21.8	Trace
366	Slice, 34 slices per loaf	1 slice	27	35	75	2	1	--	--	--	14	26	.7	Trace	.07	.05	.6	Trace
367	Slice, toasted	1 slice	23	35	75	2	1	--	--	--	14	26	.7	Trace	.07	.05	.6	Trace
	Whole-wheat bread, soft-crumb type:																	
368	Loaf, 1 lb	1 loaf	454	36	1,095	41	12	2	6	2	224	381	13.6	Trace	1.36	.45	12.7	Trace
369	Slice, 16 slices per loaf	1 slice	28	36	65	3	1	--	--	--	14	24	.8	Trace	.09	.03	.8	Trace
370	Slice, toasted	1 slice	24	24	65	3	1	--	--	--	14	24	.8	Trace	.09	.03	.8	Trace

[15] Values for iron, thiamin, riboflavin, and niacin per pound of unenriched white bread would be as follows:

	Iron Milligrams	Thiamin Milligrams	Riboflavin Milligrams	Niacin Milligrams
Soft crumb	3.2	.31	.39	5.0
Firm crumb	3.2	.32	.59	4.1

Table A-4 (continued)

Nutritive Values of the Edible Part of Foods

[Dashes in the columns for nutrients show that no suitable value could be found although there is reason to believe that a measurable amount of the nutrient may be present]

	Food, approximate measure, and weight (in grams)		Water	Food energy	Protein	Fat	Fatty acids			Carbohydrate	Calcium	Iron	Vitamin A value	Thiamin	Riboflavin	Niacin	Ascorbic acid
							Saturated (total)	Unsaturated									
								Oleic	Linoleic								
		Grams	Percent	Calories	Grams	Grams	Grams	Grams	Grams	Grams	Milligrams	Milligrams	International units	Milligrams	Milligrams	Milligrams	Milligrams
	GRAIN PRODUCTS—Continued																
	Bread—Continued																
	Whole-wheat bread, firm-crumb type:																
371	Loaf, 1 lb------- 1 loaf-------	454	36	1,100	48	14	3	6	3	216	449	13.6	Trace	1.18	0.54	12.7	Trace
372	Slice, 18 slices per loaf. 1 slice.	25	36	60	3	1	------	------	------	12	25	.8	Trace	.06	.03	.7	Trace
373	Slice, toasted------ 1 slice------	21	24	60	3	1	------	------	------	12	25	.8	Trace	.06	.03	.7	Trace
374	Breadcrumbs, dry, grated. 1 cup------	100	6	390	13	5	1	2	1	73	122	3.6	Trace	.22	.30	3.5	Trace
375	Buckwheat flour, light, 1 cup------ sifted.	98	12	340	6	1	------	------	------	78	11	1.0	0	.08	.04	.4	0
376	Bulgur, canned, seasoned. 1 cup------	135	56	245	8	4	------	------	------	44	27	1.9	0	.08	.05	4.1	0
	Cakes made from cake mixes:																
	Angelfood:																
377	Whole cake------- 1 cake------	635	34	1,645	36	1	------	------	------	377	603	1.9	0	.03	.70	.6	0
378	Piece, 1/12 of 10-in. 1 piece------ diam. cake.	53	34	135	3	Trace	------	------	------	32	50	.2	0	Trace	.06	.1	0
	Cupcakes, small, 2½ in. diam.:																
379	Without icing------ 1 cupcake---	25	26	90	1	3	1	1	1	14	40	.1	40	.01	.03	.1	Trace
380	With chocolate icing. 1 cupcake---	36	22	130	2	5	2	2	1	21	47	.3	60	.01	.04	.1	Trace
	Devil's food, 2-layer, with chocolate icing:																
381	Whole cake------1 cake------	1,107	24	3,755	49	136	54	58	16	645	653	8.9	1,660	.33	.89	3.3	1
382	Piece, 1/16 of 9-in. 1 piece------ diam. cake.	69	24	235	3	9	3	4	1	40	41	.6	100	.02	.06	.2	Trace
383	Cupcake, small, 2½ 1 cupcake--- in. diam.	35	24	120	2	4	1	2	Trace	20	21	.3	50	.01	.03	.1	Trace
	Gingerbread:																
384	Whole cake------- 1 cake------	570	37	1,575	18	39	10	19	9	291	513	9.1	Trace	.17	.51	4.6	2
385	Piece, 1/9 of 8-in. 1 piece------ square cake.	63	37	175	2	4	1	2	1	32	57	1.0	Trace	.02	.06	.5	Trace
	White, 2-layer, with chocolate icing:																
386	Whole cake------1 cake------	1,140	21	4,000	45	122	45	54	17	716	1,129	5.7	680	.23	.91	2.3	2

Cakes made from home recipes:[16]

Fruitcake, dark, made with enriched flour:

Plain sheet cake:
  Without icing:

Pound:

Sponge:

Yellow, 2-layer, without icing:

Yellow, 2-layer, with chocolate icing:

Cake icings. See Sugars, Sweets.
Cookies:
  Brownies with nuts:

No.	Food	Measure	g																
387	Piece, 1/6 of 9-in. diam. cake.	1 piece-----	71	21	250	3	8	3	3	1	45	70	.4	40	.01	.06	.1	Trace
388	Boston cream pie; piece 1/12 of 8-in. diam.	1 piece-----	69	35	210	4	6	2	3	1	34	46	.3	140	.02	.08	.1	Trace
389	Loaf, 1-lb.	1 loaf-----	454	18	1,720	22	69	15	37	13	271	327	11.8	540	.59	.64	3.6	2
390	Slice, 1/30 of 8-in. loaf.	1 slice-----	15	18	55	1	2	Trace	1	Trace	9	11	.4	20	.02	.02	.1	Trace
391	Whole cake-----	1 cake-----	777	25	2,830	35	108	30	52	21	434	497	3.1	1,320	.16	.70	1.6	2
392	Piece, 1/9 of 9-in. square cake.	1 piece-----	86	25	315	4	12	3	6	2	48	55	.3	150	.02	.08	.2	Trace
393	With boiled white icing, piece, 1/9 of 9-in. square cake.	1 piece-----	114	23	400	4	12	3	6	2	71	56	.3	150	.02	.08	.2	Trace
394	Loaf, 8 1/2 by 3 1/2 by 3 in.	1 loaf-----	514	17	2,430	29	152	34	68	17	242	108	4.1	1,440	.15	.46	1.0	0
395	Slice, 1/2-in. thick.	1 slice-----	30	17	140	2	9	2	4	1	14	6	.2	80	.01	.03	.1	0
396	Whole cake-----	1 cake-----	790	32	2,345	60	45	14	20	4	427	237	9.5	3,560	.40	1.11	1.6	Trace
397	Piece, 1/12 of 10-in. diam. cake.	1 piece-----	66	32	195	5	4	1	2	Trace	36	20	.8	300	.03	.09	.1	Trace
398	Whole cake-----	1 cake-----	870	24	3,160	39	111	31	53	22	506	618	3.5	1,310	.17	.70	1.7	2
399	Piece, 1/16 of 9-in. diam. cake.	1 piece-----	54	24	200	2	7	2	3	1	32	39	.2	80	.01	.04	.1	Trace
400	Whole cake-----	1 cake-----	1,203	21	4,390	51	156	55	69	23	727	818	7.2	1,920	.24	.96	2.4	Trace
401	Piece, 1/16 of 9-in. diam. cake.	1 piece-----	75	21	275	3	10	3	4	1	45	51	.5	120	.02	.06	.2	Trace
402	Made from home recipe with enriched flour.	1 brownie-----	20	10	95	1	6	1	3	1	10	8	.4	40	.04	.02	.1	Trace
403	Made from mix-----	1 brownie-----	20	11	85	1	4	1	2	1	13	9	.4	20	.03	.02	.1	Trace

[16] Unenriched cake flour used unless otherwise specified.

[Dashes in the columns for nutrients show that no suitable value could be found although there is reason to believe that a measurable amount of the nutrient may be present]

	Food, approximate measure, and weight (in grams)	Water	Food energy	Protein	Fat	Fatty acids Saturated (total)	Unsaturated Oleic	Unsaturated Linoleic	Carbohydrate	Calcium	Iron	Vitamin A value	Thiamin	Riboflavin	Niacin	Ascorbic acid
		Per cent	*Calories*	*Grams*	*Grams*	*Grams*	*Grams*	*Grams*	*Grams*	*Milligrams*	*Milligrams*	*International units*	*Milligrams*	*Milligrams*	*Milligrams*	*Milligrams*
	GRAIN PRODUCTS—Continued															
	Cookies—Continued															
	Chocolate chip:															
404	Made from home recipe with enriched flour. 1 cookie____ 10 Grams	3	50	1	3	1	1	1	6	4	0.2	10	0.01	0.01	0.1	Trace
405	Commercial____ 1 cookie____ 10	3	50	1	2	1	1	Trace	7	4	.2	10	Trace	Trace	Trace	Trace
406	Fig bars, commercial__ 1 cookie____ 14	14	50	1	1				11	11	.2	20	Trace	.01	.1	Trace
407	Sandwich, chocolate or vanilla, commercial. 1 cookie____ 10	2	50	1	2	1	1	Trace	7	2	.1	0	Trace	Trace	.1	0
	Corn flakes, added nutrients:															
408	Plain_____ 1 cup____ 25	4	100	2	Trace				21	4	.4	0	.11	.02	.5	0
409	Sugar-covered____ 1 cup____ 40	2	155	2	Trace				36	5	.4	0	.16	.02	.8	0
	Corn (hominy) grits, degermed, cooked:															
410	Enriched_____ 1 cup____ 245	87	125	3	Trace				27	2	.7	[17] 150	.10	.07	1.0	0
411	Unenriched____ 1 cup____ 245	87	125	3	Trace				27	2	.2	[17] 150	.05	.02	.5	0
	Cornmeal:															
412	Whole-ground, unbolted, dry. 1 cup____ 122	12	435	11	5	1	2	2	90	24	2.9	[17] 620	.46	.13	2.4	0
413	Bolted (nearly whole-grain) dry. 1 cup____ 122	12	440	11	4	Trace	1	2	91	21	2.2	[17] 590	.37	.10	2.3	0
	Degermed, enriched:															
414	Dry form_____ 1 cup____ 138	12	500	11	2				108	8	4.0	[17] 610	.61	.36	4.8	0
415	Cooked_____ 1 cup____ 240	88	120	3	1				26	2	1.0	[17] 140	.14	.10	1.2	0
	Degermed, unenriched:															
416	Dry form_____ 1 cup____ 138	12	500	11	2				108	8	1.5	[17] 610	.19	.07	1.4	0
417	Cooked_____ 1 cup____ 240	88	120	3	1				26	2	.5	[17] 140	.05	.02	.2	0
418	Corn muffins, made with enriched degermed cornmeal and enriched flour; muffin 2⅜-in. diam. 1 muffin____ 40	33	125	3	4	2	2	Trace	19	42	.7	[17] 120	.08	.09	.6	Trace

No.	Food, approximate measure, and weight (grams)		Weight	Calories	Protein	Fat	Saturated	Oleic	Linoleic	Carbohydrate	Calcium	Iron	Vitamin A	Thiamin	Riboflavin	Niacin	Ascorbic acid
419	Corn muffins, made with mix, egg, and milk; muffin 2⅜-in. diam.	1 muffin	40	130	3	4	1	2	1	20	96	.6	100	.07	.08	.6	Trace
420	Corn, puffed, presweetened, added nutrients.	1 cup	30	115	2	Trace	----	----	----	27	3	.5	0	.13	.05	.6	0
421	Corn, shredded, added nutrients.	1 cup	25	100	2	Trace	----	----	----	22	1	.6	0	.11	.05	.5	0
	Crackers:																
422	Graham, 2½-in. square	4 crackers	28	110	2	3	----	1	----	21	11	.4	0	.01	.06	.4	0
423	Saltines	4 crackers	11	50	1	1	----	1	----	8	2	.1	0	Trace	Trace	.1	0
	Danish pastry, plain (without fruit or nuts):																
424	Packaged ring, 12 ounces.	1 ring	340	1,435	25	80	24	37	15	155	170	3.1	1,050	.24	.51	2.7	Trace
425	Round piece, approx. 4¼-in. diam. by 1 in.	1 pastry	65	275	5	15	5	7	3	30	33	.6	200	.05	.10	.5	Trace
426	Ounce	1 oz	28	120	2	7	2	3	1	13	14	.3	90	.02	.04	.2	Trace
427	Doughnuts, cake type	1 doughnut	32	125	1	6	1	4	Trace	16	13	[18].4	30	[18].05	[18].05	[18].4	Trace
428	Farina, quick-cooking, enriched, cooked.	1 cup	245	105	3	Trace	----	----	----	22	147	[19].7	0	[19].12	[19].07	[19]1.0	0
	Macaroni, cooked:																
	Enriched:																
429	Cooked, firm stage (undergoes additional cooking in a food mixture).	1 cup	130	190	6	1	----	----	----	39	14	[19]1.4	0	[19].23	[19].14	[19]1.8	0
430	Cooked until tender	1 cup	140	155	5	1	----	----	----	32	8	[19]1.3	0	[19].20	[19].11	[19]1.5	0
	Unenriched:																
431	Cooked, firm stage (undergoes additional cooking in a food mixture).	1 cup	130	190	6	1	----	----	----	39	14	.7	0	.03	.03	.5	0
432	Cooked until tender	1 cup	140	155	5	1	----	----	----	32	11	.6	0	.01	.01	.4	0
433	Macaroni (enriched) and cheese, baked.	1 cup	200	430	17	22	10	9	2	40	362	1.8	860	.20	.40	1.8	Trace
434	Canned	1 cup	240	230	9	10	4	3	1	26	199	1.0	260	.12	.24	1.0	Trace
435	Muffins, with enriched white flour; muffin, 3-inch diam.	1 muffin	40	120	3	4	1	2	1	17	42	.6	40	.07	.09	.6	Trace
	Noodles (egg noodles), cooked:																
436	Enriched	1 cup	160	200	7	2	----	1	Trace	37	16	[19]1.4	110	[19].22	[19].13	[19]1.9	0
437	Unenriched	1 cup	160	200	7	2	----	1	Trace	37	16	1.0	110	.05	.03	.6	0

[17] This value is based on product made from yellow varieties of corn; white varieties contain only a trace.

[18] Based on product made with enriched flour. With unenriched flour, approximate values per doughnut are: Iron, 0.2 milligram; thiamin, 0.01 milligram; riboflavin, 0.03 milligram; niacin, 0.2 milligram.

[19] Iron, thiamin, riboflavin, and niacin are based on the minimum levels of enrichment specified in standards of identity promulgated under the Federal Food, Drug, and Cosmetic Act.

Nutritive Values of the Edible Part of Foods

[Dashes in the columns for nutrients show that no suitable value could be found although there is reason to believe that a measurable amount of the nutrient may be present]

	Food, approximate measure, and weight (in grams)	Water	Food energy	Protein	Fat	Fatty acids			Carbohydrate	Calcium	Iron	Vitamin A value	Thiamin	Riboflavin	Niacin	Ascorbic acid
						Saturated (total)	Unsaturated									
							Oleic	Linoleic								
		Per cent	Calories	Grams	Grams	Grams	Grams	Grams	Grams	Milligrams	Milligrams	International units	Milligrams	Milligrams	Milligrams	Milligrams
	GRAIN PRODUCTS—Continued															
438	Oats (with or without corn) puffed, added nutrients. 1 cup ------ Grams 25	3	100	3	1	—	—	—	19	44	1.2	0	0.24	0.04	0.5	0
439	Oatmeal or rolled oats, cooked. 1 cup ------ 240	87	130	5	2	—	—	1	23	22	1.4	0	.19	.05	.2	0
	Pancakes, 4-inch diam.:															
440	Wheat, enriched flour (home recipe). 1 cake ----- 27	50	60	2	2	Trace	1	Trace	9	27	.4	30	.05	.06	.4	Trace
441	Buckwheat (made from mix with egg and milk). 1 cake ----- 27	58	55	2	2	1	1	Trace	6	59	.4	60	.03	.04	.2	Trace
442	Plain or buttermilk (made from mix with egg and milk). 1 cake ----- 27	51	60	2	2	1	1	Trace	9	58	.3	70	.04	.06	.2	Trace
	Pie (piecrust made with unenriched flour):															
	Sector, 4-in., ⅐ of 9-in. diam. pie:															
443	Apple (2-crust) ----- 1 sector 135	48	350	3	15	4	7	3	51	11	.4	40	.03	.03	.5	1
444	Butterscotch (1-crust) - 1 sector 130	45	350	6	14	5	6	2	50	98	1.2	340	.04	.13	.3	Trace
445	Cherry (2-crust) ----- 1 sector 135	47	350	4	15	4	7	3	52	19	.4	590	.03	.03	.7	Trace
446	Custard (1-crust) ----- 1 sector 130	58	285	8	14	5	6	2	30	125	.8	300	.07	.21	.4	0
447	Lemon meringue (1-crust). 1 sector 120	47	305	4	12	4	6	2	45	17	.6	200	.04	.10	.2	4
448	Mince (2-crust) ----- 1 sector 135	43	365	3	16	4	8	3	56	38	1.4	Trace	.09	.05	.5	1
449	Pecan (1-crust) ----- 1 sector 118	20	490	6	27	4	16	5	60	55	3.3	190	.19	.08	.4	Trace
450	Pineapple chiffon (1-crust). 1 sector 93	41	265	6	11	3	5	2	36	22	.8	320	.04	.08	.4	1
451	Pumpkin (1-crust) ----- 1 sector 130	59	275	5	15	5	6	2	32	66	.7	3,210	.04	.13	.7	Trace
	Piecrust, baked shell for pie made with:															
452	Enriched flour ------ 1 shell 180	15	900	11	60	16	28	12	79	25	3.1	0	.36	.25	3.2	0
453	Unenriched flour ----- 1 shell 180	15	900	11	60	16	28	12	79	25	.9	0	.05	.05	.9	0

No.	Food, approximate measure	Measure	Grams	Water (pct)	Food energy (cal.)	Protein (g)	Fat (g)	Saturated	Oleic	Linoleic	Carbohydrate (g)	Calcium (mg)	Iron (mg)	Vitamin A (I.U.)	Thiamin (mg)	Riboflavin (mg)	Niacin (mg)	Ascorbic acid (mg)
	Piecrust mix including stick form:																	
454	Package, 10-oz., for double crust.	1 pkg.	284	9	1,480	20	93	23	46	21	141	131	1.4	0	.11	.11	2.0	0
455	Pizza (cheese) 5½-in. sector; ⅛ of 14-in. diam. pie.	1 sector	75	45	185	7	6	2	3	Trace	27	107	.7	290	.04	.12	.7	4
	Popcorn, popped:																	
456	Plain, large kernel	1 cup	6	4	25	1	Trace				5	1	.2			.01	.1	0
457	With oil and salt	1 cup	9	3	40	1	2	1	Trace	Trace	5	1	.2			.01	.2	0
458	Sugar coated	1 cup	35	4	135	2	1				30	2	.5			.02	.4	0
	Pretzels:																	
459	Dutch, twisted	1 pretzel	16	5	60	2	1				12	4	.2	0	Trace	Trace	.1	0
460	Thin, twisted	1 pretzel	6	5	25	1	Trace				5	1	.1	0	Trace	Trace	Trace	0
461	Stick, small, 2¼ inches	10 sticks	3	5	10	Trace	Trace				2	1	Trace	0	Trace	Trace	Trace	0
462	Stick, regular, 3⅛ inches.	5 sticks	3	5	10	Trace	Trace				2	1	Trace	0	Trace	Trace	Trace	0
	Rice, white:																	
	Enriched:																	
463	Raw	1 cup	185	12	670	12	1				149	44	[20]5.4	0	[20].81	[20].06	[20]6.5	0
464	Cooked	1 cup	205	73	225	4	Trace				50	21	[20]1.8	0	[20].23	[20].02	[20]2.1	0
465	Instant, ready-to-serve.	1 cup	165	73	180	4	Trace				40	5	[20]1.3	0	[20].21	[20]—	[20]1.7	0
466	Unenriched, cooked	1 cup	205	73	225	4	Trace				50	21	.4	0	.04	.02	.8	0
467	Parboiled, cooked	1 cup	175	73	185	4	Trace				41	33	[20]1.4	0	[20].19	[20]—	[20]2.1	0
468	Rice, puffed, added nutrients.	1 cup	15	4	60	1	Trace				13	3	.3	0	.07	.01	.7	0
	Rolls, enriched:																	
	Cloverleaf or pan:																	
469	Home recipe	1 roll	35	26	120	3	3	1	1	1	20	16	.7	30	.09	.09	.8	Trace
470	Commercial	1 roll	28	31	85	2	2	Trace	1	Trace	15	21	.5	Trace	.08	.05	.6	Trace
471	Frankfurter or hamburger.	1 roll	40	31	120	3	2	1	1	1	21	30	.8	Trace	.11	.07	.9	Trace
472	Hard, round or rectangular.	1 roll	50	25	155	5	2	Trace	1	Trace	30	24	1.2	Trace	.13	.12	1.4	Trace
473	Rye wafers, whole-grain, 1⅞ by 3½ inches.	2 wafers	13	6	45	2	Trace				10	7	.5	0	.04	.03	.2	0
474	Spaghetti, cooked, tender stage, enriched.	1 cup	140	72	155	5	1				32	11	[19]1.3	0	[19].20	[19].11	[19]1.5	0

[19] Iron, thiamin, riboflavin, and niacin are based on the minimum levels of enrichment specified in standards of identity promulgated under the Federal Food, Drug, and Cosmetic Act.

[20] Iron, thiamin, and niacin are based on the minimum levels of enrichment specified in standards of identity promulgated under the Federal Food, Drug, and Cosmetic Act. Riboflavin is based on unenriched rice. When the minimum level of enrichment for riboflavin specified in the standards of identity becomes effective the value will be 0.12 milligram per cup of parboiled rice and of white rice.

Table A–4 (continued)
Nutritive Values of the Edible Part of Foods

[Dashes show that no basis could be found for imputing a value although there was some reason to believe that a measurable amount of the constituent might be present]

	Food, approximate measure, and weight (in grams)	Water	Food energy	Protein	Fat	Fatty acids Saturated (total)	Unsaturated Oleic	Linoleic	Carbohydrate	Calcium	Iron	Vitamin A value	Thiamin	Riboflavin	Niacin	Ascorbic acid
		Per cent	Calories	Grams	Grams	Grams	Grams	Grams	Grams	Milligrams	Milligrams	International units	Milligrams	Milligrams	Milligrams	Milligrams
	GRAIN PRODUCTS—Continued															
	Spaghetti with meat balls, and tomato sauce:															
475	Home recipe — 1 cup — 248	70	330	19	12	4	6	1	39	124	3.7	1,590	0.25	0.30	4.0	22
476	Canned — 1 cup — 250	78	260	12	10	2	3	4	28	53	3.3	1,000	.15	.18	2.3	5
	Spaghetti in tomato sauce with cheese:															
477	Home recipe — 1 cup — 250	77	260	9	9	2	5	1	37	80	2.3	1,080	.25	.18	2.3	13
478	Canned — 1 cup — 250	80	190	6	2	1	1	1	38	40	2.8	930	.35	.28	4.5	10
479	Waffles, with enriched flour, 7-in. diam. — 1 waffle — 75	41	210	7	7	2	4	1	28	85	1.3	250	.13	.19	1.0	Trace
480	Waffles, made from mix, enriched, egg and milk added, 7-in. diam. — 1 waffle — 75	42	205	7	8	3	3	1	27	179	1.0	170	.11	.17	.7	Trace
481	Wheat, puffed, added nutrients. — 1 cup — 15	3	55	2	Trace				12	4	.6	0	.08	.03	1.2	0
482	Wheat, shredded, plain — 1 biscuit — 25	7	90	2	1				20	11	.9	0	.06	.03	1.1	0
483	Wheat flakes, added nutrients. — 1 cup — 30	4	105	3	Trace				24	12	1.3	0	.19	.04	1.5	0
	Wheat flours:															
484	Whole-wheat, from hard wheats, stirred. — 1 cup — 120	12	400	16	2	Trace	1	1	85	49	4.0	0	.66	.14	5.2	0
	All-purpose or family flour, enriched:															
485	Sifted — 1 cup — 115	12	420	12	1				88	18	[19]3.3	0	[19].51	[19].30	[19]4.0	0
486	Unsifted — 1 cup — 125	12	455	13	1				95	20	[19]3.6	0	[19].55	[19].33	[19]4.4	0
487	Self-rising, enriched — 1 cup — 125	12	440	12	1				93	331	[19]3.6	0	[19].55	[19].33	[19]4.4	0
488	Cake or pastry flour, sifted — 1 cup — 96	12	350	7	1				76	16	.5	0	.03	.03	.7	0
	FATS, OILS															
	Butter:															
	Regular, 4 sticks per pound:															
489	Stick — ½ cup — 113	16	810	1	92	51	30	3	1	23	0	[23]3,750	---	---	---	0

No.	Food, approximate measure, and weight (in grams)		Grams	Water (percent)	Food energy (calories)	Protein (g)	Fat (g)	Saturated fatty acids, total (g)	Unsaturated, oleic (g)	Unsaturated, linoleic (g)	Carbohydrate (g)	Calcium (mg)	Iron (mg)	Vitamin A (I.U.)	Thiamin (mg)	Riboflavin (mg)	Niacin (mg)	Ascorbic acid (mg)
490	Tablespoon (approx. ⅛ stick).	1 tbsp	14	16	100	Trace	12	6	4	Trace	Trace	3	0	[22]470	—	—	—	0
491	Pat (1-in. sq. ⅓-in. high; 90 per lb.).	1 pat	5	16	35	Trace	4	2	1	Trace	Trace	1	0	[22]170	—	—	—	0
	Whipped, 6 sticks or 2, 8-oz. containers per pound:																	
492	Stick.	½ cup	76	16	540	1	61	34	20	2	Trace	15	0	[22]2,500	—	—	—	0
493	Tablespoon (approx. ⅛ stick).	1 tbsp	9	16	65	Trace	8	4	3	Trace	Trace	2	0	[22]310	—	—	—	0
494	Pat (1¼-in. sq. ⅓-in. high; 120 per lb.).	1 pat	4	16	25	Trace	3	2	1	Trace	Trace	1	0	[22]130	—	—	—	0
	Fats, cooking:																	
495	Lard.	1 cup	205	0	1,850	0	205	78	94	20	0	0	0	0	0	0	0	0
496		1 tbsp	13	0	115	0	13	5	6	1	0	0	0	0	0	0	0	0
497	Vegetable fats.	1 cup	200	0	1,770	0	200	50	100	44	0	0	0	—	0	0	0	0
498		1 tbsp	13	0	110	0	13	3	6	3	0	0	0	—	0	0	0	0
	Margarine:																	
	Regular, 4 sticks per pound:																	
499	Stick.	½ cup	113	16	815	1	92	17	46	25	1	23	0	[22]3,750	—	—	—	0
500	Tablespoon (approx. ⅛ stick).	1 tbsp	14	16	100	Trace	12	2	6	3	Trace	3	0	[22]470	—	—	—	0
501	Pat (1-in. sq. ⅓-in. high; 90 per lb.).	1 pat	5	16	35	Trace	4	1	2	1	Trace	1	0	[22]170	—	—	—	0
	Whipped, 6 sticks per pound:																	
502	Stick.	½ cup	76	16	545	1	61	11	31	17	Trace	15	0	[22]2,500	—	—	—	0
	Soft, 2 8-oz. tubs per pound:																	
503	Tub.	1 tub	227	16	1,635	1	184	34	68	68	1	45	0	[22]7,500	—	—	—	0
504	Tablespoon.	1 tbsp	14	16	100	Trace	11	2	4	4	Trace	3	0	[22]470	—	—	—	0
	Oils, salad or cooking:																	
505	Corn.	1 cup	220	0	1,945	0	220	22	62	117	0	0	0	0	0	0	0	0
506		1 tbsp	14	0	125	0	14	1	4	7	0	0	0	0	0	0	0	0
507	Cottonseed.	1 cup	220	0	1,945	0	220	55	46	110	0	0	0	0	0	0	0	0
508		1 tbsp	14	0	125	0	14	4	3	7	0	0	0	0	0	0	0	0
509	Olive.	1 cup	220	0	1,945	0	220	24	167	15	0	0	0	0	0	0	0	0
510		1 tbsp	14	0	125	0	14	2	11	1	0	0	0	0	0	0	0	0
511	Peanut.	1 cup	220	0	1,945	0	220	40	103	64	0	0	0	0	0	0	0	0
512		1 tbsp	14	0	125	0	14	3	7	4	0	0	0	0	0	0	0	0
513	Safflower.	1 cup	220	0	1,945	0	220	18	37	165	0	0	0	0	0	0	0	0
514		1 tbsp	14	0	125	0	14	1	2	10	0	0	0	0	0	0	0	0
515	Soybean.	1 cup	220	0	1,945	0	220	33	44	114	0	0	0	0	0	0	0	0
516		1 tbsp	14	0	125	0	14	2	3	7	0	0	0	0	0	0	0	0

[19] Iron, thiamin, riboflavin, and niacin are based on the minimum levels of enrichment specified in standards of identity promulgated under the Federal Food, Drug, and Cosmetic Act.

[21] Year-round average.

[22] Based on the average vitamin A content of fortified margarine. Federal specifications for fortified margarine require a minimum of 15,000 I.U. of vitamin A per pound.

Table A–4 (continued)
Nutritive Values of the Edible Part of Foods

[Dashes in the columns for nutrients show that no suitable value could be found although there is reason to believe that a measurable amount of the nutrient may be present]

	Food, approximate measure, and weight (in grams)	Water	Food energy	Protein	Fat	Fatty acids Saturated (total)	Unsaturated Oleic	Unsaturated Linoleic	Carbohydrate	Calcium	Iron	Vitamin A value	Thiamin	Riboflavin	Niacin	Ascorbic acid
		Grams	Per cent	Calories	Grams	Grams	Grams	Grams	Grams	Grams	Milligrams	Milligrams	International units	Milligrams	Milligrams	Milligrams	Milligrams
	FATS, OILS—Continued															
	Salad dressings:															
517	Blue cheese 1 tbsp.	15	32	75	8	2	2	4	1	12	Trace	30	Trace	0.02	Trace	Trace
	Commercial, mayonnaise type:															
518	Regular 1 tbsp.	15	41	65	Trace	6	1	1	3	2	2	Trace	30	Trace	Trace	Trace
519	Special dietary, low-calorie 1 tbsp.	16	81	20	Trace	2	Trace	Trace	1	1	3	Trace	40	Trace	Trace	Trace
	French:															
520	Regular 1 tbsp.	16	39	65	Trace	6	1	1	3	3	2	.1	---	---	---	---
521	Special dietary, low-fat with artificial sweeteners 1 tbsp.	15	95	Trace	Trace	Trace	---	---	Trace	Trace	2	.1	---	---	---	---
522	Home cooked, boiled 1 tbsp.	16	68	25	1	2	1	1	Trace	2	14	.1	80	.01	.03	Trace	Trace
523	Mayonnaise 1 tbsp.	14	15	100	Trace	11	2	2	6	Trace	3	.1	40	Trace	.01	Trace	---
524	Thousand island 1 tbsp.	16	32	80	Trace	8	1	2	4	3	2	.1	50	Trace	Trace	Trace	Trace
	SUGARS, SWEETS															
	Cake icings:															
525	Chocolate made with milk and table fat. 1 cup	275	14	1,035	9	38	21	14	1	185	165	3.3	580	.06	.28	.6	1
526	Coconut (with boiled icing). 1 cup	166	15	605	3	13	11	1	Trace	124	10	.8	0	.02	.07	.3	0
527	Creamy fudge from mix with water only. 1 cup	245	15	830	7	16	5	8	3	183	96	2.7	Trace	.05	.20	.7	Trace
528	White, boiled 1 cup	94	18	300	1	0	---	---	---	76	2	Trace	0	0	.03	Trace	0
	Candy:															
529	Caramels, plain or chocolate. 1 oz.	28	8	115	1	3	2	1	Trace	22	42	.4	Trace	.01	.05	.1	Trace
530	Chocolate, milk, plain. 1 oz.	28	1	145	2	9	5	3	Trace	16	65	.3	80	.02	.10	.1	Trace
531	Chocolate-coated peanuts. 1 oz.	28	1	160	5	12	3	6	2	11	33	.4	Trace	.10	.05	2.1	Trace

No.	Food, approximate measure, and weight (in grams)		Water (percent)	Food energy (cal.)	Protein (g)	Fat (g)	Saturated fat (g)	Unsaturated Oleic (g)	Unsaturated Linoleic (g)	Carbohydrate (g)	Calcium (mg)	Iron (mg)	Vitamin A (I.U.)	Thiamin (mg)	Riboflavin (mg)	Niacin (mg)	Ascorbic acid (mg)
532	Fondant; mints, uncoated; candy corn.	1 oz. 28	8	105	Trace	1	—	—	—	25	4	.3	0	Trace	Trace	Trace	0
533	Fudge, plain.	1 oz. 28	8	115	1	4	2	1	Trace	21	22	.3	Trace	.01	.03	.1	Trace
534	Gum drops.	1 oz. 28	12	100	Trace	Trace	—	—	—	25	2	.1	0	0	Trace	Trace	0
535	Hard.	1 oz. 28	1	110	0	Trace	—	—	—	28	6	.5	0	0	0	0	0
536	Marshmallows.	1 oz. 28	17	90	1	Trace	—	—	—	23	5	.5	0	0	Trace	Trace	0
	Chocolate-flavored sirup or topping:																
537	Thin type.	1 fl. oz. 38	32	90	1	1	Trace	Trace	Trace	24	6	.6	Trace	.01	.03	.2	0
538	Fudge type.	1 fl. oz. 38	25	125	2	5	3	2	Trace	20	48	.5	60	.02	.08	.2	Trace
539	Chocolate-flavored beverage powder (approx. 4 heaping teaspoons per oz.): With nonfat dry milk.	1 oz. 28	2	100	5	1	Trace	Trace	Trace	20	167	.5	10	.04	.21	.2	1
540	Without nonfat dry milk.	1 oz. 28	1	100	1	1	Trace	Trace	Trace	25	9	.6	—	.01	.03	.1	0
541	Honey, strained or extracted.	1 tbsp. 21	17	65	Trace	0	—	—	—	17	1	.1	0	Trace	.01	.1	Trace
542	Jams and preserves.	1 tbsp. 20	29	55	Trace	Trace	—	—	—	14	4	.2	Trace	Trace	.01	Trace	Trace
543	Jellies.	1 tbsp. 18	29	50	Trace	Trace	—	—	—	13	4	.3	Trace	Trace	.01	Trace	1
	Molasses, cane:																
544	Light (first extraction).	1 tbsp. 20	24	50	—	—	—	—	—	13	33	.9	—	.01	.01	Trace	—
545	Blackstrap (third extraction).	1 tbsp. 20	24	45	—	—	—	—	—	11	137	3.2	—	.02	.04	.4	—
	Sirups:																
546	Sorghum.	1 tbsp. 21	23	55	—	—	—	—	—	14	35	2.6	—	—	.02	Trace	—
547	Table blends, chiefly corn, light and dark.	1 tbsp. 21	24	60	0	0	—	—	—	15	9	.8	0	0	0	0	0
	Sugars:																
548	Brown, firm packed.	1 cup. 220	2	820	0	0	—	—	—	212	187	7.5	0	.02	.07	.4	0
	White:																
549	Granulated.	1 cup. 200	Trace	770	0	0	—	—	—	199	0	.2	0	0	0	0	0
550		1 tbsp. 11	Trace	40	0	0	—	—	—	11	0	Trace	0	0	0	0	0
551	Powdered, stirred before measuring.	1 cup. 120	Trace	460	0	0	—	—	—	119	0	.1	0	0	0	0	0

MISCELLANEOUS ITEMS

No.	Food, approximate measure, and weight (in grams)		Water (percent)	Food energy (cal.)	Protein (g)	Fat (g)	Saturated fat (g)	Unsaturated Oleic (g)	Unsaturated Linoleic (g)	Carbohydrate (g)	Calcium (mg)	Iron (mg)	Vitamin A (I.U.)	Thiamin (mg)	Riboflavin (mg)	Niacin (mg)	Ascorbic acid (mg)
552	Barbecue sauce.	1 cup. 250	81	230	4	17	2	5	9	20	53	2.0	900	.03	.03	.8	13
	Beverages, alcoholic:																
553	Beer.	12 fl. oz. 360	92	150	1	0	—	—	—	14	18	Trace	—	.01	.11	2.2	—
	Gin, rum, vodka, whiskey:																
554	80-proof.	1½ fl. oz. jigger. 42	67	100	—	—	—	—	—	Trace	—	—	—	—	—	—	—
555	86-proof.	1½ fl. oz. jigger. 42	64	105	—	—	—	—	—	Trace	—	—	—	—	—	—	—
556	90-proof.	1½ fl. oz. jigger. 42	62	110	—	—	—	—	—	Trace	—	—	—	—	—	—	—

Table A–4 (continued)

Nutritive Values of the Edible Part of Foods

[Dashes in the columns for nutrients show that no suitable value could be found although there is reason to believe that a measurable amount of the nutrient may be present]

	Food, approximate measure, and weight (in grams)		Water	Food energy	Pro-tein	Fat	Fatty acids			Carbo-hy-drate	Cal-cium	Iron	Vita-min A value	Thia-min	Ribo-flavin	Niacin	Ascor-bic acid
							Satu-rated (total)	Unsaturated									
								Oleic	Lin-oleic								
		Grams	*Per-cent*	*Calo-ries*	*Grams*	*Grams*	*Grams*	*Grams*	*Grams*	*Grams*	*Milli-grams*	*Milli-grams*	*Inter-national units*	*Milli-grams*	*Milli-grams*	*Milli-grams*	*Milli-grams*
	MISCELLANEOUS ITEMS—Continued																
	Beverages, alcoholic—Continued																
	Gin, rum, vodka, whiskey—Con.																
557	94-proof — 1½ fl. oz. jigger.	42	60	115	—	—				Trace							
558	100-proof — 1½ fl. oz. jigger.	42	58	125	—	—				Trace							
	Wines:																
559	Dessert — 3½ fl. oz. glass.	103	77	140	Trace	0				8	8			.01	.02	.2	
560	Table — 3½ fl. oz. glass.	102	86	85	Trace	0				4	9	.4		Trace	.01	.1	
	Beverages, carbonated, sweetened, nonalcoholic:																
561	Carbonated water — 12 fl. oz.	366	92	115	0	0				29			0	0	0	0	0
562	Cola type — 12 fl. oz.	369	90	145	0	0				37			0	0	0	0	0
563	Fruit-flavored sodas and Tom Collins mixes. 12 fl. oz.	372	88	170	0	0				45			0	0	0	0	0
564	Ginger ale — 12 fl. oz.	366	92	115	0	0				29			0	0	0	0	0
565	Root beer — 12 fl. oz.	370	90	150	0	0				39			0	0	0	0	0
566	Bouillon cubes, approx. ½ in. 1 cube.	4	4	5	1	Trace				Trace							
	Chocolate:																
567	Bitter or baking — 1 oz.	28	2	145	3	15	8	6	Trace	8	22	1.9	20	.01	.07	.4	0
568	Semi-sweet, small pieces. 1 cup.	170	1	860	7	61	34	22	1	97	51	4.4	30	.02	.14	.9	0
	Gelatin:																
569	Plain, dry powder in envelope. 1 envelope.	7	13	25	6	Trace				0							
570	Dessert powder, 3-oz. package. 1 pkg.	85	2	315	8	0				75							
571	Gelatin dessert, prepared with water. 1 cup.	240	84	140	4	0				34							

No.	Food, approximate measure	Measure	Grams	Water (%)	Food energy (cal.)	Protein (g)	Fat (g)	Saturated (total) (g)	Oleic (g)	Linoleic (g)	Carbohydrate (g)	Calcium (mg)	Iron (mg)	Vitamin A (I.U.)	Thiamin (mg)	Riboflavin (mg)	Niacin (mg)	Ascorbic acid (mg)
572	Olives, pickled: Green	4 medium or 3 extra large or 2 giant.	16	78	15	Trace	2	Trace	2	Trace	Trace	8	.2	40	—	—	—	—
573	Ripe: Mission	3 small or 2 large.	10	73	15	Trace	2	Trace	2	Trace	Trace	9	.1	10	Trace	Trace	Trace	—
	Pickles, cucumber:																	
574	Dill, medium, whole, 3¾ in. long, 1¼ in. diam.	1 pickle	65	93	10	1	Trace	—	—	—	1	17	.7	70	Trace	.01	Trace	4
575	Fresh, sliced, 1½ in. diam., ¼ in. thick.	2 slices	15	79	10	Trace	Trace	—	—	—	3	5	.3	20	Trace	Trace	Trace	1
576	Sweet, gherkin, small, whole, approx. 2½ in. long, ¾ in. diam.	1 pickle	15	61	20	Trace	Trace	—	—	—	6	2	.2	10	Trace	Trace	Trace	1
577	Relish, finely chopped, sweet.	1 tbsp.	15	63	20	Trace	Trace	—	—	—	5	3	.1					—
	Popcorn. See Grain Products.																	
578	Popsicle, 3 fl. oz. size	1 popsicle	95	80	70	0	0	—	0	0	18	0	Trace	0	0	0	0	0
	Pudding, home recipe with starch base:																	
579	Chocolate	1 cup	260	66	385	8	12	7	4	Trace	67	250	1.3	390	.05	.36	.3	1
580	Vanilla (blanc mange)	1 cup	255	76	285	9	10	5	3	Trace	41	298	Trace	410	.08	.41	.3	2
581	Pudding mix, dry form, 4-oz. package.	1 pkg.	113	2	410	3	2	1	1	Trace	103	23	1.8	Trace	.02	.08	.5	0
582	Sherbet	1 cup	193	67	260	2	2	—	—	—	59	31	Trace	120	.02	.06	Trace	4
	Soups: Canned, condensed, ready-to-serve: Prepared with an equal volume of milk:																	
583	Cream of chicken	1 cup	245	85	180	7	10	3	3	3	15	172	.5	610	.05	.27	.7	2
584	Cream of mushroom	1 cup	245	83	215	7	14	4	4	5	16	191	.5	250	.05	.34	.7	1
	Prepared with an equal volume of water:																	
585	Tomato	1 cup	250	84	175	7	7	3	2	1	23	168	.8	1,200	.10	.25	1.3	15
586	Bean with pork	1 cup	250	84	170	8	6	2	2	2	22	63	2.3	650	.13	.08	1.0	3
587	Beef broth, bouillon consomme.	1 cup	240	96	30	5	0	—	—	—	3	Trace	.5	Trace	Trace	.02	1.2	
588	Beef noodle	1 cup	240	93	70	4	3	1	1	1	7	7	1.0	50	.05	.07	1.0	Trace
589	Clam chowder, Manhattan type (with tomatoes, without milk).	1 cup	245	92	80	2	3	—	—	—	12	34	1.0	880	.02	.02	1.0	—
590	Cream of chicken	1 cup	240	92	95	3	6	2	3	Trace	8	24	.5	410	.02	.05	.5	Trace
591	Cream of mushroom	1 cup	240	90	135	2	10	3	5	Trace	10	41	.5	70	.02	.12	.7	Trace
592	Minestrone	1 cup	245	90	105	5	3	—	—	—	14	37	1.0	2,350	.07	.05	1.0	—

Table A–4 (continued)

Nutritive Values of the Edible Part of Foods

[Dashes in the columns for nutrients show that no suitable value could be found although there is reason to believe that a measurable amount of the nutrient may be present]

	Food, approximate measure, and weight (in grams)	Water	Food energy	Protein	Fat	Fatty acids Saturated (total)	Fatty acids Unsaturated Oleic	Fatty acids Unsaturated Linoleic	Carbohydrate	Calcium	Iron	Vitamin A value	Thiamin	Riboflavin	Niacin	Ascorbic acid
		Percent	Calories	Grams	Grams	Grams	Grams	Grams	Grams	Milligrams	Milligrams	International units	Milligrams	Milligrams	Milligrams	Milligrams
	MISCELLANEOUS ITEMS—Continued															
	Soups—Continued															
	Canned, condensed, ready-to-serve—Con.															
	Prepared with an equal volume of water—Con.															
593	Split pea _____ 1 cup _____ 245 Grams	85	145	9	3	1	2	Trace	21	29	1.5	440	0.25	0.15	1.5	1
594	Tomato _____ 1 cup _____ 245	90	90	2	3	Trace	1	1	16	15	.7	1,000	.05	.05	1.2	12
595	Vegetable beef __ 1 cup _____ 245	92	80	5	2	----	----	----	10	12	.7	2,700	.05	.05	1.0	----
596	Vegetarian ____ 1 cup _____ 245	92	80	2	2	----	----	----	13	20	1.0	2,940	.05	.05	1.0	----
	Dehydrated, dry form:															
597	Chicken noodle (2-oz. package). 1 pkg _____ 57	6	220	8	6	2	3	1	33	34	1.4	190	.30	.15	2.4	3
598	Onion mix (1½-oz. package). 1 pkg _____ 43	3	150	6	5	1	2	1	23	42	.6	30	.05	.03	.3	6
599	Tomato vegetable with noodles (2½-oz. pkg.). 1 pkg _____ 71	4	245	6	6	2	3	1	45	33	1.4	1,700	.21	.13	1.8	18
	Frozen, condensed:															
	Clam chowder, New England type (with milk, without tomatoes):															
600	Prepared with equal volume of milk. 1 cup _____ 245	83	210	9	12	----	----	----	16	240	1.0	250	.07	.29	.5	Trace
601	Prepared with equal volume of water. 1 cup _____ 240	89	130	4	8	----	----	----	11	91	1.0	50	.05	.10	.5	----
	Cream of potato:															
602	Prepared with equal volume of milk. 1 cup _____ 245	83	185	8	10	5	3	Trace	18	208	1.0	590	.10	.27	.5	Trace
603	Prepared with equal volume of water. 1 cup _____ 240	90	105	3	5	3	2	Trace	12	58	1.0	410	.05	.05	.5	----

No.	Food	Measure																
	Cream of shrimp:																	
604	Prepared with equal volume of milk.	1 cup	245	82	245	9	16	--	--		15	189	.5	290	.07	.27	.5	Trace
605	Prepared with equal volume of water.	1 cup	240	88	160	5	12	--	--		8	38	.5	120	.05	.05	.5	--
	Oyster stew:																	
606	Prepared with equal volume of milk.	1 cup	240	83	200	10	12	--	--		14	305	1.4	410	.12	.41	.5	Trace
607	Prepared with equal volume of water.	1 cup	240	90	120	6	8	--	--		8	158	1.4	240	.07	.19	.5	--
608	Tapioca, dry, quick-cooking.	1 cup	152	13	535	1	Trace	--	--		131	15	.6	0	0	0	0	0
	Tapioca desserts:																	
609	Apple.	1 cup	250	70	295	1	Trace	--	--		74	8	.5	30	Trace	Trace	Trace	Trace
610	Cream pudding.	1 cup	165	72	220	8	8	4	3	Trace	28	173	.7	480	.07	.30	.2	2
611	Tartar sauce.	1 tbsp.	14	34	75	Trace	8	1	1	4	3	3	.1	30	Trace	Trace	Trace	Trace
612	Vinegar.	1 tbsp.	15	94	Trace	Trace	0	--	--		1	1	.1	0	Trace	Trace	Trace	--
613	White sauce, medium.	1 cup	250	73	405	10	31	16	10	1	22	288	.5	1,150	.10	.43	.5	2
	Yeast:																	
614	Baker's, dry, active.	1 pkg.	7	5	20	3	Trace	--	--		3	3	1.1	Trace	.16	.38	2.6	Trace
615	Brewer's, dry.	1 tbsp.	8	5	25	3	Trace	--	--		3	17	1.4	Trace	1.25	.34	3.0	Trace
	Yoghurt. See Milk, Cheese, Cream, Imitation Cream.																	

Table A-5

Weight-Height-Age Table for Boys and Girls of School Age *

	Boys				Girls			
Age years	*Average Weight lb*	*Range† in Weight lb*	*Average Height in.*	*Range† in Height in.*	*Average Weight lb*	*Range† in Weight lb*	*Average Height in.*	*Range† in Height in.*
4	38.2	33.7– 42.7	40.9	39.0–42.8	37.3	32.5– 42.1	40.9	39.0–42.8
5	43.2	37.7– 48.7	43.9	41.9–45.9	42.0	36.1– 47.9	43.6	41.6–45.6
6	47.6	41.3– 53.9	46.1	44.0–48.2	46.4	39.6– 53.2	45.8	43.7–47.9
7	52.5	45.4– 59.6	48.2	46.0–50.4	51.2	43.7– 58.7	47.9	45.7–50.1
8	58.2	49.5– 66.9	50.4	48.1–52.7	56.9	47.5– 66.3	50.0	47.7–52.3
9	64.4	54.6– 74.2	52.4	50.0–54.8	63.0	51.9– 74.1	52.0	49.6–54.4
10	70.7	59.2– 82.2	54.3	51.8–56.8	70.3	57.1– 83.5	54.2	51.6–56.8
11	77.6	64.5– 90.7	56.2	53.6–58.8	79.0	63.5– 94.5	56.5	53.7–59.3
12	85.6	69.8–101.4	58.2	55.3–61.1	89.7	71.9–107.5	59.0	56.1–61.9
13	95.6	77.4–113.8	60.5	57.3–63.7	100.3	82.3–118.3	60.6	58.0–63.2
14	107.9	87.8–128.0	63.0	59.6–66.4	108.5	91.3–125.7	62.3	59.6–64.7
15	121.7	101.1–142.3	65.6	62.5–68.7	115.0	98.8–131.2	63.2	60.9–65.6
16	131.9	113.0–150.8	67.3	64.5–70.1	117.6	101.7–133.5	63.5	61.3–65.7
17	138.3	119.5–157.1	68.2	65.6–70.8	119.0	103.5–134.5	63.6	61.4–65.8

* From "Basic Body Measurements of School Age Children," Washington, D.C.: Office of Education, U.S. Department of Health, Education, and Welfare, 1953. This table is a compilation of heights and weights of 296,498 children (152,191 boys and 144,307 girls) from 17 states and the District of Columbia. No data reported before 1930 were included. The measurements were made on subjects wearing light indoor clothing with shoes removed.
† The ranges given include the cases which fell within the middle two thirds of those in the sample.

Index

Acid-base balance, *see* Electrolyte balance

Acid and base products of metabolism, 329

Acidosis and alkalosis, 331, 332

Adolescence, basal metabolism in, 40: body composition in relation to sex, 380: important in relation to reproduction, 389: intake and/or need for ascorbic acid, 250, 386; for calcium and phosphorus, 126, 133, 138, 383; for calories, 39, 50, 382; for copper, 175; for folic acid, 387; for iodine, 165, 167; for iron, 148, 153, 385; for magnesium, 181; for niacin, 285, 386; for protein, 382; for riboflavin, 273, 274, 386; for thiamin, 263, 386; for vitamin A, 211, 386; for vitamin B_6, 292, 387; for vitamin B_{12}, 387; for vitamin D, 223, 386; for vitamin E, 387: MDR, 431: obesity during, 55, 390: quality of diet, 389: RDA, 432: special problems during, 389: teenage pregnancies, 334, 389: water requirement, 387: weight control during, 55, 390

Aging, *see* Later years

AID, 2

Alcoholism, 255, 264

Aldosterone, 185, 342

Algae, 112

Alkali reserve, 331

Alkaline phosphatase, 219, 220, 342, 397

Amino acids, absorption and metabolism, 95: aromatic, and ascorbic acid, 363: balance studies on women, 98: body reserve, 91: during pregnancy, 338: essential and nonessential, 92: essential, signs of lack, 92: essential, studies on human subjects, 98, 102: functions, 93: imbalance, 101: in plasma, 102: intake, 110: limiting, 101: needs in later years, 395; of children, 100; of infants, 100, 356; of lactating women, 100; of men and women, 98, 100, 110; of pregnant women, 100, 338: nonessential, functions, 92: nonessential, needs in relation to synthesis, 93: patterns used in evaluation, 102–106: ratio of nonessential to essential, 93: relation to nonspecific nitrogen, 93: relation to riboflavin function, 267: sources, 103–105: supplementary values, 100, 409

Anemia, color index in, 144, 150: hemorrhagic, 144–146, 149, 150: hypochromic, 149: in adolescence, 142, 154, 385: in infancy, 149, 151, 359, 361, 363: in lactation, 349: in later years, 397: in pellagra, 278: in pregnancy, 142, 344, 345: nutritional, 144, 146, 154: pernicious, 144, 150, 295, 298, 300, 301: prevalence in men *vs.* women, 142, 153: prevalence throughout the world, 410: related to blood donation, 142, 149, 150, 154; to copper, 147, 174, 183; to folacin, 150, 278, 295, 296; to infection, 149; to molybdenum, 183; to riboflavin, 269; to vitamin B_6, 147, 290, 293; to vitamin B_{12}, 147, 150, 298, 300; to vitamins C and E, 147, 227, 245; to zinc, 189, 411: symptoms of hypochromic, 149: treatment, 146, 147, 150

Anorexia, related to thiamin lack, 257

Antibiotics, 302, 308

Anticoagulants, 231

Antigray hair factors, 304, 305, 309

Antioxidants, used in food processing, 77, 199, 224, 415

Antivitamins, *see* Vitamin antagonists

Appetite, factors affecting, in children, 393: relation to calorie intake, 31, 52, 55: to pellagra, 275; to thiamin, 251

Arachidonic acid, 79, 81, 304

Arginine, function of, 127

Ascorbic acid, antagonist, 243: chemical nature, 242: chemical structure, 242: diseases related to lack, 245–251: effect of food processing on, 248; of light on, 246; of soda on, 248: excretion, 243, 249: forms, 242: